Exam-Oriented
MICROBIOLOGY
(Questions & Answers)

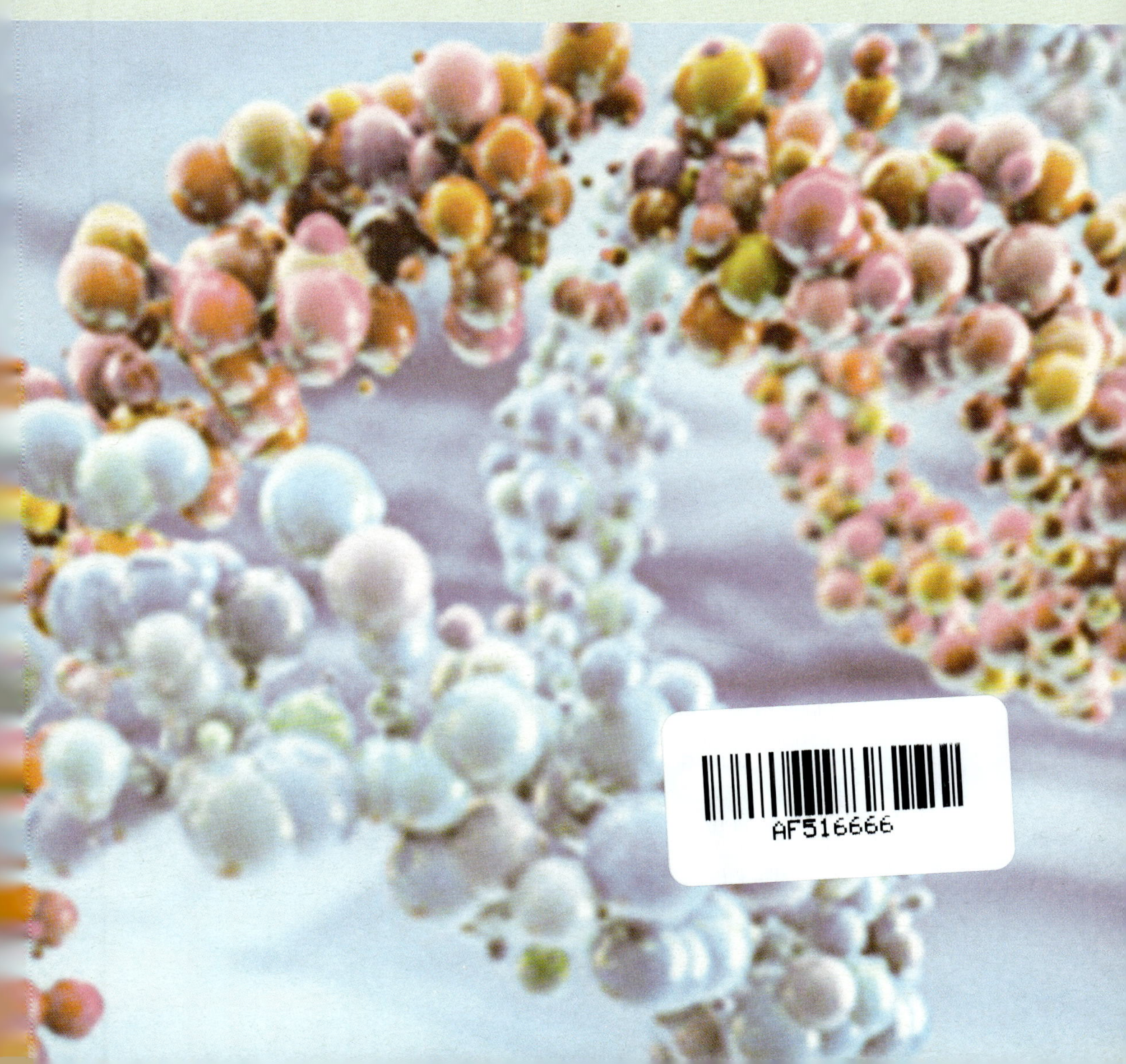

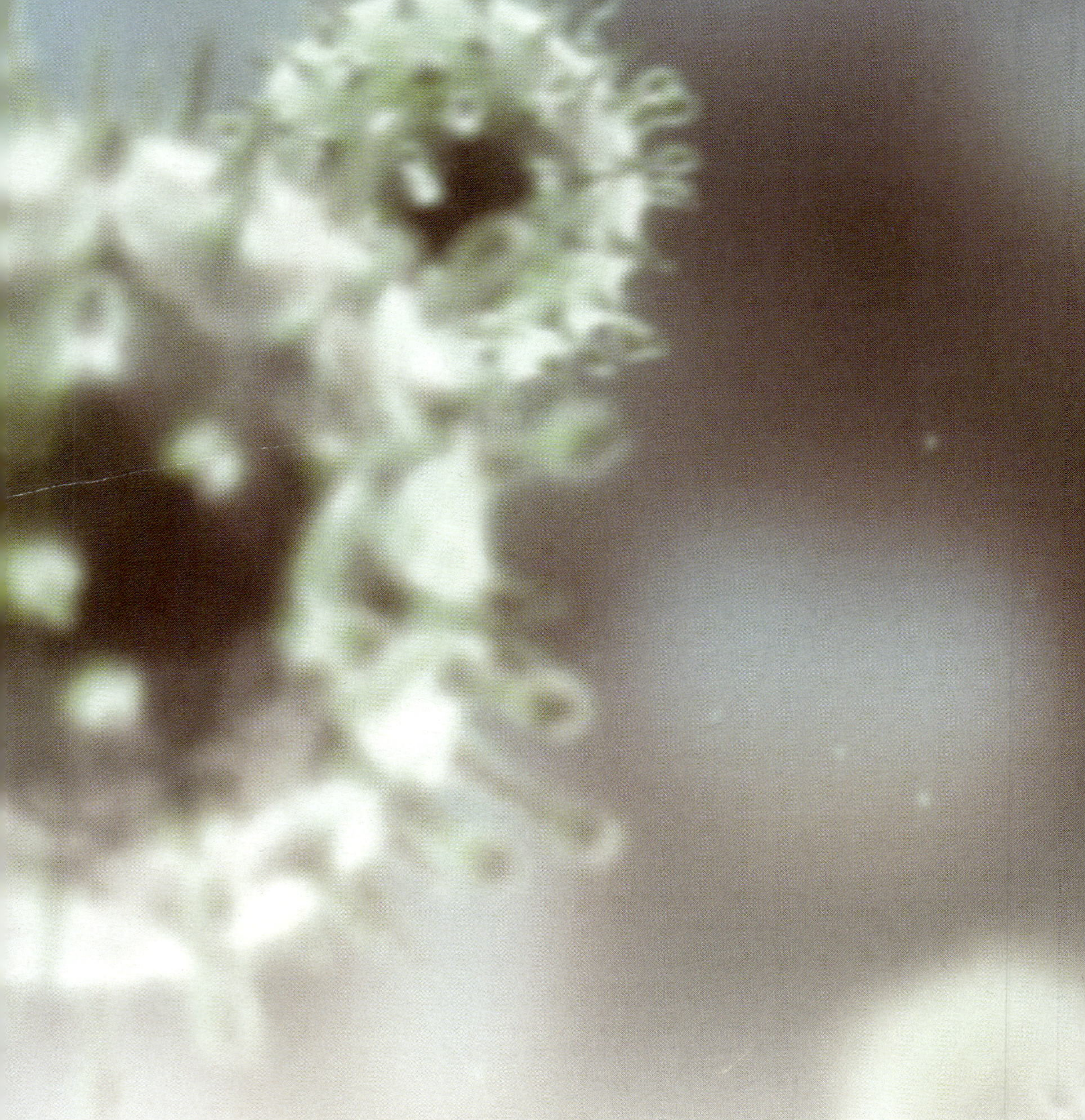

Other Books by Dr. D.R. Arora

- Textbook of Microbiology, 5/e
- Textbook of Microbiology for Dental Students, 4/e
- Medical Parasitology, 4/e
- Medical Mycology
- Essentials of Microbiology for B.Sc. Nursing Students
- Practical Microbiology
- Practical Microbiology for Dental Students
- MCQs in Microbiology — with explanation (In Press)

Exam-Oriented
MICROBIOLOGY
(Questions & Answers)

Dr. D.R. Arora M.D., Ph.D., M.N.A.M.S.

Ex-Professor & Head, Department of Microbiology,
Postgraduate Institute of Medical Sciences, Rohtak, Haryana (India), and
Maharaja Agarsen Medical College, Agroha, Haryana (India)

Ex-Professor & Head, Department of Microbiology,
Medical Superintendent, and Dean Faculty of Allied Health Sciences,
SGT University, Gurgaon, Haryana (India)

Ex-W.H.O. Fellow; and Visiting Professor, University of Mauritius

Lead Assessor and Member, Accreditation Committee,
National Accreditation Board for Testing and Calibration Laboratories (NABL),
Gurgaon, Haryana (India)

Principal Assessor, National Accreditation Board for Hospitals &
Healthcare Providers (NABH), New Delhi (India)

Assessor, National Accreditation Board for
Education and Training (NABET), New Delhi (India)

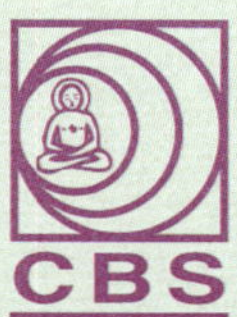

CBS Publishers & Distributors Pvt. Ltd.

New Delhi • Bengaluru • Chennai • Kochi • Kolkata • Mumbai

Hyderabad • Nagpur • Patna • Pune • Vijayawada

ISBN: 978-93-86310-92-7

First Edition: 2017

Published by **Satish Kumar Jain** and produced by **Varun Jain** for
CBS Publishers & Distributors Pvt. Ltd.,
4819/XI Prahlad Street, 24 Ansari Road, Daryaganj, New Delhi - 110002
delhi@cbspd.com, cbspubs@airtelmail.in • www.cbspd.com
Ph.: 23289259, 23266861, 23266867 • Fax: 011-23243014

Corporate Office: 204 FIE, Industrial Area, Patparganj, Delhi - 110 092
Ph: 49344934 • Fax: 011-49344935
E-mail: publishing@cbspd.com • publicity@cbspd.com

Branches:
- ***Bengaluru:*** 2975, 17th Cross, K.R. Road, Bansankari 2nd Stage, Bengaluru - 70 • Ph: +91-80-26771678/79 • Fax: +91-80-26771680 E-mail: cbsbng@gmail.com, bangalore@cbspd.com
- ***Chennai:*** No. 7, Subbaraya Street, Shenoy Nagar, Chennai - 600030 Ph: +91-44-26681266, 26680620 • Fax: +91-44-42032115 E-mail: chennai@cbspd.com
- ***Kochi:*** Ashana House, 39/1904, A.M. Thomas Road, Valanjambalam, Ernakulum, Kochi • Ph: +91-484-4059061-65 Fax: +91-484-4059065 • E-mail: cochin@cbspd.com
- ***Kolkata:*** 6-B, Ground Floor, Rameshwar Shaw Road, Kolkata - 700014 Ph: +91-33-22891126/7/8 • E-mail: kolkata@cbspd.com
- ***Mumbai:*** 83-C, Dr. E. Moses Road, Worli, Mumbai - 400018 Ph: +91-9833017933, 022-24902340/41 • E-mail: mumbai@cbspd.com

Representatives:
- Hyderabad: 0-9885175004
- Patna: 0-9334159340
- Vijayawada: 0-9000660880
- Nagpur: 0-9021734563
- Pune: 0-9623451994

Printed at:
Goyal Offset Printers, Delhi (India)

Dedicated to the
Sweet Memories of

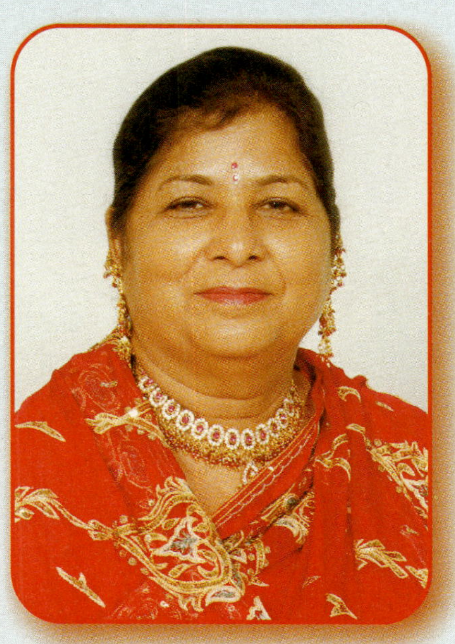

Dr. Brij Bala Arora

(4.3.1947 – 21.11.2014)

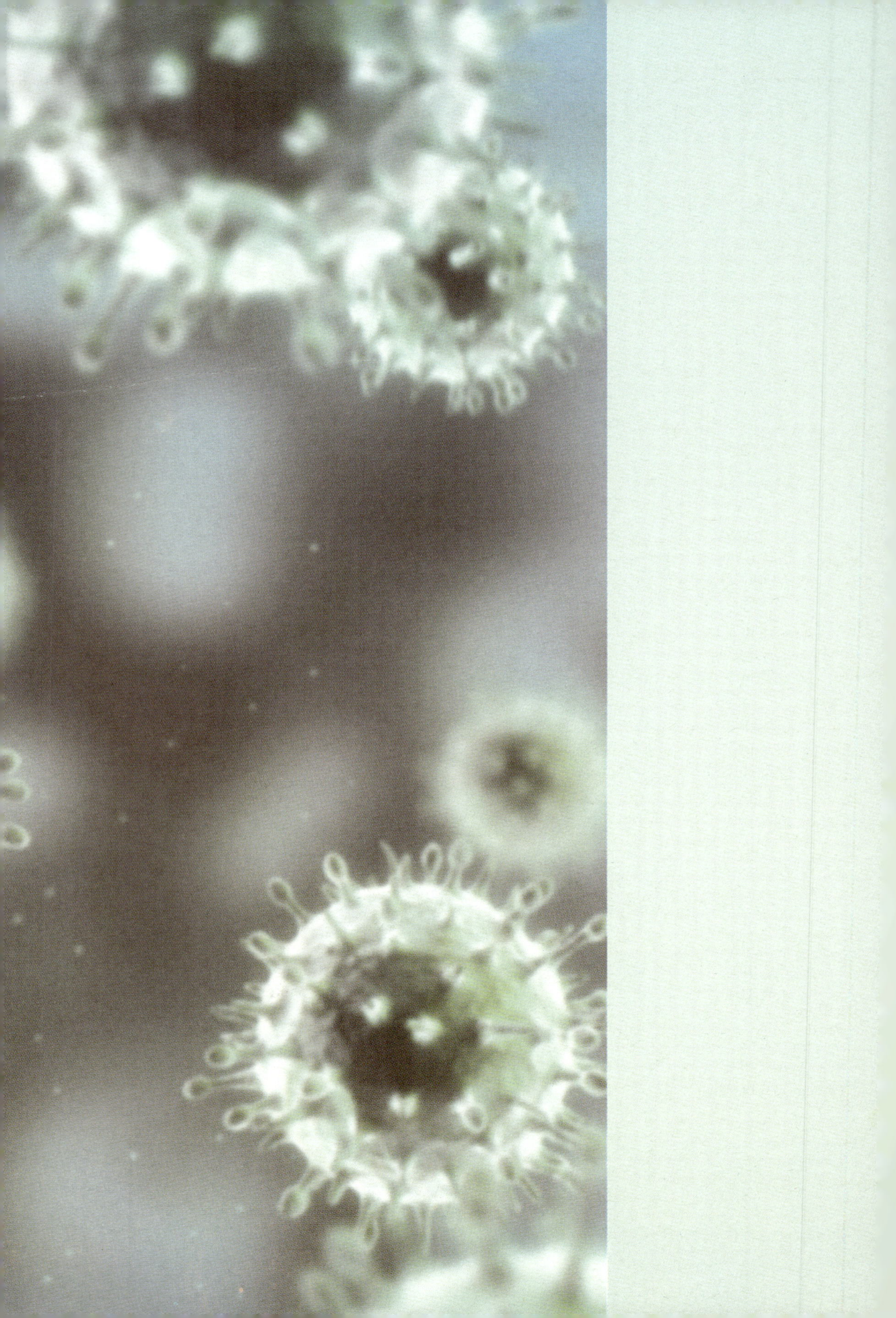

PREFACE

Human history is full of examples of major devastations caused by bacteria and viruses. Infectious diseases account for 26% of total deaths in the world and this percentage is higher in the developing world including India. Microorganisms are always one step ahead of us. We develop means (an antibiotic/ a vaccine) to control/eradicate the pathogenic microorganisms and they develop genes/mechanisms to resist these means. New agents of infectious diseases continue to be recognized. On the top of that, microorganisms are being used as weapons of war. Biotechnology and genetic engineering have added new dimension to the threat whereby scientists/terrorists can alter strains of bacteria to cause atypical symptoms, acute fatal disease, increased transmissibility, and make microorganisms resistant to usual antibiotics. In the future, study of space microbiology may help to reveal if there is life on other planets.

Rapidly increasing information in medical science is a big burden on the students. Quite often a student is not sure about the exact answers of the questions asked in the examination. Therefore, question-answer format has been adopted throughout the book in order to acquaint the students with the kind of questions asked in the examination and appropriate answers to be given by the students. Both long and short answer questions, as are asked in the examination, have been given.

The text has been presented in a simple and lucid manner for the students to help them to thoroughly imbibe the basics of the subject. A picture speaks more than a thousand words. Keeping this in mind, every chapter has been well illustrated with relevant fully coloured diagrams, clinical photographs and photomicrographs to enhance the understanding of the students. I am thankful to Dr. P.S. Gill, Professor of Microbiology, Postgraduate Institute of Medical Sciences, Rohtak, for drawing the figures. I am grateful for valuable professional help and support provided by Mr. B.M. Singh and other staff at CBS Publishers & Distributors. I honestly acknowledge the most sincere and dedicated support and advice of Mr. Dharmvir.

This book will be highly useful to the exam-going UG and PG students. The readers are requested to send suggestions for the improvement of the book at *draroradr@rediffmail.com*. The suggestions and changes will be incorporated in subsequent editions.

D.R. Arora

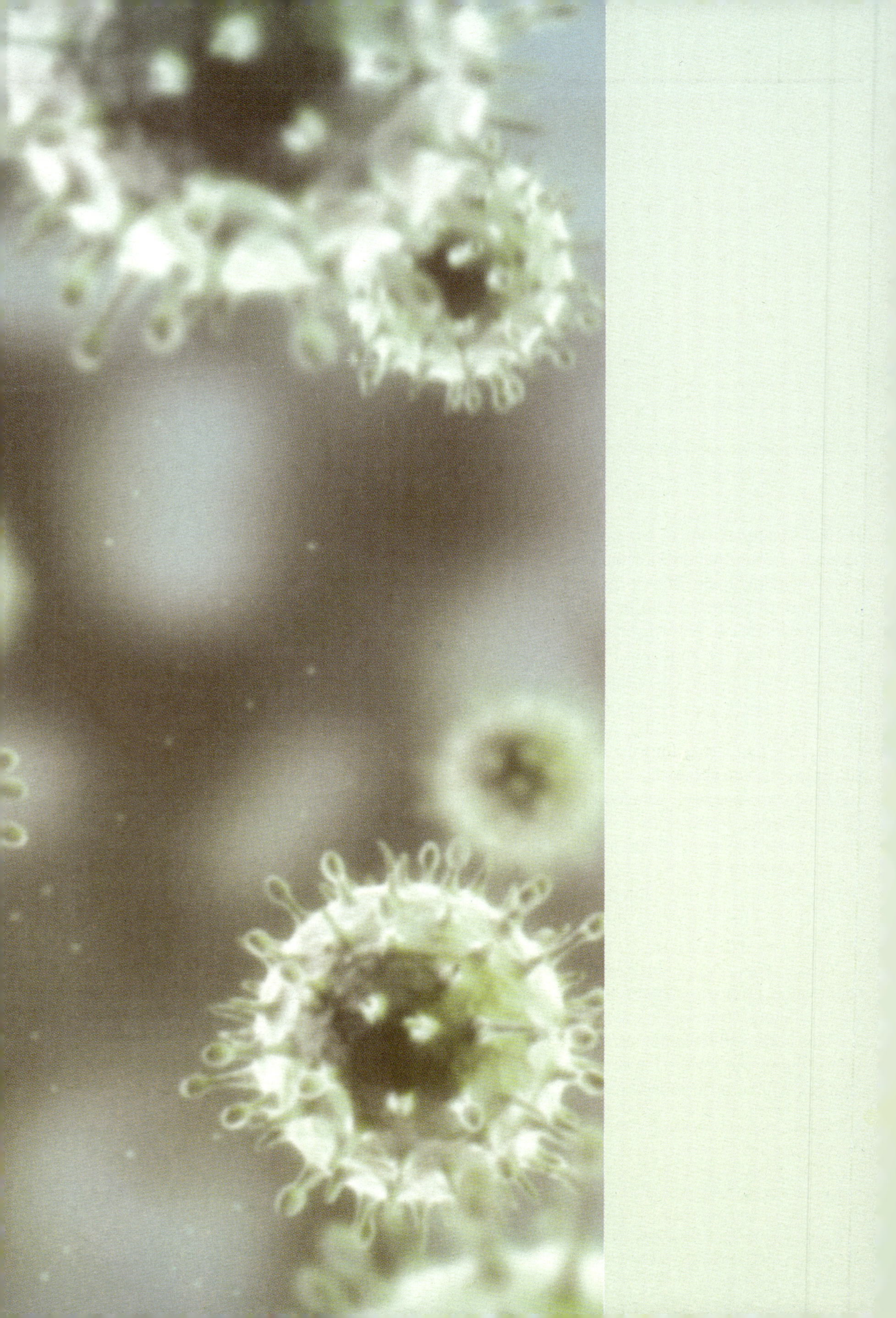

CONTENTS

1

INTRODUCTION

Q. 1. Define microbiology and discuss Koch's postulates. Name microorganisms which do not meet the criteria of Koch's postulates.

Ans. **Microbiology** is the study of living organisms of microscopic size. This term was introduced by French chemist Louis Pasteur, who demonstrated that fermentation was caused by the growth of bacteria and yeasts.

Medical microbiology is the study of microbes that infect humans, the disease they cause, and their diagnosis, prevention and treatment. It also deals with the response of the human host to microbial infection. Although the primary interest is in the diseases caused by the microorganisms, it must also be appreciated that microorganisms play a critical role in human survival.

Koch's postulates

A microorganism can be accepted as the causative agent of an infectious disease only if following postulates, known as Koch's postulates, are satisfied (Fig. 1.1):

1. The microorganism must be present in the lesions in every case of the infectious disease.
2. It should be possible to isolate the microorganism in pure culture from the lesions.
3. Inoculation of the pure culture by a suitable route into a suitable laboratory animal should produce a similar disease.
4. It should again be possible to re-isolate the microorganism in pure culture from the lesions produced in the experimental animals.

A fifth criterion introduced subsequently states that specific antibodies to the organism should be demonstrable in the serum of the patient suffering from the disease. These postulates have proved extremely useful in confirming the authenticity of doubtful claims made regarding the causative agents of infectious diseases.

Microorganisms which do not meet the criteria of Koch's postulates

Koch's postulates have remained a mainstay of microbiology; however, many microorganisms that do not meet the criteria of postulates have been shown to cause disease. For example, *Treponema pallidum* and *Mycobacterium leprae*, causative agents of syphilis and leprosy respectively, cannot be grown *in vitro*; however, there are animal models of infection with these agents. In another example, *Neisseria gonorrhoeae*, which causes gonorrhoea, there is no animal model even though the bacteria can readily be cultured *in vitro*.

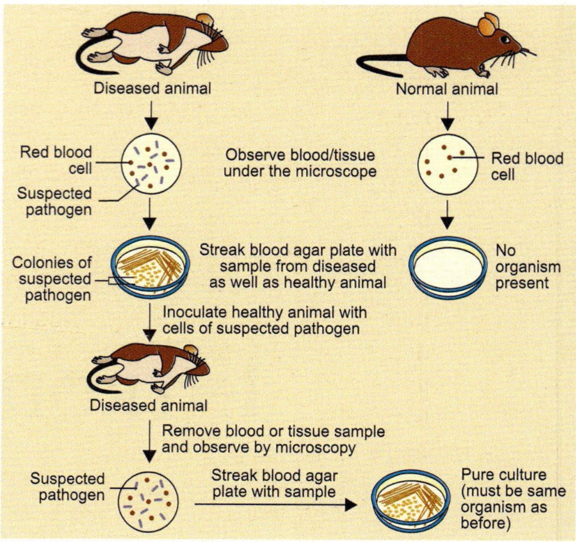

Fig. 1.1. Koch's postulates.

Q. 2. List contributions of Louis Pasteur in the field of medical microbiology.

Ans. Louis Pasteur (1822–1895) was born in the village of Dole, France on December 27, 1822 the son of humble parents. His father was a tanner. He was originally trained as a chemist, but his studies on fermentation led him to take interest in microorganisms. His discoveries revolutionized medical practice, although he never studied medicine.

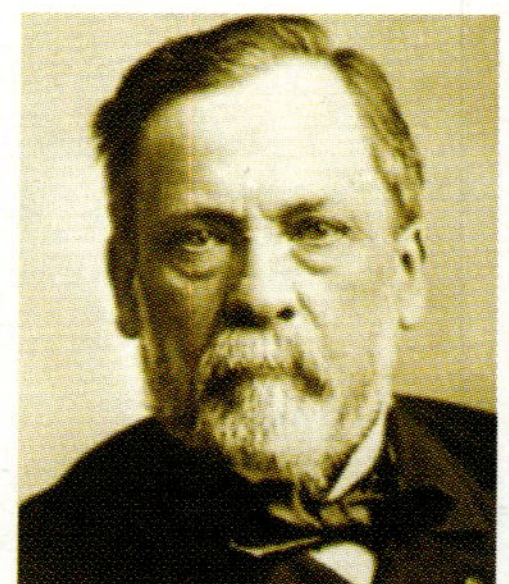

1. The term **microbiology**, as the study of living organisms of microscopic size, was coined by Pasteur.
2. He also coined the term **vaccine**.
3. He used various forms of nutrient fluid to grow microorganisms and showed that a medium suitable for one might be unsuitable for another, so for successful cultivation it was necessary to discover a suitable growth medium and to establish optimal conditions of temperature, acidity or alkalinity, and oxygen tension.
4. He showed that some organisms were not destroyed by boiling. For the sterilization of fluids he advocated heating to 120°C under pressure and for glassware the use of dry heat at 170°C. He showed that cotton plugs (a primitive air-filtration device) could prevent microbes from reaching otherwise air-exposed sterile broths.
5. In 1860-61, he disapproved the **theory of spontaneous generation**.
6. In 1860–64, he gave experimental evidence that fermentation and putrefaction are effects of microbial growth.
7. In 1863–65, he devised the process of destroying bacteria, known as **pasteurization**. This process is employed throughout the civilized world today to preserve milk and certain other perishable foods.

8. In 1877, Koch and Pasteur demonstrated that anthrax is caused by bacteria. Pasteur grew the organisms in sterilized yeast water and kept them in the laboratory for several months, transferring them frequently to new culture fluid, in which they multiplied readily, and showed that these cultures would always cause anthrax when inoculated into healthy animals.
9. In 1880, he prevented chicken cholera by injection of live attenuated culture. He found that pure cultures of the germ of this disease which had been kept in the laboratory for some time would not kill his animals as fresh cultures did, but would merely cause a passing illness from which the chickens recovered. Then he discovered that the animals that had recovered from a previous inoculation of weakened germs were immune, and did not succumb to the disease. Pasteur immediately perceived that it might be possible to make individuals resistant by inoculating them with the weakened (and therefore harmless) germs of a particular disease.
10. In 1880, he first cultured staphylococci in liquid medium and produced abscesses by inoculating them into rabbits.
11. In 1881, he developed **live attenuated anthrax vaccine**.
12. In 1881, pneumococci were first noticed by Pasteur and Sternberg independently.
13. The crowning achievement of Pasteur was the successful application of the principle of vaccination to the prevention of rabies, or hydrophobia, in human beings and developed **Pasteur rabies vaccine** in 1885. He did not find the germs of this disease under his microscope (now known as rabies virus) but he was able to propagate them by artificial inoculation into the brains of dogs and rabbits. Finally he developed a system of vaccination with weakened virus which prevented the development of this fatal disease if the inoculations are given soon after the bite of the rabid animal. He gave the first treatment for rabies in 1885 to a young boy bitten by a rabid dog.
14. In 1887, Pasteur and Joubert first described *Clostridium septicum* and called it *Vibrion septique*.

Q. 3. Describe important contributions of Robert Koch in the field of medical microbiology.

Ans. A bacteriologist second only to Louis Pasteur was Robert Koch (1843–1910). He was born on December 11, 1843 in Germany. In 1866, he took his degree in Medicine and began a general practice in a small country town. In 1872, he took a diploma in Public Health. He became interested in microscopical studies. With a microscope given as a birthday present by his wife he set up a primitive laboratory and started his studies on microbes in relation to diseases. His contributions to microbiology are variegated and enormous:

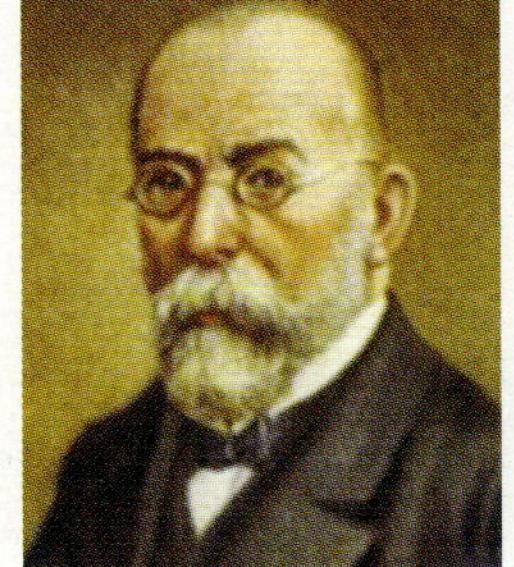

1. In 1876, Robert Koch reported the isolation of anthrax bacillus in pure culture, formation and germination of its spores and the proof of its infectiousness. This agent as the sole cause of anthrax was confirmed by Pasteur.
2. In 1877, he introduced the method of making smears of bacteria on glass slides, and of staining them with the aniline dyes. He was also the first to employ in bacteriological work the improved compound microscope of Abbe.

3. In 1878, his studies of wound infections explored the role of animal experimentation in establishing the cause of bacterial infections.
4. In 1881, he described means of cultivating bacteria on solid media, thus making it possible to obtain pure cultures by transferring material from a single colony.
5. The **hanging-drop method** of studying bacteria as used today is a product of his genius.
6. In 1882, Koch startled the world by announcing his discovery of **tubercle bacillus** (*Mycobacterium tuberculosis*), the causative agent of tuberculosis. He described a special staining method for detection of this organism and grew it in pure cultures in the laboratory. He showed that animals would develop tuberculosis when inoculated with pure cultures of this organism, and recovered the identical organisms from the diseased tissues of the animals. The discovery of the tubercle bacillus made him internationally famous and the bacillus was called **Koch's bacillus** and tuberculosis, **Koch's disease**.
7. In 1883, he discovered the causative agents of cholera (*Vibrio cholerae*), Egyptian ophthalmia (pink eye) and Koch Weeks bacillus.
8. In 1884, Koch expounded the postulates or laws by which an organism may be proved to be the cause of a particular disease. These are known as **Koch's postulates**.
9. Koch continued his work on tuberculosis and in 1890–91 he showed how a normal guinea-pig and an already infected guinea-pig behaved differently to an infection with tubercle bacillus. This is known as **Koch's phenomenon**.
10. From 1885–90, Koch studied various organisms present in water, soil and air and their relation in prevention of disease.
11. He invented the **hot air oven** and **steam sterilizer**, basic tools in any microbiology laboratory.

Q. 4. What are important contributions of Antonie van Leeuwenhoek in the field of medical microbiology?

Ans. Antonie van Leeuwenhoek (1632–1723), a citizen of Delft, Holland, was not a man of great learning, but he was very ingenious. He became expert in the grinding of simple magnifying lenses. He made these lenses of small bits of glass, polished them very carefully, and mounted each separately between two brass, copper, silver, or gold plates, to which he fastened an adjustable holder for the object to be examined. He constructed many of these 'microscopes' each containing a single lens ground by himself. The best of lenses magnified about 200 times. His microscopes were superior to any of that time. He observed, drew and measured a large number of living organisms including bacteria and protozoa in materials such as rain water, pond and well water, and saliva and the intestinal contents of healthy subjects and communicated them to the Royal Society of London in 1683. He was the first to accurately describe different shapes of bacteria (coccal, bacillary and spiral) and picture their arrangement in infected material.

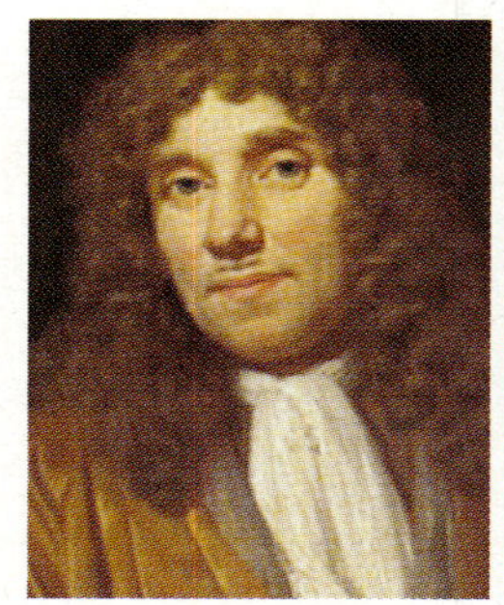

Leeuwenhoek observed that very large numbers of bacteria appeared in watery infusions of animals or vegetable matter which were left to stand for a week or two at room temperature. He believed that these huge populations were the progeny of a few parental organisms, or seeds, that were originally present in the materials of the infusion or had entered it from the air. The significance of these observations was not realized then and to Leeuwenhoek the world of 'little animalcules' represented only a curiosity of nature. Their importance in medicine and other areas of biology came to be recognized two centuries later.

Q. 5. Describe contribution of Edward Jenner in the field of medical microbiology.

Ans. Edward Jenner (1749–1823) was born in Berkeley in 1749. Orphaned before he was 5-years-old, his brothers and sisters set him on a career of medicine. He completed his training with the great surgeon John Hunter in London. *He introduced the modern method of vaccination to prevent smallpox.* He observed that milkmaids who contracted cowpox or vaccinia while milking were subsequently immune to smallpox. On May 14,1796, he devised a brave experiment. He performed a vaccination against smallpox by transferring material from a cowpox pustule on the hand of a milkmaid, Sarah Nelmes, to the arm of a small boy named James Phipps, his gardener's son. *The terms vaccine and vaccination were first used by Pasteur out of deference to Jenner.*

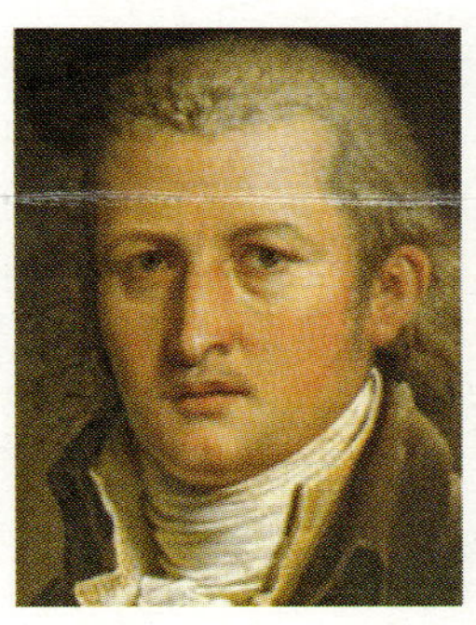

Edward Jenner's discovery has now been developed into one of the most important parts of modern medicine – **Immunology**. This science helps us to treat many infectious diseases, and to understand transplantation, allergies and diseases such as rheumatoid arthritis and AIDS.

Q. 6. Write important contributions of Paul Ehrlich in the field of medical microbiology.

Ans. Paul Ehrlich (1854–1915), an outstanding German scientist and genius of extraordinary activity, added a great mass to our knowledge of medical science, and a large number of technical methods he proposed are now in daily use in microbiological and chemical laboratories.

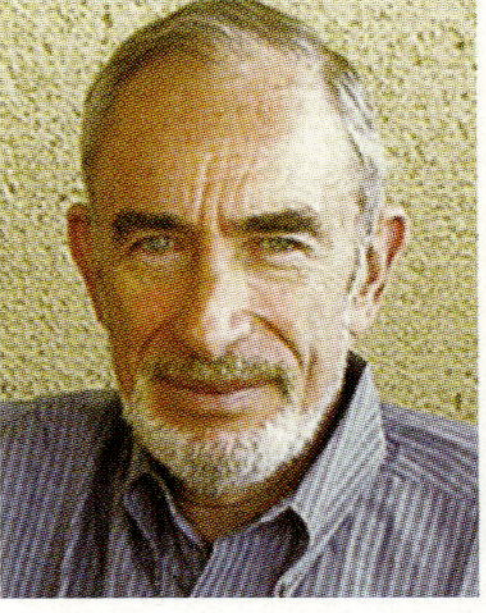

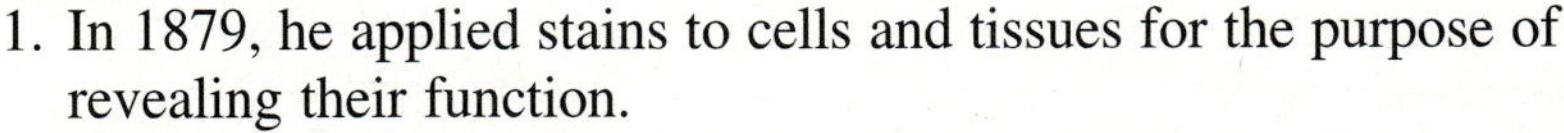

1. In 1879, he applied stains to cells and tissues for the purpose of revealing their function.
2. In 1882, he reported the *acid-fastness* of tubercle bacillus.
3. From 1890–1900 he did important research in immunology. He soon found that the specific effect of immune serum could be demonstrated *in vivo* and *in vitro* and introduced methods of standardizing toxin and antitoxin. To him goes the credit of *minimum lethal dose.*
4. In 1898, he proposed *side chain theory of antibody production.*
5. In 1909, he introduced salvarsan, an arsenical compound, sometimes called the '*magic bullet*'. It was capable of destroying the spirochaete of syphilis with only moderate toxic effects. He continued his experimentation until 1912 when he announced the discovery of neosalvarsan. Thus he created a new branch of medicine known as **chemotherapy**.

2

Morphology of Bacteria

Q. 1. Tabulate differences between prokaryotes and eukaryotes.

Ans. Differences between prokaryotes and eukaryotes are given in Table 2.1.

Table 2.1. Comparison of prokaryotes and eukaryotes

Characteristic	Prokaryotes	Eukaryotes
Major groups	Bacteria and blue-green algae	Other algae, fungi, protozoa, plants and animals
Genetic material		
Location	Free in the cytoplasm attached to a structure called a mesosome located in the cell membrane	Contained within a membrane-bound nucleus inside the cell
Form	A single circular piece of DNA	Multiple chromosomes, which are surrounded by basic proteins called histones
Nucleolus	Absent	Present
Replication	By binary fission	By mitosis and meiosis
Extrachromosomal DNA	Plasmids – small circular pieces of DNA containing accessory information, present in the cytoplasm	In mitochondria
Protein production site	No endoplasmic reticulum; ribosomes – free in the cytoplasm or attached to the cell membrane	• Rough endoplasmic reticulum, a membrane covered with ribosomes, where protein is made • Smooth endoplasmic reticulum or Golgi complex, where secreted proteins are packaged and transported to the cell surface

(*Contd.*)

Characteristic	Prokaryotes	Eukaryotes
Ribosomes	70S in size, consisting of a 50S and 30S subunits	80S in size, consisting of a 60S and 40S subunits
Energy production site	Electron transport chain located in the cell membrane; no mitochondria present	Within membrane-bound mitochondria
Intracellular organelles (lysosomes)	Absent	Contain hydrolytic enzymes
Cytoplasmic membrane	With the exception of *Mycoplasma*, bacterial cytoplasmic membrane lacks sterols	Does contain sterols
Cell wall	Present; is a complex structure containing peptidoglycans, protein, and lipids	Usually absent except in fungi, which contain chitin in the cell wall

Q. 2. Classify bacteria on the basis of their shape and describe their group patterns.

Ans. **Shape of bacteria**

Bacteria exist in different shapes as under (Fig. 2.1):

1. **Cocci** (from *kokkos* meaning berry) are round or oval cells.
2. **Bacilli** (from *baculus* meaning rod) are rod or stick-shaped. In some of the bacilli the length of the cells may be equal to width. Such bacillary forms are known as **coccobacilli**. The latter have to be carefully differentiated from cocci.
3. **Vibrios** are curved or comma-shaped rods.
4. **Spirilla** are non-flexuous spiral forms with one to three fixed curves in their rigid bodies.
5. **Spirochaetes** (from *spira* meaning coil and *chaite* meaning hair) are slender and flexuous spiral forms.
6. **Mycoplasmas** are cell wall deficient organisms. Therefore, they do not possess stable morphology. They occur as round or oval bodies or as interlacing filaments.

Group patterns

The most frequent method of reproduction among bacteria is asexual binary fission, that is, each cell splits in half, forming two new cells. As they increase in number they form distinct groups. Cocci that split along one plane only tend to arrange themselves in pairs (**diplococci**) or in chains (**streptococci**). When the division occurs alternatively in each of two planes, groups of four (**tetrads**) or eight (**octads**) are formed. Haphazard splitting in several planes results in the formation of clusters of cocci (Fig. 2.1).

Bacilli split only across their short axes, therefore, the patterns formed by them are limited. They may appear as end to end pairs (**diplobacilli**), or chains (**streptobacilli**) (Fig. 2.1). In some instances, there occurs incomplete separation of the daughter cells after binary fission. The bacilli remain attached to each other at various angles, resembling the letters V or L. This is called **Chinese letter arrangement** and is characteristic of *Corynebacterium diphtheriae*.

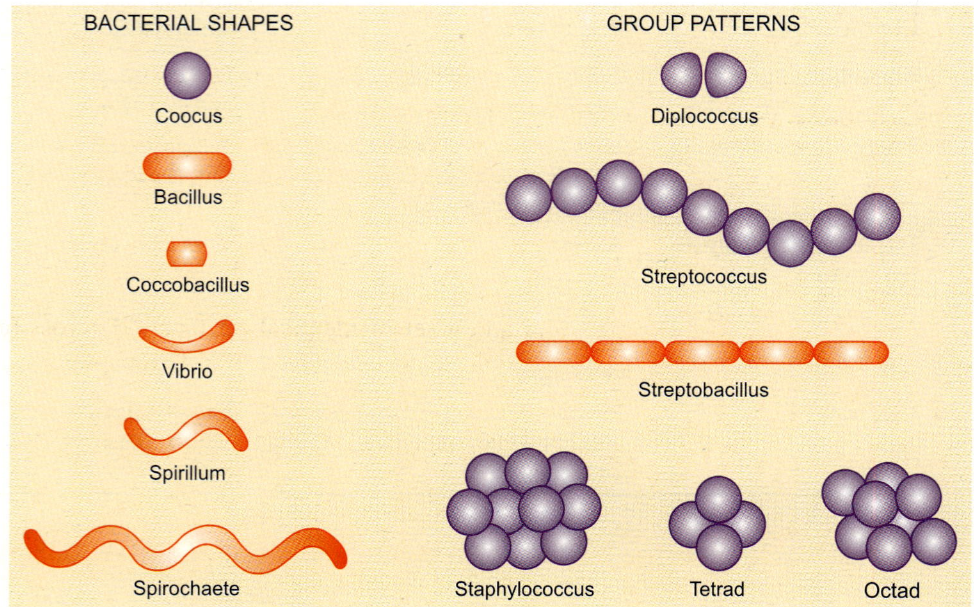

Fig. 2.1. Shapes and group patterns of bacteria.

Q. 3. Draw a labelled diagram of anatomy of a bacterial cell.

Ans. Fig. 2.2 shows the anatomy of a bacterial cell.

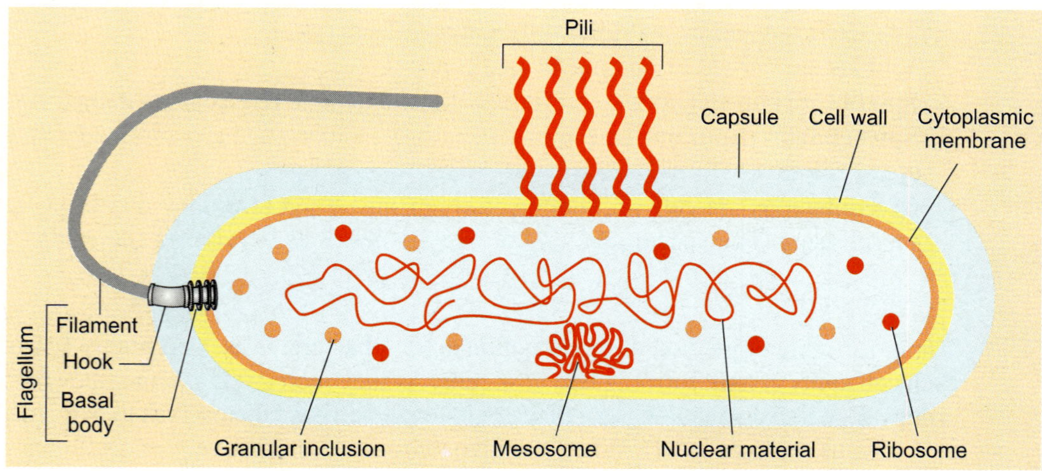

Fig. 2.2. Anatomy of a bacterial cell.

Q. 4. Describe the functions and structure of Gram-positive, Gram-negative and acid-fast bacterial cell wall. Tabulate difference between cell walls of Gram-positive and Gram-negative bacteria. Mention steps for demonstration of bacterial cell wall.

Ans. Functions of bacterial cell wall

- It is a complex rigid structure which gives bacteria their definite shape.

- It is permeable to passage of liquid nutrient material into the cell, and to outward passage of substances produced within the cell.
- It is about 10–20 nm in thickness and constitutes 20–30% of dry weight of the cell.
- The cell walls of Gram-positive bacteria are generally thicker than those of Gram-negative bacteria.
- The strength of the bacterial cell wall is due to the presence in it of a substance referred to as **peptidoglycan**, mucopeptide or murein.

Peptidoglycan consists of three parts – a backbone, composed of alternating *N*-acetylglucosamine and *N*-acetylmuramic acid; a set of identical tetrapeptide side chains attached to *N*-acetylmuramic acid and a set of identical pentapeptide cross-bridges (Fig. 2.3). In all bacterial species the backbone is the same, however, tetrapeptide side chains and pentapeptide cross-bridges vary from species to species.

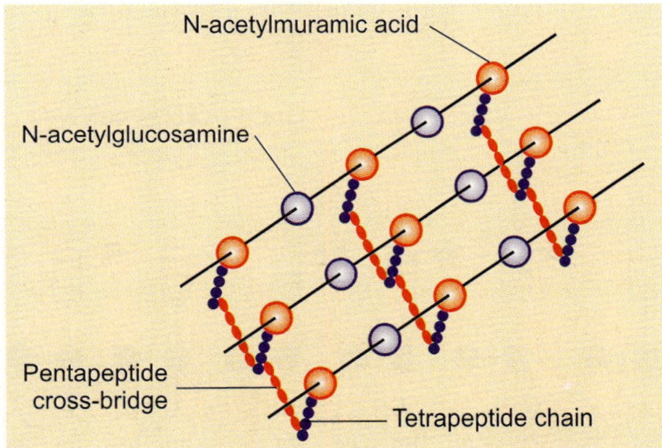

Fig. 2.3. Chemical structure of peptidoglycan.

Structure of Gram-positive bacterial cell wall

- The Gram-positive bacterial cell wall (Fig. 2.4) is 16–80 nm thick and is composed mostly of several layers of **peptidoglycan**.
- It constitutes **50–90%** of the dry weight of the wall.
- In addition to peptidoglycan, Gram-positive cell wall also contains teichoic acids and polysaccharides. There are two types of teichoic acids – cell wall teichoic acid, covalently linked to peptidoglycan; and membrane teichoic acid, covalently linked to cytoplasmic membrane.

Structure of Gram-negative bacterial cell wall

- The cell wall of Gram-negative bacteria (Fig. 2.5) is thinner (2 nm) than that of Gram-positive bacteria but is structurally more complex. It consists of peptidoglycan, lipoprotein, outer membrane, and lipopolysaccharide.
- Peptidoglycan layer is a single-unit thick. It constitutes 5–10% of the dry weight of the wall of Gram-negative bacteria.
- Outside the thin peptidoglycan layer is the outer membrane. In this membrane are embedded various large molecules like outer membrane protein and porin protein. Large antibiotic

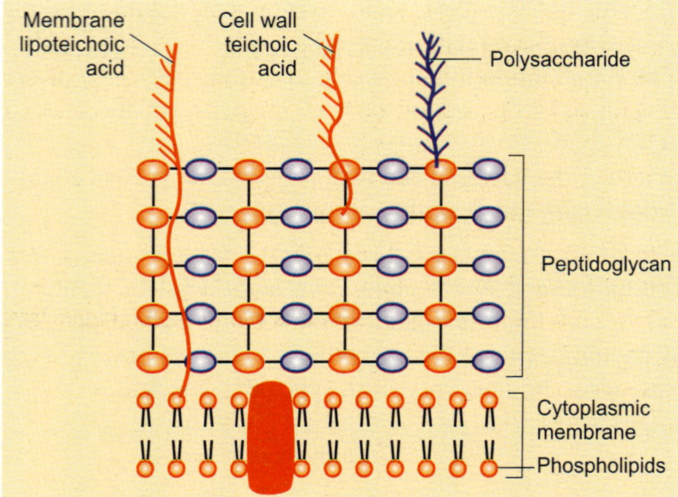

Fig. 2.4. Gram-positive cell wall.

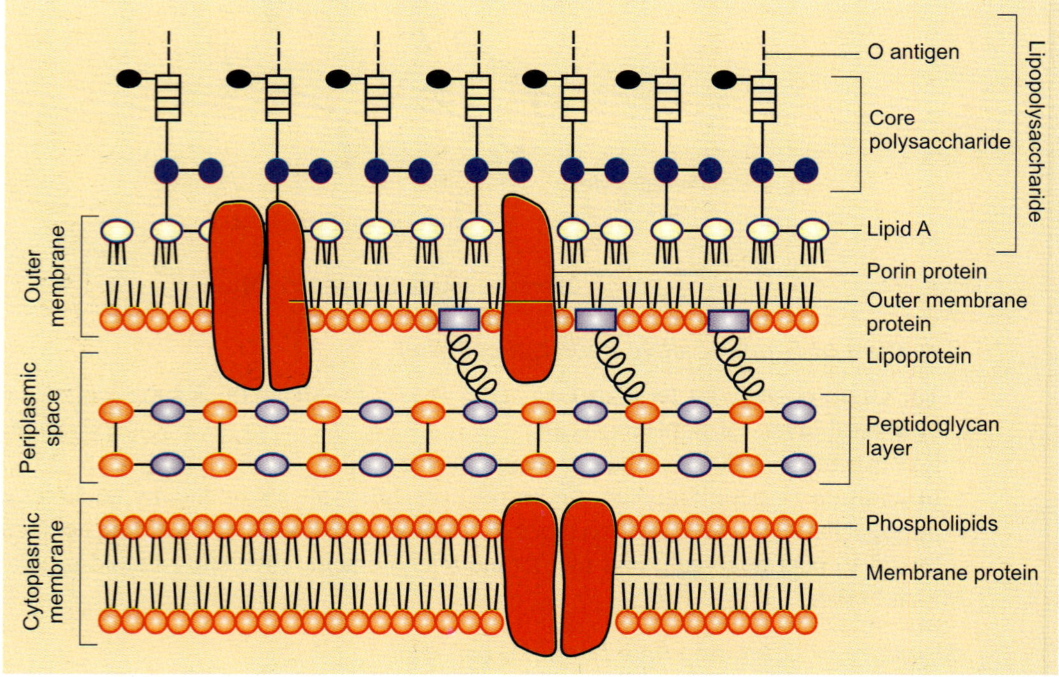

Fig. 2.5. Gram-negative cell wall.

molecules penetrate outer membrane relatively slowly, which accounts for the relatively high antibiotic resistance of Gram-negative bacteria. Outer membrane is anchored to the peptidoglycan layer by strongly lipophilic lipoprotein.

- A structural component that is unique to the Gram-negative outer membrane is **lipopolysaccharide (LPS)**. It consists of a complex lipid, called lipid A, to which is attached a core polysaccharide. From core polysaccharide extends outward O polysaccharide. It has several peculiar sugars and varies in composition between bacterial strains, conferring species-specific antigen specificity. It represents a major surface antigen of the bacterial cell. It is known as **O antigen**. Bacteria carrying LPS containing O antigen form smooth colonies in bacteriological media in contrast to those lacking O antigen, which form rough colonies. LPS is firmly bound to the cell surface and is released only when the cells are lysed. It is, therefore, known as **endotoxin** and is extremely toxic to animals. All the toxicity of the endotoxin is due to lipid A.

- The space between the inner membrane (cytoplasmic membrane) and outer membrane is known as **periplasmic space**. It contains the peptidoglycan layer and a gel-like solution of proteins.

The differences between cell walls of Gram-positive and Gram-negative bacteria are given in Table 2.2.

Table 2.2. Differences between cell walls of Gram-positive and Gram-negative bacteria

No.	Character	Gram-positive cell wall	Gram-negative cell wall
1.	Thickness	Thicker	Thinner
2.	Peptidoglycan	Thick layer (16–80 nm)	Thin layer (2 nm)
3.	Lipid content	2–5%	15–20%
4.	Techoic acid	Absent	Present
5.	Porin proteins	Absent	Present
6.	Variety of amino acids	Few	Several
7.	Periplasmic space	Absent	Present
8.	Endotoxic activity	Absent	Present

Acid-fast cell wall

Certain genera (*Mycobacterium* and *Nocardia*) have a Gram-positive cell wall structure but, in addition, contain a waxy layer of glycolipids and fatty acids (**mycolic acid**) bound to the exterior of the cell wall. This makes *Mycobacterium* species difficult to stain with the Gram stain. The mycobacteria and nocardiae can be stained with an acid-fast stain, in which the bacteria are stained with carbol fuchsin, followed by treatment with sulphuric acid or acid alcohol as decolourizer. Other bacteria are decolourized, whereas mycobacteria and nocardiae retain the stain. They are, therefore, known as **acid-fast bacteria**.

Demonstration of cell wall

The cell wall cannot be seen by light microscopy and does not stain with simple dyes. It can be demonstrated by:

- plasmolysis,
- microdissection,
- exposure to specific antibody,
- mechanical rupture of the cell,
- differential staining procedure, and
- electron microscopy.

Q. 5. Write short note on protoplasts and spheroplasts.

Ans. **Protoplast**

When a Gram-positive bacterium is treated with lysozyme in a hypotonic solution it lyses. If the osmotic strength of the solution is raised to balance the internal osmotic pressure of the cell, a free protoplast is liberated consisting of cytoplasmic membrane and its contents.

Spheroplast

When Gram-negative bacteria are treated with lysozyme, the outer membrane of the cell wall prevents access of lysozyme unless disrupted by an agent such as ethylenediamine tetraacetic acid (EDTA). Lysozyme-EDTA treated bacteria result in the formation of spheroplasts which still possess remnants of the complex Gram-negative cell wall.

Removal of the bacterial cell wall may also be accomplished by growing the organisms in the presence of a substance such as penicillin, bacitracin or cycloserine that blocks peptidoglycan biosynthesis. A similar result may be obtained by growing the organisms on a medium lacking nutrients like diaminopimelic acid, lysine or hexosamine which are essential for cell wall synthesis. If maintained on osmotically protective medium, protoplasts metabolize and grow in size but they do not multiply. Spheroplasts, on the other hand, when kept on osmotically protective agar medium containing cell wall inhibitor such as penicillin, may multiply by fission or budding and reproduce through many serial subcultures.

Because spheroplasts retain a residual cell wall, therefore, they are osmotically less sensitive than protoplasts and are often capable of growing on an ordinary agar medium. Spheroplasts are capable of reverting to parent bacterial form when cell wall inhibitor is removed from the culture medium. Protoplasts perhaps cannot do so. Because of their resemblance with L forms of bacteria, spheroplasts may be called **unstable L forms**.

Q. 6. Describe briefly cytoplasmic membrane.

Ans. Bacterial cytoplasmic membrane, also called cell membrane, limits the bacterial protoplast externally. It is thin (5–10 nm), elastic and consists of a phospholipid bilayer in which various constituent proteins are embedded (Figs. 2.4 and 2.5). With the exception of *Mycoplasma*, bacterial cytoplasmic membrane lacks sterols. **It acts as a semipermeable membrane controlling the inflow and outflow of metabolites to and from the protoplasm.** It permits the passive diffusion inward and outward of water and other small molecular substances, but it actively effects the selective transport of specific nutrients into the cell and that of waste products out of it. This is mediated through specific enzymes (permeases) present in the cytoplasmic membrane.

Q. 7. Write briefly about cytoplasm. How does it differ from that of eukaryotic organisms?

Ans. Cytoplasm of the bacterial cell is a viscous watery solution of soft gel, containing a variety of organic and inorganic solutes. It contains all biosynthetic components required by the bacterium for the growth and cell division, together with genetic material. The cytoplasm of bacteria differs from that of higher eukaryotic organisms in not containing endoplasmic reticulum, Golgi apparatus, mitochondria, lysosomes and in not showing signs of internal mobility, e.g., cytoplasmic streaming, the formation, migration and disappearance of vacuoles and amoeboid movement. Cytoplasm contains ribosomes, mesosomes and intracytoplasmic inclusion bodies (Fig. 2.2).

Q. 8. Write short note on ribosomes. How do they differ from host cell ribosomes?

Ans. Ribosomes are composed of ribosomal RNA (rRNA) and ribosomal proteins and are designated by their sedimentation coefficient (S or Svedberg unit). They are slightly smaller than those of eukaryotic cells. They measure 10–20 nm in diameter and have a sedimentation coefficient of 70S. Each 70S particle is composed of a 30S and a 50S subparticle. Each cell contains thousands of ribosomes strung together on strands of messenger RNA (mRNA) to form polysomes and it is at this site that code of mRNA is translated into peptide sequences. There are certain considerable differences between bacterial and host cell ribosomes. This allows us to use antibacterial agents such as streptomycin which interfere with bacterial metabolism at the ribosomal level without unduly upsetting human ribosomal function.

Q. 9. Write short note on mesosomes.

Ans. These are convoluted or multilaminated membranous bodies which develop by invagination of cytoplasmic membrane into the cytoplasm (Fig. 2.2). They provide increased membrane surface and are principal sites of respiratory enzymes in bacteria. They are analogous to mitochondria of eukaryotes and are more prominent in Gram-positive bacteria. They are often seen in relation to the nuclear body and the site of synthesis of cross-wall septa, suggesting that they coordinate nuclear and cytoplasmic division during binary fission.

Q. 10. Write short note on bacterial nucleus.

Ans. The genetic information of a bacterial cell is contained in a single, circular, double-stranded molecule of DNA. It is often accompanied by a smaller extrachromosomal DNA known as **plasmid**. It is 1000 μm or more in length, about 1000 times the length of the cell. Therefore, it occurs tightly coiled like a skein of woollen thread. Since it is not bound to proteins, therefore, it does not stain like a eukaryotic chromosome. **Bacterial nucleus does not possess nuclear membrane, nucleolus, deoxyribonucleoprotein and does not divide by mitosis.**

Q. 11. Write briefly about bacterial capsule and slime layer. Mention procedures for demonstration of capsule, and enumerate functions of capsule.

Ans. Cell wall in many bacteria is enclosed by a protective gelatinous covering layer. If it is easily washed off and does not appear to be associated with the cell in any definite fashion it is referred to as a **slime layer**, on the other hand if it appears as discrete, thickened gel around each cell, it is called a **capsule** (Fig. 2.6). If capsule is too thin to be seen with light microscope, it is called **microcapsule**. In most species it is made up of a complex polysaccharide (e.g., pneumococcus), though in some species its main constituent is polypeptide (e.g., anthrax bacillus). When slime forming bacteria are grown on a solid culture medium, the slime remains around the bacteria as a matrix in which they are embedded and its presence confers on growth a **mucoid** character.

Demonstration of capsule

- Capsule cannot be stained with ordinary stains like Gram staining.

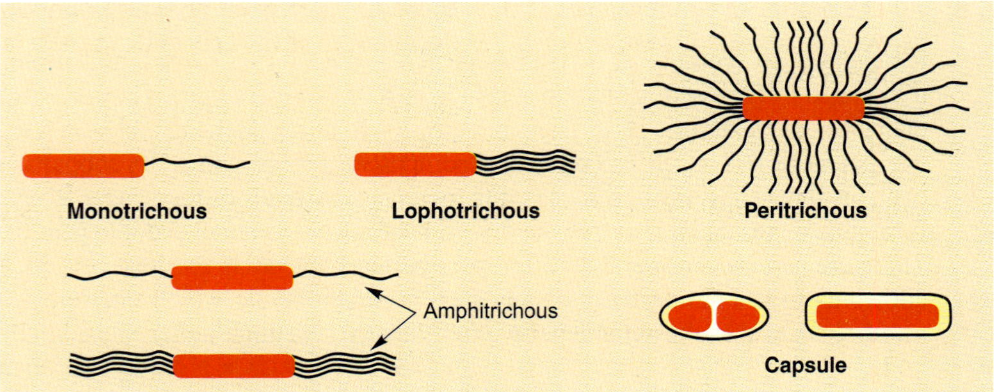

Fig. 2.6. Arrangement of flagella and capsule.

- It can be visualized by suspending the organisms in India ink and observing microscopically the exclusion of the colloidal ink particles from the area around the cell that is occupied by the capsule.
- It may also be visualized by reaction with specific antibody which causes a characteristic swelling of the capsule. It is known as **Quellung reaction**. This phenomenon is seen in and allows rapid identification of capsular serotypes of *Streptococcus pneumoniae*, *Neisseria meningitidis*, several groups of streptococci, *Klebsiella* and *Haemophilus influenzae*.

Functions

- Capsules protect the bacteria from antibacterial agents such as lytic enzymes found in nature.
- They inhibit phagocytosis thus contributing to the virulence of the bacteria.
- The capsular antigen is specific for bacteria, therefore, it can be used for identification and typing of bacteria.

Loss of capsule by mutation may render the bacterium avirulent. Bacteria tend to lose capsules on repeated subcultures *in vitro*.

Q. 12. Discuss structure, arrangement and procedure for demonstration of flagella.

Ans. A large number of bacteria including a few coccal forms, about one half of bacilli and almost all of the spirilla and vibrios are motile by means of flagella. Flagella are long, hollow, helical filaments usually several times the length of the cell. They are 10–20 nm in diameter, 3–20 μm in length and are found on both Gram-positive and Gram-negative bacteria. Their number varies from 1 to 20 flagella per bacterial cell.

Arrangement of flagella

There are four types of arrangement of flagella (Fig. 2.6).

1. **Monotrichous:** These organisms have a single polar flagellum.
2. **Lophotrichous:** They have a tuft of flagella at one pole.
3. **Amphitrichous:** They have single polar flagella or tuft of flagella at both poles.
4. **Peritrichous:** Flagella are distributed all round the cell.

The motility in spirochaetes is due to one or more pairs of axial filaments which run between **outer membrane and peptidoglycan layer of the cell wall, and are anchored by knobs at both poles**.

Flagella consist mainly of a protein called flagellin which belongs to the same chemical group as myosin – the contractile protein of muscle. Though flagella of different genera of bacteria have the same chemical composition, they are antigenically different. Flagellar antigens induce specific antibodies in high titres. These antibodies are non-protective but are useful in serodiagnosis.

Structure of flagellum

The flagellum consists of three parts – the **filament**, the **hook** and the **basal body**. The basal body, anchored in the cytoplasmic membrane, comprises a rod and two or more sets of encircling rings. In Gram-negative bacteria four types of rings (M, S, P and L) are seen. Through ring M it attaches to the cytoplasmic membrane, ring S is located just above cytoplasmic membrane and through rings P and L it is attached to peptidoglycan and outer lipopolysaccharide membrane respectively (Fig. 2.7). Rings P and L are absent in Gram-positive bacteria.

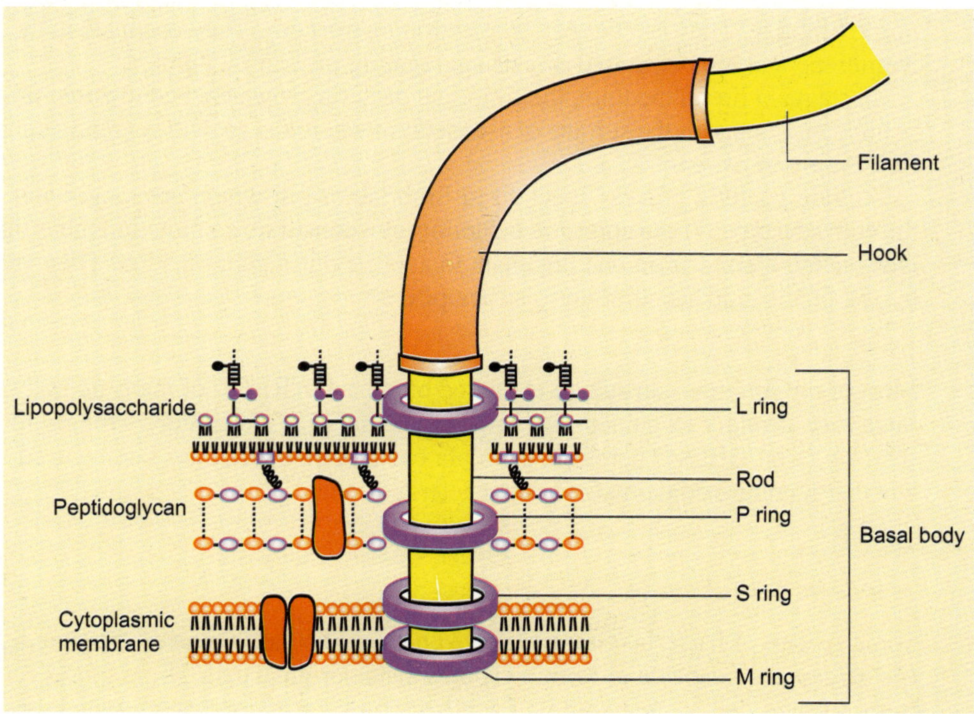

Fig. 2.7. Structure of flagellum.

Demonstration of flagella

- Flagella can be demonstrated by ordinary light microscope by special staining techniques in which their thickness is increased by mordanting. In some instances, they can be seen with dark-ground microscopy. However, they can be easily visualized under electron microscope. In routine, their presence is inferred by the motility of the bacteria. The latter may be observed either microscopically or by the occurrence of spreading growth in semisolid agar medium.

- On microscopic examination of wet films, motile bacteria are seen swimming in different directions across the field with darting (*V. cholerae*), very active (*Proteus* spp.), active (*Escherichia coli*), sluggish and tumbling (*Listeria monocytogenes*) motility. True motility should be differentiated from Brownian movement which is a rapid oscillation of the bacterium within a very limited area due to bombardment by the water molecules.

Q. 13. Write short note on fimbriae.

Ans. They are hair-like microfibrils 1–1.5 µm in length and 4–8 nm in diameter. They are straighter, thinner and shorter than flagella (Fig. 2.2). They are present on many Gram-negative cells and provide a means for adherence to other cells, either bacterial or animal. They are an example of a class of surface structures termed **adhesins** that allow attachment of bacterial cell to cell surfaces (organelles of adhesion). Therefore, they are very important for bacterial survival in an animal host. They occur in both flagellated and non-flagellated bacteria and are far more numerous than flagella. Each bacterium possesses 100–500 peritrichously-borne fimbriae. They can be seen by electron microscopy. They originate in the cytoplasmic membrane and are composed of self-aggregating protein monomers.

In stagnant liquid medium, the fimbriate bacteria grow attached together in the form of a pellicle that floats on the surface of the medium where the growth is greatly enhanced by the free supply of oxygen.

Certain bacteria possess specialized fimbriae or pili which are longer and thinner than the common type. These appear to be hollow and constitute conjugation tubes through which DNA is transferred from one organism to another during conjugation. They are determined by sex factors and are referred to as **sex pili**.

Detection of fimbriae

Most of the fimbriae can adhere to the red blood cells (RBCs) of many animal species. They bind very strongly to guinea-pig, fowl, horse and pig; moderately strongly to human; and scarcely to ox RBCs. Therefore, a simple haemagglutination test can be used to determine whether a culture contains fimbriate bacteria or not.

Q. 14. Discuss bacterial spore, sporulation, shape and position, resistance, germination and demonstration of bacterial spores.

Ans. Some species of bacteria (Gram-positive only), particularly those of the genera *Bacillus* and *Clostridium*, are capable of forming spores inside original cell. These spores can be released from original cell as free spores. Each bacterium forms one spore which on germination forms a single vegetative cell. Sporulation in bacteria, therefore, is a method of preservation and not of reproduction.

Spores are small, highly resistant, metabolically dormant structures which develop as a response to starvation. They are not formed as long as conditions continue to favour maximal vegetative growth. Formation of spores occurs over a period of 4–8 hours after the cells stop growing upon depletion of their carbohydrate supply.

Sporulation

It develops from a portion of protoplasm near one end of the cell. This part of the bacterial cell is known as **forespore** and the remaining part as **sporangium** (Fig. 2.8). Bacterial DNA replicates and partitions into two halves and one of them, which is equivalent to one genome of the cell, is incorporated into forespore. A transverse septum derived from the cytoplasmic membrane is then formed by a process of invagination which divides forespore and sporangium. The forespore is subsequently completely encircled by dividing septum as a double layered membrane.

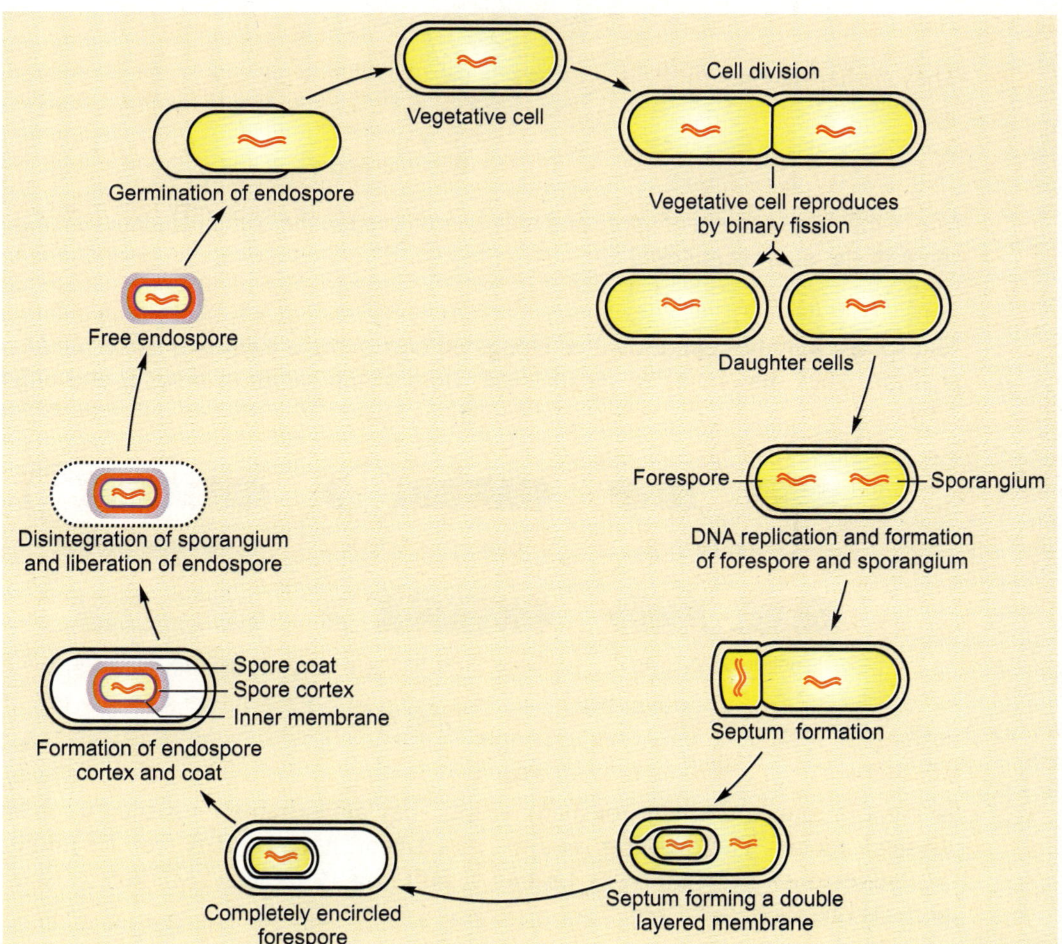

Fig. 2.8. Morphological events in sporulation.

The two spore membranes now engage in active synthesis of various layers of the spore. The inner layer becomes the **inner membrane**. Between the two layers is laid **spore cortex** and outer layer is transformed into **spore coat** which consists of several layers. In some species from outer layer also develops **exosporium** which bears ridges and folds (Fig. 2.9). Finally exosporium disintegrates and the endospore is freed. Mesosomes appear to play a

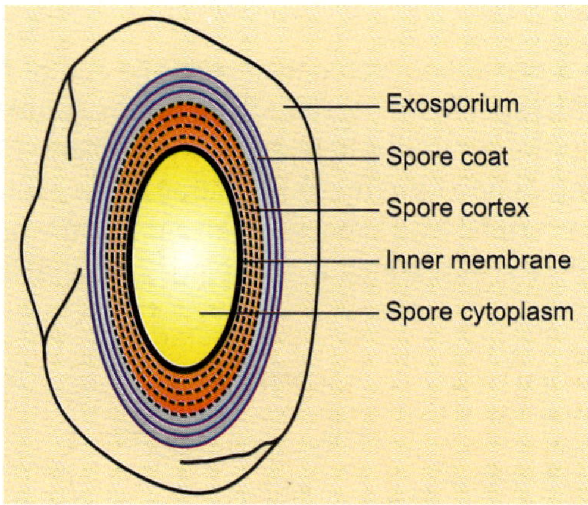

Fig. 2.9. Bacterial spore.

role in the development of spore and may be involved in the compartmentation of the spore's share of the nuclear material.

Shape and position

The spores may be round, oval or elongated occupying a terminal, subterminal or central position. They may be narrower than the width of the bacilli or broader and bulging (Fig. 2.10).

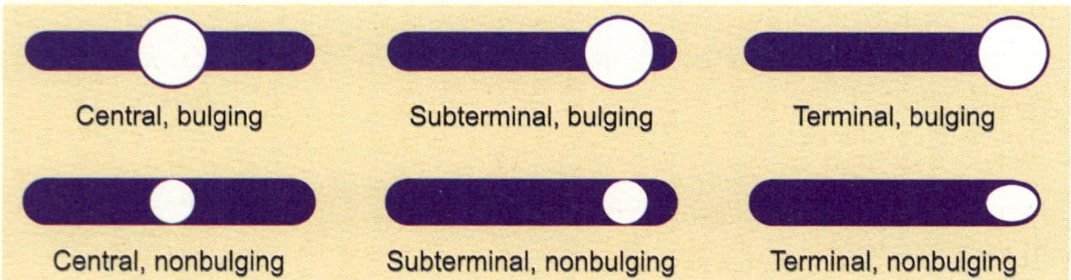

Fig. 2.10. Types of spores.

Resistance

Spores can remain dormant for many years. They are extremely resistant to chemical and physical agents. Their killing requires moist heat at 100–120°C for 10 minutes while vegetative cells can be killed by heating at 60°C for 10 minutes. Marked resistance of the spores is due to:

- the impermeability of their cortex and outer coat,
- their high content of calcium and dipicolinic acid,
- their low content of water, and
- their very low metabolic and enzymatic activity.

Germination

Spores are able to **germinate** when the external conditions become favourable to growth by access to moisture and nutrients particularly trigger nutrients such as a particular amino acid, pyrimidine or sugar in a suitable aqueous environment. Within a short period of time spore loses its heat resistance, refractility, dipicolinic acid and calcium. It then swells and absorbs water, after which the spore coat ruptures, and a new vegetative cell grows out.

Demonstration

- In unstained preparations, the spore is recognized within the parent cell by its greater refractility. In simple stains like Gram it remains unstained and appears as a clear space within the stained cell protoplasm (Fig. 2.11).
- They are slightly acid-fast and may be demonstrated by modified Ziehl-Neelsen staining.

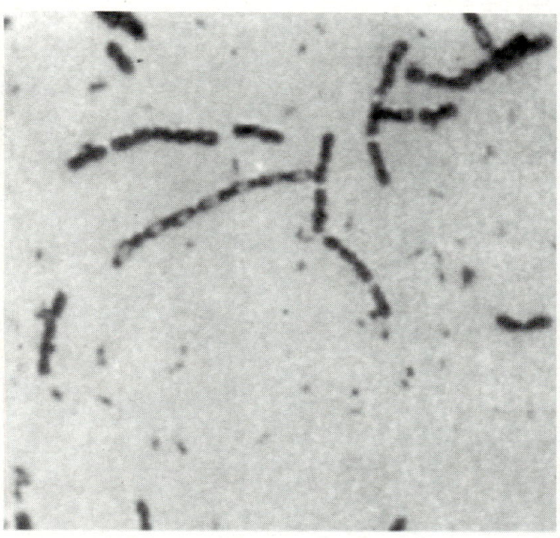

Fig. 2.11. Gram-stained smear of *Bacillus subtilis* showing Gram-positive bacilli in chains with spores which appear as unstained areas within the bacilli.

Q. 15. Describe briefly L-forms of bacteria.

Ans. L-forms (after Lister Institute, London) of bacteria are cell wall deficient bacteria derived by variation, usually in the laboratory, from bacteria of normal morphology. They are stable in the sense that special conditions of culture, such as presence of penicillin, are not required to prevent their reversion to the parental bacterial forms. They lack regular size and shape. They may be spherical or disc-like and measure 0.1–20 μm in diameter.

Cultural characteristics

L-forms are difficult to grow and usually require a medium that is solidified with agar as well as having the right osmotic strength. L-forms are produced more readily with penicillin than with lysozyme.

Colonies of L-forms of bacteria on agar medium show a characteristic **'fried-egg'** appearance with a dark thick centre, where many of the organisms embed themselves and grow within the agar, and a lighter periphery consisting of organisms lying on the surface of the agar. In liquid medium they grow in the form of clumps. Some L-forms are capable of reverting to normal bacillary forms upon removal of the inducing stimulus. Other L-forms are, however, stable and never revert. Presence of residual peptidoglycan is essential for reversion. It acts as a primer in its own biosynthesis.

3

GROWTH AND NUTRITION OF BACTERIA

Q. 1. Describe bacterial growth curve.

Ans. When a bacterium is inoculated into a suitable culture medium and incubated, its growth follows a characteristic course. If both total and viable counts are made at different intervals and plotted in relation to time, then a characteristic growth curve is obtained. A typical growth curve contains four major phases (Fig. 3.1).

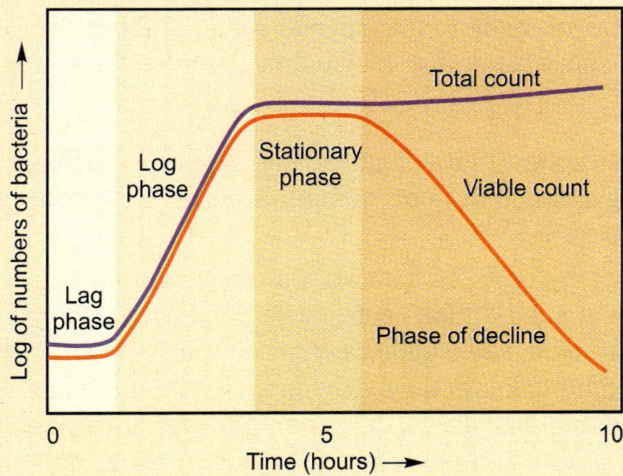

Fig. 3.1. Bacterial growth curve.

1. Lag phase

When bacteria are seeded into fresh medium, multiplication usually does not begin immediately. The period between inoculation and beginning of multiplication is known as lag phase. **During this period the organisms adapt themselves to growth in fresh medium**

and increase in size and metabolic activity. Therefore, lag phase is regarded as a period not of rest but of intense metabolic activity.

2. Log or exponential growth phase

During this phase the bacteria are multiplying at their maximum rate and their number increases exponentially or by geometric progression with time. If logarithm of bacterial count is plotted against time a straight line is obtained. **In the log phase, the bacterial cells are smaller and stain uniformly.** Exponential phase is of limited duration because of:

- exhaustion of nutrients,
- accumulation of toxic metabolic end products,
- rise in cell density,
- change in pH, and
- decrease in oxygen tension (in case of aerobic organisms).

3. Stationary phase

Due to above reasons exponential growth slows down and the bacterial population enters the stationary phase in which the number of viable cells remains constant. There is almost a balance between the bacterial reproduction and bacterial death. **During this phase, bacteria become Gram-variable, show irregular staining and spores start forming in spore-forming bacteria.**

4. Phase of decline

Stationary phase is followed eventually by the phase of decline because rate of death exceeds the rate of reproduction and the number of viable cells declines. **Finally, after a variable period, all the cells die and culture becomes sterile.**

Q. 2. Classify culture media. Describe these giving suitable examples.

Ans. Culture media may be classified into basal media, enriched media, selective media, enrichment media, indicator or differential media, transport or holding media, storage media, sugar media and anaerobic media.

Basal media

These include peptone water and nutrient broths which form the basis of most media used in the study of the common pathogenic bacteria.

Meat extract broth is most commonly used. It can be made solid by addition of 1–2% agar. If the concentration of agar is reduced to 0.2–0.5%, it is called **semisolid agar**. If its concentration is raised to 6%, it is called **hard agar**. In semisolid agar the motile organisms show growth in entire medium, and on surface of hard agar swarming of *Proteus* is inhibited.

Enriched media

These are prepared to meet the nutritional requirements of fastidious organisms by addition of substances such as blood, serum and egg to a basal medium. Important examples of enriched media are blood agar for isolation of *Streptococcus*, chocolate agar for isolation of *Neisseria* and *Haemophilus*, and Loeffler's serum slope for the isolation of *Corynebacterium diphtheriae*.

Selective media

When a substance is added to a solid medium which inhibits the growth of unwanted bacteria but permits the growth of wanted bacteria in the form of colonies it is known as selective medium. Important examples of this type of media are MacConkey agar for *E. coli*, deoxycholate citrate agar (DCA) for *Salmonella* and *Shigella*, Wilson and Blair's medium for *Salmonella*, Lowenstein-Jensen medium for *Mycobacterium tuberculosis*, and blood tellurite agar medium for isolation of *Corynebacterium diphtheriae*.

Enrichment media

When a substance is added to a liquid medium which inhibits the growth of unwanted bacteria and favours the growth of wanted bacteria it is known as enrichment medium. Important examples of this type of media are tetrathionate and selenite broth for *Salmonella* and *Shigella*, and alkaline peptone water for *Vibrio cholerae*.

Indicator media or differential media

When a substance is added into a medium which would produce a visible change in the medium following the growth of a particular organism, it is designated as indicator or differential medium. For example, MacConkey medium contains lactose and neutral red. Lactose-fermenting organisms after growth on this medium produce acid and in acidic pH neutral red becomes red in colour. Thus *E. coli* which is lactose fermenter produces red or pink colonies on this medium.

Christensen's medium contains urea and phenol red. When urease producing organisms like *Proteus* and *Klebsiella* grow on this medium, urea is split up into ammonia and carbon dioxide. Ammonia makes the medium alkaline and in alkaline pH the medium becomes pink in colour (in alkaline pH phenol red is pink in colour). Enriched media can also be differential on the basis of certain growth characteristics evident on the medium. Blood agar is considered both an enriched and differential medium because it differentiates organisms based on whether they are α-, β- or γ-haemolytic.

Transport or holding media

When the clinical sample is being transported from the hospital to the laboratory, delicate organisms like *Neisseria gonorrhoeae* may not survive or the normal flora (*E. coli*) may overgrow pathogenic flora (*Salmonella*, *Shigella* and *V. cholerae*). Transport media maintain the viability of microorganisms present in a specimen without supporting the growth of any organism. These maintain the organisms in a state of suspended animation so that no organism overgrows another or dies out. These media typically contain only buffers and salts. They lack carbon, nitrogen and organic growth factors, hence do not facilitate microbial multiplication. Stuart's transport medium and Amies transport medium are examples of transport media.

Storage media

Bacteria are best preserved and stored by lyophilization. But for preservation and storage for a few months or so, they can be stab inoculated on semisolid agar or on Dorset egg medium followed by incubation. When growth appears they can be stored in refrigerator.

Sugar media

For the identification of most of the organisms, sugar fermentation reactions are carried out. Glucose, lactose, sucrose and mannitol are widely used sugars. For the preparation of sugar media, 1% of the concerned sugar is added to peptone water with a suitable indicator. Durham's tube (a small tube) is kept inverted in the tube containing this medium to detect gas production. For fastidious organisms like *C. diphtheriae* and pneumococci, Hiss's serum peptone water medium is used.

Anaerobic media

For the growth of anaerobes, the media used contain reducing substances. These include thioglycollate broth and cooked meat broth. The sterile muscle tissue, in cooked meat broth, contains reducing substances, particularly glutathione, which permit the growth of many strict anaerobes. In addition to its reducing effect, the meat provides a variety of nutritional substances for bacterial growth. In this medium, saccharolytic clostridia rapidly produce acid and gas but do not digest the meat. The cultures may have slight sour smell and the meat is often reddened. The proteolytic clostridia produce blackening of the meat, decomposing it and reducing it in volume with the formation of foul-smelling products.

Q. 3. Describe anaerobic culture methods.

Ans. A variety of methods are available for the culture of anaerobic organisms in the clinical laboratory. Exclusion of oxygen from the medium is the simplest method, and is effected by growing the organisms within the culture medium such as freshly steamed liquid media and deep nutrient agar with 0.5% glucose and minimal shaking and solidified rapidly by placing the tube in cold water.

Liquid media soon become aerobic unless a reducing agent such as glucose 0.5–1.0%, ascorbic acid 0.1%, cysteine 0.1%, sodium thioglycollate 0.1%, or particles of meat in cooked meat broth are added. Liquid media should be prereduced by holding in a boiling water bath for 10 minutes to drive off dissolved oxygen, then quickly cooled to 37°C just before use.

Cooked meat broth, **CMB** (original medium known as 'Robertson's bullock-heart medium') has a special place in anaerobic bacteriology; and thioglycollate broth and its modifications are also very useful. CMB is suitable for growing anaerobes in air and also for the preservation of stock cultures of aerobic organisms. The inoculum is introduced deep in the medium in contact with the meat. Meat particles are placed in 30 ml bottles to a depth of about 2.5 cm and covered with about 15 ml broth.

Anaerobic jars

When an oxygen-free or anaerobic atmosphere is required for obtaining surface growths of anaerobes, anaerobic jars provide the method of choice. The most reliable and widely used anaerobic jar is the **McIntosh-Fildes' anaerobic jar**. It is a cylindrical vessel made of glass or metal with a metal lid which is held firmly in place by a clamp (Fig. 3.2). The lid has two tubes with taps, one acting as gas inlet and the other as the outlet. On its undersurface it carries a gauze sachet carrying alumina pellets coated with palladium. It acts as a room temperature catalyst for the conversion of hydrogen and oxygen into water. It acts as a catalyst, as long as the sachet is kept dry.

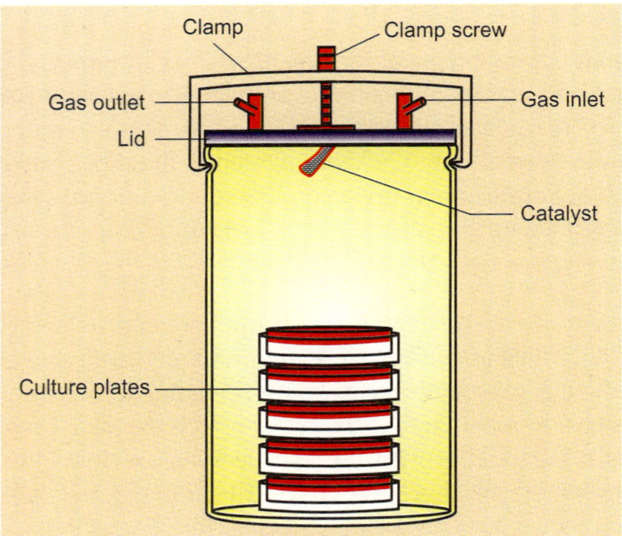

Fig. 3.2. Anaerobic jar.

Inoculated culture plates are placed inside the jar and the lid clamped tight. The outlet tube is connected to a vacuum pump and the air inside is evacuated. The outlet tap is then closed and the inlet tube connected to a hydrogen supply. Hydrogen is drawn in rapidly. As soon as this inrush of gas has ceased the inlet tap is also closed. After about 5 minutes inlet tap is again opened. There occurs again an immediate inrush of hydrogen since the catalyst creates a reduced pressure within the jar due to the conversion of hydrogen and left over oxygen into water. If there is no inrush of hydrogen, it means the catalyst is inactive and must be replaced. The jar is left connected to the hydrogen supply for about 5 minutes, then the inlet tap is closed and the jar is placed in the incubator, catalysis will continue until all the oxygen in the jar has been used up.

The **GasPak** is now the method of choice for preparing anaerobic jar. The GasPak is commercially available as a disposable envelope containing chemicals which generate hydrogen and carbon dioxide on the addition of water. After the inoculated plates are kept in the jar, the GasPak envelope with water added, is placed inside and the lid screwed tight. Hydrogen and carbon dioxide are liberated and the presence of a cold catalyst in the envelope permits the combination of hydrogen and oxygen to produce an anaerobic environment. The outstanding feature of the GasPak system is the disposable gas generator envelope, which does away with the need for a vacuum pump and cylinders of compressed gas; the operation of the jar is consequently very quick and simple. As the standard GasPak jar is not evacuated before use a relatively large volume of water is formed during catalysis.

An **indicator** should be used for verifying the anaerobic condition in the jar. Methylene blue is generally used for this purpose. When it is placed in an anaerobic environment it is reduced from its coloured oxidized form to a colourless reduced leuco-compound.

In addition to, or instead of, using a chemical indicator, some workers include in the jar a plate inoculated with a known strict anaerobe such as *Clostridium tetani* or *Bacteroides fragilis*, and a strict aerobe, such as *Pseudomonas aeruginosa*. This method is quite reliable if the indicator anaerobe grows and the aerobe does not.

Anaerobic chamber

This is an ideal anaerobic incubation system, which provides oxygen-free environment for inoculating media and incubating cultures. Identification and susceptibility tests can also be performed in anaerobic chambers.

Anaerobic chambers may be fitted with airtight rubber gloves to insert hands and manipulate specimens, plates, tubes or they may be gloveless where airtight rubber sleeves fit tightly against user's bare forearms. All anaerobic chambers contain a catalyst, dessicant, H_2 gas (5–10%), CO_2 gas (5–10%), N_2 gas (80–90%) and an indicator.

Anaerobic bags or pouches

These bags are available commercially and one or two inoculated plates are placed into a bag and an oxygen removal system is activated and the bag is sealed and incubated. Plates can be examined for growth without removing the plates from bag, thus without exposing the colonies to oxygen. But as with anaerobic jar, plates must be removed from the bags in order to work with the colonies at the bench. These bags are also useful in transport of biopsy specimen for anaerobic cultures.

Incubation

Inoculated plates should be incubated at 37°C for at least 48 hours, and reincubated for another 2–4 days to allow slow-growing organisms (certain species of *Actinomyces* and *Eubacterium*) to form colonies.

4

IDENTIFICATION OF BACTERIA AND TAXONOMY

Q. 1. Describe method, uses and mechanism of Gram staining.

Ans. *Method of Gram staining*

- Prepare smear from clinical specimen, culture smear of colony or broth culture on a clean glass slide by spreading thinly on the slide.
- Allow it to dry in air and fix it by passing the dried side, film downwards, three times slowly through the flame.
- Cover the smear with crystal violet (primary stain) for one minute. Other pararosaniline dyes such as methyl violet or gentian violet may also be used as primary stain.
- Pour Gram's iodine over the slide for two minutes.
- Decolorize with alcohol or acetone for 10–30 seconds.
- Counterstain with dilute carbol fuchsin or safranin for 30 seconds.
- Wash thoroughly with water; blot and dry in air.
- Examine under oil-immersion lens.

On the basis of their reaction to the Gram stain, bacteria can be divided into two groups, i.e., Gram-positive and Gram-negative. Both Gram-positive and Gram-negative bacteria take up violet colour with pararosaniline dyes. After treatment with decolorizing agent, Gram-positive bacteria retain this dye and violet colour while Gram-negative lose the dye and become colourless. They then take up counterstain and appear red in colour.

Uses of Gram staining

The Gram stain is useful in two ways:

1. In the identification of many bacteria.
2. In influencing the choice of antibiotic.

Mechanism of Gram staining

The exact mechanism of Gram reaction is not known. It may, however, be attributed to:

- Gram-positive bacteria have a more acidic protoplasm, which may account for their retaining the basic primary dye more strongly than Gram-negative bacteria.
- The violet basic dye and the iodine form a dye-iodine complex inside both Gram-positive and Gram-negative bacteria but during alcohol or acetone wash, cell membranes (outer membrane of cell wall and cytoplasmic membrane) are dissolved. However, dye-iodine complex is retained in Gram-positive cells by the thick peptidoglycan mesh, whereas it is readily washed out through the very thin peptidoglycan layer remaining in Gram-negative cells after both membranes have been dissolved.
- Gram-positive organisms that have lost cell wall integrity because of antibiotic treatment, old age, or action of autolytic enzymes may allow crystal violet to wash out with the decolorizing step and may appear Gram-variable, with some cells staining pink and others staining violet. However, for identification purposes these organisms are considered Gram-positive. On the other hand, Gram-negative bacteria rarely, if ever, retain crystal violet if staining procedure has been properly performed. Host cells, such as red and white blood cells, allow the crystal violet stain to wash out with decolorization and appear red.

Q. 2. Describe uses, method, result and principle of Ziehl-Neelsen stain.

Ans. *Uses*

Next to Gram stain, this is the method most frequently used in diagnostic bacteriology. It is of value in distinguishing a few bacterial species, e.g., tubercle bacilli, atypical mycobacteria, lepra bacilli and *Nocardia* from all others. Tubercle bacilli, atypical mycobacteria and lepra bacilli are relatively impermeable to simple stains but when stained with hot concentrated carbol fuchsin, subsequently resist decolorization by 20%, 20% and 5% sulphuric acid respectively. Decolorized non-acid-fast organisms are counterstained with methylene blue. However, *Nocardia* which resists decolorization with 0.5% sulphuric acid, can be easily stained with Gram stain and is Gram-positive. Modified Ziehl-Neelsen staining is used for detection of parasites such as *Cryptosporidium*, *Isospora*, *Cyclospora* and microsporidia.

Method

- Cover the slide with filtered carbol fuchsin and heat until steam rises. Allow the preparation to stain for 5 minutes, heat being applied at intervals to keep the stain hot. The stain must not be allowed to evaporate and dry on the slide. If necessary, pour more carbol fuchsin to keep the whole slide covered with carbol fuchsin.
- Wash with water.
- The stained smear is decolorized with 20% sulphuric acid and washed with water. This step is repeated till the film is only very faintly pink.
- Wash the slide well with water.
- Counterstain it with 2% methylene blue for 15–20 seconds.
- Wash, blot, dry and examine under oil-immersion lens.

Result

Acid-fast bacilli stain bright red, while the tissue cells and other organisms are stained blue.

Principle of acid-fastness

Acid-fastness has been attributed to the high content of lipids, fatty acids and higher alcohols found in acid-fast bacteria. Of the lipids, mycolic acid, a high molecular weight hydroxy acid wax containing carboxyl groups, is most important because it is acid-fast even in free state.

Q. 3. Describe briefly use, method and result of Albert staining.

Ans. This method is useful for identification of *Corynebacterium diphtheriae*.

Method

- Prepare the film, dry in air, and fix by heat.
- Cover slide with Albert's stain and allow to act for 3–5 minutes.
- Wash in water and blot dry.
- Cover the slide with Albert's iodine, allow to act for one minute.
- Wash in water and blot dry.

Result

The granules and the protoplasm of *C. diphtheriae* are bluish-black and green respectively.

Q. 4. Write short note on indole production.

Ans. Certain bacteria which possess enzyme **tryptophanase**, degrade amino acid tryptophan to indole, pyruvic acid and ammonia. Indole production is detected by inoculating the test organism into peptone water and incubating it at 37°C for 48–96 hours. Then add 0.5 ml of Kovac's reagent and shake gently. A **red colour** in the alcohol layer indicates a positive reaction.

Q. 5. Write short note on methyl red (MR) test.

Ans. This test detects the production of sufficient acid by fermentation of glucose so that pH of the medium falls and it is maintained below 4.5. Inoculate the test organism in glucose phosphate broth and incubate at 37°C for 2–5 days. Then add five drops of 0.04% solution of methyl red, mix well and read the result immediately. Positive tests are bright red (indicating a low pH) and negative are yellow. If the test is negative after 2 days repeat it after 5 days.

Q. 6. Write short note on Voges-Proskauer (VP) test for acetoin production.

Ans. Many bacteria ferment carbohydrates with the production of acetyl methyl carbinol (acetoin). In the presence of potassium hydroxide and atmospheric oxygen, acetoin is converted to diacetyl, and α-naphthol serves as a catalyst to form a red complex. This test is usually done in conjunction with the methyl red test. *An organism of the family Enterobacteriaceae is usually either methyl red positive and Voges-Proskauer negative or methyl red negative and Voges-Proskauer positive.*

Inoculate test organism in glucose phosphate broth and incubate at 37°C for 48 hours. Then add 1 ml potassium hydroxide and 3 ml of 5% solution of α-naphthol in absolute alcohol. A positive reaction is indicated by the development of **pink colour** in 2–5 minutes and crimson in 30 minutes.

Q. 7. Write short note on citrate utilization.

Ans. This test is used to study the ability of an organism to utilize citrate as a sole source of carbon for the growth. Liquid (Koser's) and solid (Simmon's) media containing citrate as a sole source of carbon can be used. A part of colony is picked up with a straight wire and inoculated into either of these media. The ability of an organism to utilize citrate as a sole source of carbon is detected by the **production of turbidity** (due to growth) in liquid medium. Solid medium also contains bromothymol blue as indicator, therefore, on the solid medium the **appearance of growth and blue colour** is positive, and original green colour and no growth is negative.

The blue colour is due to the alkaline pH that results from utilization of citrate. It turns the indicator in the medium from **green to blue**. It is important to keep the inoculum light, since dead organisms can be a source of carbon, producing a false positive reaction.

Q. 8. Write short note on sugar fermentation.

Ans. The ability of an organism to ferment various sugars is tested by inoculation of the test organism in different sugar media containing Andrade's indicator. A small inverted tube (**Durham's tube**) completely filled with liquid and containing no air bubbles is usually included in each culture tube. Production of acid is indicated by the change in the colour of the medium to red or pink, and gas, if produced, collects in Durham's tube.

Q. 9. Write short note on nitrate reduction.

Ans. This test detects the production of enzyme **nitrate reductase** which reduces nitrate to nitrite. *All the organisms of the family Enterobacteriaceae are positive for this test.* Inoculate test organism in 5 ml medium containing potassium nitrate, peptone and distilled water. Incubate it at 37°C for 96 hours. Then add 0.1 ml test reagent which consists of equal volumes of 0.8% sulphanilic acid and 0.5% α-naphthylamine in 5 N acetic acid mixed just before use. A **red colour** developing within a few minutes indicates the presence of nitrite and hence the ability of test organism to reduce nitrate to nitrite.

If no colour develops, this may indicate that nitrate has not been reduced (a true negative reaction) or that nitrate has been reduced beyond nitrite to nitrogen gas (N_2), nitric oxide (NO), or nitrous oxide (N_2O). Because the test reagents detect only nitrites, the latter process would lead to a false negative reading. Thus it is necessary to add a small quantity of zinc dust to all negative reactions. Zinc ions reduce nitrate to nitrite, and the development of a red colour after adding zinc dust indicates the presence of residual nitrates and confirms a true negative reaction.

Q. 10. Write short note on urease test.

Ans. This test detects the ability of an organism to produce urease enzyme. The test organism is inoculated on the entire slope of Christensen's medium which contains urea and phenol red indicator in addition to other constituents including agar. It is incubated at 37°C and examined after 4 hours and after overnight incubation. Development of **purple-pink** colour indicates production of urease. The latter in the presence of water converts urea into ammonia and carbon dioxide. Ammonia makes the medium alkaline and phenol red indicator changes to purple-pink in colour.

Q. 11. Write short note on hydrogen sulphide production.

Ans. Some organisms produce hydrogen sulphide from sulphur containing amino acids. It may be detected by suspending strips of filter paper impregnated with lead acetate between the cotton plug and the tube. Blackening of the paper indicates hydrogen sulphide production. It has variable sensitivity. When cultured in media containing lead acetate or ferric ammonium citrate or ferrous acetate they turn them black or brown. This method is more sensitive than lead acetate strip method.

Q. 12. Write short note on potassium cyanide test.

Ans. This tests the ability of an organism to grow in the presence of potassium cyanide. Inoculate buffered peptone water medium, containing 1 in 13,000 concentration of potassium cyanide, with test organism. Incubate at 37°C for 24–48 hours. Development of **turbidity** in the medium indicates the ability of the organism to grow in the presence of potassium cyanide.

Q. 13. Write short note on catalase production.

Ans. The enzyme catalase mediates the breakdown of hydrogen peroxide into oxygen and water. This principle is used for the detection of catalase enzyme in a bacterial isolate. Put a loopful of 10% hydrogen peroxide on colonies of the test organism on nutrient agar. Alternatively, pick up a few colonies of the test organism with platinum loop from nutrient agar plate and dip it in a drop of 10% hydrogen peroxide on a clean glass slide. The production of **gas bubbles** from the culture indicates a positive reaction. A false positive result may be obtained if the growth is picked up from medium containing catalase, e.g., blood agar or if an iron wire loop is used.

Q. 14. Write short note on oxidase test.

Ans. This test depends on the presence, in bacteria, of certain oxidases that catalyze the oxidation of reduced tetramethyl-*p*-phenylenediamine dihydrochloride (oxidase reagent) by molecular oxygen. Put a drop of freshly prepared 1% solution of oxidase reagent on a piece of filter paper. Then rub a few colonies of test organism on it. If it is oxidase-positive, it will produce a **deep purple** colour within 10 seconds. Alternatively, pour oxidase reagent over the colonies of the test organism on the culture plate. The colonies of oxidase-positive organisms rapidly develop a deep purple colour.

Various species of *Neisseria*, *Pseudomonas*, *Aeromonas*, *Vibrio*, *Alcaligenes* and *Campylobacter* are oxidase-positive. All the members of the family Enterobacteriaceae are oxidase-negative.

Q. 15. Write short note on motility test medium.

Ans. The motility test medium has agar concentration of 0.4% or less, to allow free spread of organisms. Inoculation is done by a single stab into the medium. After overnight incubation, movement away from the stab line or a hazy appearance throughout the medium indicates a motile organism.

Q. 16. Write short note on phenylalanine deaminase test.

Ans. Phenylalanine deaminase determines whether the organism possesses the enzyme phenylalanine deaminase that deaminates phenylalanine to phenylpyruvic acid, which reacts with ferric salts to give a green colour. Agar slants of the medium containing DL-phenylalanine is inoculated with a single colony of the test organism. After incubation at 37°C for 18–24 hours, 4 or 5 drops of 10% solution of ferric chloride reagent are added directly to the surface of the agar. If the test is positive, a green colour will develop in the fluid and in the slope. This test is useful in initial differentiation of *Proteus*, *Morganella*, and *Providencia* from the rest of the Enterobacteriaceae.

Q. 17. Write short note on animal pathogenicity.

Ans. Various experimental models used in diagnostic microbiology laboratory are mouse, rat, guinea-pig, rabbit, nine-banded armadillo and monkey. Various routes of inoculation are intradermal, subcutaneous, intramuscular, intraperitoneal, intracerebral and intravenous. Oral and nasal routes can also be used. The identification of the organism is carried out on the basis of clinical and postmortem findings, and cultural characteristics.

Q. 18. Discuss bacterial taxonomy.

Ans. The taxonomy of bacteria refers to three basic concepts – classification, nomenclature and identification.

Classification

It can be defined as the arrangement of organisms into taxonomic groups (taxa) on the basis of genotypic (genetic) and phenotypic (observable) similarities and differences. It allows the orderly grouping of microorganisms. For bacterial classification, three main approaches are usually followed. These include phylogenetic, Adansonian, genetic and intraspecies classification.

Phylogenetic classification

It is a hierarchial classification. It represents a branching tree-like arrangement, one characteristic being employed for division at each branch or level. This system is called phylogenetic because it denotes an evolutionary arrangement of species. Here some characteristics are given special weightage. For example, Gram staining, spore formation, lactose fermentation, etc. are used to differentiate major groups, whereas less important properties such as nutritional requirements for growth of bacteria, production of certain enzymes by bacteria, etc. are employed to distinguish minor groups such as genera and species.

The formal levels of classification, in successive smaller subsets, are kingdom, phylum or division, class, order, family, tribe, genus and species. At present no standard classification of bacteria is universally accepted and applied although **Bergey's Manual of Systematic Bacteriology** is widely used as authoritative source.

Adansonian classification

Adansonian classification makes no phylogenetic assumption but merely takes into account all the characteristics expressed at the time of study. Hence it is called **phonetic system**. It gives equal weight to all measurable features, and groups the organisms on the basis of similarities of several characteristics. The availability of computers has extended the scope of phonetic classification by permitting comparison of very large number of properties of several organisms at the same time. This is known as **numerical taxonomy**.

Genetic classification

This is based on homology of DNA base sequences of the microorganisms. DNA relatedness is determined by studying the nucleotide sequence of DNA by DNA hybridization or recombination methods. The study of messenger RNA and ribosomal RNA also provides useful information on genetic relatedness among bacteria. Genetic classification has been used more with viruses than with bacteria.

Intraspecies classification

Intraspecies classification is based on biochemical properties (biotypes), antigenic properties (serotypes), susceptibility to bacteriophages (phage types), resistance to various chemicals (resistotypes), or production of bacteriocins (colicin types).

Nomenclature

It refers to the naming of microorganisms. It is governed by the *International Committee on Systematic Bacteriology* and published as *Approved List of Bacterial Names* in the *International Journal of Systematic Bacteriology*. By accepted taxonomic convention, order names have the endings -ales (i.e., the order Eubacteriales), family names have the latinized ending -aceae (e.g., the family Enterobacteriaceae), and tribe names end in -eae (e.g., the tribe Proteae). The order, family and tribe names are capitalized. The genus name is also capitalized followed by species name which is not capitalized. If typed, the genus and species names should be italicized. If written, they should be underlined. Species should not be capitalized even when derived from the name of the person who discovered it. Often, the genus name is abbreviated by using the first letter of the genus followed by a period and the species epithet (name) (e.g., *E. coli*). The genus name followed by the word species (e.g., *Staphylococcus* species) may be used to refer to the genus as a whole. Species abbreviated sp. (singular) or spp. (plural) is used when the species is not specified. When the bacteria are referred to as a group, their names are neither capitalized nor underlined (e.g., staphylococci).

Identification

Suitable criteria for the purpose of identification include cell shape, Gram reaction and the presence or absence of specialized structures such as spores or flagella. Staining procedures such as Gram stain can provide reliable assessment of the nature of cell surfaces. Some bacteria produce characteristic pigments and others can be differentiated on the basis of their complement of extracellular enzymes (e.g., haemolysins). Tests such as oxidase test can be used to distinguish organisms on the basis of the presence of a respiratory enzyme, cytochrome C.

The traditional method of placing an organism into a particular genus and species is based on the similarity of all members in a number of phenotypic characteristics. This is accomplished by testing each bacterial culture for a variety of metabolic characteristics and comparing the results with those listed in established charts.

In rapid identification systems, a numerical taxonomy (also called computer taxonomy, phenetics, or taxometrics) is used. Numerical classification schemes use a large number (frequently 100 or more) of taxonomically useful characteristics. All these characteristics are assigned numerical value. The computer clusters different strains at selected levels of overall similarity (usually 80% at the species level) on the basis of the frequency with which they share traits.

5

STERILIZATION & DISINFECTION

Q. 1. Define the terms sterilization, disinfection and antisepsis.

Ans. **Sterilization**

It is defined as the process by which an article, a surface or a medium is freed of all microorganisms including viruses, bacteria, their spores and fungi, both pathogenic and non-pathogenic.

Disinfection

It is a process of destruction or removal of organisms capable of giving rise to infection. A **disinfectant** is a chemical or physical agent that is applied to inaninate objects to kill microbes. Disinfectants are capable of killing vegetative bacteria, fungi, viruses and rarely bacterial spores. Therefore, disinfection must never be used when sterilization is possible.

Antisepsis

It is the destruction or inhibition of microorganisms in living tissues thereby limiting or preventing the harmful effects of infection. A disinfectant that is applied to living tissue, to kill microbes, is referred to as an **antiseptic**. Note that not all disinfectants are antiseptics because an antiseptic additionally must not be so harsh that it damages living tissue.

Q. 2. Describe physical methods of sterilization.

Ans. Following physical methods are employed for sterilization:

1. Sunlight

Sunlight possesses ultraviolet rays which along with heat rays are responsible for appreciable germicidal activity. These rays, however, cannot penetrate through glass, i.e., window panes. This is one of the natural methods of sterilization of water in tanks, rivers and lakes.

2. Drying

Water constitutes 80% of the weight of the bacteria and is also essential for the growth of bacteria. Therefore, drying has deleterious effect on many bacteria. However, spores are unaffected by drying.

3. Heat

Heat is the most reliable, certain and rapid method of sterilization. It can be easily controlled and unlike chemical disinfection, leaves no potentially harmful residue. Unless the material to be sterilized is heat-sensitive, this method should be preferred. The time required for sterilization by heat is inversely proportional to the temperature of exposure, i.e., higher the temperature shorter the time of exposure.

Factors influencing sterilization by heat

- Number of microorganisms and spores present in the specimen.
- Species, strain and spore-forming ability of the microorganisms.
- Nature of the material in which microorganisms are heated.

Types of heat and principle

There are two types of heat – dry heat and wet heat.

Dry heat

It is believed to kill microorganisms by causing destructive oxidation of essential cell constituents. Dry heat at 100°C for 60 minutes and 115°C for 60 minutes can kill all vegetative bacteria and fungal spores respectively. Bacterial spores can be killed by dry heat at 160°C for one hour or 180°C for 20 minutes. On the whole dry heat is less efficient sterilization process than moist heat.

Moist heat

It causes denaturation and coagulation of proteins. When steam condenses on cooler surface, it releases its latent heat and raises the temperature of its surface. If spores are present, steam condenses on them and increases their water content leading to hydrolysis and breakdown of bacterial proteins. Most vegetative bacteria are killed by moist heat at 50–65°C in 10 minutes. Resistance of bacterial spores varies with different strains of the same species. For example, spores of most strains of *Clostridium tetani* are killed by boiling at 100°C for 10 minutes. However, some strains resist boiling for 1–3 hours. The spores of some strains of *C. botulinum* resist boiling at 100°C up to 8 hours. However, all spores are killed by autoclaving at 121°C for 10–30 minutes.

I. Sterilization by dry heat

A. Red heat

Inoculating wires and loops, points of forceps and spatulas are sterilized by holding them almost vertical in a bunsen burner flame until red hot (Table 5.1).

B. Flaming

Scalpel blades, needles, mouths of culture tubes, glass slides and cover slips are sterilized by passing the article through the bunsen flame without allowing them to become red hot.

Table 5.1. Sterilization by dry heat

Mode of sterilization	Instrument	Temperature and time	Sterilization of	Advantages/ disadvantages
Red heat	Bunsen burner	Till red hot	Inoculating wire loops, forceps and spatulas	Sterilization is rapid and thorough.
Flaming	Bunsen burner	Waving through the flame	Scalpel blades, glass slides, mouth of culture tubes and bottles	1. Surface sterilization is possible. 2. Rapid method.
Hot air	Hot air oven	160°C for 1 hour or 180°C for 20 minutes	Glassware, sealed materials like oils, greases, dry powder, etc.	Can be used for loads that cannot be penetrated by steam.

These items may be immersed in spirit in a tray and then burning off the spirit. However, it does not produce sufficient heat and destroys only vegetative organisms.

C. Incineration

This is an efficient method for rapidly destroying contaminated materials such as soiled dressings and pathological materials, etc.

D. Hot air oven

It is a method of choice for sterilization of glassware such as assembled all glass syringes, test tubes, petri dishes, pipettes and flasks; metal instruments such as forceps, scissors and scalpels; sealed materials such as oils, jellies and powders which are impervious to steam; and swab sticks packed in test tubes. It is not suitable for materials like fabrics which may be damaged by heat.

Hot air oven is electrically heated and is fitted with a thermostat that maintains the chamber air at a chosen temperature and a fan that distributes hot air in the chamber (Fig. 5.1). It must not be overloaded and spaces must be left for circulation of air through the load. Holding time for sterilization in hot air oven is **one hour at 160°C** or **20 minutes at 180°C**. It is timed as beginning when the thermometer first shows 160°C or 180°C respectively.

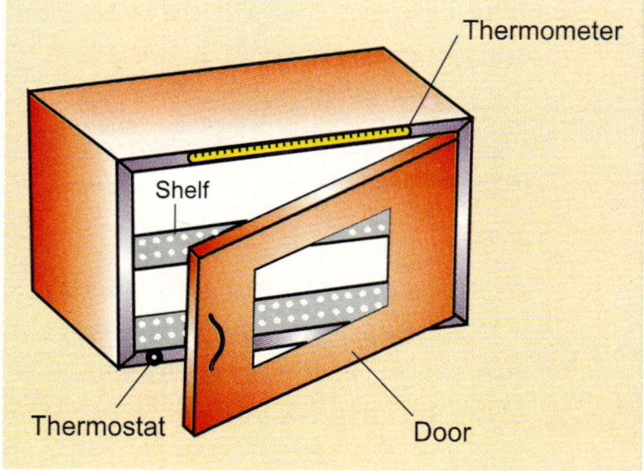

Fig. 5.1. Hot air oven.

Sterilization controls

Two types of controls are available:

1. Biological control

An envelope containing a filter paper strip impregnated with 10^6 spores of *Bacillus subtilis* subsp. *niger* (NCTC 10075 or ATCC 9372) is placed within the load (Table 5.2). After

Table 5.2. Biological controls of different sterilization methods

Method of sterilization	Biological control
Hot air oven	*Bacillus subtilis* subsp. *niger*
Autoclave	*Bacillus stearothermophilus*
Low temperature steam-formaldehyde	*Bacillus stearothermophilus*
Ethylene oxide	*Bacillus globigi* (a red-pigmented variant of *Bacillus subtilis*)
Ionizing radiations	*Bacillus pumilis*
Filtration	*Serratia marcescens*, *Pseudomonas diminuta*

sterilization is over, the strip is removed and inoculated into tryptone soy broth and incubated anaerobically at 37°C for five days. No growth of *B. subtilis* subsp. *niger* indicates proper sterilization.

2. Chemical control

A Browne's tube containing red solution is placed within the load. A change of colour of the solution from **red to green** indicates proper sterilization.

II. Sterilization by moist heat

Sterilization by moist heat means killing of the microorganisms with hot water or steam. Moist heat is divided into 3 forms (Table 5.3):

A. At temperatures below 100°C.
B. At a temperature of 100°C.
  (a) Boiling water
  (b) Free steam
C. At temperature above 100°C.

Table 5.3. Sterilization by moist heat

Mode of sterilization	Instrument	Temperature and time	Sterilization of	Advantages/disadvantages
Below 100°C	Water bath	56°C for 1 hour or 65–75°C for 10 min.	Serum, body fluids, vaccines and spatulas	May be used for disinfection. Most vegetative mesophilic bacteria are killed.
At 100°C	Boiling water bath	100°C for 10–20 min.	Glass, metal and rubber items	Kills all vegetative bacteria and some spores.
Steaming at 100°C	Arnold steamer	100°C for 20 min. on 3 successive days	Culture media containing sugar and gelatin	Prevents decomposition of media. *Spores of thermophilic bacteria may escape killing.*
Above 100°C	Autoclave	121°C for 15–20 min.	Culture media and other aqueous solutions, dressing material, linen, gloves, etc.	Most reliable method of sterilization.

A. Moist heat at temperatures below 100°C

Heat-labile fluids may be disinfected (not sterilized) by heating at temperatures below 100°C. Such treatment is sufficient to kill mesophilic vegetative bacteria. This includes:

- **Pasteurization** of milk and butter. The temperature employed is either **63°C for 30 minutes** (holder method) or **72°C for 20 seconds** (flash method) followed by rapid cooling to 13°C or lower. By this method non-sporing organisms such as mycobacteria, *Brucella* and salmonellae are destroyed. However, *Coxiella burnetii*, causative agent of Q fever, may survive pasteurization of milk by holder method and is at borderline of inactivation by the flash method.

  The flash method is preferable for pasteurization of milk because it is less likely to change the flavour and nutrient content, and it is more effective against resistant pathogens such as *C. burnetii*. Although pasteurization inactivates most viruses and vegetative stages of 97–99% of bacteria and fungi, they do not kill endospores and thermoresistant species (mostly nonpathogenic lactobacilli, micrococci and yeasts). Therefore, milk is not sterile after regular pasteurization, which explains why even an unopened carton of milk will eventually spoil on prolonged storage. Newer techniques have now been used to produce sterile milk that has a storage of 3 months. In this method, the milk is processed with **ultrahigh temperature of 134°C for 1–2 seconds**.
- **Heat-labile fluids** such as serum may be disinfected by heating at 56°C for one hour. If temperature rises above 59°C it will coagulate.
- **Vaccines** prepared from non-sporing bacteria may be inactivated in a water bath at 60°C for one hour.
- **Household utensils** and **patient's clothing** may be disinfected by washing in water at 70–80°C for several minutes.
- Media such as Lowenstein-Jensen and Loeffler's serum slope are rendered sterile by heating at 80–85°C for half an hour on three successive days in an inspissator.
- Items which cannot withstand heat at 100°C may be disinfected by steam at sub-atmospheric pressure at a temperature of 75°C with formaldehyde vapour. This is known as **low temperature steam-formaldehyde (LTSF) sterilization.**

Bacillus stearothermophilus (NCTC 10003 or ATCC 7953) has been used to test the efficacy of LTSF sterilizers (Table 5.2).

B. Moist heat at a temperature of 100°C

(a) **Boiling at 100°C:** Boiling at 100°C for 10–30 minutes kills all vegetative bacteria and some bacterial spores. Therefore, it is not recommended for sterilization of instruments for surgical procedures.

(b) **Free steam at 100°C:** Steam at normal atmospheric pressure is at 100°C. But, in addition, it has latent heat which on condensing on the article to be sterilized releases its latent heat. A **Koch** or **Arnold steam sterilizer** consists of a vertical metal cylinder with a removable conical lid having a small opening for the escaping steam. Water is added on the bottom and there is a perforated shelf above water level (Fig. 5.2). On this shelf articles to be sterilized are placed.

One single exposure to steam for 90 minutes ensures complete sterilization but for media containing sugar and gelatin, which may get decomposed on long heating, an exposure of **100°C for 20 minutes on three consecutive days** is employed. This is known as **tyndallization** or **intermittent sterilization**. First exposure to steam kills all vegetative bacteria, and any spores present being in a favourable medium, will germinate and will be killed on the subsequent occasions. Therefore, non-nutrient media cannot be sterilized by this method.

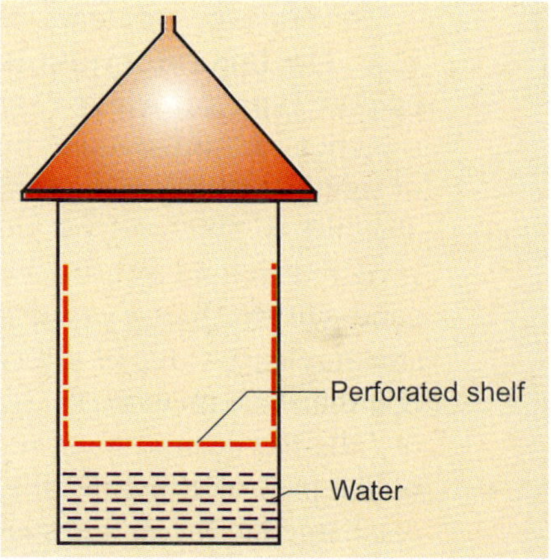

C. Moist heat at temperature above 100°C

Steam above 100°C or saturated steam is a more efficient sterilizing agent than hot air because:

Fig. 5.2. Steam sterilizer.

- it provides greater lethal action of moist heat,
- it is quicker in heating up the exposed articles, and
- it can penetrate easily porous material such as cotton wool stoppers, paper and cloth wrappers, bundles of surgical linen, and hollow apparatus.

When the steam meets the cooler surface of the article, it condenses into a small volume of water and liberates its considerable latent heat to that surface, for example, 1600 ml of steam at 100°C, i.e., at atmospheric pressure condenses into 1 ml of water at 100°C liberating 518 calories of heat. The large contraction in volume brings more steam to the same site and the process continues until the temperature of the article is raised to that of steam. The water of condensation ensures moist conditions for killing of the exposed microorganisms. Pure steam must be used and the presence of air avoided since air hinders penetration by the steam.

Water boils when its pressure equals the pressure of the surrounding atmosphere. When the atmospheric pressure is raised then the boiling temperature is also raised. At normal pressure water boils at 100°C but when it is boiled in a closed vessel at increased pressure the temperature at which it boils and that of the steam it forms rises above 100°C. This principle has been exploited in autoclave and pressure cooker.

Sterilization by **steam under pressure (autoclaving)** is suitable for culture media and aqueous solutions (since atmosphere of steam prevents evaporation during heating), dressing material, linen, gloves, etc. Satisfactory sterilization can be achieved at 15 pounds per square inch (psi) pressure equivalent to **121°C in 15–20 minutes**. In fact the only practical and dependable method of sterilization is steam under pressure using different types of autoclaves. *However, the autoclave is ineffective for sterilizing substances that repel moisture (oils, waxes or powders).* All the air must be removed from the autoclave chamber and the articles to be sterilized so that the latter are exposed to pure steam. There are three reasons for this:

- The admixture of air with steam results in lower temperature being achieved.
- Air hinders penetration of steam into the interstices of porous materials, surgical dressings, syringes, etc.
- The air being denser forms a separate and cooler layer in the lower part of the autoclave, so it prevents adequate heating of articles there.

Several types of steam sterilizers are available. The **laboratory autoclave** or **pressure cooker type autoclave** (Fig. 5.3) consists of a vertical or horizontal cylinder of gun metal or stainless steel in a supporting frame or case. The lid is fastened by screw clamps and rendered air tight by asbestos gasket. Lid bears a tap for discharge of air and steam, and a steam release valve or safety valve. The latter opens and closes when the steam pressure rises or falls the desired level respectively. On its upper part of the side, the autoclave has a discharge tap for air and steam, and an air and steam release knob. Heating is done by electricity. Water is added on the bottom of the autoclave. Above this is a perforated shelf on which articles to be sterilized are placed.

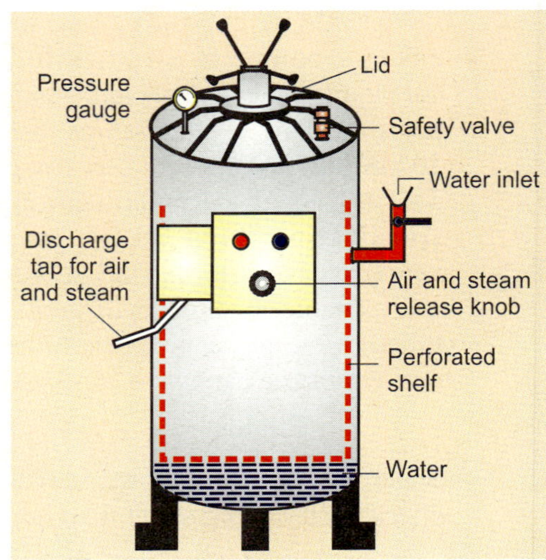

Fig. 5.3. Autoclave.

The lid is closed, discharge tap is opened and safety valve is adjusted to the required pressure. As heating continues, the steam and air mixture escapes. To know when all the air inside the autoclave has escaped the discharge tap is connected with one end of a rubber tube and the other end of it is placed in water. When the air bubbles stop coming it indicates that all the air from inside the autoclave has been removed. The discharge tap is now closed. Steam pressure rises inside and when it reaches the desired set level (15 psi) the safety valve opens and excess steam escapes. From this point the **holding time** (15 minutes) is counted.

When the holding time is over, the heating is stopped and autoclave allowed to cool till pressure gauze indicates that inside pressure has reached to the atmospheric pressure. The discharge tap is now opened and air is allowed to enter the autoclave. The lid is now opened and the sterilized articles removed. If the tap or lid is opened when the pressure inside is high, the liquid media boil violently and may explode. On the other hand, if the articles are not removed for a long time after the normal atmospheric pressure has reached inside the autoclave, an excessive amount of water will be evaporated and lost from the media.

Sterilization controls

Two types of controls are available:

1. Biological control

An envelope containing a filter paper strip impregnated with 10^6 spores of *Bacillus stearothermophilus* (NCTC 10003 or ATCC 7953) is placed with the load in the coolest and least accessible part of the autoclave chamber (Table 5.2). After sterilization is over the strip is removed and inoculated into tryptone soy broth and incubated at 56°C for 5 days. No growth of *B. stearothermophilus* indicates proper sterilization. Spores of this organism withstand 121°C for up to 12 minutes and this has made the organism ideal for testing autoclaves.

2. Chemical control

A Browne's tube containing red solution is placed within the load. A change of colour of the solution from **red to green** indicates proper sterilization.

Q. 3. Name and describe various types of bacterial filters. Mention their uses and limitations.

Ans. Types of filters

1. Earthenware filters

Important examples are earthenware filters made from kieselguhr (a fossil diatomaceous earth), and chamberland filters made of unglazed porcelain. They are made in the form of hollow candles with different grades of porosity. The fluid to be sterilized is passed through the candle. After use they can be sterilized by scrubbing with stiff brush followed by boiling and autoclaving.

2. Asbestos (Seitz) filters

They are made up of a disc of asbestos (magnesium trisilicate). It is supported on a perforated metal disc within a metal funnel. The latter with filter disc fitted is sterilized by autoclaving. It is then fitted onto a sterile flask through a silicone rubber bung. The fluid to be sterilized is put into the funnel and flask connected to the exhaust pump through its side tap. Sterilized fluid is collected from the flask and filter disc is discarded after use. These discs are available with different grades of porosity.

3. Sintered glass filters

These are made of finely ground glass fused together. These are available in different pore sizes. They are also available in the form of a disc fused into a glass funnel. After use they are washed with running tap water in reverse direction and cleaned with warm, strong sulphuric acid.

4. Membrane filters

These are made up of cellulose esters and are widely used now-a-days for sterilization of heat-labile fluids. These are also known as millipore filters. They are available as discs of pore size varying from 0.015–12 μm. The 0.22 μm filter is the most commonly used because the pore size is smaller than that of bacteria. They can also be used for bacterial counts of water. A known amount of water is filtered through the membrane filter disc. The upper side of the disc is then placed on an appropriate moist culture medium and incubated. The colonies that develop can be counted and viable count calculated.

5. Syringe filters

Syringes fitted with membranes of 13 mm and 25 mm diameter are available. The fluid to be sterilized is forced through the disc by pressing the piston of the syringe.

6. Air filters

Large volumes of air may be rapidly freed from infection by passage through high efficiency particulate air (HEPA) filters.

Uses of bacterial filters

Liquids such as sera and solutions of heat-labile substances such as sugars and urea, used for preparation of media, can be sterilized by filtration. Filtration does not kill microbes, it separates them out. This method is also useful for:

- sterilization of pharmaceutical substances,
- separation of bacteriophages and bacterial toxins from bacteria, and
- isolation of organisms which are scanty in fluids.

The filter disc retains the organisms which can then be cultured.

Limitations of bacterial filters

Mycoplasma and viruses, which are very small, cannot be kept back by the bacterial filters, therefore, serum sterilized by filtration cannot be employed for clinical use. *Serratia marcescens* and *Pseudomonas diminuta* have been used to test the efficacy of different filters (Table 5.2).

Q. 4. Describe non-ionizing and ionizing radiations. What are their advantages and disadvantages?

Ans. Two types of radiations (Table 5.4) are used:

- Non-ionizing.
- Ionizing.

Table 5.4. Sterilization by radiation

Type of radiation	Instrument	Dose	Application	Advantages/ disadvantages
Ionizing	Cobalt 60	2.5 Mrad	Sterilization of antibiotics, hormones, sutures and pre-packed disposable items such as plastic syringes, transfusion sets, catheters, cannulas, culture plates, etc.	Excellent sterilizing agent, penetrates deep into objects, produces less heat, can be used for heat sensitive items. But it is expensive.
Non-ionizing (UV radiation)	UV lamps, commercial UV units and mercury vapour lamps	250–260 nm wavelength for 30 min.	Disinfection of clear surfaces like inoculation hoods, laboratories, wards, operation theatres, etc.	Destroys micro-organisms only on exposed surfaces. Hazardous for eyes and skin.

Non-ionizing radiations

These include infrared and ultraviolet radiations:

Infrared rays

Infrared rays bring about sterilization by generation of heat. Articles to be sterilized are placed in a moving conveyor belt and passed through a tunnel that is heated by infrared radiators to a temperature of 180°C. The articles are exposed to that temperature for a period of 7.5 minutes. Articles sterilized include metallic instruments and glassware. It is mainly used in central sterile supply department. Efficiency can be checked by using Browne's tube No. 4 (blue spot).

Ultraviolet (UV) radiations

Ultraviolet (UV) radiations in the range of 250–260 nm wavelength are highly effective. Low pressure mercury vapour lamps emit over 95% of radiations with the wavelength of 253.7 nm. Most vegetative bacteria are susceptible to UV radiations. Spores are highly resistant and susceptibility of viruses is variable. **Human immunodeficiency virus is not inactivated by UV radiations.** UV radiations induce thymine dimers in DNA and this interferes with DNA replication. They can penetrate only a few mm into liquids and not at all into solids. Therefore, their use is best restricted to disinfection of clean surfaces like *inoculation hoods*, *laboratories*, *wards*, and *operation theatres*. Source of UV radiations must be shielded to prevent the radiations falling on eyes and skin because it may damage them.

Ionizing radiations

These include *X-rays*, *gamma rays* and *cosmic rays*. These have very high penetrative power and are highly lethal to all cells including bacteria. They damage DNA by various mechanisms. Spores are more resistant than vegetative bacteria. Large commercial plants use gamma radiations for sterilization of prepacked disposable items such as *plastic syringes*, *transfusion sets*, *catheters*, *cannulas*, *culture plates*, etc. that are unable to withstand heat because there is no appreciable increase in the temperature. Therefore, this method is known as **cold sterilization**. High cost of installation limits its use commercially. *Bacillus pumilis* has been used to test the efficacy of ionizing radiations (Table 5.2).

Q. 5. Describe phenols and phenol derivatives, and halogens as agents of sterilization and disinfection.

Ans. Phenols

Lister, the father of antiseptic surgery, introduced the use of phenol (carbolic acid) in surgery. These are obtained by distillation of coal tar and have a powerful microbicidal action. They cause cell membrane damage thus releasing cell contents and causing cell lysis. They are resistant to inactivation by organic matter and are active against Gram-positive and Gram-negative bacteria, moderately active against mycobacteria, and have little activity against spores and viruses. They are used mainly for *discarded cultures*, *contaminated pipettes and other infected material*. Phenol is bactericidal at a concentration of 1%. At a concentration of 0.5% it is used for preservation of sera and vaccines.

Phenol derivatives

Certain phenol derivatives like cresols, chlorhexidine, chloroxylenol and hexachlorophane are commonly used as disinfectants:

- **Cresols:** Cresols are obtained by distillation of coal tar, are emulsified with green soap and sold under the trade names of *Lysol* and *Creolin*. They are active against a wide range of organisms. They are most commonly used for sterilization of infected glasswares, cleaning floors and disinfection of excreta. They are not inactivated by the presence of organic matter.
- **Chlorhexidine:** It is a relatively non-toxic skin disinfectant. It is most active against Gram-positive organisms, and fairly effective against Gram-negative ones. Aqueous solutions are used in the treatment of wounds.

- **Chloroxylenol (Dettol):** It is less toxic and less irritant, and is also less active. It is readily inactivated by organic matter. It is inactive against *Pseudomonas*.
- **Hexachlorophane:** It is more active against Gram-positive than Gram-negative bacteria. It is applied on skin for prophylaxis against staphylococcal infections. It is bacteriostatic at very high dilutions. It is potentially toxic and should be used with care.

Halogens

Halogens are oxidizing agents. They cause damage by oxidation of essential sulfhydryl groups of enzymes. Chlorine and iodine are the halogens which are used as disinfectants. They are bactericidal and sporicidal. They are active in very high dilutions and their action is very rapid. In addition to chlorine itself there are three types of chlorine compounds, the hypochlorites, and the inorganic and organic chloramines. **The disinfectant action of all the chlorine compounds is due to release of free chlorine.** When elemental chlorine or hypochlorites are added to water, the chlorine reacts with water to form hypochlorous acid. It is a strong oxidising agent and effective disinfectant. The activity of chlorine is markedly influenced by the presence of organic matter. Sodium hypochlorite, chloramine and bleaching powder are most widely used for disinfection of HIV infected material. Hypochlorite solution decays rapidly, therefore, it should be prepared daily.

- **Chlorine** has a special place in the treatment of water supply and combinations of hypochlorite and detergents are useful for cleansing and disinfection in food and dairy industry. Hypochlorites have a wide spectrum of activity against viruses and very little activity against tubercle bacilli. They are available in liquid or powder form as salts of calcium, lithium and sodium.
- **Iodine** in alcoholic and aqueous solutions is used almost exclusively as a skin disinfectant (antiseptic). Like chlorine, it is also inactivated by organic matter. It is also active against tubercle bacilli and a number of viruses. Mixtures of iodine with various surface active agents that act as carriers for iodine are known as **iodophores**, an example of this is **betadine**. It can be used as a **bactericidal antiseptic for intact skin** and for disinfection of superficial wounds. It is also active against fungi and *Trichomonas*.

Q. 6. Describe aldehydes, alcohols and dyes as agents of sterilization and disinfection.

Ans.

Aldehydes

Two aldehydes (formaldehyde and glutaraldehyde) are currently of considerable importance, although others also possess antimicrobial activity. They act through alkylation of amino, carboxyl or hydroxyl groups, and probably damage nucleic acids.

Formaldehyde

It is an irritant, water-soluble gas. It is highly lethal to bacteria and their spores, fungi and viruses. However, **it is not active against prions**. It is cheap and can be used for *sterilization of rooms*, *furniture* and a wide variety of articles liable to be damaged by heat, such as *clothing*, *woollen blankets*, *mattresses*, *respirators*, *heat-sensitive instruments*, etc. It may be used in gaseous form or an aqueous solution. It combines readily with proteins and is less effective in the presence of organic matter. Irritant residues of formaldehyde may be removed by exposure of the disinfected articles to ammonia vapour. *Formaldehyde is a suspected carcinogen. It must, therefore, be stored and used in a fume-hood or well-ventilated area.*

Glutaraldehyde

It is more effective and less irritant than formaldehyde. It possesses high microbicidal activity against bacteria and their spores, mycelial and spore forms of fungi, and various types of viruses, including human immunodeficiency viruses and enteroviruses. Two per cent alkaline buffered solution is used for sterilization of heat-sensitive instruments like *cystoscopes, bronchoscopes, thermometers*, etc. *Gluteraldehyde is toxic and irritant to skin and mucous membranes, therefore, contact with it must be avoided. It must be used in a fume-hood or in well ventilated area.*

Alcohols

Several alcohols possess antimicrobial activity. The antimicrobial activity of alcohols can be attributed to their ability to denature proteins. Alcohol solutions containing 60–70% alcohol are most effective, and higher concentrations are less potent because proteins are not denatured easily in the absence of water. They are active against vegetative bacteria including tubercle bacilli, fungi and lipid-containing viruses but not against spores. Their action on nonlipid viruses is variable.

- **Isopropyl alcohol** is preferred over ethyl alcohol as it is a better fat solvent, more bactericidal and less volatile. It is commonly used for *disinfection of clinical thermometers*.
- **Methyl alcohol** is effective against fungal spores.
- **Alcohol-based hand-rubs** are recommended for the decontamination of highly soiled hands in situations where proper hand-washing is inconvenient or not possible. However, it must be remembered that alcohol is ineffective against spores and may not kill all types of nonlipid viruses.

Alcohols are volatile and flammable and must not be used near open flames. Working solutions should be stored in proper containers to avoid evaporation of alcohol.

Dyes

Two groups of dyes, the aniline dyes and the acridines have been used extensively as skin and wound antiseptics. Both groups are bacteriostatic in high dilution but have low bactericidal activity. They are much more active against Gram-positive than Gram-negative bacteria.

- **Aniline dyes** include brilliant green, malachite green and crystal violet. Their activity is inhibited by the presence of organic matter like pus. **They have no activity against tubercle bacilli, therefore, addition of malachite green to Lowenstein-Jensen medium makes it selective for the isolation of tubercle bacilli.** They interfere with the synthesis of the peptidoglycan component of the cell wall.
- **Acridine dyes** include acriflavine, proflavine, euflavine and aminacrine. They are little, if at all, affected by the presence of organic matter. Acridine dyes interfere with the synthesis of nucleic acids and proteins in both bacterial and mammalian cells.

Q. 7. Describe briefly vapour-phase disinfectants.

Ans. Two most important vapour-phase disinfectants are ethylene oxide and formaldehyde.

Ethylene oxide

It is a colourless gas soluble in water. It is highly lethal to all kinds of microbes including spores and tubercle bacilli. It is useful for sterilization of articles liable to be damaged by heat, e.g., *plastic and rubber articles, blankets, pharmaceutical products (crude drugs and powders) and complex apparatus such as heart-lung machines.*

It is highly effective sterilizing agent because it rapidly penetrates packing materials, even plastic wraps. It forms explosive mixture when more than 3% is present in air. This hazard can be overcome by using a mixture of 10% ethylene oxide in carbon dioxide. **It has an alkylating action on proteins.** Inhibition produced by it is irreversible, resulting in enzyme modification and inhibition of enzyme activity. *Bacillus globigi*, a red-pigmented variant of *B. subtilis*, has been used to test ethylene oxide sterilizers (Table 5.2).

Formaldehyde gas

It is liberated by spraying or heating of formalin, by addition of formalin to potassium permanganate or by volatilization of paraformaldehyde. Its antimicrobial activity depends upon several factors. The atmosphere must have a high relative humidity (more than 60% and preferably 80 to 90%) and a temperature of at least 18°C.

It is used for fumigation of operation theatres, wards and laboratories. After sealing the windows and other outlets, formaldehyde gas is generated by adding 150 g of potassium permanganate to 280 ml formalin for every 1000 cubic feet of room volume. The rooms are left unopened for 48 hours. Then open the doors and windows to allow vapours to disperse and neutralise any residual formaldehyde with ammonia by exposing 250 ml of SG 880 ammonia per litre of formalin used.

Beta-propiolactone (BPL) is a condensation product of ketone and formaldehyde. **It is an alkylating agent that acts through alkylation of carboxyl and hydroxyl groups.** It is active against all microorganisms including viruses. In the liquid form it is used to sterilize vaccines and sera. It is more efficient than formaldehyde for fumigation purpose. BPL destroys microorganisms more readily than ethylene oxide but does not penetrate materials well and **may be carcinogenic. For these reasons, BPL has not been used as extensively as ethylene oxide.**

Hydrogen peroxide fogging

This is a better method replacing fumigation. It is done by fogging machine using hydrogen peroxide as disinfectant. It has the advantage of short cycle time and is non-toxic.

Q. 8. Write short note on surface active disinfectants.

Ans. Substances that alter the energy relationships at interfaces leading to reduction of surface or interfacial tension, are known as **surface active agents** or **surfactants**. They possess both hydrophobic (water-repelling) and hydrophilic (water-attracting) groups. On the basis of charge or the absence of ionization of the hydrophilic group, these surfactants are classified into anionic, cationic, non-ionic and amphoteric compounds. Non-toxic surfactants do not have antimicrobial activity.

Cationic compounds such as quarternary ammonium compounds are the most important surfactants. **These act on phosphate groups of cell membrane phospholipids and also enter the cell.** This leads to loss of membrane semipermeability and leakage from the cell of nitrogen and phosphorus containing compounds. The agent which enters the cell, denatures its proteins. They possess strong bactericidal but weak detergent properties. They are essentially bacteriostatic and are more active against Gram-positive than Gram-negative bacteria. *Pseudomonas aeruginosa* is particularly resistant to these agents.

They are also fungistatic and active against viruses with lipid envelopes (e.g., herpes and influenza) and much less against nonenveloped viruses (e.g., enteroviruses). Commercially available preparations of cationic compounds include cetrimide (cetavalon), benzalkonium chloride and laurodin. These compounds are most active in alkaline pH. Antimicrobial activity is affected greatly by acidic pH, organic matter and anionic surface active agents such as ordinary soaps.

Anionic surfactants such as common soaps usually have strong detergent but weak antimicrobial properties. These agents are most active at acid pH and effective against Gram-positive organisms but are relatively ineffective against Gram-negative organisms. These compounds cause gross disruption of lipoprotein framework of the cell membrane.

Amphoteric agents such as tego compounds possess detergent properties of anionic and antimicrobial activity of cationic compounds. They are active over a wide range of pH but their activity is markedly reduced by organic matter. At a concentration of 1% in water they are effective against a wide range of Gram-positive and Gram-negative organisms and some viruses.

Q. 9. Define biomedical waste, infectious waste and hazardous waste. Describe briefly waste segregation. Tabulate biomedical waste categories and their segregation, collection, treatment, processing and disposal options.

Ans. Biomedical waste (BMW)

It is a broader term applied to waste generated in the diagnosis, treatment or immunization of human beings or animals, in research or in the production or testing of biological products. It also includes waste coming out of medical treatment given at home.

Infectious waste

Medical waste which has the potential to transmit viral, bacterial or parasitic diseases. It includes both human and animal infectious waste and waste generated in laboratories, and veterinary practice. Infectious waste is hazardous in nature.

Hazardous waste

Waste which has a potential to pose a threat to human health and life. The persons most at risk are the staff of hospitals particularly nurses and waste handlers. In countries such as India, scavengers and ragpickers are at serious risk.

Waste segregation

The biomedical waste shall be segregated into containers or bags at the point of generation, since 80% of the waste is non-hazardous and can be disposed of easily into the municipal bin. It is important that hazardous waste component is separated from non-hazardous waste. Mixing of waste will render the entire waste potentially hazardous. Waste should be segregated in bags of different colours to facilitate appropriate treatment and disposal. Table 5.5 shows biomedical waste categories and their segregation, collection, treatment, processing and disposal options.

Table 5.5. Biomedical waste categories and their segregation, collection, treatment, processing and disposal options

Category	Type of waste	Type of bag or container to be used	Treatment and disposal options
Yellow	(a) **Human anatomical waste:** Human tissues, organs, body parts and fetus below the viability period (as per the Medical Termination of Pregnancy Act 1971, amended from time to time).	Yellow-coloured non-chlorinated plastic bags	Incineration or plasma pyrolysis or deep burial*.
	(b) **Animal anatomical waste:** Experimental animal carcasses, body parts, organs, tissues, including the waste generated from animals used in experiments or testing in veterinary hospitals or colleges or animal houses.		
	(c) **Soiled waste:** Items contaminated with blood, body fluids like dressings, plaster casts, cotton swabs and bags containing residual or discarded blood and blood components.		Incineration or plasma pyrolysis or deep burial*. In absence of above facilities, autoclaving or microwaving/ hydroclaving followed by shredding or mutilation or combination of sterilization and shredding. Treated waste to be sent for energy recovery.
	(d) **Expired or discarded medicines:** Pharmaceutical waste like antibiotics, cytotoxic drugs including all items contaminated with cytotoxic drugs along with glass or plastic ampoules, vial, etc.	Yellow-coloured non-chlorinated plastic bags or containers	Expired cytotoxic drugs and items contaminated with cytotoxic drugs to be returned to the manufacturer or supplier for incineration at temperature > 1200°C or to common bio-medical waste treatment facility or hazardous waste treatment, storage and disposal facility for incineration at > 1200°C or encapsulation or plasma pyrolysis at >1200°C.

(Contd.)

Category	Type of waste	Type of bag or container to be used	Treatment and disposal options
			All other discarded medicines shall be either sent back to manufacturer or disposed by incineration.
	(e) **Chemical waste:** Chemicals used in production of biologicals and used or discarded disinfectants.	Yellow-coloured containers or non-chlorinated plastic bags	Disposed of by incineration or plasma pyrolysis or encapsulation in hazardous waste treatment, storage and disposal facility.
	(f) **Chemical liquid waste:** Liquid waste generated due to use of chemicals in production of biologicals and used or discarded disinfectants, silver X-ray film developing liquid, discarded formalin, infected secretions, aspirated body fluids, liquid from laboratories and floor washings, cleaning, housekeeping and disinfecting activities, etc.	Separate collection system leading to effluent treatment system	After resource recovery, the chemical liquid waste shall be pre-treated before mixing with other waste water.
	(g) Discarded linen, mattresses, beddings contaminated with blood or body fluid.	Non-chlorinated yellow plastic bags or suitable packing material	Non-chlorinated chemical disinfection followed by incineration or plasma pyrolysis or for energy recovery. In absence of above facilities, shredding or mutilation or combination of sterilization and shredding. Treated waste to be sent for energy recovery or incineration or plasma pyrolysis.
	(h) **Microbiology, biotechnology and other clinical laboratory waste:** Blood bags, laboratory cultures, stocks or specimens of microorganisms, live or attenuated vaccines, human and animal cell cultures used in research, industrial laboratories, production of biologicals, residual toxins, dishes and devices used for cultures.	Autoclave-safe plastic bags or containers	Pre-treat to sterilize with non-chlorinated chemicals on-site as per National AIDS Control Organisation or World Health Organisation guidelines thereafter for incineration.
Red	**Contaminated waste (Recyclable):** Wastes generated from disposable items such as tubings, bottles, intra-venous tubes and sets, catheters, urine bags, syringes (without needles and fixed needle syringes) and vaccutainers with their needles cut) and gloves.	Red-coloured non-chlorinated plastic bags or containers	Autoclaving or microwaving/ hydroclaving followed by shredding or mutilation or combination of sterilization and shredding. Treated waste to be sent to registered or authorized recyclers or for energy recovery or plastics to diesel or fuel oil or for road making, whichever is possible. Plastic waste should not be sent to landfill sites.

(*Contd.*)

Category	Type of waste	Type of bag or container to be used	Treatment and disposal options
White (Trans-lucent)	**Waste sharps including metals:** Needles, syringes with fixed needles, needles from needle tip cutter or burner, scalpels, blades, or any other contaminated sharp object that may cause puncture and cuts. This includes both used, discarded and contaminated metal sharps.	Puncture-proof, leak-proof, tamper-proof containers	Autoclaving or dry heat sterilization followed by shredding or mutilation or encapsulation in metal container or cement concrete; combination of shredding-cum-autoclaving; and sent for final disposal to iron foundries (having consent to operate from the State Pollution Control Boards or Pollution Control Committees) or sanitary landfill or designated concrete waste sharp pit.
Blue	(a) **Glassware:** Broken or discarded and contaminated glass including medicine vials and ampoules except those contaminated with cytotoxic wastes. (b) **Metallic body implants**.	Cardboard boxes with blue-coloured marking Cardboard boxes with blue-coloured marking	Disinfection (by soaking the washed glass waste after cleaning with detergent and sodium hypochlorite treatment) or through autoclaving or microwaving or hydroclaving and then sent for recycling.

* Disposal by deep burial is permitted only in rural or remote areas where there is no access to common biomedical waste treatment facility. This will be carried out with prior approval from the prescribed authority and as per the Standards specified in Schedule-III. The deep burial facility shall be located as per the provisions and guidelines issued by Central Pollution Control Board from time to time.

Other questions which may also be asked in the examination

Write short notes on:

(a) hot air oven,
(b) autoclave.

For answers see page 36 for (a) and pages 39–40 for (b).

6

CHEMOTHERAPY

Q. 1. Define the terms antimicrobial agent, chemotherapeutic agent and antibiotic. Describe mechanism of action of antimicrobial agents giving suitable examples.

Ans.
- **Antimicrobial agent** is a chemical substance inhibiting the growth or causing the death of a microorganism. Many chemicals have this property if sufficiently high concentrations are used.
- **Chemotherapeutic agent** is a chemical substance used to kill or inhibit the growth of microorganisms already established in the tissues of the body.
- The term **antibiotic** is defined as a substance produced wholly or partially by chemical synthesis that is capable of inhibiting the growth or causing death of other microorganisms in low concentrations.

Mechanisms of action of antimicrobial agents

Since bacterial metabolism is different in many ways from the human metabolism, their metabolic pathways are chosen as targets for inhibition by antimicrobial agents. Penicillin and related compounds inhibit peptidoglycan synthesis, but since such a metabolic pathway is non-existent in humans, antibiotic agent poses no toxicity (excluding hypersensitivity and other drug reactions). Mechanisms of action of antimicrobial agents can be placed under four headings (Table 6.1):

1. Inhibition of cell wall synthesis.
2. Inhibition of cytoplasmic membrane function.
3. Inhibition of nucleic acid synthesis.
4. Inhibition of protein synthesis.

1. Inhibition of cell wall synthesis

Bacteria are surrounded by a rigid cell wall. It maintains the shape of the microorganisms and protects them from osmotic and mechanical trauma. Injury to the cell wall (e.g., by

Table 6.1. Antimicrobial agents

Inhibitors of cell wall synthesis	Inhibitors of cytoplasmic membrane function	Inhibitors of nucleic acid synthesis	Inhibitors of protein synthesis
• Penicillins • Cephalosporins • Vancomycin • Bacitracin • Cycloserine • Caspofungin • Isoniazid	• Polymyxin B • Amphotericin B • Azoles	• Sulfonamides • Trimethoprim • Quinolones • Rifampicin	• Aminoglycosides • Chloramphenicol • Tetracyclines • Macrolides • Clindamycin • Fusidic acid

lysozyme) or inhibition of its formation may lead to lysis of the cell. The antibiotics which inhibit cell wall synthesis are β-lactam antibiotics (penicillins and cephalosporins), vancomycin, bacitracin, cycloserine, caspofungin and isoniazid.

Penicillins and cephalosporins are called β-lactam antibiotics because they possess an intact β-lactam ring, essential for antimicrobial activity. **β-lactam antibiotics are inactive against organisms devoid of peptidoglycan cell wall such as *Mycoplasma*, protozoa, fungi and viruses.** Penicillins and cephalosporins are usually bactericidal. Cephalosporins tend to be more resistant than the penicillin to inactivation by β-lactamases produced by some bacteria.

2. Inhibition of cytoplasmic membrane function

A group of polypeptide antibiotics act on the cytoplasmic membrane, the best example being polymyxin B, which acts essentially as a cationic detergent binding specifically to the membrane. As a result of this, the property of semipermeability is lost and essential low molecular weight intermediates and coenzymes pass into environment causing cell death. Because polymyxin will also combine with the membranes of eukaryotic cells, its selective toxicity is not great and it has to be used with caution.

Amphotericin B and azoles such as ketoconazole, fluconazole, itraconazole and clotrimazole are frequently used antifungal drugs. They show selective toxicity against fungi because cell membrane of fungi contains ergosterol, whereas human cell membrane has cholesterol. Bacteria with the exception of *Mycoplasma* do not have sterols in their cell membranes, hence they are resistant to the action of these drugs. Amphotericin B acts against the fungi by disrupting the cell membrane by binding at the site of ergosterol in the membrane. Azole inhibits synthesis of ergosterol.

3. Inhibition of nucleic acid synthesis

Sulphonamides, trimethoprim, quinolones and rifampicin inhibit nucleic acid synthesis.

4. Inhibition of protein synthesis

Bacteria have 70S ribosomes, whereas mammalian cells have 80S ribosomes. The subunits of each type of ribosomes, their chemical composition, and their functional specificities are sufficiently different to explain why antimicrobial drugs can inhibit protein synthesis in bacterial ribosomes without having a major effect on mammalian ribosomes. They interfere with different stages of the process of protein synthesis.

Each 70S bacterial ribosome is composed of a 30S and a 50S ribosomal subunits. Aminoglycosides and tetracyclines act at the level of 30S ribosomal subunits, whereas macrolides (erythromycin, roxithromycin and oleandomycin), chloramphenicol and clindamycin act at the level of 50S ribosomal subunits.

7

BACTERIAL GENETICS

Q. 1. Define genetics. Describe briefly central dogma of molecular biology.

Ans. Genetics is the study of genes, their structure and function, heredity and variation. Like other organisms, bacteria too obey the laws of genetics and breed true. However, a small proportion of their progeny exhibits variations in some properties.

The genetic information in bacteria, as in other cells, is contained in the specific sequence of nucleotides in the cell's deoxyribonucleic acid (DNA). The DNA acts as a template for its own replication so that at the time of cell division two copies are available. It also acts as a template for transcription of messenger RNA (mRNA) which is then translated, by ribosomes into particular polypeptide (DNA → RNA → polypeptide). This is the **central dogma of molecular biology**. DNA is the storehouse of all information for protein synthesis. However, in 1970, Baltimore and Temin showed that the retroviruses (RNA viruses) encode an RNA-dependent deoxyribonucleic acid polymerase (reverse transcriptase) and replicate through a DNA intermediate. The DNA copy of the viral genome is then integrated into the host chromosome to become a cellular gene.

Q. 2. Write brief account of codon, cistron or gene, locus and genome.

Ans. Genetic information is stored in DNA as a code. The unit of code is known as **codon**. It consists of a sequence of three bases. Therefore, code is triplet. Each codon specifies or codes for a single amino acid, but more than one codon may exist for a single amino acid. Thus codon AGA codes for arginine but the codons AGG, CGU, CGC, CGA and CGG also code for the same amino acid. Therefore, code is **degenerate**. Three codons UAA, UAG and UGA do not code for any amino acid and are known as **nonsense codons**. They act as punctuation marks, terminating the message for synthesis of a polypeptide.

A segment of DNA carrying a number of codons specifying for a particular polypeptide is known as **cistron** or **gene**. A large number of genes constitute a **locus** and a large number of loci constitute cell **genome**. Therefore, DNA can be compared with a book of information. Letters represent nucleotides, words represent codons, sentences represent genes, paragraphs represent loci and entire book as DNA molecule or **cell genome**.

Most bacteria contain enough DNA to code for 1,000–3,000 different types of polypeptide chains, i.e., 1,000–3,000 genes. DNA molecule of *Escherichia coli* is 1,000–1,300 μm long. Since it is much longer than the length of the bacteria, therefore, it is coiled and tightly packed up in a bundle resembling a skein of woollen thread. The length of DNA is usually expressed as kilobases (1 kb = 1,000 base pairs).

Q. 3. Write short note on plasmid.

Ans. In addition to chromosomal DNA, bacteria may also possess extrachromosomal genetic material known as plasmid. It may be defined as a small extrachromosomal piece of genetic material that can replicate autonomously (independent replicans) and can maintain in the cytoplasm of a bacterium for many generations. It consists of a circular piece of double-stranded DNA. It is not essential for the normal life and function of the host bacterium though it may confer on it additional properties such as drug resistance, bacteriocin production, toxigenicity, etc. which may confer on the host bacterium survival advantage under appropriate conditions. In addition, it may contain genetic information for controlling its own replication and ensuring segregation of one copy into each daughter cell at cell division. Plasmid contains 50–100 genes. By their ability to transfer genes from one cell to another, plasmids have become important vectors in genetic engineering.

Q. 4. Write short note on episome.

Ans. Plasmid DNA (extrachromosomal) may get integrated into host cell genome. In this state it is often known as episome. But both these terms are frequently used synonymously. Some plasmids confer on the host cell maleness or ability to conjugate (bacterial equivalent of sexual mating in higher organisms). Following conjugation, the recipient acquires the plasmid and in turn becomes male or donor cell.

Q. 5. What is meant by genotypic and phenotypic variations. Give suitable examples.

Ans. The characteristics expressed by a cell in a given environment are referred to as its **phenotype** (phaeno; display) and the collection of genes encoding these characteristics, the **genotype**. Bacteria, in general, are very adaptable and may alter their phenotype in response to environmental change while the genotype remains unchanged. Not all the genes of the bacterial cell are expressed all the time. For example, typhoid bacillus is normally flagellated but when grown on phenol agar, the flagella are not synthesized, but when subcultured from phenol agar into nutrient broth flagellated cells appear.

Another example of environmental influence is the synthesis of an enzyme β-galactosidase, necessary for lactose fermentation to its constituent sugars – glucose and galactose, in *Escherichia coli*. This organism possesses genetic information for synthesis of the enzyme, but it is produced by the bacteria only when lactose is present in the growth medium. This enzyme is not synthesized if *E. coli* is grown in medium containing glucose only. Such enzymes, which are synthesized only when induced by substrate, are called

induced enzymes, while those enzymes, which are synthesized both in the presence or absence of the substrate, are known as **constitutive enzymes**. Regulation of enzyme induction illustrates the economy of nature, the enzyme being produced only when appropriate substrates are present.

Phenotypic variations are influenced by environment, are temporary and are not heritable. **Genotypic variations** are stable, heritable and are not influenced by the environment. These are due to mutation or by any of the methods of genetic transfer such as transformation, transduction, lysogenic conversion and conjugation.

Q. 6. Describe briefly Lac operon.

Ans. Operon concept was proposed by Jacob and Monod. Lactose fermentation requires three enzymes – β-galactosidase, galactoside permease and transacetylase coded by structural genes *Lac-z*, *Lac-y* and *Lac-a* of Lac operon respectively (Fig. 7.1). Regulatory gene in this case is *Lac-i* which codes for a repressor. It is a protein molecule which can combine with either operator region on the chromosome or with the inducer (lactose). Between *Lac-i* and structural *Lac* genes lie promoter and operator regions. For transcription of mRNA for enzyme synthesis, the RNA polymerase has to attach to promoter region and travel along structural genes sequence. Operator region lies between the promoter and structural genes.

In resting stage when lactose (inducer) is not present in the medium, repressor molecule is bound to the operator, preventing the passage of RNA polymerase from promoter to the structural genes. The repressor molecule has an affinity for lactose, in the presence of which it leaves the operator region free enabling the transcription to take place. Lactose thus acts both as an inducer and the substrate for β-galactosidase. When lactose present is completely metabolized, the repressor again attaches to the operator, switching off transcription.

Q. 7. What do you understand by mutation? Discuss different types of mutation. What is the practical importance of bacterial mutation.

Ans. It is a random, undirected, heritable variation caused by an alteration in the nucleotide sequence at some point of the DNA of the cell, which may be due to addition, deletion or substitution of one or more bases. Mutations occur spontaneously at fairly constant rates, usually in the range of one per 10^2–10^{10} cell divisions. A large colony of bacteria contains about 10^9 cells, all derived from a single organism by repeated cell divisions. It may be realized that after 10^9 cell divisions, many thousands of different mutations will have occurred, affecting many of the genes in the cell. Similarly, in every infected patient, a variety of mutants arise spontaneously.

Mutants will outnumber and overgrow, if their new character makes them better fitted to grow under the prevailing conditions in the culture medium or host tissue than the parental bacteria. This is known as **selection of mutants**. An antibiotic resistant mutant will outgrow the sensitive parental bacteria in a culture medium containing antibiotic or in the body of the patient receiving antibiotic therapy. **A mutant with altered surface antigens will escape deleterious effect of immunity developed previously.**

Though mutation occurs spontaneously, its frequency can be artificially increased by several mutagenic agents such as nitrogen mustard, acriflavine, mitomycin-C, 5-bromouracil and 2-aminopurine.

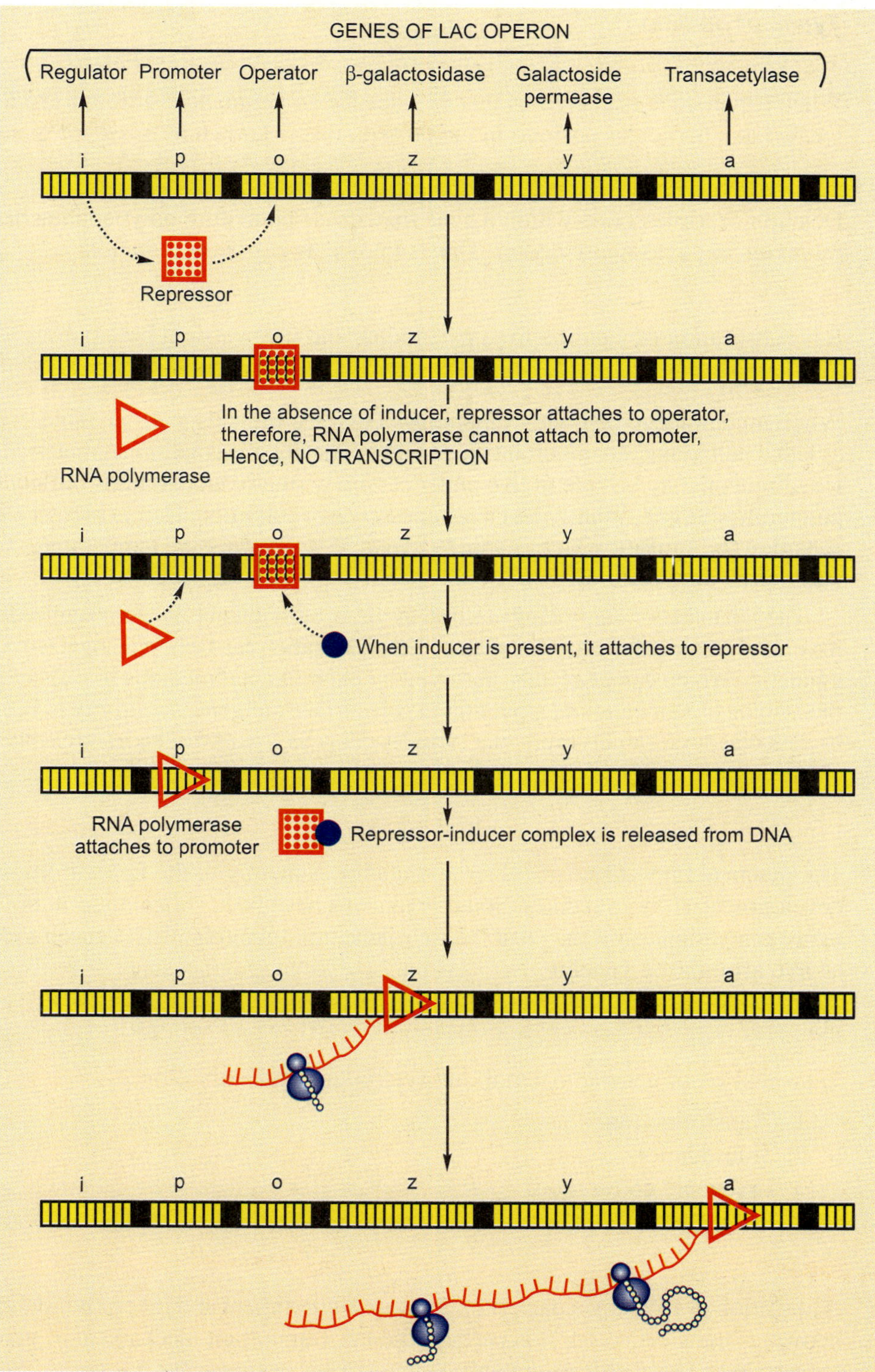

Fig. 7.1. The lac operon of *Escherichia coli.*

Types of mutation

Missense mutation

When triplet code is altered so that it codes for an amino acid different from that normally located at a particular position in the protein, this is known as missense mutation.

Nonsense mutation

Deletion of a nucleotide within a gene may cause premature polypeptide chain termination by producing a nonsense codon. This is known as nonsense mutation.

Transversion

It is substitution of a purine for a pyrimidine and vice versa in base pairing.

Conditional lethal mutation

When mutations involve vital functions so that the mutants are nonviable, these are known as lethal mutations. An important type of lethal mutation is conditional mutation. A conditional lethal mutant may be able to live under certain permissive conditions but not under other or nonpermissive conditions. The commonest type of conditional lethal mutant is **temperature-sensitive (ts) mutant** which is able to live at 35°C (permissive temperature) but not at 39°C (restrictive temperature).

Though mutations are taking place all the time, most mutants go unrecognized as the mutation may involve minor function or it may be lethal. Mutation can be best recognized when it involves a function which can be readily observed by experimental methods like alteration in colonial morphology, pigmentation, alteration in cell surface antigens, sensitivity to bacteriophages or bacteriocins, loss of ability to produce capsule or flagella, loss of virulence and change in biochemical characters.

Practical importance of bacterial mutation

The practical importance of bacterial mutation is mainly in the field of drug resistance and development of live vaccines. Some organisms have been subcultured in the laboratory for many generations until they lost their virulence for man (e.g., BCG vaccine). This is known as **live attenuated vaccine**.

Q. 8. Name various methods of acquisition of new genes. Discuss in detail transformation.

Ans. Transmission of genetic material, in bacteria, may take place by:

1. Transformation
2. Transduction
3. Lysogenic conversion
4. Conjugation

Transformation

Acquisition of DNA by a bacterium from its environment and incorporation in its genome is known as transformation. It is perhaps the most important mechanism of genetic exchange for certain bacterial species, notably *Streptococcus pneumoniae*, *S. sanguis*, *Bacillus subtilis*, *Haemophilus influenzae* and *Neisseria gonorrhoeae*. For transformation to occur DNA must have been derived from a closely related strain, since a piece of DNA can undergo recombination with chromosome only when there is adequate nucleic acid homology. Transformation was first demonstrated by Griffith in 1928. *S. pneumoniae* in capsulated form is an extremely virulent organism for mice, whereas non-capsulated variants are avirulent. The virulence of the organism is due to polysaccharide capsule.

Mutant pneumococci that have lost their ability to synthesize this capsule arise spontaneously. These show rough (R) colonies on blood agar as compared to smooth (S) colonies of capsulated form of pneumococcus. Griffith mixed live non-capsulated cells that had originally produced a capsule of one antigenic type with heat-killed smooth cells of a different capsular type. Neither preparation alone caused disease in mice, but mixture of the two preparations was lethal and Griffith was able to isolate from blood of the mice live pneumococci having a capsule of the same antigenic type as that of heat-killed cells. It was later shown that **DNA was the transforming principle** that was released from the heat-killed bacteria and was able to confer upon a live recipient cell the ability to produce a new type of capsule. The DNA that was taken up by the rough cells supplied the genetic information needed to make the missing enzyme needed for capsule synthesis.

Q. 9. Describe briefly transduction, lysogenic conversion and abortive transduction.

Ans. Transfer of a portion of DNA from one bacterium to another by bacteriophages (phages) is known as **transduction**. It may be generalized when it involves any segment of donor DNA or it may be restricted when a specific bacteriophage transduces only a particular portion of DNA.

Generalized transduction

Phages are viruses that multiply in bacteria. They carry their genetic information inside a protein coat. During assembly each phage head is normally filled with a phage genome, but sometimes an occasional phage particle is formed at a frequency of 1 in 10^6 whose head has been accidentally filled with a similar length of host cell DNA. This is known as **'packing error'**. When such a particle attaches to a second cell the DNA that enters the cell is not phage DNA capable of replicating and lysing the cell but a short segment of chromosome from first host, thus bacterial genes have been transduced by the phage into a second cell.

Since these phages pick up any portion of the host chromosome, they can transduce any gene. Each transducing phage can pick up a piece of bacterial DNA about the same size as its normal phage genome. Genes can be transduced only between fairly closely related strains because bacteriophage attacks a limited range of organisms with the same surface receptors. Transduction is not confined to transfer of chromosomal DNA. Plasmids or episomes may also be transduced. **The plasmid determining penicillin resistance in staphylococci is transferred from cell to cell by transduction.**

Restricted transduction

Bacteriophages that lyse the host cell are known as **virulent phages**, however, **temperate phage** may get incorporated into the host genome and divide with it. These cells are known as **lysogenic**. Molecular basis of lysogeny has been extensively studied in λ phage of *E. coli*. When infected with this phage majority of the cells go into lytic cycle while in a small proportion of them, they get incorporated into host cell genome (**lysogeny**). In some lysogenic cells lytic cycle is resumed. The **prophage** (integrated phage DNA) is excised and codes for viral proteins and DNA. In a small proportion of cells prophage is excised inaccurately so that a neighbouring portion of bacterial DNA is also removed.

Since phage head can contain only a standard amount of DNA, a transducing phage contains a few bacterial genes at one end of its DNA and lacks a few phage genes at the other end, i.e., **phage genome is defective**. When such a piece of DNA is transduced into a second cell the defective phage can still integrate into its normal site on the chromosome. The added bacterial genes are reproduced in the progeny of the recipient bacterium. Since the temperate phage has a specific insertion site it can pickup and transduce only a short length of DNA containing a few genes on either side of this site. This is known as restricted transduction. λ phage is always inserted between the genes for galactose utilization (*gal*) and biotin synthesis (*bio*) and thus can transduce either *gal* or *bio* genes.

Lysogenic conversion

In the lysogenic bacteria the prophage behaves as an additional segment of the bacterial chromosome, coding for new characters. This process by which prophage DNA confers additional genetic information to the host cell is known as **lysogenic or phage conversion**. An important example of lysogenic conversion is of *Corynebacterium diphtheriae* by β-phage. Only those organisms which are lysogenic produce diphtheria toxin because ***tox* gene** coding for the production of **diphtheria toxin** is present on the phage DNA. The cells that lose the phage, lose toxin production. Another example of lysogenic conversion is the production of **dick toxin** by *Streptococcus pyogenes*.

Abortive transduction

Sometimes transduced DNA fragment does not integrate into the recipient chromosome, perhaps because of the presence of only a limited degree of homology. However, the transduced fragment can express its genetic information but cannot replicate. They remain only in one progeny cells following division. This process is known as abortive transduction.

Q. 10. Describe conjugation in bacteria.

Ans. It is the transfer of DNA that occurs during contact between bacterial cells. This mechanism is much more efficient than transformation or transduction. Transfer of DNA by conjugation is very common among Gram-negative bacteria, but it is rare in Gram-positive bacteria. **It is a major mechanism of transfer of drug resistance and can occur among unrelated genera.**

Conjugation was first described by Lederberg and Tatum in 1946 in *E. coli* K12 strain and has been most extensively studied in this strain. The donor status of a bacterial cell is determined by the presence of a plasmid which codes for **sex pilus**. It is 1–2 μm in length. The tip of the pilus attaches to the surface of a recipient cell and holds the two cells together. The two strands of plasmid separate. One strand enters the recipient bacterium, probably along the sex pilus, while one strand remains in the donor. Each strand then makes a complementary copy (Fig. 7.2). It is probable, but not absolutely certain, that transfer actually occurs through the pilus. Alternately, the pilus could act as a mechanism by which the donor and recipient cells are drawn together. As donor ability is dependent upon having a copy of the plasmid, therefore, the recipient strain becomes converted into a donor. It can, in turn, conjugate with other recipient cells.

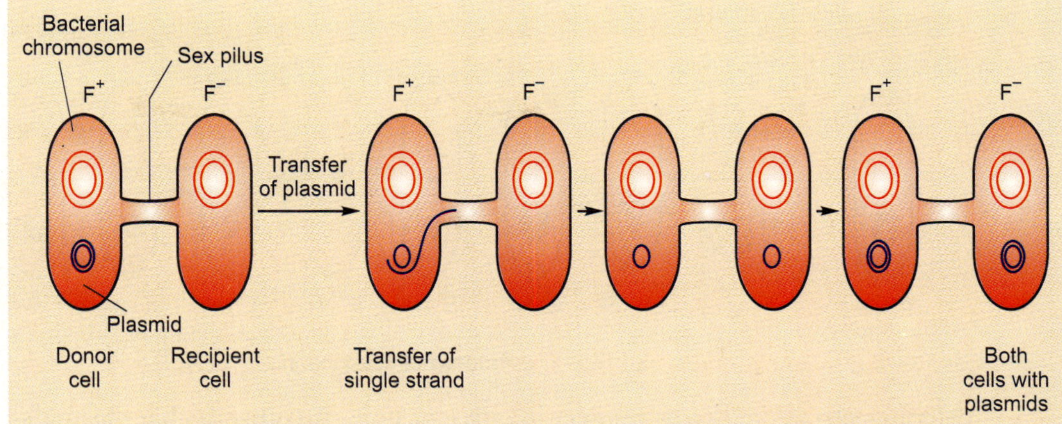

Fig. 7.2. Process of conjugation.

Stability of inheritance of plasmids varies from one plasmid to another. Some are lost very easily while others are very stable indeed and rarely, if ever, lost. Some plasmids can be eliminated from the host cell artificially (cured) by treatment with one of a variety of chemical agents (**curing agents**). These include acridine orange, sodium dodecyl sulphate and ethidium bromide.

Q. 11. Write short note on F plasmid.

Ans. F plasmid or F factor is a transfer factor that contains the genetic information necessary for the synthesis of the sex pilus and for self transfer but it does not possess other identifiable genetic markers such as drug resistance. Cells that possess one or more copies of the F plasmid are called **F$^+$** and the cells lacking the F plasmid are called **F$^-$**. F$^+$ cells have no distinguishing features other than their ability to mate with F$^-$ cells and render them F$^+$.

Certain *E. coli* strains contain an F plasmid that has become permanently integrated into the cell's chromosome. Such cells are able to transfer chromosomal genes to recipient cell with high frequency and are known as **Hfr (high frequency recombinant) cells**. F plasmid may revert from Hfr state to free state. Sometimes it may carry with it some chromosomal genes from near the site of its attachment leaving a part of its own DNA from other end in the donor chromosome (Fig. 7.3). Such F factor possessing chromosomal genes is known as **F′ (F prime) factor**. When an F′ cell mates with a recipient cell, it transfers, along with the F factor, the host genes incorporated with it. This process of transfer of host genes through F factor resembles transduction and is known as **sexduction**.

Q. 12. Describe briefly resistance (R) plasmid.

Ans. It consists of two parts – resistance transfer factor and resistance determinants (RTF + *r*). RTF is responsible for conjugal transfer and *r* determinants code for resistance against various drugs. As many as eight or more *r* determinants may be carried on each plasmid. Therefore, resistance to eight or more drugs may be transferred simultaneously. Sometimes RTF dissociates from *r* determinants. Those plasmids which lack RTF, i.e., possess only *r*

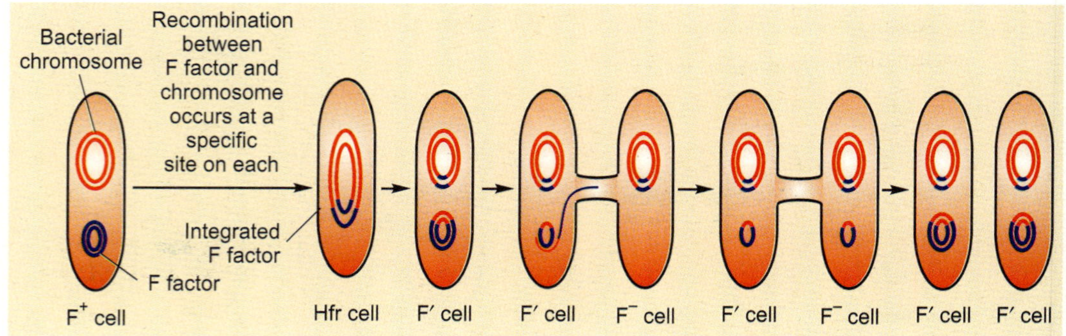

Fig. 7.3. Process of sexduction.

determinants are known as **non-conjugative** or **nonself-transmissible plasmids** but they still code for drug resistance. Those plasmids which possess both RTF and *r* determinants are known as **conjugative** or **self-transmissible plasmids**. Non-conjugative plasmids can, however, be transferred by adding another strain possessing transfer factor like colicin plasmid (Col I) or by bacteriophages.

Q. 13. Write short note on colicins.

Ans. Several strains of coliform bacteria produce colicins. These are antibiotic-like substances that are specifically and selectively lethal to other enterobacteria. Since similar substances are also produced by other than coliforms, e.g., pyocin by *Pseudomonas aeruginosa* and diphthericin by *Corynebacterium diphtheriae*, therefore, the name bacteriocin has been given to this group of substances. The specificity of action of bacteriocins enables intraspecies classification of certain bacteria, e.g., colicin typing (*Shigella sonnei*), klebocin typing (*Klebsiella* spp.), proticin typing (*Proteus* spp.), and pyocin typing (*Pseudomonas* spp.).

Colicin and klebocin production is known to be mediated by col and klebocin plasmids, respectively.

Q. 14. Discuss in detail antibiotic resistance.

Ans. Antibiotic resistance in bacteria may either be intrinsic or acquired. **Intrinsic resistance** means that the bacteria were resistant to the antibiotic even before the antibiotic was introduced. **Acquired resistance** means that a bacterium that was previously sensitive to an antibiotic has now turned resistant. It is the acquired resistance that is of great importance because it would result in treatment failure as well as potential dissemination of resistance to other bacteria.

The physiological mechanisms of antibiotic resistance include:

- Inactivation of the antibiotic by enzymes produced by the bacteria.
- Alteration of target proteins such that the antibiotic does not bind or binds with decreased affinity.
- Alteration of the membrane which decreases the permeability of the antibiotic.
- Active efflux of the antibiotic.
- Development of alternate metabolic pathway to bypass the action of antibiotic.

With antibiotics, as previously with sulphonamides, resistance began to arise. At first, organisms were encountered with low-level resistance to penicillin, and infections caused by these could be treated with larger doses of the antibiotics, because the low-level resistance was due to mutation which decreases the cell permeability to the antimicrobial agent and if larger doses are given then effective concentration of the drug can enter the bacterial cell. In time, however, highly resistant strains emerged which could not be therapeutically controlled.

Genetic basis of resistance

The initial low-level resistant microbial strains carried genes for resistance on the **chromosome**. These were soon replaced by higher-level resistant types, principally harbouring **plasmids**. Plasmid-mediated drug resistance is seen in various pathogenic and commensal bacteria of man and animals, e.g., *E. coli*, *Klebsiella pneumoniae*, *Proteus*, *Salmonella*, *Shigella* and *Pseudomonas*. Transfer of drug resistance occurs readily *in vitro*. It also occurs *in vivo* but in normal intestines it is inhibited by several factors like anaerobic conditions, bile salts, alkaline pH and abundance of anaerobic Gram-positive bacteria minimising the chances of contact between donor cells and suitable recipient cells. But in intestines of persons on oral antibiotic therapy, transfer occurs readily due to the destruction of the sensitive normal flora and the selection pressure provided by the drug.

Transferable drug resistance involves all antibiotics in common use. Bacteria containing R plasmid can spread from animal to man. Therefore, indiscriminate use of antibiotics in man and animals or in animal feed can increase the spread of plasmid-mediated drug resistance in the community. Because of the misuse and overuse of antibiotics in the hospitals it is said '*hospital is the heaven for drug resistant bacteria*'.

Some chromosomal-mediated resistances remain a therapeutic problem, namely, those responsible for resistance to methicillin, rifampicin, nalidixic acid and isoniazid. However, most resistances of concern are associated with R plasmids. While plasmids may be the vectors of the resistance genes, the genes may themselves be located on discrete movable DNA elements called **transposons**. These are very often on plasmids, but have the ability to 'hop' from plasmid to plasmid or from plasmid to chromosome. In many bacteria, such as staphylococci, bacteriophages may also be important vectors for transposon spread.

Transposons may carry single or multiple resistances. The transposon can enter and remain stable in different species even if its entry vector (e.g., plasmid or phage) is lost, since the resistance transposon can be incorporated in a stable resident plasmid or the chromosome of the new host. The discovery of transposable resistance provided the basis for understanding the rapid spread of resistance markers throughout the bacterial kingdom and helped to explain why different genera seemed to have 'evolved' similar genes of resistance.

Bacteria resist antimicrobial agents by various mechanisms. **Chromosomal resistance**, except when resulting from transposon insertions, is generally mediated by a single low-level, non-enzymatic mechanism. In many organisms, these resistances seem related to decreased permeability, e.g., resistance in meningococci, mycobacteria, pneumococci and methicillin resistance in *S. aureus*. Exceptions are the chromosomally located degradative enzymes for the β-lactam antibiotics and the chromosomal-mediated resistance to rifampicin (via resistant RNA polymerases) and nalidixic acid (via resistant DNA gyrases).

In general, **the plasmid- or transposon-mediated** resistances are of higher level and involve more active processes. Some plasmid-mediated resistance to penicillin and to chloramphenicol seems to involve decreased permeability, but the exact mechanism is not yet defined. Many plasmid-mediated resistances involve extracellular inactivation of the drug by enzymatic modification or degradation of its active element. In this category are the enzymes (β-lactamases) which destroy the β-lactam ring of the penicillins and cephalosporins, and those which inactivate chloramphenicol.

In clinical practice, resistance acquired by mutation is very important in tuberculosis. If a patient is put on streptomycin alone then initially organisms die in large numbers but soon resistant mutants appear which multiply in number while sensitive parents may be eliminated. If two or more drugs are used and if a mutant appears which is resistant to one of the drugs then it will be killed by other drug/s. **The chance of a mutant developing resistance to more than one drug at one time is remote.** This is the rationale of combined therapy in tuberculosis.

R plasmid-mediated resistance is usually to multiple drugs, therefore, there is no use of combined therapy. Table 7.1 shows important differences between mutational drug resistance and plasmid-mediated drug resistance. Acquisition of resistance by transduction is common in staphylococci. The penicillinase plasmids, which are transmitted by transduction, may also carry determinants of resistance to mercuric chloride and erythromycin.

Table 7.1. Mutational and plasmid-mediated drug resistance

Mutational drug resistance	Plasmid-mediated drug resistance
1. It is due to decreased permeability to drug, development of alternate metabolic pathways and development of enzymes inactivating the drug.	It is due to the development of degrading enzymes.
2. Involves resistance to one drug at one time.	Involves many drugs at one time.
3. Degree of resistance is usually low, therefore, infection may be treated by giving higher doses of the antibiotics.	Degree of resistance is usually high, therefore, higher doses of antibiotics do not help.
4. Development of drug resistance can be prevented by treatment with combination of drugs.	Development of drug resistance cannot be prevented by treatment with combination of drugs.
5. Resistance is not transferable to other organisms.	Resistance is transferable to other organisms.
6. Resistant mutants are usually metabolically defective.	They are metabolically normal.
7. Virulence of resistant mutants may be lowered.	Virulence usually not decreased. It may rather be increased by acquisition of virulence plasmids.

Q. 15. Describe briefly transposable genetic elements.

Ans. Lederberg, in 1960, described an unusual class of *Gal*-mutants in *E. coli* caused by insertion of extra pieces of DNA called **insertion sequences** or **IS elements** at the point of mutation. Since then a large number of IS elements have been described in a wide variety of bacteria. They are common in bacterial plasmids and are common components of many, if not all, bacterial chromosomes. They are also **cryptic** in the sense that they do not confer on the host bacterium a predictable phenotype. Their presence is usually indicated by mutation. IS elements possess ability to transpose, i.e., they can insert into different sites on the same or on different DNA molecules.

In 1974, the discovery of a new type of transposable element that encoded a recognizable gene product (β-lactam antibiotic resistance) was reported. It was termed a **transposon (tn)**. Since then many others carrying a variety of resistance and other genes have been identified. Because of the ability of transposable elements to move from one plasmid to another or to a phage or to the bacterial chromosome they have assumed the popular name of **jumping genes**. **Unlike plasmids, transposons do not contain genetic information necessary for their own replication**, and their replication, therefore, depends on their physical integration with a bacterial replicon.

IS elements are small (1–2 kb) and cryptic, whereas transposons are larger (4–25 kb) and encode at least one function that alters cell phenotype. Therefore, **transposon may be defined as a segment of DNA with one or more genes in the centre and the two ends carrying inverted repeat sequences of nucleotides – nucleotide sequences complementary to each other but in the reverse order**. Because of this feature each strand of the transposon can form a single-stranded loop carrying the gene/genes and a double-stranded stem formed by hydrogen bonding between the inverted repeat sequences (Fig. 7.4).

The transfer of genetic material from one DNA molecule to another is known as **transposition**. It does not need genetic homology between transposable element and its site of insertion. It is, therefore, different from recombination. Insertion of a transposon leads to the acquisition of new characteristics by the recipient DNA molecule. **It has been suggested that R plasmids may have evolved as collections of transposons each carrying a gene that confers resistance to one or more antibiotics.**

Q. 16. Describe briefly principle of genetic engineering and its applications.

Ans. Insertion of a foreign DNA molecule into DNA of a vector, which can replicate autonomously in a suitable host, is known as recombinant DNA (rDNA) technology or genetic engineering. This technique makes it possible to isolate any gene coding for any desired protein from microorganisms or from cells of higher forms of life including human beings, and their introduction into suitable microorganisms in which genes would be functional, directing the production of specific protein. Such cloning of genes in microorganisms enables the preparation of the desired protein in pure form, in large quantities and at a reasonable cost.

Applications of genetic engineering

- Genetic engineering is a useful tool for the **production of vaccines** (for prevention of disease) **and antigens** (for the diagnosis of disease).
- Yeast derived recombinant vaccine against hepatitis B is now commercially available.
- Genes coding for gp120 of human immunodeficiency virus (HIV) have been inserted into vaccinia virus. Inoculation of this hybrid-live virus (gp120/vaccinia hybrid vaccine) elicits both antibody-mediated and cell-mediated immunity against HIV.
- Vaccinia virus has also been used for the development of hybrid live vaccine against hepatitis B.

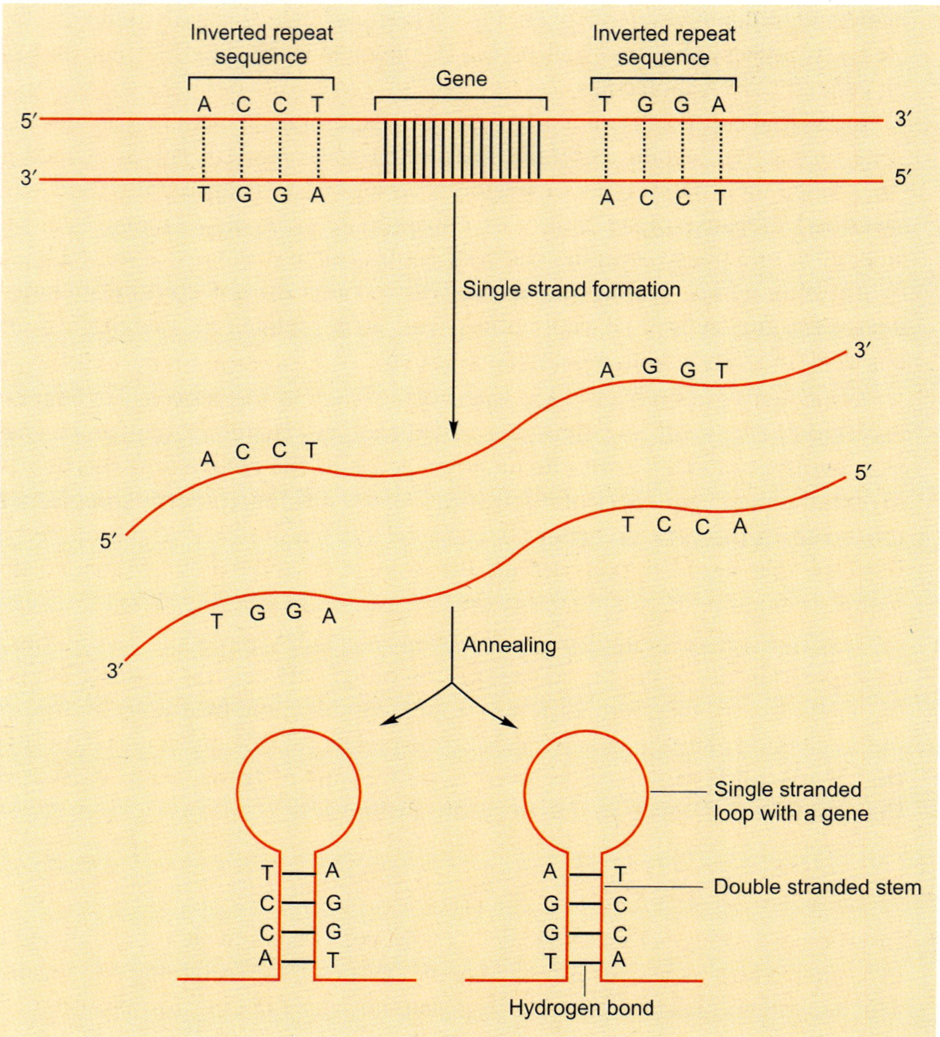

Fig. 7.4. Structure of transposon.

- Recombinant DNA technology has also been used for the **production of proteins** of therapeutic interest. These include human growth hormone, human insulin, erythropoietin, factor VIII, tissue plasminogen activator, interferons, tumour necrosis factor, interleukin-2, granulocyte colony stimulating factor, epidermal growth factor and fibroblast growth factor.
- An important application of recombinant technology is gene therapy. Normal genes can be introduced into the patient so that genetic diseases can be cured.

Q. 17. What are DNA probes? Describe briefly development and applications of DNA probes.

Ans. DNA probes are radiolabelled or chromogenically labelled pieces of single-stranded DNA which can be used for the detection of homologous DNA by hybridization.

Development of DNA probe

All microorganisms, simple or complex, contain some unique sequences of nucleic acid within their genome that distinguish them from all other organisms. The method of developing a DNA probe is to cut or isolate those sequences from the nucleic acid of the cell using a set of enzymes known as restriction endonucleases, reproduce them in large quantities and attach a reporter molecule to them so that they can be incorporated into a hybridization reaction. **Hybridization** is the process whereby two single strands of nucleic acid come together to form a stable double-stranded molecule. However, they will bind and stay together only if the sequences of bases along each stretch of nucleic acid are complementary (adenine opposite thymine and cytosine opposite guanine).

Hybridizations are accomplished in tubes or by spotting the unknown organisms on a filter paper such as nitrocellulose paper, lysing them to release the DNA, and denaturing in mild alkali to single strands. The probe can then be added and after thorough washing to remove any unbound probe, the tube or probe is examined for evidence of hybridization. Formalin-fixed, paraffin-embedded tissues can also be probed particularly for viral DNA sequences. DNA probes can also be designed that bind to RNA and this procedure has been used particularly to locate ribosomal RNA.

Applications of DNA probes

- In the diagnostic laboratory, DNA probes are being used for culture confirmation as an alternative to conventional, time-consuming or labour-intensive methods. For example, DNA hybridization makes it possible to rapidly identify *Mycobacterium tuberculosis*, *M. kansasii*, *M. avium* complex, and *M. gordonae* isolated in culture, significantly reducing the time for reporting of the species of the isolate.
- Probe technology may also be used for detection of fastidious organisms directly in clinical specimens. Examples are *Neisseria gonorrhoeae* and *Chlamydia trachomatis*.

Q. 18. Describe briefly polymerase chain reaction. What are the applications of the same?

Ans. Kary Mulis invented this method in 1989. He was awarded Nobel Prize in 1993. Polymerase chain reaction is a primer-mediated, temperature-dependent technique for the enzymatic amplification of a specific sequence (target sequence) to such an extent that it can be detected. The technique can be used to detect very small amounts of specific nucleic acid material in clinical specimens where bacterial, viral or fungal agents are thought to play a causative role. The fundamental basis of this technology is that each pathogenic organism possesses a unique 'signature sequence' in its DNA or RNA composition by which it can be identified. It is based on repeated cycles of high temperature template denaturation, oligonucleotide primer annealing, and polymerase mediated extension (Fig. 7.5).

To multiply a strip of genetic material, four ingredients are placed together in a small vial:

1. Target DNA.
2. Short strands of DNA called primers which tag the section to be copied.
3. Polymerase – an enzyme that promotes gene replication in all living cells.
4. Nucleotides – the building blocks for making DNA.

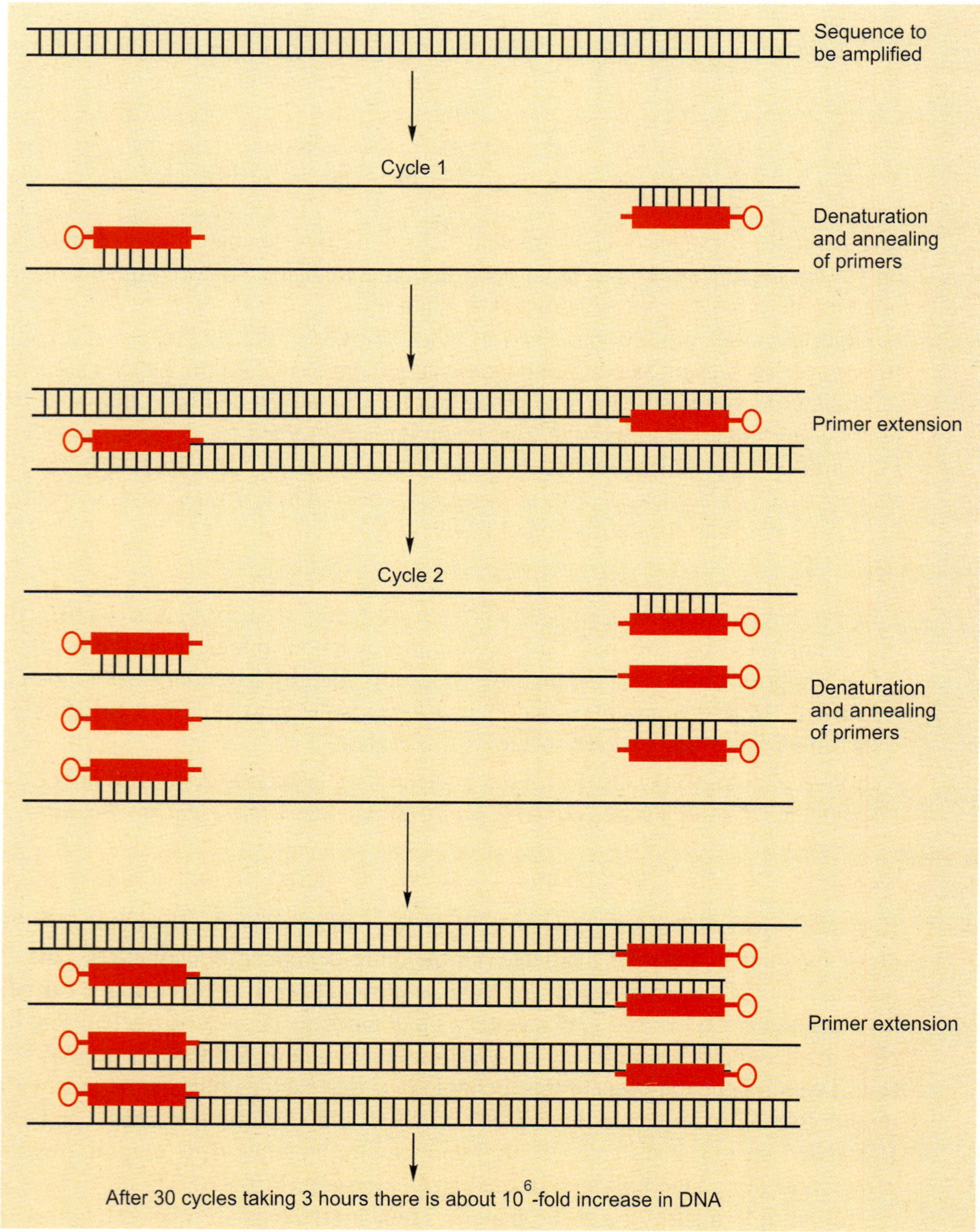

Fig. 7.5. Polymerase chain reaction.

PCR is carried out in three steps:

1. Heat at 94°C is applied to the target DNA, breaking the bonds that hold the strands together. This is known as **denaturation**.

2. The temperature is then reduced to 55°C, promoting the primers to attach themselves to either end of the target strip. This is known as **annealing of primers**.
3. Then polymerase enzyme triggers the formation of new DNA strand from the nucleotides. Extension of the primers is done by a thermostable *Taq* polymerase (purified from *Thermus aquaticus*, a thermophilic bacterium that lives in hot springs at temperatures of 70–75°C). This is known as **primer extension**. When the temperature is again raised the new strands separate and the process begins again.

These three steps are repeated again and again by manipulating the temperature, a process that is automated by the PCR machine (Table 7.2). A cycle takes about 3–5 minutes and after 30 cycles, taking about 3 hours, a single copy of DNA can be increased up to 1,000,000 copies, a sharp contrast to the days required by conventional amplification method (culture).

Table 7.2. Programming of cycles in polymerase chain reaction

Step	Temperature	Time	Cycle
Initial denaturation	94°C	5 minutes	First cycle
Denaturation	94°C	30 seconds	30 cycles
Annealing of primers	55°C	1 minute	
Primer extension	72°C	1 minute	
Final primer extension	72°C	7 minutes	Last cycle

Amplified sequences of target DNA can be detected by a variety of methods. If enough amplified DNA is present, it can be visualized by:

1. Gel electrophoresis and ethidium bromide staining.
2. Southern blot and dot-blot analysis with either radioactive or nonradioactive probes.
3. Oligomer restriction.
4. Oligomer hybridization.
5. Reverse dot-blot.

Applications of PCR

The development of PCR or gene amplification method is a major methodological breakthrough in molecular biology. Within a short span, this method has found its way into nearly every type of laboratory from forensic to ecology and from diagnosis to pure research. Applications of PCR in clinical laboratory are given in Table 7.3.

- ***In diagnosis of inherited disorders:*** The PCR technology is being widely used to amplify gene segments that contain known mutations for diagnosis of inherited diseases such as sickle cell anaemia, β-thalassaemia, cystic fibrosis, etc. PCR is especially useful for prenatal diagnosis of inherited diseases, where cells obtained from the foetus by amniocentesis are very few.
- ***In cancer detection:*** Identification of mutations in oncosuppressor genes such as retinoblastoma gene can help to identify individuals at high risk of cancer.
- ***In medicolegal cases:*** PCR allows DNA in a single cell, hair follicle or sperm to be amplified enormously and analyzed. The pattern obtained is then compared with that of various suspects.

Table 7.3. Applications of PCR in clinical laboratory

Diagnosis of infections due to:

A. ***Viruses:*** HIV-1, HIV-2, HTLV-1, cytomegalovirus, human papillomavirus, herpes simplex viruses, hepatitis B virus, HCV, HDV, HEV, rubella virus, Epstein-Barr virus, varicella-zoster virus, human herpesvirus 6 and 7, parvovirus B19, enteroviruses, coxsackieviruses, echoviruses, rhinoviruses, measles virus, rotavirus, adenovirus, respiratory syncytial virus

B. ***Bacteria:*** *Mycobacterium tuberculosis*, *Mycobacterium avium* complex, *Legionella pneumophila*, *Chlamydia trachomatis*, *Mycoplasma pneumoniae*, *Helicobacter pylori*, *Burkholderia pseudomallei*, *Campylobacter* spp., *Corynebacterium diphtheriae*, *Leptospira interrogans*, *Streptococcus pyogenes*, *Streptococcus pneumoniae*, *Yersinia enterocolitica*

C. ***Fungi:*** *Candida* spp., *Cryptococcus neoformans*, *Aspergillus* spp., *Pneumocystis jiroveci*

D. ***Protozoa:*** *Toxoplasma gondii*, *Trypanosoma cruzi*, *Enterocytozoon bieneusi*, *Encephalitozoon hellem*, *Plasmodium* spp.

Other question which may also be asked in the examination

Tabulate differences between mutational and plasmid-mediated drug resistance.

For answer see page 64.

8

BACTERIA IN HEALTH & DISEASE

Q. 1. Describe sources of infection.

Ans. Infections may be endogenous, due to the organisms of the normal flora, and exogenous, due to the organisms derived from a source outside the body.

Endogenous infections

These are also referred to as autoinfections. Organisms of normal flora are usually non-pathogenic but occasionally they may lead to infection. The most important autoinfections are:

1. **Viridans streptococci** are the normal flora of the mouth but when there is abnormality of the heart, like rheumatic heart disease and injury to the oral cavity like tooth extraction or fractured mandible, these organisms enter into the blood stream and settle down on the heart leading to infective endocarditis. In both the above examples, two conditions are fulfilled – the organism initiating infection does so in an area of the body remote from its normal habitat and infection develops only where there is some tissue abnormality lowering local tissue resistance.
2. ***E. coli*** **and** ***Enterococcus faecalis***, which are the normal flora of the intestines, may cause urinary tract infection particularly when there is some abnormality of the urinary tract like congenital malformation, urinary calculi and ureteric and prostatic obstruction. These conditions lower the local tissue resistance.

Exogenous infections

Most of the infections are exogenous in origin. The sources of exogenous infections are as under:

1. Human cases and carriers.
2. Animal cases and carriers.
3. Insects.
4. Environment.

1. Human cases and carriers

The commonest source of human infection is man himself who may be a patient or a carrier. Infections due to some organisms are acquired mainly or exclusively from ill persons, e.g., AIDS, syphilis, gonorrhoea, pulmonary tuberculosis, leprosy, whooping cough, hepatitis B and C, measles, mumps, influenza, poliomyelitis, etc.

A **carrier** is a person who harbours the pathogenic microorganisms without suffering from it. There are several types of carriers:

- *Healthy carrier:* One who harbours the pathogen but has never suffered from the disease caused by it.
- *Convalescent carrier:* One who has recovered from the disease but continues to harbour the pathogen on his body.
- *Temporary carrier:* When carrier state lasts for less than six months.
- *Chronic carrier:* When carrier state lasts for years or may be for the life of the patient.
- *Paradoxical carrier:* Who acquires the organisms from another carrier.
- *Contact carrier:* Who acquires the organisms from a patient.

Carriers are very important source of infection. For example, a person acquires organisms from a patient of meningococcal meningitis and becomes a contact carrier. He is then a source of infection for other persons (patient → carrier → patient).

2. Animal cases and carriers

Certain pathogens are capable of causing infection in both man and animals. Therefore, animals may act as a source of infection of such organisms. The infection may be acquired by contact with the animal, animal bite and ingestion of milk or meat. Infection in animals may be asymptomatic and these animals may serve as reservoir for human infections. These are known as **reservoir hosts**. Infectious diseases transmitted from animals to man are known as **zoonoses**. For example:

- *Bacterial:* Bovine tuberculosis, bubonic plague, *Salmonella* food poisoning, anthrax.
- *Viral:* Rabies, yellow fever.
- *Protozoal:* Leishmaniasis.
- *Helminthic:* Hydatid disease.
- *Fungal: Microsporum canis, Trichophyton verrucosum.*

In these infections man is generally an end host and there is rarely any secondary spread from the patient to other persons or back to animals. **Important exceptions** are man to man spread of pneumonic plague which may supervene on bubonic plague contracted by man from rat, and arbovirus infections such as yellow fever in which man to man spread may supervene on infection of man from an animal host.

3. Insects

Blood-sucking insects such as mosquitoes, ticks, mites, flies, and lice act as a source of a number of human and animal infections. Insects transmitting pathogens are known as **vectors**.

4. Environment

This includes soil, water and food. A few infective diseases of man are caused by saprophytic microbes derived from soil and vegetation. Some pathogens can survive in the environment for very long periods. For example, spores of tetanus and gas gangrene bacilli remain viable in the soil for several decades and serve as a source of infection. The normal habitat of these organisms is the human and animal intestines and they enter the soil through their faeces.

Fungi causing mycetoma, sporotrichosis and histoplasmosis survive in soil and cause human infection. Eggs of parasites like roundworms and hookworms survive and develop in the soil and cause human infection. Water contaminated with *Shigella*, *Salmonella*, *Vibrio cholerae*, poliovirus, hepatitis A and E viruses and cyclops containing larvae of guinea worm acts as a source of these infections.

Contaminated food acts as a source of organisms causing food poisoning, gastroenteritis, diarrhoea and dysentery.

Q. 2. Describe modes of spread of infection.

Ans. Pathogenic organisms can spread from one host to another by a variety of mechanisms. These include:

1. Inhalation

Respiratory infections such as common cold, influenza, measles, mumps, tuberculosis and whooping cough are acquired by inhalation. These organisms are shed into the environment by patients in secretions of nose or throat during sneezing, coughing, talking and other forceful expiratory activities. These activities expel a spray of droplets. **Large droplets** more than 0.1 mm in diameter fly forwards and downwards from the mouth to the distance of a few feet and they reach the floor within a few seconds or they may fall on the eyes, face, mouth and clothes of the person standing in front of the producer of the spray. Small droplets, less than 0.1 mm in diameter, evaporate immediately to become minute residue or **droplet nuclei** and remain airborne and may be inhaled into the nose, throat or lungs.

2. Ingestion

Intestinal infections like enteric fever, cholera, dysentery, food poisoning, poliomyelitis, hepatitis A and E, and most of the parasitic infections are acquired by ingestion. The source of these infections is the faeces of the patients or carriers. The faeces containing pathogens may contaminate food and drinks.

3. Contact

Infection may be acquired by direct or indirect contact with the patient. Sexually transmitted diseases (STD) such as syphilis, gonorrhoea, lymphogranuloma venereum, lymphogranuloma inguinale, trichomoniasis, herpes simplex type 2, hepatitis B and C, and AIDS are acquired by direct contact. The term **contagious disease** may be used for the disease acquired by direct contact, and disease acquired by other modes, through inanimate objects, as **infectious disease**.

4. Contamination of wounds

The infections may be caused by:

- Organisms present in the nose or throat of the patient himself or of nurses or doctors. Pathogenic staphylococci and streptococci derived from respiratory tract are important causes of wound and burn infection.
- Airborne spread of organisms from the infected wounds of other patients.

- Contact with infected hands, clothing or other articles.
- In some instances pathogens may be inoculated directly into the tissues of the host, for example, rabies virus which is present in the saliva of a rabid animal, usually dog, is inoculated directly into the host tissue.
- Spores of *Clostridium tetani* and *C. perfringens* are present in the soil. These get inoculated into the host tissue following severe wounds leading to tetanus and gas gangrene respectively.

5. Blood-sucking arthropods

In some diseases, blood-sucking insects play an important role in the spread of infection from one individual to another. Table 8.1 shows common arthropods and diseases transmitted by them.

Insects normally become infected by biting a human or animal host in whose blood the causative organism is present. After this there is an interval, known as **extrinsic incubation period**, during which the insect is incapable of transmitting the infection. During this period the organisms multiply in the body of the insect. *Ticks which transmit certain rickettsial and*

Table 8.1. Common arthropods and diseases transmitted by them

Arthropod	Diseases transmitted
1. **Mosquitoes**	
• Anopheles	Malaria, filariasis
• Culex	Filariasis, Japanese encephalitis, West Nile fever
• Aedes	Yellow fever, dengue, chikungunya haemorrhagic fever, Rift Valley fever, filariasis
• Mansonia	Brugian filariasis
2. **Flies**	
• House fly	Typhoid and paratyphoid fever, diarrhoea, dysentery, cholera, gastroenteritis, amoebiasis
• Sand fly	Kala-azar, oriental sore, espundia, oroya fever
• Tsetse fly	African trypanosomiasis
3. Louse	Epidemic typhus, relapsing fever, trench fever
4. Rat flea	Bubonic plague, endemic typhus, *Hymenolepis diminuta* infestation
5. Black fly	Onchocerciasis
6. Reduviid bug	Chagas' disease
7. **Ticks**	
• Hard ticks	Spotted fever group, viral encephalitis, Colorado tick typhus, tularaemia, human babesiosis
• Soft ticks	Q fever, relapsing fever, Kyasanur Forest disease
8. **Mites**	
• Trombiculid mite	Scrub typhus
• Gamasid mite	Rickettsial pox
• Itch mite	Scabies
9. Body and head lice	Epidemic typhus, relapsing fever
10. Cyclops	Dracunculosis, diphyllobothriasis
11. Cockroaches	Same as in case of house fly

arbovirus infections, and mites which transmit scrub typhus are unusual in that the infective agent can be transmitted from one generation of the insect to the next through the ovum.

Arthropods transmit infection in four ways:

1. The infective agent gains access to the salivary glands of the insect and the organisms enter into the wound caused by the insect bite along with the saliva, e.g., transmission of malaria by female anopheles mosquito.
2. The infective agent multiplies in the intestinal tract of the insect and during feeding it is regurgitated into the wound, e.g., transmission of bubonic plague by rat flea.
3. The agent multiplies in the intestinal tract and is excreted in the faeces. These are deposited by the insect besides the wound when it bites and due to irritation caused by insect bite, are scratched by the victim into the wound, e.g., transmission of rickettsial diseases.
4. The infective agent multiplies in the coelomic cavity of the insect and infection is due to contamination of the wound of bite with the coelomic fluid of an insect that has been crushed in its vicinity by the victim, e.g., transmission of louse-borne relapsing fever.

6. Iatrogenic and laboratory infections

If meticulous care in asepsis is not taken, infections like AIDS, and hepatitis B, C and D may sometimes be transmitted during therapeutic and investigative procedures such as injections, lumbar puncture, blood transfusion, dialysis, and heart and kidney transplant surgery. These are known as **iatrogenic or physician-induced infections**. Laboratory personnel handling infectious material and doing mouth-pipetting are particularly at risk.

7. Congenital

Some microorganisms like *Toxoplasma*, rubella virus, cytomegalovirus, herpes simplex virus, *Treponema pallidum*, human immunodeficiency virus, malaria parasites, etc. can cross the placental barrier and infect the foetus in utero. This is known as **vertical transmission**. This may result in abortion, miscarriage or stillbirth. Live infants may be born with manifestations of the disease.

Another form of transmission from mother to infant occurs by contact during birth with organisms such as group B streptococci, *Chlamydia trachomatis* and *Neisseria gonorrhoeae* which colonize the vagina. Herpes simplex virus, cytomegalovirus and human immunodeficiency virus may be present in the genital secretions and infant may acquire these during birth. Cytomegalovirus and human immunodeficiency virus may be transmitted by breast milk, a third mechanism of vertical transmission.

Q. 3. Define pathogenicity and virulence. Describe determinants of virulence.

Ans. **Pathogenicity** denotes the ability of a microbial species to cause disease, while the term **virulence** refers to the same property in a strain of the species.

Determinants of virulence

1. Adhesion

Many bacteria possess on their surface colonization factors or adhesins. These usually occur on fimbriae. Through adhesins bacteria attach specifically on the receptors present on the host cells. They are, therefore, responsible for tissue tropism. Adhesion is necessary to avoid innate host defence mechanisms such as peristalsis in the gut and the flushing action of mucus, saliva and urine which remove nonadherent bacteria. Loss of adhesins may render a strain avirulent.

2. Invasion of tissues

Invasiveness signifies the ability of an organism to penetrate a tissue after it adheres to a cell surface. Some bacteria can invade tissues in the absence of physical injury, e.g., *N. meningitidis* in nasal epithelium and salmonellae in intestinal epithelium. These organisms are endocytosed by epithelial cells, transported across these cells within vacuoles and released into the submucosal space, from which they invade the underlying tissues. *Shigella* and enteroinvasive *E. coli* are also endocytosed by intestinal epithelial cells but do not penetrate the basement membrane.

3. Capsules

Cell wall in many bacteria is enclosed by a protective gelatinous covering layer known as capsule. It contributes to the virulence of the bacteria by inhibiting phagocytosis. Virtually all the pathogens associated with meningitis and pneumonia including *H. influenzae*, *N. meningitidis*, and *S. pneumoniae* are capsulated, and noncapsulated variants usually exhibit much reduced virulence. Some bacterial surface antigens such as Vi antigen of *S.* Typhi and K antigen of *E. coli* also help the bacteria to withstand phagocytosis and the lytic activity of complement.

4. Streptococcal M protein

The M protein present on the surface of *S. pyogenes* binds both fibrinogen and fibrin to the bacterial cell wall thus masking the bacterial receptors from complement.

5. Bacterial toxins

These are substances produced by or present in bacteria, which have a direct toxic action on tissue cells. Two major types of toxin have been described – endotoxins and exotoxins (Table 8.2).

Endotoxins

They are components of the outer membrane of Gram-negative bacteria. They are lipopolysaccharide (LPS) in nature and are released from the bacterial surface by natural lysis of the bacteria or by disintegration of the organisms *in vitro*. The endotoxic activity of LPS resides in its lipid A moiety. The latter is not destroyed by autoclaving, hence infusion of a sterile solution containing endotoxin can cause serious illness. They are poor antigens and the toxicity is not completely neutralized by the homologous antibodies. They cannot be toxoided. Endotoxins exert a wide spectrum of effects on the host, the most dramatic of which are fever and the shock syndrome associated with Gram-negative bacterial sepsis. Man is particularly sensitive to minute amounts of endotoxins and often a mild Gram-negative bacterial infection will cause fever. Larger amounts of endotoxin may cause irreversible shock seen in association with a fulminating Gram-negative bacteraemia.

Exotoxins

They are produced extracellularly by both Gram-positive and Gram-negative bacteria. They are highly potent even in small amounts and constitute some of the most poisonous substances known. **Botulinum toxin is the most poisonous followed by tetanus toxin.** Minimum lethal dose for botulinum toxin for a mouse is 0.03 ng and for humans may be 1 μg. It has been estimated that 3 kg of this toxin can kill all the inhabitants of the world. Exotoxins are heat-labile, protein in nature and have enzymatic activity. Some exotoxins can be partially denatured by treatment with formaldehyde to generate toxoids which lack toxicity but retain antigenicity inducing protective immunity when used as vaccines. Some exotoxins like diphtheria toxin, and enterotoxins of cholera vibrio and *E. coli* consist of two fragments A and B. The toxin binds to the specific receptors, on the host cell surface, through fragment B (binding) and then toxic or enzymatic A fragment causes cell damage.

6. Resistance to killing by phagocytic cells

Some pathogens like tubercle bacilli can be readily ingested (phagocytosed) by macrophages and other phagocytes but they resist intracellular killing by preventing fusion of phagosome with lysosome. These organisms rather multiply inside these cells. Other bacteria such as *S. aureus* and *N. gonorrhoeae* are able to resist the action of lysosomal components following fusion.

Q. 4. Tabulate differences between exotoxins and endotoxins.

Ans. Differences between exotoxins and endotoxins are given in Table 8.2.

Table 8.2. Differences between exotoxins and endotoxins

Exotoxins	Endotoxins
1. Proteins with high molecular weight ranging from 10,000 to 900,000.	Lipopolysaccharide in nature. Lipid A portion is probably responsible for the toxicity.
2. Heat-labile. The toxicity is destroyed by heating above 60°C.	Heat-stable; can withstand heat over 60°C without losing toxicity.
3. Highly antigenic; stimulate formation of antitoxin which neutralizes toxin.	Weakly antigenic; do not stimulate the formation of antitoxin. Antibodies against only polysaccharide component are raised.
4. Actively secreted by the cells; diffuse into the surrounding medium.	Form integral part of the cell wall; do not diffuse into surrounding medium. These can be obtained only by cell lysis.
5. Converted into toxoid by formaldehyde.	Cannot be toxoided.
6. Action often enzymic.	No enzymic action.
7. Specific pharmacological effect for each exotoxin.	Non-specific action of all endotoxins.
8. Highly specific for particular tissue, e.g., tetanus toxin for CNS.	Non-specific in action.
9. Very high potency (one mg of botulinum or tetanus toxin can kill more than one million guinea-pigs).	Low potency (one mg of extracted somatic antigen can kill one mouse).
10. Do not produce fever in the host.	Usually produce fever in the host.
11. Produced by both Gram-positive bacteria and Gram-negative bacteria.	Produced by Gram-negative bacteria only.
12. Frequently controlled by extrachromosomal genes (e.g., plasmids).	Synthesis directed by chromosomal genes.

9

IMMUNITY

Q. 1. Define and classify immunity.

Ans. **Immunity** is defined as state of resistance of a host to pathogens and their toxic products. It is of two types:

1. **Innate immunity**
   - (a) Non-specific
   - (b) Specific

   ] Species, Racial, Individual

2. **Acquired immunity**
   - (a) *Active*
     - Natural
     - Artificial
   - (b) *Passive*
     - Natural
     - Artificial

Q. 2. What is innate immunity due to? Describe briefly different types of innate immunity.

Ans. Innate immunity is due to genetic and constitutional make-up of an individual. Prior contact with microorganisms or their products is not essential. It may be specific against a particular organism or non-specific. Innate immunity may be further divided into species, racial or individual immunity.

Species immunity

It is total or relative resistance to a pathogen shown by all the members of a species. For example, all human beings are resistant to plant pathogens and many animal pathogens. Rat is strikingly resistant to diphtheria whilst guinea-pig and man are highly susceptible. This is due to physical and biochemical differences between the tissues of different host species which determine if a pathogen can multiply in them.

Racial immunity

Within a species, there may be marked racial differences in resistance to infection, e.g., Algerian sheep is highly resistant to anthrax as compared to European sheep. In the USA, Negroes are more susceptible to tuberculosis than whites. Racial differences in immunity are known to be genetic in origin. A hereditary (genetic) abnormality of red blood cells (sickling) confers immunity to infection by *Plasmodium falciparum* because such RBCs cannot be parasitized by these parasites. This may provide survival advantage to such individuals in malaria-infested areas.

Individual immunity

Different individuals in a race differ in their resistance to microbial infections. The genetic basis of individual immunity is apparent from the observation that if one homozygous twin develops tuberculosis, there is a 75% chance that the other twin will develop overt tuberculosis. In contrast, for heterozygous twins, there is only 33% chance that the second twin will contract overt disease.

Q. 3. Describe factors influencing innate immunity.

Ans. Following factors influence innate immunity:

1. Age

In general, very young and very old are more susceptible to infectious diseases than persons in other age groups. This appears to be due to the immaturity of immune system in very young and gradual waning of immune response in very old. Foetus in utero is protected from maternal infection by placental barrier. But some pathogens such as HIV cross this barrier leading to foetal infection, while others like *Toxoplasma gondii*, rubella and cytomegalovirus lead to congenital malformations.

Newborn animals are more susceptible to experimental infection than adult animals, e.g., coxsackievirus causes fatal infection in suckling mice but not in adult mice. On the other hand, in many diseases such as measles, mumps, poliomyelitis and chickenpox, the clinical illness is more severe in adults than in children. This may be due to more active immune response which leads to greater tissue damage.

2. Hormonal influences and sex

There is an increased susceptibility to infection in endocrine disorders such as diabetes mellitus, hypothyroidism and adrenal dysfunction. The reason for this increased susceptibility is not known but it may be related to hormone activity. For example, glucocorticoids are anti-inflammatory agents. They inhibit the ability of phagocytes to ingest foreign particles. Staphylococcal, streptococcal and certain fungal infections such as candidiasis, aspergillosis and mucormycosis occur more frequently in diabetics. Pregnant women are more susceptible to microbial infections due to increased steroid levels during pregnancy. In general, incidence and death rate from infectious diseases is greater in males than in females. However, in case of hepatitis A and whooping cough, morbidity and mortality is higher in females than in males.

3. Nutritional factors

Both antibody-mediated and cell-mediated immunity are lowered in malnutrition. Protein calorie malnutrition:

- lowers C3 and factor B of the complement system,
- decreases the interferon response, and
- inhibits neutrophil activity.

Similarly, deficiency of vitamin A, vitamin C, folic acid and zinc predisposes to certain infections. Experimental studies have also shown that inadequate diet may be correlated with increased susceptibility to a variety of bacterial infections associated with decreased phagocytic activity and leucopenia.

Q. 4. Describe mechanism of innate immunity.

Ans. Innate immunity employs the following mechanisms:

1. Mechanical barriers and surface secretions

The intact skin and the mucous membranes provide a high degree of protection against pathogens. If skin is damaged, as in case of injury or burns, infections may be a serious problem. Skin is a very effective barrier because of unusual structure of outermost epithelial layer which is composed mainly of keratin which is indigestible by most microorganisms, and thus protects the living cells of the epidermis from microorganisms and their toxins.

Even more important than this are the **fatty acids secreted by the sebaceous glands**, **propionic acid produced by the normal flora of the skin** and **high salt concentration in drying sweat**. Secretions from sebaceous glands contain both saturated and unsaturated fatty acids that kill many bacteria and fungi. The protective ability of these secretions varies at different stages of life. For example, ringworm of scalp caused by *Microsporum* and *Trichophyton* is difficult to cure in children, but after puberty it disappears without treatment. This appears to be due to change in amount and kind of fatty acids secreted by the sebaceous glands. Normal bacterial flora of skin and mucous surfaces help to prevent colonisation by pathogens.

We have a **specialized epithelial lining in our respiratory and gastrointestinal tract to minimize infection**. Mucous membrane is composed of specialized epithelial cells which secrete a sticky substance called mucus. This traps dust. In respiratory tract there are also ciliated cells, which move the dust-laden mucus up and out of respiratory tract (**mucociliary escalator**) enabling it to be swallowed or coughed out. When swallowed they are destroyed in the stomach's highly acidic environment and digestive juices. Should a pathogen survive in stomach, it usually cannot penetrate mucous membrane lining the entire gastrointestinal tract and if it escapes the respiratory mucociliary escalator, it would be met by phagocytes lining the alveoli.

The mouth is constantly bathed in **saliva** which has an inhibitory effect on many microorganisms. Nevertheless viruses, bacteria, fungi and protozoa have developed strategies to circumvent these defences. Influenza virions, for example, have haemagglutinins on their surfaces. With the help of these they attach to the receptors on epithelial cells. Influenza virions also possess neuraminidase spikes on their surface. Neuraminidase splits up neuraminic acid of mucus thus helping them to establish contact of haemagglutinins with the receptors on epithelial cells because mucus forms a barrier between epithelial cells and microparasites. Nicotine from cigarettes can paralyse the mucociliary escalator. This exposes cigarette smokers to bacterial infection leading to chronic bronchitis.

Gastrointestinal tract

Four factors protect gastrointestinal tract from infection:

1. **Physical barrier** produced by mucus-secreting epithelial cells.
2. **Secretory IgA antibodies** produced here.
3. **Highly acidic environment** of stomach may hydrolyze microbial invaders.
4. Already established **normal flora** such as *Escherichia coli* serves to inhibit invasion and repopulation by pathogenic microorganisms. However, normal flora is a double-edged weapon. If body resistance is lowered it may lead to opportunistic infections.

Urogenital tract

Kidneys produce sterile urine which travels down the ureter to the bladder and passes out through the urethral opening. Although urethra has normal flora, invading microorganisms usually do not gain access to the bladder. It is mainly due to frequent flushing of urethra by sterile urine. However, if organisms have mechanism to attach to epithelial cells lining the tract even frequent flushing might not evacuate them. Because of short urethra, bladder infection is more common in females than in males.

An interesting relation exists between lactobacilli and *Candida* in vagina. Both normally colonize vagina and keep each other's growth under check. Both are able to use glycogen present in vagina. Lactobacilli produce lactic acid which lowers the pH, thereby inhibiting the growth of *Candida*. On the other hand, *Candida* inhibits growth of lactobacilli by limiting the food supply. Administration of broad-spectrum antibiotics kills lactobacilli releasing *Candida* from growth restraints.

Conjunctiva

Conjunctiva is continually being assaulted by microbe-laden dust. Whenever the dust hits the conjunctiva we blink and tears are produced. Tears mechanically wash away the particles and a hydrolytic enzyme, lysozyme, destroys most viruses and bacteria. However, some microorganisms such as chlamydiae have a special ability to attach to the conjunctival surface. In addition to tears, lysozyme is present in tissue fluids and in nearly all secretions except CSF, sweat and urine.

2. Humoral defence mechanisms

Many microbicidal substances are present in the tissues and body fluids. These are non-specific. There is no specific recognition of the microorganism and the response is not enhanced by re-exposure to the same antigen. They are responsible for innate immunity. Following are the bactericidal substances present in the tissues and body fluids:

Lysozyme

This is a basic protein of low molecular weight (approximately 20,000 daltons) found in high concentrations in polymorphonuclear leucocytes as well as in most tissue fluids except CSF, sweat and urine. It functions as a mucolytic enzyme, splitting sugars of the structural mucopeptide of the cell wall of many Gram-positive bacteria leading to their lysis. It may also play a role in the intracellular destruction of some Gram-negative bacteria.

Basic polypeptides

Several basic proteins, derived from tissues and blood cells, possess antibacterial activity. These include spermine and spermidine which can kill tubercle bacilli and some staphylococci. Other antibacterial substances include arginine and lysine-containing proteins, protamine and histone. Basic polypeptides such as leukins extracted from leucocytes and plakins from platelets have antibacterial effect.

Complement

(See Chapter 12)

Interferons

These are a family of antiviral agents produced by cells stimulated by live or killed viruses and certain other inducers. A number of molecules have been described. α and β interferons are part of innate immunity, and γ interferon is produced by T cells as part of acquired immunity.

3. Cellular defence mechanisms

Microparasites that penetrate the physical barriers are confronted, in addition to humoral defence mechanism, by non-specific cellular defences. Cellular defence against microparasites is provided by **phagocytes** and a subpopulation of lymphocytes known as **natural killer (NK) cells**. Phagocytes are classified into microphages and macrophages. **Microphages** are polymorphonuclear leucocytes and **macrophages** consist of histiocytes which are the wandering amoeboid cells seen in tissues, fixed reticuloendothelial cells and monocytes of blood. In connective tissue they are known as histiocytes, in kidneys as mesangial cells, in bones as osteoclast, in brain as microglial cells, in lungs as alveolar macrophages, in liver as Kupffer cells, and in spleen, lymph nodes and thymus as sinus lining macrophages.

Phagocytic cells reach the site of inflammation in large numbers. They engulf, kill and digest bacteria. On the other hand, viral invasion is countered by NK cells. Residing in the peripheral lymphoid organs, NK cells recognize virus-infected cells, bind to them and subsequently lyse them. NK cells have also been implicated in host defence against cancers. They are thought to recognize the changes in the cell membranes of transformed cells in a mechanism similar to that used to combat virus infection. Fungi are confronted by polymorphonuclear leucocytes, macrophages and NK cells.

Phagocytic cell engulfs microparasite by extending pseudopodia around it. These fuse and microorganism is internalized into a vacuole (**phagosome**) which fuses with lysosomes found in the cell to form **phagolysosome** (Fig. 9.1). Microparasites are subjected to the lytic enzymes in the phagolysosome and are destroyed. The macrophages present in the walls of capillaries and vascular tissues in spleen, liver, lungs and bone marrow serve a very important role in clearing the blood stream of foreign particulate material such as bacteria. Some microorganisms such as **mycobacteria and brucellae resist intracellular digestion and may actively multiply inside the phagocyte**. Phagocytosis in such instances may help to disseminate infection to different parts of the body. However, these organisms can be digested by activated macrophages.

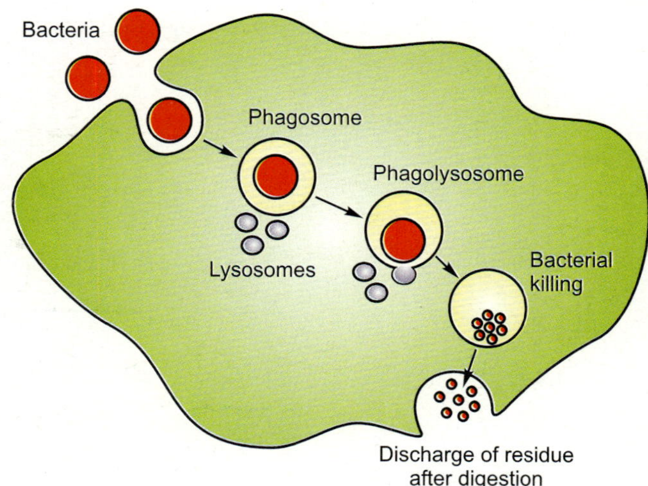

Fig. 9.1. Events of phagocytosis.

Eosinophils are polymorphonuclear leucocytes with cytoplasmic granules and bilobed nucleus. Their number in the blood of normal individuals is 3–5%. But **in patients with parasitic infections and allergies their number increases**. They are not efficient phagocytic cells. However, their granules possess molecules that are toxic to parasites. Large parasites such as helminths cannot be internalized. Therefore, they must be killed extracellularly. Eosinophils possess Fc receptors (that bind to the Fc fragment of different classes and subclasses of immunoglobulins) and complement receptors that bind the antibody and complement coated parasites. The granule contents of the eosinophils are then released into the space between the cell and the parasite. Eosinophil granules contain enzymes and toxic molecules that are active against helminths.

4. Fever

A rise in temperature following infection is a natural defence mechanism. It inhibits or kills the infecting organisms. Before penicillin era, therapeutic induction of fever was employed for destruction of *Treponema pallidum* in patients suffering from syphilis. Fever also stimulates production of interferon and helps in recovery from virus infection.

5. Inflammation

It is the cellular and vascular response to injury such as invasion by an infectious agent, exposure to a noxious chemical or physical trauma. The signs of inflammation are redness, swelling, heat, pain and disturbed or altered functions. Inflammation leads to vasodilation, increased vascular permeability and cellular infiltration. **Polymorphonuclear leucocytes** escape into the tissues by diapedesis and accumulate in large numbers attracted by the chemotactic substances released at the site of injury. They then phagocytose microorganisms and their products. Because of increased vascular permeability, there is an **outpouring of plasma** which helps to dilute the toxic products present. In addition, plasma contains a number of non-specific (complement, properdin, beta lysin, leukins and plakins) and specific (antibodies) inhibitors.

Q. 5. Define and classify acquired immunity.

Ans. The resistance that an individual acquires during his life-time is known as acquired immunity. It is antigen-specific and may be antibody-mediated or cell-mediated. It is of two types – active immunity and passive immunity (Table 9.1 and Fig. 9.2).

Both active and passive immunity may be further divided into natural and artificial.

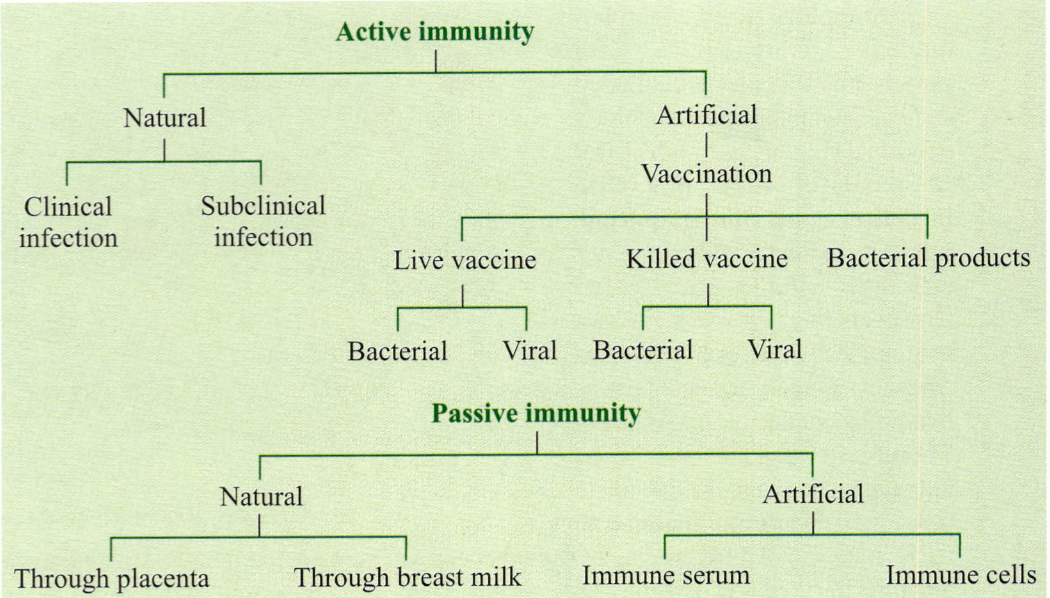

Fig. 9.2. Types of immunity.

Q. 6. Tabulate differences between active and passive immunity.

Ans. Differences between active and passive immunity are given in Table 9.1.

Table 9.1. Differences between active and passive immunity

Active immunity	Passive immunity
• Produced actively by host's immune system as a result of antigenic stimulation.	• Received passively by the host. No participation of host's immune system.
• Induced by infection or by contact with antigens.	• Conferred by administration of antibodies.
• Long lasting.	• Transient.
• Immunity effective only after a lag period, i.e., time required for generation of antibodies and immunocompetent cells.	• Immunity effective immediately.
• During development of active immunity there is often a negative phase during which the level of measurable immunity may actually be lower than before antigenic stimulus. This is due to antigen combining with the pre-existing antibodies and lowering its level.	• No negative phase.
• Immunological memory present, therefore, subsequent challenge (secondary response) is more effective.	• No immunological memory. Subsequent administration of antibodies is less effective due to immune elimination.
• More effective and confers better protection.	• Less effective and provides inferior immunity.
• Not applicable in immunodeficient individuals.	• Applicable in immunodeficient individuals.

Q. 7. What is meant by active immunity? Briefly describe natural active and artificial active immunity.

Ans. Active immunity

This involves the active involvement of the person's own immune apparatus leading to the synthesis of antibodies and/or the production of immunocompetent cells (ICCs). It appears only after a **lag (latent) period**, i.e., the time required for generation of antibodies and ICCs. During development of active immunity there is often a negative phase during which the level of measurable immunity may actually be lower than before antigenic stimulus. This is due to antigen combining with pre-existing antibodies and lowering its level.

If an individual who has been actively immunized against an antigen, experiences the same antigen subsequently, the immune response occurs more quickly and more abundantly than during the first encounter. This is known as **secondary response**.

Immune system is able to retain the memory of a prior antigenic exposure for long periods and produces a secondary type response when encountered with the same antigen. This is known as **immunological memory**.

Natural active immunity

Natural active immunity results either from a subclinical or clinical infection. A large majority of adults in the developing countries possess natural active immunity to poliomyelitis due to repeated subclinical infections with poliovirus during childhood. Some infections like diphtheria, whooping cough, measles and mumps induce long-lasting immunity. Others such as common cold and influenza confer immunity which lasts for a short time.

- In case of influenza, short-lived immunity is due to the ability of influenza virus to undergo antigenic variation, so that immunity following first infection is not effective against second infection due to an antigenically different virus.
- In common cold the apparent lack of immunity is because the same clinical picture can be produced by infection with a large number of different viruses. In general, immunity following bacterial infections is generally less permanent than that following viral infections.
- In some infections like syphilis and malaria, immunity lasts only till original infection remains active. This is known as **concomitant immunity** (previously called **premunition** or **infection-immunity**). Once the disease is cured the patient becomes susceptible again. In chancroid, caused by *Haemophilus ducreyi*, there does not appear to be any effective immunity as the patient may develop lesions following reinfection even while the original infection is active.

Artificial active immunity

This is the resistance induced by vaccines which are preparations of live or killed microorganisms or their products.

Q. 8. Write short note on vaccines.

Ans. Bacterial and viral vaccines are as follows:

Bacterial vaccines

1. *Live:*
   - B.C.G. for tuberculosis
   - Ty 21a for typhoid
2. *Killed:*
   - TAB for enteric fever.
   - Cholera
   - Pertussis
3. *Bacterial products*
   - Tetanus toxoid
   - Diphtheria toxoid
   - Capsular polysaccharide of meningococci
   - Capsular polysaccharide of *Haemophilus influenzae* type b

Viral vaccines

1. *Live:*
   - Sabin vaccine for poliomyelitis or oral polio vaccine (OPV)
   - 17D vaccine for yellow fever
   - MMR vaccine for measles, mumps, rubella
   - Varicella-zoster
2. *Killed:*
   - Salk vaccine for poliomyelitis
   - Neural and non-neural vaccines for rabies
   - Influenza
   - Hepatitis A
   - Hepatitis B
   - Japanese encephalitis

DPT (diphtheria, pertussis, tetanus), DT (diphtheria, tetanus), TT (tetanus toxoid) and typhoid vaccines, and also diluents need to be stored in the refrigerator part having a temperature of 4–10°C. These vaccines should never be allowed to freeze. OPV, MMR and rabies vaccines, which are highly heat labile need to be stored in the freezer compartment having a temperature of 0°C. Storing OPV in deep freezer with a temperature of –20°C enhances the life of the vaccine from 3 months to 1 year.

Live vaccines initiate a sort of mini infection without causing disease. The immunity following vaccination, therefore, parallels that following natural infection. However, it is of lower order than that induced by infection. Since live vaccines undergo limited multiplication in the body, therefore, number of organisms required in a dose is less; single doses may be sufficient and they are relatively cheaper. Live vaccines may be administered orally (e.g., Sabin vaccine for poliomyelitis). They provide more effective and more lasting immunity than killed vaccines. Some of them can be given as combined vaccines, e.g., measles, mumps, rubella (MMR) vaccine.

Killed vaccines have the advantage of stability and safety. These can be given in combination in polyvalent vaccines, e.g., diphtheria, pertussis, tetanus (DPT) vaccine. These are generally less immunogenic than live vaccines and protection lasts only for a short period.

Therefore, they have to be administered repeatedly. At least two doses are required. First dose is known as **primary** and subsequent doses as **booster doses**. In killed vaccines since the organisms are killed, therefore, larger number of these are required in each dose. Oral route for killed vaccines is generally not effective. Antibody response to killed vaccines is improved by addition of adjuvants, for example, aluminium phosphate adjuvant vaccine for cholera.

Q. 9. What is passive immunity? Briefly describe natural passive and artificial passive immunity. Enumerate indications of passive immunization.

Ans. Passive immunity

The immunity that is transferred to a recipient in a ready-made form is known as passive immunity. Here the recipient's immune system plays no active role. There is no lag or latent period, the immunity is effective immediately after passive immunization. There is no negative phase. It confers only transient immunity lasting usually for days or weeks till the antibodies are metabolized and eliminated. There is no secondary type response. Rather subsequent administration of antibodies is less effective due to **immune elimination**.

Following first injection of antibody, its elimination is only by metabolic breakdown but during subsequent injections its elimination is much quicker because metabolic breakdown is combined with immune elimination as it combines with antibodies to horse serum that would have been produced following first injection. This happens when horse (foreign) serum is used. Immune elimination is not a problem when human serum is used. Because of its immediate action it is employed where instant immunity is required as in case of protection against tetanus, gas gangrene and diphtheria following exposure.

Natural passive immunity

This is the resistance transferred from mother to foetus through placenta. IgG antibodies can cross placental barrier to reach the foetus. After birth, immunoglobulins are passed to the newborn through the breast milk. Human colostrum is rich in IgA antibodies which are resistant to digestion in stomach and small intestine, hence confers immunity in the neonate up to three months of age. Human foetus acquires some ability to synthesize IgM antibodies from twentieth week of gestation, but its immunological capacity is still inadequate at birth. It is only by the age of three months that the infant acquires a satisfactory level of immunological independence. Until then, maternal antibodies give passive protection against infectious diseases of the infant.

Transport of antibodies across placenta is an active process, therefore, the concentration of antibodies in foetal blood may sometimes be higher than that seen in the mother. These antibodies are generally against all common infectious diseases in the locality. Therefore, most paediatric infections are commoner after the age of three months when maternal immunoglobulins disappear. By active immunization of mother during pregnancy the immune status of the neonate can be improved. Therefore, immunization of pregnant women with tetanus toxoid is recommended in countries where neonatal tetanus is common.

Artificial passive immunity

This is the immunity transferred passively to the recipient by administration of antibodies. This is done by administration of hyperimmune sera of man or animals. For example, tetanus antitoxin is prepared in horses by active immunization of horses with tetanus toxoid, bleeding them and separating the serum. Similarly, diphtheria antitoxin and gas gangrene antitoxin are also prepared. However, since these antitoxins are foreign proteins and are liable to cause serious or even fatal hypersensitivity reactions, these should be administered only after testing for hypersensitivity. After first administration, it is removed by metabolism and following subsequent injections by metabolism and immune elimination. Therefore, immunity conferred is short-lived.

Sera collected from patients convalescing from infectious diseases contain high levels of specific antibodies. Convalescent sera have, therefore, been employed for passive immunization against viral infections such as measles and rubella. Sera of healthy adults contain antibodies against infectious agents prevalent in a community. Therefore, sera from a large number of individuals can be collected and used for passive immunization. Placenta provides a convenient source of human immunoglobulins. Human immune serum does not lead to any hypersensitivity reaction, there is no immune elimination and its half-life is more than that of animal sera. However, with human serum there is a grave risk of transmission of human immunodeficiency virus and hepatitis B, C and D viruses.

Indications of passive immunization

- To provide immediate protection to a non-immune individual exposed to an infection, when there is insufficient time for active immunization, e.g., administration of tetanus antitoxin and gas gangrene antitoxin to a non-immune individual with crushing road-side injury, and administration of diphtheria antitoxin to a non-immune child exposed to diphtheria.
- Administration of anti-Rh(D) IgG to Rh-negative mother, bearing Rh-positive baby at the time of delivery to prevent Rh isoimmunization.
- For suppression of active immunity, when it is injurious, for example, administration of antilymphocytic serum for suppression of lymphocytes in transplantation surgery to suppress the immune response towards the transplant.

Q. 10. Write a short note on combined active and passive immunization.

Ans. A person exposed to tetanus may be injected tetanus antitoxin on one arm and tetanus toxoid on the other with separate syringes followed by full course of tetanus toxoid. Diphtheria antitoxin and diphtheria toxoid can also be practised similarly. This is known as combined active and passive immunization.

Q. 11. Write short note on adoptive immunity.

Ans. Injection of immunologically competent lymphocytes is known as adoptive immunity. Instead of whole lymphocytes, an extract of immunologically competent lymphocytes known as transfer factor can be used. This has been attempted in the treatment of lepromatous leprosy.

Q. 12. Describe briefly local immunity.

Ans. This means immunity at a particular site, generally the site of invasion and multiplication of pathogen. For example, in case of poliomyelitis, parenteral vaccine provides systemic immunity. The antibodies neutralize virus only after blood invasion. It does not prevent multiplication of the virus at the site of entry, the gut mucosa, and its faecal excretion. However, when live oral vaccine is given it leads to local immunity. Similarly, live influenza vaccine administered intranasally provides local immunity while killed influenza vaccine evokes humoral antibody response. Local immunity is conferred by secretory IgA antibodies produced locally by plasma cells present on mucosal surfaces or in secretory glands.

Q. 13. Write short note on herd immunity.

Ans. Overall level of immunity in a community is known as herd immunity. When a large number of individuals in a community (herd) are immune to a pathogen the herd immunity to a pathogen is said to be satisfactory. When herd immunity is low, epidemics are likely to occur on the introduction of the pathogen. This is due to the fact that a larger number of individuals are susceptible.

10

Antigens

Q. 1. Explain what are antigens.

Ans. Antigens (*anti*body *gen*erators) are substances that can stimulate an immune response and, given the opportunity, react specifically by binding with the effector molecules (antibodies) and effector cells (lymphocytes) produced. Most antigens are proteins, but some are carbohydrates, lipids or nucleic acids. Some antigens are more immunogenic or capable of eliciting an immune response, than others. Some antigens such as proteins may possess a number of small chemical groups that are called antigenic determinants or **epitopes** which can bind specifically to antigen binding site (**paratope**) of the antibody molecule (Fig. 10.1) and T cell receptors. Each determinant can stimulate the formation of a particular kind of antibody or effector cell. Thus a pure protein antigen may give rise to many distinct antibodies and effector cells. The size of epitope is around 25–35 Å and a molecular weight of 400–1000.

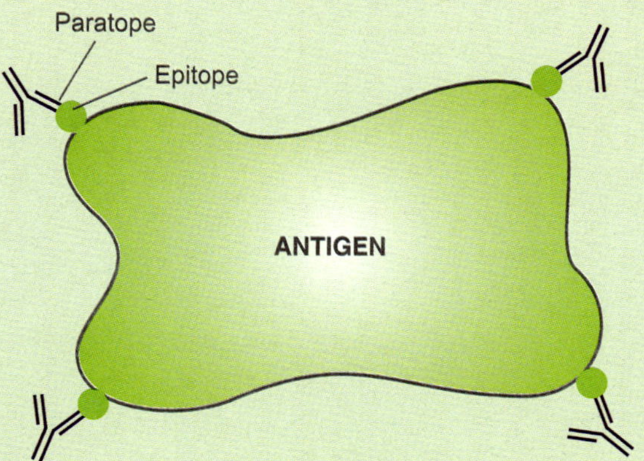

Fig. 10.1. Epitopes of antigen and paratopes of antibody.

Q. 2. Write short note on hapten.

Ans. This is a chemical substance of low molecular weight that cannot induce an immune response by itself. Nevertheless, haptens can induce a response if combined with larger molecules (normally proteins) which serve as carriers. This response requires assistance from T helper (Th) lymphocytes. In contrast to complete antigens, haptens contain a single epitope. In response to hapten carried on carrier particle, antibodies are produced not only against the hapten but also against the carrier particle. Haptens are of two types:

1. Complex haptens

These can combine with specific antibodies to form precipitate, e.g., capsular polysaccharide of pneumococci.

2. Simple haptens

These combine with specific antibodies but no precipitate is formed (non-precipitating). This is due to univalent character of simple hapten, whereas complex haptens are polyvalent, since it is assumed that precipitation requires the antigens to have two or more antibody combining sites.

Q. 3. Enumerate and briefly describe determinants of antigenicity.

Ans. Following are determinants of antigenicity:

1. Size

Antigenicity depends upon the molecular weight. Generally, molecules with a molecular weight less than 5,000 are nonantigenic or feebly so. Low molecular weight substances may be rendered antigenic by absorbing them on large inert particles such as bentonite or kaolin. Some low molecular weight substances such as picryl chloride and penicillin may be antigenic when applied on the skin, probably by combining with tissue proteins.

2. Foreignness

Only antigens which are foreign to the individual (non-self) induce an immune response because host distinguishes self from non-self and normally does not respond to self. The healthy body is immunologically tolerant to nearly all self antigens, that would be immunogenic in a foreign host. However, under certain circumstances tolerance may be broken leading to **autoimmunity**. *Antigenicity of a substance is related to the degree of its foreignness*. Antigens from other individuals of the same species are less antigenic than those from other species.

3. Chemical nature

Proteins and polysaccharides are most antigenic. Lipids and nucleic acids are less antigenic. Their antigenicity is enhanced by combination with proteins. However, all proteins are not antigenic. A well-known exception is gelatin. The presence of an aromatic radical appears to be essential for antigenicity and the absence of aromatic amino acids such as tyrosine in gelatin is responsible for its nonantigenicity.

4. Susceptibility to tissue enzymes

Only those substances which can be metabolized and are susceptible to the action of tissue enzymes behave as antigens. Antigens introduced into the body are degraded by the host into the fragments of appropriate size containing antigenic determinants. Phagocytosis and intracellular enzymes appear to play an essential role in breaking down antigens into immunogenic fragments. Substances insusceptible to tissue enzymes such as polystyrene latex and synthetic polypeptides which are not metabolized in the body, are not antigenic.

Q. 4. What are heterophile antigens? Describe briefly tests based on the principle of heterophile antigens.

Ans. Same or closely related antigens occurring in different biological species, classes and kingdoms are known as heterogenetic or heterophile antigens. The best example of such heterophile antigens is the **Forssman antigen** which is a lipid carbohydrate complex widely distributed in man, animals, birds, plants and bacteria. It is absent in rabbits, therefore, anti-Forssman antibody can be prepared in these animals. Examples of tests based on the principle of heterophile antigens used in diagnostic serology are as under:

1. Weil-Felix reaction

It is an agglutination test in which patient sera are tested for agglutinins to O antigens of non-motile strains of *Proteus* OX2, OX19 and OXK. Cross reaction between O antigen of these strains of *Proteus* and certain rickettsial antigens is the basis of this test.

2. Paul-Bunnell test

In patients with infectious mononucleosis heterophile antibodies appear in the serum of the patient. These antibodies agglutinate sheep erythrocytes. This test is known as Paul-Bunnell test.

3. Cold agglutinin test

Agglutination of human O group erythrocytes at 4°C by the sera of patients suffering from primary atypical pneumonia.

4. Agglutination of Streptococcus MG

Agglutination of *Streptococcus* MG by the sera of the patients of primary atypical pneumonia.

Q. 5. Write short note on tolerogens.

Ans. Antigens do not always exhibit immunogenicity or evoke antibody formation. In some instances an antigen presented at one concentration might induce specific immunological unresponsiveness or tolerance, while at another concentration it might promote immunity. **An antigen that induces tolerance is referred to as tolerogen.** One important manifestation of tolerance occurs during foetal development. Therefore, an individual's immune system does not normally react against self antigens. Burnet suggested that during foetal life a large number of lymphocytes capable of reacting with different antigens are formed. But cells with immunological reactivity with self antigens are eliminated. This process is known as **clonal deletion**. Their persistence or development in later life leads to **autoimmunity**.

Q. 6. What are superantigens? List various superantigens.

Ans. Superantigens is a class of molecules that can interact with antigen-presenting cells (APCs) and T cells in non-specific manner. This activity does not involve the endocytic processing required for typical antigen presentation but instead occurs by concurrent association with MHC class II molecules of the APCs and the Vβ domain of the T cell receptor (Fig. 10.2). This interaction activates a large number of T cells (10%) than conventional antigens (about 1%), explaining the massive cytokine expression and immunomodulation. Various superantigens include:

- Staphylococcal enterotoxins,
- Staphylococcal toxic shock syndrome toxin,
- Staphylococcal exfoliative toxin,
- Streptococcal pyrogenic exotoxin, and
- Some viral proteins.

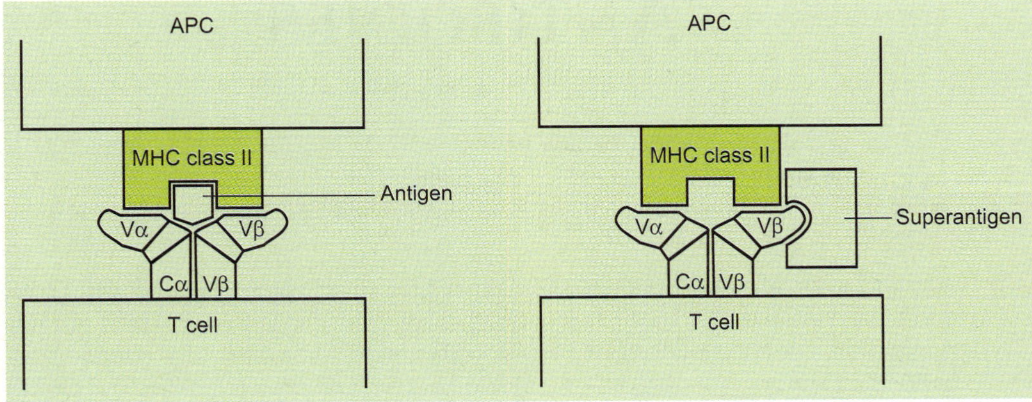

Fig. 10.2. Binding of antigen and superantigen by MHC and T cell receptor.

11

ANTIBODIES

Q. 1. What are antibodies? Name various classes of antibody and describe antibody structure with illustration.

Ans. Antibodies or immunoglobulins (Igs) are γ globulins which are produced in response to antigenic stimulation. These react specifically with the antigens which stimulated their production. Igs are produced by plasma cells and to some extent by lymphocytes also. All antibodies are Igs, but all Igs (e.g., myeloma proteins) are not antibodies. On the basis of physicochemical and antigenic structure Igs can be divided into five distinct classes or isotypes namely IgG, IgA, IgM, IgD and IgE. They differ from each other in size, charge, carbohydrate content and amino acid composition. Within certain classes there are subclasses that show slight differences in structure and function from other members of the class. If injected into animals they induce the formation of antibodies that can be used to differentiate between the different isotypes serologically.

The first antibodies produced following infection (primary response) are immunoglobulins of the IgM class, becoming detectable about 1 week after infection and persisting for about 6 weeks. About 2 weeks after infection, IgG antibody is produced and is long-lasting. IgG antibody is the main antibody formed in a secondary response.

Antibody structure

IgG has been studied extensively and serves as a model of basic structural unit of all Igs. It is a Y-shaped four polypeptide chain molecule. Of the four chains, two each are light (L) and heavy (H). These are held together by disulphide bonds (Fig. 11.1). L chain has a molecular weight of 25,000 daltons and H chain 50,000 daltons. H chains are structurally and antigenically distinct for each class and are designated with Greek letters α (alpha), δ (delta), ε (epsilon), γ (gamma) and μ (mu) in IgA, IgD, IgE, IgG and IgM respectively. L chains are of two types – κ (kappa) and λ (lambda). A molecule of Ig may have either κ or λ chains but never both together. κ and λ chains occur in a ratio of about 2 : 1 in human serum.

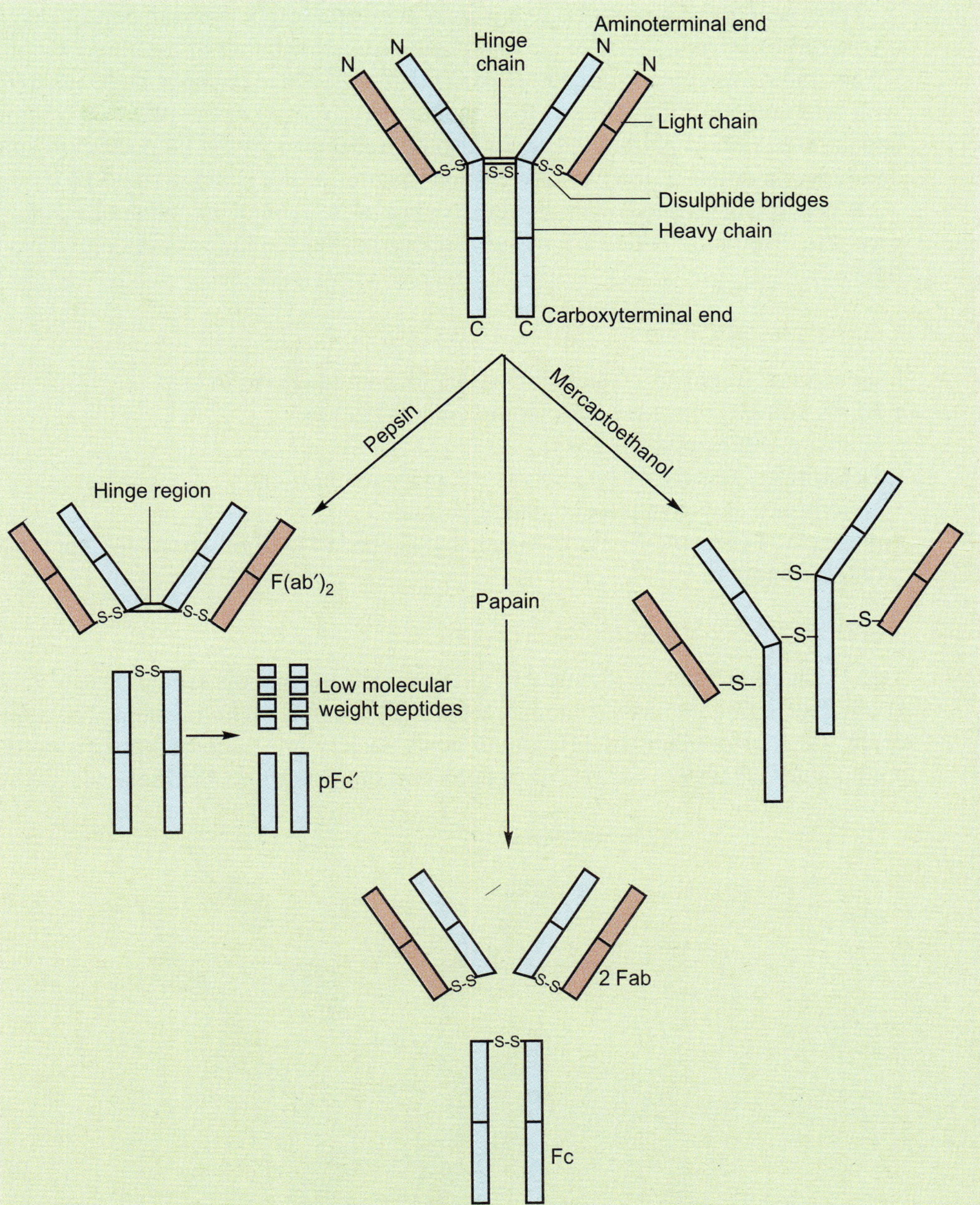

Fig. 11.1. Basic immunoglobulin structure.

IgG when treated with proteolytic enzyme papain in the presence of cysteine cleaves it into three fragments. Two identical fragments (45,000 daltons each) still possess the antigen-binding sites and are thus named **fragment antigen binding (Fab)**. These two fragments represent bivalency of IgG molecule. The third fragment (50,000 daltons) which lacks the ability to bind to antigen can be crystallized. It is, therefore, known as **fragment crystallizable (Fc)**.

Treatment of the IgG antibody molecule with proteolytic enzyme pepsin cleaves H chains on the carboxyterminal side of the interchain disulphide bonds of the hinge region. Therefore, 2 Fab fragments remain united (100,000 daltons). This fragment is designated as **F(ab′)$_2$** with two antigen-binding sites. It is about 10% larger than the two Fab fragments from a papain digestion of antibody. Pepsin also degrades part of the Fc portion to small peptides and leaves a dimer of the carboxyterminal quarter of the chain, termed **pFc′**.

When IgG is treated with reducing agent such as mercaptoethanol in the presence of urea, the disulphide bonds are reduced releasing four peptide chains – two heavy and two light.

Q. 2. Enumerate functions of fragment crystallizable (Fc) of immunoglobulin.

Ans. Functions of fragment crystallizable (Fc) of immunoglobulin are:

- Binds complement leading to complement fixation.
- Binds to cell receptors (FcRs).
- Determines passage of IgG across the placental barrier.
- Determines skin fixation and catabolic rate.
- Antigenic determinants that distinguish one class of antibody from another are also located on Fc fragment.

Q. 3. Describe briefly immunoglobulin domains.

Ans. Two H chains are always identical in a given molecule and the same is true of L chains. Each H chain of IgG contains 440 amino acids while each L chain contains 220 amino acids. H chain has four domains of 110 amino acids each, while L chain has two domains of 110 amino acids each (Fig. 11.2). The antigen combining sites of the molecule are at its amino-

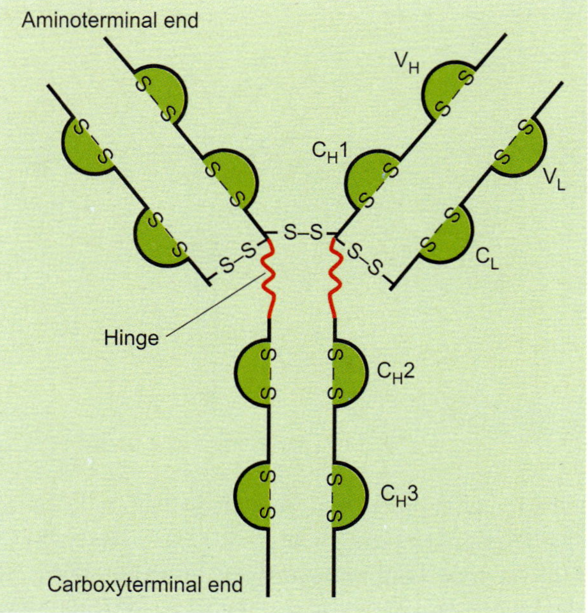

Fig. 11.2. Variable and constant domains of immunoglobulin molecule.

terminal end. These are composed of both H and L chains. Of the 220 amino acids, those that constitute carboxyterminal half of L chain occur in a constant sequence. This part of the chain is called **constant region** (C_L). Only two sequence patterns are seen in constant region of κ and λ chains. On the other hand, amino acid sequence in aminoterminal half of the L chain is highly variable; the variability determines the immunological specificity of the antibody molecule. It is, therefore, called **variable region** (V_L).

A similar pattern is seen in H chains. The variable region of H chain, however, is only 25% as long as constant region. The variable region of H chain like that of L chain has highly variable sequence of amino acids and is known as V_H. The constant region of H chain is divided into three portions C_H1, C_H2 and C_H3. The infinite range of specificity of Igs depends upon the variability of amino acid sequences at the variable regions of H and L chains which form antigen combining sites.

Q. 4. Write short note on Fd piece of immunoglobulins.

Ans. Fd piece is the portion of H chains present in Fab fragment. H chains carry a carbohydrate moiety which is distinct for each class of immunoglobulins. Each Ig peptide chain has internal disulphide links in addition to interchain disulphide bonds which bridge H and L chains. These intrachain disulphide bonds form loops in the peptide chain and each of the loops is completely folded to form a globular domain and each domain has its separate function. Variable region domains V_L and V_H are responsible for the formation of a specific antigen-binding site. C_H2 region in IgG binds C1q in the classical complement sequence and C_H3 domain mediates adherence to monocyte surface. The area of H chain in the C region between C_H1 and C_H2 is the **hinge region**. It is more flexible and is more exposed to enzymes and chemicals.

Q. 5. Describe briefly immunoglobulin G, its subclasses, catabolism and immunological activities.

Ans. This is the most abundant class of Ig in the body constituting approximately 75% of the total Igs. This is distributed equally within the intravascular and extravascular pools. Very little IgG is produced during the early stages of the primary response to antigen, but it is the major form of antibody produced during the secondary response. It is not synthesized by the foetus in any significant amount. IgG is also most commonly seen **myeloma protein**. It has a half-life of 21 days. The normal serum concentration of IgG is about 12 mg/ml. It is a glycoprotein with a molecular weight of 150,000 daltons.

There are **four subclasses** of human IgG (IgG1, IgG2, IgG3 and IgG4). Each subclass possesses a distinct type of γ chain which can be identified with specific antiserum. They constitute about 59%, 30%, 8% and 3% respectively of the total human IgG. All normal humans possess all four subclasses of IgG, just as they possess all classes of Igs. IgG binds complement in classical pathway. IgG3 is most effective in binding complement followed by IgG1 and IgG2. It can bind to protein A (from *Staphylococcus aureus*) and protein G (from group G streptococci). *IgG is the only class of Igs that can cross the placenta and is responsible for the protection of the infant during first few months of life. However, subclass IgG2 does not cross the placenta.* IgG is also found, along with IgA, in milk during the first few weeks after birth, providing additional protection if the infant is breast-fed.

Macrophages and monocytes bear Fc receptors (FcRs) which bind to the Fc portion of IgG1 and IgG3 in C_H3 domain. Such binding permits these cells to exhibit antibody-dependent cellular toxicity. IgG usually exhibits high affinity for antigens leading to efficient neutralization of toxins. Among null cells, a distinct subpopulation of cytotoxic cells has been recognized which also possesses FcRs for Fc part of IgG. They are capable of lysing or killing target cells sensitized with IgG. They are known as **killer cells**. They are responsible for **antibody-dependent cell-mediated cytotoxicity (ADCC)**. Platelets also possess FcRs for Fc portion of IgG leading to aggregation, degranulation and release of histamine. IgG is the only Ig which has the property of fixing to guinea-pig skin.

Catabolism of IgG is unique in that it varies with its serum concentration. When its level is raised, as in chronic malaria, kala-azar or myeloma, the IgG synthesized against a particular antigen will be catabolised rapidly and may result in the particular antibody deficiency. Conversely, in hypogammaglobulinaemia, the IgG given for treatment will be catabolised slowly.

IgG participates in most immunological reactions such as complement fixation, precipitation and neutralization of toxins and viruses. Passively administered IgG suppresses the homologous antibody synthesis by a feedback process. This property is utilized for prevention of isoimmunization of Rh-negative mother bearing Rh-positive baby by administration of anti-Rh (D) IgG at the time of delivery.

Q. 6. Describe briefly structure and biological activities of immunoglobulin M.

Ans. It is so named because it is a macroglobulin at least five times larger than IgG. It is a glycoprotein with molecular weight of 900,000–1,000,000 daltons (millionaire molecule). It is present on the surface of virtually all uncommitted B cells. About 10% of normal serum Igs consist of this class. The normal serum level of IgM is 1.2 mg/ml. It has a half-life of about 5 days. IgM normally exists as a pentamer, consisting of 5 Ig subunits (Fig. 11.3).

In contrast to IgG, IgM remains almost exclusively in the serum and is not usually found extravascularly in body cavities or secretions. Therefore, IgM is believed to be responsible for protection against blood invasion by microorganisms. Pentameric IgM is apparently too large to cross the placenta. The Hμ chain has four C_H domains rather than three as seen in H chains of IgG. H chains are held together by disulphide bonds. There is an additional peptide chain called the **joining (J) chain**. The J chain may be largely responsible for the polymerization process, which occurs shortly before the molecule is secreted by plasma cell.

IgM contains 10 Fab fragments, and thus 10 antigen-binding sites. Therefore, theoretically it can bind to 10 antigen molecules. However, it appears that many antigens are so large that when bound to one site, they physically prevent the binding of another antigen molecule to an adjacent binding site. Thus, generally, IgM is capable of binding as few as five molecules of antigen.

Phylogenetically IgM is the oldest Ig class. It is usually the first antibody to appear following stimulation by an antigen. However, IgM synthesis is usually not prolonged, and IgG antibodies soon become the most prevalent class. IgM is also the earliest to be synthesized by foetus beginning by about **20 weeks of gestation**. As it cannot cross the placental barrier, the presence of IgM in the foetus or newborn indicates intrauterine

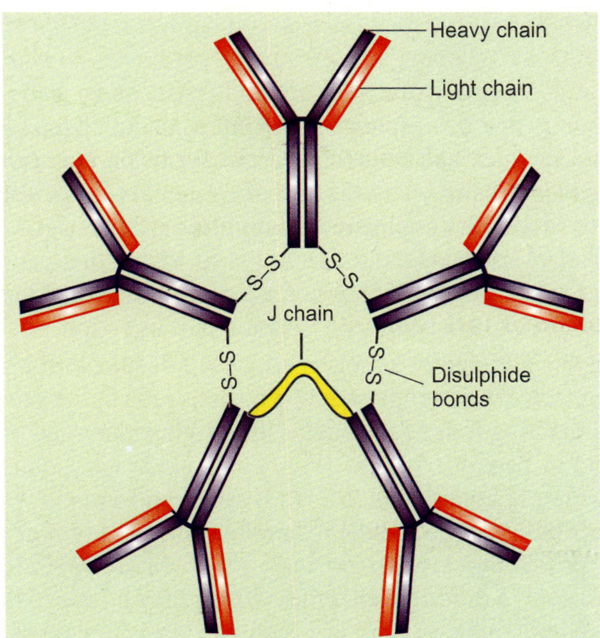

Fig. 11.3. IgM immunoglobulin.

infection. Its detection is, therefore, useful for the diagnosis of congenital syphilis, rubella, HIV infection and toxoplasmosis. IgM antibodies are relatively short-lived, hence their demonstration in the serum indicates recent infection. Treatment of serum with 0.12 M 2-mercaptoethanol selectively destroys IgM without affecting IgG antibodies. This provides a simple method for differential estimation of IgG and IgM antibodies.

IgM is much more efficient than IgG in its ability to fix complement, promoting lysis and death of most Gram-negative bacteria. This greater efficacy is due to the fact that complement may bind to several Fc regions of pentameric IgM simultaneously thus initiating complement cascade and target cell lysis with a single molecule.

Isohaemagglutinins (anti-A and anti-B), and antibodies to *Salmonella* Typhi O antigen and Wassermann reaction antibodies in syphilis are usually IgM. In certain disease states such as lupus erythematosus and rheumatoid arthritis, IgM may occur in monomeric form in high concentration. Monomeric IgM has lower avidity for antigen than does the pentameric form. A single molecule of IgM can bring about haemolysis, whereas 1000 IgG molecules are required for the same effect. IgM is also more effective than IgG in opsonization, bactericidal action and in bacterial agglutination. However, in neutralization of toxins and viruses, it is less active than IgG.

Q. 7. Describe briefly structure and biological activities of immunoglobulin A.

Ans. The basic structure of IgA is similar to that of IgG. It contains two identical light chains (either κ or λ) and two heavy α chains. It is the second most abundant class, constituting about 15% of human serum Igs where it exists as a monomeric Ig. More important form is the dimeric form, known as **secretory IgA (sIgA)**. It is the predominant class of Igs in secretions such as milk, tears, nasal secretions, saliva, perspiration, genitourinary secretions and seromucous secretions.

On mucus surfaces sIgA form an antibody paste and is believed to play an important role in local immunity against respiratory and intestinal pathogens. sIgA is relatively resistant to the digestive enzymes and reducing agents. Many infectious organisms cause disease by attaching to glycoproteins on the surface of epithelial cells of secretory gland. If this adhesion is sufficiently strong, the organism will divide, establish a colony and cause disease by any of a number of mechanisms, e.g., secretion of toxins that cause local and systemic injury. Secretory IgA when present in the secretions prevents attachment of organisms to epithelial cells thus preventing adhesion, colonization and infection.

Serum IgA is principally a monomeric 7S molecule with a molecular weight of 160,000 daltons. Secretory IgA is synthesized by plasma cells in the subepithelial tissue and secreted as a dimer containing four heavy chains, four light chains and one J chain which is similar to J chain found in pentameric IgM (Fig. 11.4). sIgA also possesses an additional structural unit called secretory component (SC). It is synthesized not in lymphoid cells but in epithelial cells of glands of intestine, and the respiratory tract and is attached to IgA molecules at their Fc portions producing 11S dimer with a molecular weight of 385,000 daltons. sIgA is relatively resistant to digestive enzymes, which may be due to the secretory component. IgA does not fix complement in classical pathway but can activate the alternative complement pathway. It promotes phagocytosis and intracellular killing of microorganisms.

There are two subclasses of IgA in humans – IgA1 and IgA2. In serum, IgA1 constitutes 80% to 90% of IgA while sIgA consists of about equal amounts of the two subclasses.

Certain streptococci and pathogenic *Neisseria* produce proteases that specifically cleave the heavy chain of IgA1. IgA2 is resistant to such cleavage because it has a shorter hinge region and lacks the proline-rich site cleaved by the proteases.

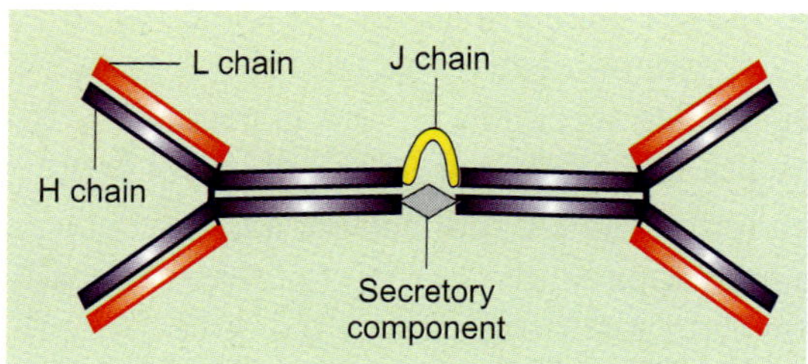

Fig. 11.4. Secretory IgA.

Q. 8. Describe briefly structure and biological activities of immunoglobulin D.

Ans. Like other monomeric antibodies IgD is composed of two light and two heavy chains. The latter are designated as δ chains. It contains about 13% carbohydrate. Its molecular weight is 180,000 daltons. It does not bind complement. It does not cross placenta and does not bind to cells via Fc region. IgD is present on the surface of B lymphocytes which are destined to differentiate into antibody-producing plasma cells and its serum concentration is very low (0.03 mg/ml). Reaction of antigen with surface immunoglobulin may lead to cell differentiation and antibody synthesis.

Q. 9. Write short note on immunoglobulin E.

Ans. Immunoglobulin E resembles IgG structurally. Its molecular weight is 190,000 daltons. Its half-life is about two days. It does not fix complement or cross placental barrier. In contrast to other Igs it is heat-labile and gets inactivated by heating it at 56°C for 30 minutes. It is susceptible to 2-mercaptoethanol. It is chiefly produced in the linings of the respiratory and intestinal tracts. It is present in extremely low concentrations (0.00004 mg/ml) in the serum. But raised serum levels are seen in atopic (type I hypersensitivity) conditions like asthma and hay fever.

Most of a person's IgE is fixed to the surface of mast cells and basophils and when a specific antigen binds with IgE bound to mast cell or basophil membrane, the reaction results in the release of pharmacologically active substances such as histamine and serotonin which dilate capillaries, increase vascular permeability and cause bronchial constriction. Fc portion of IgE binds to the Fc receptors present on the surface of mast cells and basophils leaving antigen-binding sites free to react with specific antigen.

So far, no beneficial effect of IgE has been identified. It has been observed that IgE levels may rise following infections with parasites especially helminths. It has been suggested that mast cell-bound IgE reacts with antigens on the parasite followed by release of histamine. This results in increased vascular permeability followed by influx of plasma and cells (particularly eosinophils) and destruction of parasite. IgE mediates Prausnitz-Kustner reaction.

Q. 10. Tabulate properties of various immunoglobulin classes.

Ans.

Table 11.1. Properties of various immunoglobulin classes

	IgG	IgA	IgM	IgD	IgE
1. Molecular weight in kDa	150	160,385*	900–1,000	180	190
2. Sedimentation coefficient	7	7, 11	19	7	8
3. Carbohydrate content (%)	3	8	12	13	12
4. Heavy chain	$\gamma_1, \gamma_2, \gamma_3, \gamma_4$	α_1, α_2	μ	δ	ε
5. Light chain	κ or λ	κ or λ	κ or λ	κ or λ	κ or λ
6. Serum concentration (mg/ml)	12	2	1.2	0.03	0.00004
7. Half-life (days)	21	6	5	3	2
8. Complement binding	Classical pathway	Alternative pathway	Classical pathway	None	None
9. Binding to tissue	Hetero-logous	None	None	None	Homo-logous
10. Secretion from serous membranes	No	Yes*	No	No	Yes
11. Placental passage	Yes	No	No	No	No
12. Heat stability (56°C)	Yes	Yes	Yes	Yes	No

* Secretory IgA.

12

THE COMPLEMENT SYSTEM

Q. 1. Name different protein components of complement and discuss classical pathway of complement activation.

Ans. The term **complement** (C) is applied to a system of components present in the serum of man and animals. It consists of nine different proteins denoted C1–C9. The fraction C1 occurs in serum as calcium ion dependent complex, which on chelation with EDTA yields three protein subunits called C1q, C1r and C1s. Thus C is made up of 11 different proteins. Complement proteins differ in their electrophoretic mobility and molecular weight having sedimentation coefficient ranging from 4S to 11S. These differences permit their separation by physical methods. Though some of its components are stable, C as a whole is heat-labile undergoing spontaneous denaturation slowly at room temperature and in 30 minutes at 56°C. Serum deprived of C activity by heating it at 56°C for 30 minutes is said to be inactivated.

Classical pathway of complement activation

Activation of classical pathway of complement requires the presence of antibody, either IgM or IgG, bound to cell surface antigen or as an antigen-antibody immune complex. All the 11 proteins of the complement comprise the classical complement pathway. All are designated by C followed by the number of the component (complement's protein). Inactive components are described as C1, C2, C3 and so on. Activated forms are designated by placing a bar over the number, for example, $C\overline{2}$ represents activated C2 which is actually C2b.

The classical pathway (Fig. 12.1) is initiated when C1 interacts with the Fc portion of either cell-bound Ig (IgG or IgM) or immune complex. This interaction results in the sequential activation of C4, C2 and C3 and leads to the formation of complex cleaving enzymes. Activation of C5, C6, C7, C8 and C9 then completes the cascade and results in the formation of the **C5 to C9 membrane attack complex (MAC)**, which can lyse the cell. C1 is composed of one molecule of C1q, and two molecules each of C1r and C1s. C1q binds to Fc portion of

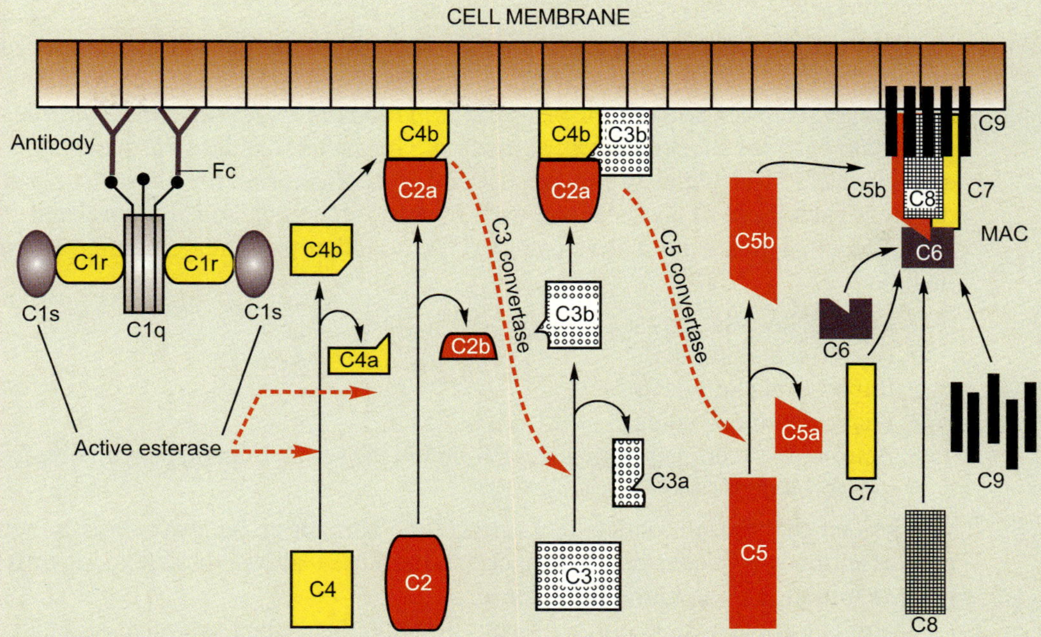

Fig. 12.1. Classical pathway of complement activation.

the antibody molecule. Binding of this component of C1 causes a conformational change in the C1 complex that leads to the autoactivation of C1r.

This then converts C1s into an active esterase that acts on C4 to produce C4a and a reactive C4b. C4a is released and less than 1% of the C4b becomes attached to the cell membrane. Unbound molecules of C4b are rapidly inactivated. C1s also cleaves C2 into two components – C2a, larger component, and C2b, smaller component. C2a attaches itself to membrane-bound C4b to form a new active protease, $\overline{C4b2a}$, which is called C3 convertase since it can bind and cleave the next inactive complement component in the sequence, C3.

The newly formed C3 convertase, $\overline{C4b2a}$ cleaves C3 into two fragments, C3a and C3b. The larger C3b fragment attaches to both the cell membrane and $\overline{C4b2a}$ complex, while the smaller fragment, C3a, is released to the body fluids. C3a has chemotactic and anaphylatoxic properties. $\overline{C4b2a3b}$ is termed C5 convertase. It cleaves C5 into two products, C5a and C5b. C5a which is a powerful chemotactant of neutrophils and monocytes and has anaphylatoxic activity is released when formed and C5b attaches to the cell membrane. The binding of $\overline{C5b}$ leads to the uncovering of a binding site for C6 and C7 on the molecule, producing a stable complex $\overline{C5b67}$.

This trimolecular complex attaches to the membrane surface and enables C8 to join. C8 then binds several C9 molecules. About 10–18 protein units of C9 attach to $\overline{C5b678}$ base to form a long hollow tube. This is a stable complex and is referred to as membrane attack complex (MAC). This creates a membrane pore or lesion, that is 100 Å in diameter leading to cell death. Pores in the cell membrane created by MAC may also permit degradative enzymes in the area to enter and destroy cellular organelles contributing to target cell death.

Q. 2. Describe alternative or properdin pathway of complement activation.

Ans. This pathway does not require the presence of specific antibodies. C3 is the major component of C. In the classical pathway, activation of C3 is achieved by the C3 convertase ($\overline{C4b2a}$). *The activation of C3, without the prior participation of C142, is known as the alternative or properdin pathway of complement activation.* The overall result of this pathway is the same as that of classical pathway but the C3 and C5 convertases for alternative pathway are different from those of classical pathway. A wide range of chemically unrelated substances are known to activate alternative pathway. These (other than antigen-antibody complexes) include:

- Yeast cell walls.
- Bacterial endotoxins.
- Rabbit (not sheep) RBCs.
- Snake venom proteins.
- A protein termed 'nephritic factor' found in the serum of patients with diseases such as glomerulonephritis.

The fact that these products can activate the alternative pathway directly, without the need of antibody is of considerable importance because it allows for defence against infection prior to initiation of an immune response.

There are at least three normal serum proteins that, when activated together with C3, form a functional C3 convertase and a C5 convertase. These are factor B, factor D and properdin. These are normal serum proteins, and the alternative pathway is routinely being activated in the absence of any stimulus. In the absence of initiators, the initial complexes of the alternative pathway are rapidly destroyed. In the presence of the initiators, such complexes are stabilized and complement is activated to form the MAC as in case of classical pathway.

Intrinsically, C3 undergoes a low level of hydrolysis of an internal thioester bond to generate C3b. Nonimmune activators, such as repeating polysaccharide units or the lipopolysaccharide found on the cell walls of some microbes split up C3 into C3a and C3b. There are a wide variety of pathogens that can be recognized within minutes after they come in contact with plasma. Organisms sensitive to attack by the alternative pathway include bacteria, fungi, certain viruses, virus-infected cells, parasites and certain tumour cells. C3b, in the presence of Mg^{++}, binds to these foreign surfaces and interacts with plasma protein factor B forming C3bB (Fig. 12.2).

The factor B portion of C3bB complex is split by factor D into two fragments, Ba and Bb. Ba is released during reaction and Bb remains bound to C3b forming C3bBb. The newly formed $\overline{C3bBb}$ is a C3 convertase of alternative pathway. $\overline{C3bBb}$ splits more C3 to C3a and C3b. The newly formed C3b binds more factor B. This continues until the membrane surface is saturated with $\overline{C3bBb}$. The result is opsonization of the cell or particle by neutrophils. The soluble C3a, that is released upon cleavage of C3, has chemotactic and anaphylatoxic activity, which can initiate an inflammatory response. C3 convertase ($\overline{C3bBb}$) can bind additional C3b to produce C5 convertase ($\overline{C3bBb3b}$). This activates terminal lytic complement sequence, C5 to C9.

Thus activation of either classical or alternative pathway leads to the formation of C3 convertases ($\overline{C4b2a}$ or $\overline{C3bBb}$). These cleave C3 into C3a and C3b. The latter combines with C3 convertases forming C5 convertases ($\overline{C4b2a3b}$ or $\overline{C3bBb3b}$). These split C5 into

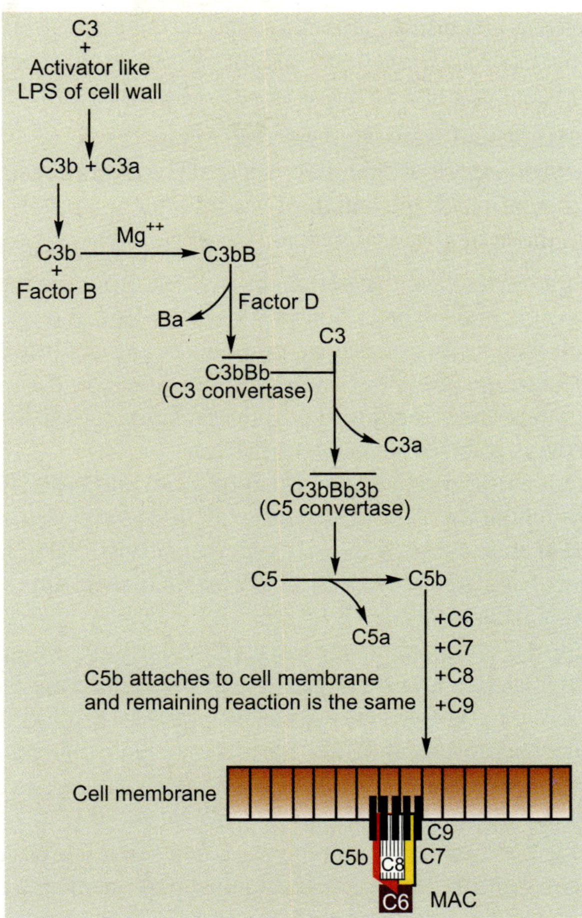

Fig. 12.2. Alternative pathway of complement activation.

C5a and C5b. C5b then binds C6, C7, C8 and several molecules of C9 to form MAC which initiates lysis of target cells in both pathways.

Q. 3. Describe biological effects of complement.

Ans. 1. Complement mediates **immunological membrane damage.** This results in bacteriolysis and cytolysis. Different cells vary in their susceptibility to complement-mediated lysis. Gram-negative bacteria are generally sensitive to lysis, while Gram-positive are killed without lysis. Neutralization of certain viruses requires the participation of C, e.g., neutralization of herpes virus by IgM antibody requires the binding of C1, C4 and possibly C3 too.

2. C fragments released during cascade reaction help in **amplifying the inflammatory response.** Proteolytic cleavage of C3 and C5, in either the classical or alternative pathway, generates two potent mediators of inflammation, C3a and C5a. Mast cells and basophils possess receptors for C3a and C5a. Binding of C3a or C5a to these receptors causes these

cells to release histamine. This may lead to contraction of the uterus, trachea, arteries, atrium of the heart and intestines, and increased vascular permeability leading to oedema. C5a, in addition exerts a series of unique effects on white blood cells. These include:

- Degranulation and lysosomal enzyme release.
- Promotes adherence of granulocytes to the endothelium.
- Induces chemotactic migration of granulocytes.

$C\overline{5b67}$ is also chemotactic. C4a has weak anaphylatoxic activity. It is weakly spasmogenic and increases vascular permeability. Therefore, redness, pain, swelling and heat of inflammation is due to the action of C4a, C3a, C5a and histamine.

3. Phagocytes such as macrophages, monocytes and neutrophils possess surface receptors for C3b. If immune complexes have activated the complement system, the C3b bound to them facilitates their recognition and ingestion by these phagocytes. This facilitated phagocytosis is referred to as **opsonization**.
4. Complement participates in **type II (cytotoxic)** and **type III (immune complex) hypersensitivity** reactions. The destruction of erythrocytes, following incompatible blood transfusion is an example of type II hypersensitivity. Participation of C is required for the production of immune complex diseases such as serum sickness and Arthus reaction (type III hypersensitivity).
5. Several serum C components are lowered in many autoimmune diseases such as systemic lupus erythematosus and rheumatoid arthritis. These may, therefore, be involved in the pathogenesis of autoimmune diseases. C plays a major role in the pathogenesis of autoimmune haemolytic anaemia, paroxysmal nocturnal haemoglobinuria and hereditary angioneurotic oedema.
6. C3 and C6 participate in coagulation process.
7. C bound to antigen-antibody complexes adheres to erythrocytes. This is known as **immune adherence**. It contributes to defence against pathogenic microorganisms as such adherent particles are rapidly phagocytosed. C3 and C4 are necessary for immune adherence.

13

Antigen-Antibody Reactions

Q. 1. Define antigen-antibody reaction, precipitation and flocculation. Describe briefly zone phenomenon.

Ans. When an antigen is mixed with its specific antibody, in the presence of electrolytes at a suitable temperature and pH, they combine with each other in an observable manner.

Precipitation

When a soluble antigen is mixed with its specific antibody in the presence of electrolytes at a suitable temperature and pH, the antigen-antibody complex forms an insoluble precipitate. This precipitate usually settles down at the bottom of the tube. Precipitation can take place in liquid media and in gels such as agar, agarose and polyacrylamide. The process of precipitation can be hastened by electrically driving the antigen and antibody.

Flocculation

When, instead of sedimenting, the precipitate remains suspended as floccules, the reaction is called flocculation.

Zone phenomenon

If a series (10–12) of tubes is set up (Fig. 13.1), each containing a constant amount of antiserum, and increasing amounts of antigen are added to the tubes in the row, precipitation will be found to occur most rapidly and abundantly in one of the middle tubes, in which antigen and antibody are in optimal or equivalent proportion. In the preceding tubes, in which the antibody is in excess, and in the later tubes, in which the antigen is in excess, the precipitation will be weak or absent. Therefore, the amount of precipitation will be seen to increase along the row, reaching a maximum and then falling off with higher antigen concentration.

If the amounts of precipitate in different tubes are plotted on a graph, the resulting curve will have **three phases** – an ascending part (**prozone** or **zone of antibody excess**), a peak

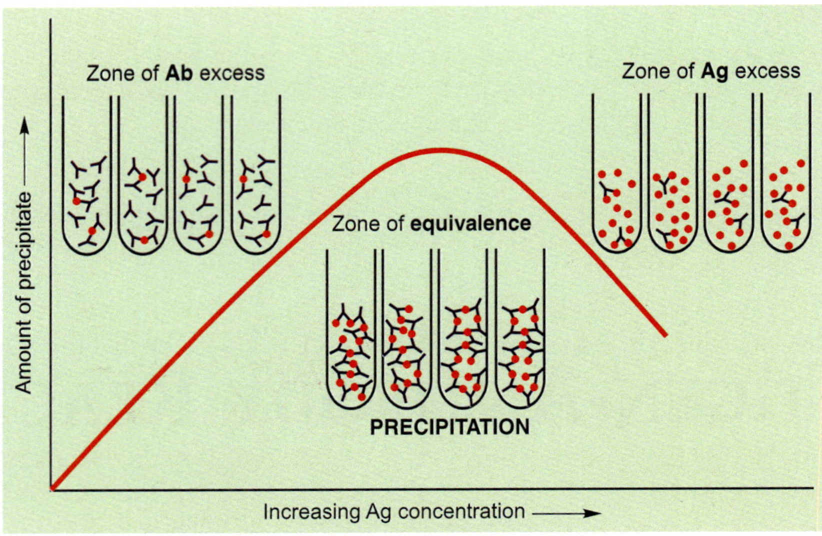

Fig. 13.1. Zone phenomenon.

(**zone of equivalence**), and a descending part (**postzone** or **zone of antigen excess**). This is called **zone phenomenon.** Assay of supernatant solution will show that those tubes containing too little antigen still contain free antibody and in the tubes with antigen excess, little precipitate forms, although soluble immune complexes and free antigens are present in the supernatant fluid. Only in tubes of maximum precipitation is all antibody removed from solution. *The prozone is of importance in clinical serology, as sera rich in antibody may sometimes give a false negative result, unless several dilutions are tested.*

If immune complexes form in serum, monocytes, neutrophils and eosinophils attempt to remove them. Complexes formed at equivalence or antibody excess are easily removed. However, small, soluble complexes formed in antigen excess are more difficult to remove. These might gain entrance to tissues, such as glomeruli of kidneys or become deposited within vessel walls causing varying degree of damage.

Q. 2. Discuss applications of precipitation and flocculation reactions.

Ans. The precipitation test may be carried out for both qualitative and quantitative determination of both antigen and antibody. It is a very sensitive test for detecting antigens and is relatively less sensitive for detection of antibodies. The precipitation test is capable of detecting as little antigen proteins as 1 μg. It can be used for identification of blood and seminal stains and food adulterants. Some of the precipitation and flocculation tests which have application in diagnostic bacteriology are as under:

Ring test

This test is done by layering antigen solution over a column of antiserum in a capillary tube. After a short while a ring of precipitate forms at the interface. *Typing of streptococci and pneumococci*, *C-reactive protein test* and *Ascoli's thermoprecipitin test* for the diagnosis of anthrax, are some of the uses of ring test. This technique is also used in *detection of adulteration of foodstuffs.*

Slide test

This is an example of flocculation test. When a drop each of antigen and antiserum are placed on a slide and mixed by shaking, floccules appear. *VDRL, a most widely used test* for the diagnosis of syphilis, is an example of slide flocculation test.

Tube test

Flocculation test can be carried out in the tubes also. *Kahn test* for the diagnosis of syphilis, and *standardization of toxins and toxoids* are examples of tube flocculation.

Immunodiffusion (precipitation in gel)

When an antibody and its antigen are placed in an agar gel they diffuse towards each other and form an opaque band of precipitation at the junction of their diffusion front. Precipitation in gel has several advantages over precipitation in liquid medium:

- The reaction appears as a distinct band of precipitation which can be stained for better visibility and preservation.
- Since each antigen-antibody reaction gives rise to one line of precipitation, therefore, different number of antigens in a mixture can be detected.
- This technique also indicates *identity*, *cross-reaction* and *nonidentity* between different antigens.

Types of immunodiffusion tests

1. Single diffusion in one dimension (Oudin procedure)

Antibody is incorporated in agar gel in a test tube. Antigen solution is then layered over it. The antigen diffuses downwards and wherever it reaches in optimum concentration with antibody a line of precipitation is formed (Fig. 13.2A). As more antigen diffuses, the line of precipitation moves downwards. Number of lines of precipitation indicates the number of antigens and antibodies present.

2. Double diffusion in one dimension (Oakley-Fulthorpe procedure)

Antibody is incorporated in agar gel in a test tube. Above this is placed a column of plain agar which in turn is overlaid with antigen, either as liquid or incorporated into agar (Fig. 13.2B). Antigen and antibody diffuse (double diffusion) towards each other (in one dimension) through the intervening column of plain agar and form a band of precipitation where they meet in optimum concentration.

3. Single diffusion in two dimensions (radial immunodiffusion)

This method is used to quantitate the amount of a specific antigen present in a sample and can be used for many antigens. The most widely used diagnostic application of this procedure is to measure the amount of various Ig classes (IgG, IgA, IgM, IgD and IgE) in patient serum.

Here monospecific antiserum (antiserum containing only antibody against the antigen which is to be assayed) is incorporated in agar gel. It is poured on a glass slide or a petri dish and a number of wells are punched into it, and different dilutions of the antigen are placed into various wells. As the antigen diffuses from the well, a ring of precipitate forms at that position where antigen and antibody are in optimal proportions. Larger the concentration of antigen, the farther it diffuses to be in optimal proportions with the antibody incorporated in

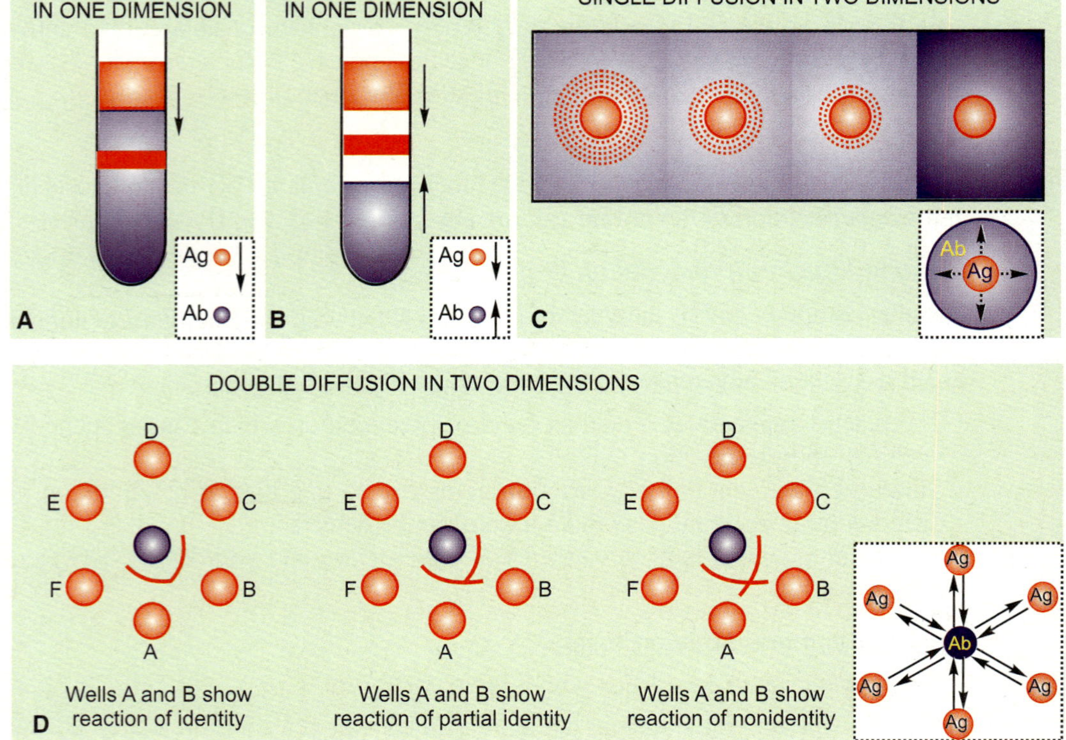

Fig. 13.2. Immunodiffusion tests.

the gel. Therefore, the diameter of the ring gives the estimate of the concentration of the antigen (Fig. 13.2C).

Using known concentrations of the antigen in question, one can prepare a standard curve by plotting the diameter of the precipitin ring versus antigen concentration. With this standard plot, one needs only to measure the diameter of the precipitin ring formed with the unknown antigen to calculate its concentration. Radial immunodiffusion is used for the laboratory diagnosis of multiple myeloma or agammaglobulinaemia.

4. Double diffusion in two dimensions (Ouchterlony procedure)

Agar is poured on the slide and wells, usually seven, are punched in it using a template. The known antiserum is placed in the central well and different antigens in surrounding wells. One of these contains known positive antigen. It acts as a positive control. This technique is also useful for comparing different antigens for the presence of identical or cross-reacting components. The samples are placed in adjacent wells, and the corresponding antibody is placed in the central well.

1. **Reaction of identity:** If two precipitin bands fuse completely (Fig. 13.2D), the pattern is termed reaction of identity. It indicates that the antigens in the adjoining wells are identical.
2. **Reaction of nonidentity:** If unrelated antigens are placed in adjacent wells, they diffuse towards central well containing antibodies for both, the two precipitin bands form independently and cross each other. This is known as reaction of nonidentity.

3. **Reaction of partial identity:** If the antigens in the two adjacent wells are cross-reacting (partial identity), the precipitation bands fuse but form a spurlike projection. This is known as reaction of partial identity.

A special variety of double diffusion in two dimensions is the **Elek's test** for toxigenicity of diphtheria bacilli (see chapter 21).

5. Immunoelectrophoresis

Immunoelectrophoresis combines electrophoresis and immunodiffusion (immune precipitation in gel). This method can be used for analyzing complex antigens in biological fluids. A glass slide is covered with molten agar or agarose. A well for antigen and a trough for antiserum is cut on it (Fig. 13.3). Antigen well is filled with antigen mixture (human serum). The slide is then placed in an electric field for about an hour to allow for the electrophoretic migration of various antigens. Different antigens will migrate at different rates or even in different directions, depending upon their size and charge and the conditions of electrophoresis.

After the completion of electrophoresis, antiserum trough is filled with appropriate antiserum (antiserum to whole human serum). Antigens and antibodies diffuse towards each other, resulting in the formation of precipitin bands, for individual antigens and antibodies, whenever they are both in zones of optimal proportions, in 18–24 hours. Because immunoelectrophoresis uses electric charge in addition to diffusion, it is more likely to separate antigen than is simple diffusion alone. By this method, over 30 different antigens can be identified in human serum. This technique is useful for detection of normal and abnormal serum proteins.

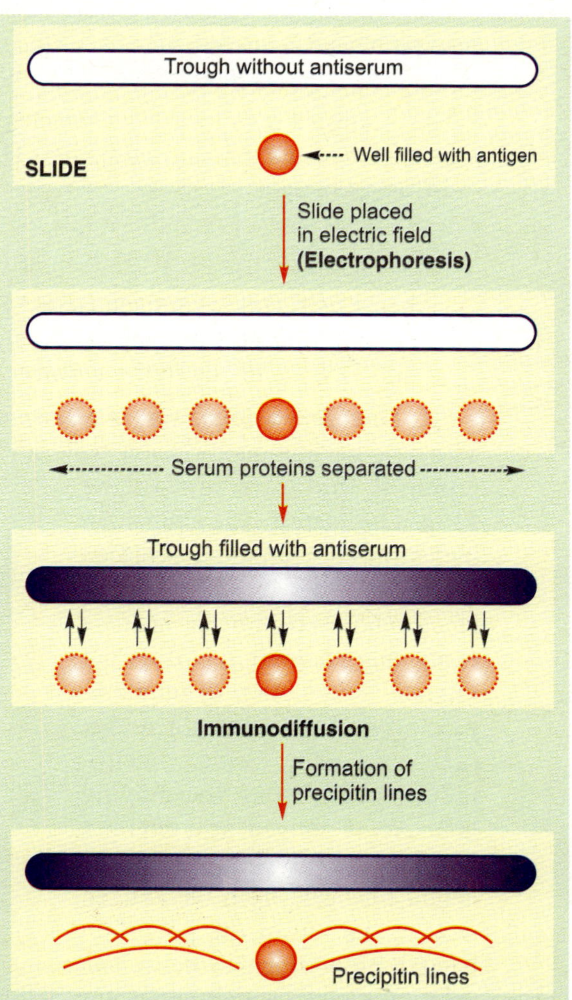

Fig. 13.3. Immunoelectrophoresis.

6. Electroimmunodiffusion

Immunodiffusion is a slow process. The development of precipitin lines can be speeded up by electrically driving antigens and antibodies in a gel, rather than simply allowing them to come in contact by diffusion. Of these, one dimensional double electroimmunodiffusion and one-dimensional single electroimmunodiffusion are used frequently in the clinical laboratory.

I. ***One dimensional double electroimmunodiffusion (counter-immunoelectrophoresis or CIE):*** This method can be used for those antigens and antibodies that migrate in opposite directions in electric field. The wells are punched about 1 cm apart in an agar slab on a glass plate. Antigen and antibody solutions are placed in wells towards cathode and anode sides respectively. Electric field is then applied electrophoresing both antigens and antibodies from separate wells. The antigen migrates towards antibody and antibody migrates towards antigen. A precipitin band is formed, in between the two wells, where they meet in optimum proportions (Fig. 13.4). This method has several advantages over simple diffusion in agar:

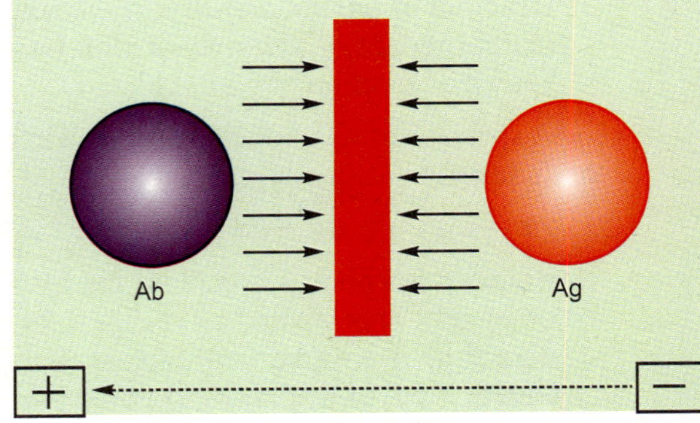

Fig. 13.4. Counterimmunoelectrophoresis.

- The electrophoresis focuses the reactants into a small area allowing the detection of small quantities of antigens and antibodies. Therefore, **it is 10 times more sensitive than simple diffusion in agar**.
- It is a rapid assay. Precipitin bands may form in just 30 minutes.

This method is used for detection of various antigens such as:
- hepatitis B surface antigen (HBsAg) and alpha-fetoprotein in serum;
- meningococcal and cryptococcal antigens in CSF; and
- anti-DNA antibody in the serum of patients with several autoimmune disorders.

II. ***One dimensional single electroimmunodiffusion (rocket electrophoresis):*** As in case of radial immunodiffusion, wells are cut in an agarose gel slab on a glass plate. Agarose contains the antiserum to the antigen of interest. The antigen, in increasing concentrations, is placed in wells. The antigen is then electrophoresed into the agarose containing antibody that does not migrate. The pattern of immuno-precipitation resembles a rocket (hence the name), since precipitation occurs along the moving boundary of antigen, as it migrates into the agarose (Fig. 13.5). The height (distance from the antigen well to the top of the precipitin band) is proportional to the antigen concentration. The main application of this technique, therefore, is for quantitative estimation of antigen.

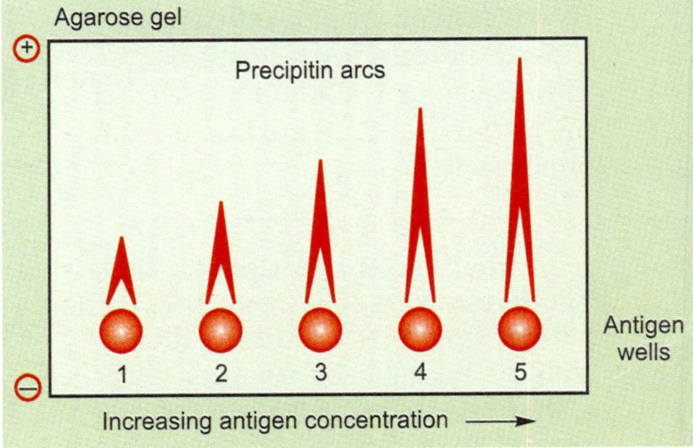

Fig. 13.5. Rocket electrophoresis.

Q. 3. Define agglutination reactions, prozone phenomenon and blocking antibodies. Describe briefly applications of agglutination reactions.

Ans. Agglutination reactions

When a particulate antigen or an antigen present on the surface of a cell (red cell or bacterium) or an inorganic particle (e.g., polystyrene latex coated with antigen) is mixed with its antibody in the presence of electrolytes at a suitable temperature and pH, the particles are clumped or agglutinated. This reaction is analogous to precipitation reaction, in that antibody merely acts as a bridge to form a lattice network of antibody and cells or inorganic particles coated with antigen. Because cells or particles are much larger than soluble antigen, therefore, they aggregate into clumps. Agglutination reaction is more sensitive than precipitation for detection of antibodies.

Prozone phenomenon

False negative agglutination reactions can occur with some antisera in antibody excess (first few dilutions). This is known as prozone phenomenon. Unagglutinated cells in prozone actually have antibody molecules adsorbed on their surface, with both sites of bivalent antibody attached to the same cell resulting into poor or no lattice formation.

Blocking antibodies

Occasionally, antibodies (e.g., anti-Rh and anti-*Brucella*) are formed that react with the antigenic determinants on a cell but do not cause agglutination. Such antibodies are called blocking antibodies, because they inhibit agglutination by complete antibody added subsequently.

Applications of agglutination reactions

Slide agglutination

A drop of saline is placed on a clean glass slide and a small amount of culture from a solid medium is emulsified in it by means of inoculating loop. It is then examined through a hand lens or low-power microscope that the suspension is even and bacteria are not auto-agglutinable. Then with a platinum loop a drop of specific antiserum is placed on the slide near the bacterial suspension. The serum and the bacterial suspension are then mixed and examined with naked eye or with hand lens or under low-power microscope for the evidence of agglutination within a minute. Slide agglutination test is rapid and convenient, but in order to obtain rapid agglutination serum is used undiluted or in low dilutions.

Uses:

- Identification of bacterial isolates (e.g., *Salmonella* spp., *Shigella* spp.) and *Vibrio cholerae* from clinical specimens. This method is practicable only when clumping of organisms occurs instantaneously or within a minute because clumping occurring after a minute may be due to drying of the fluid.
- Blood grouping and cross matching.

Tube agglutination

This is done in round-bottomed test tubes or perspex plates with round-bottomed wells. A fixed volume of a particulate antigen suspension is added to an equal volume of serial dilutions of the patient serum in test tubes or perspex plates. Following several hours of incubation at 37°C, agglutination is seen at the bottom of the tubes. **The titre of the serum is given as the reciprocal of the highest dilution that causes clumping.** Thus the serum that agglutinates at a dilution of 1 : 256 is reported to have a titre of 256 and if the test has been carried out in 1 ml volumes, the titre of the serum is 256 units/ml of serum.

Uses:

Serological diagnosis of:

- Enteric fever (Widal test)
- Brucellosis
- Typhus fever (Weil-Felix reaction)
- *Streptococcus* MG agglutination
- Cold agglutination
- Paul-Bunnell test

In the **Widal test** used for the diagnosis of enteric fever, two types of antigens are used – the flagellar (H) antigen and somatic (O) antigen. H antigen is a formolised suspension of the organisms which on combination with antibody, forms large, loose and fluffy clumps resembling wisps of cotton-wool. For H agglutination conical (Dreyer's) tubes are used. O antigen is prepared by treating the bacterial suspension with alcohol. On combination with antibody it forms fine granular deposit resembling chalk powder at the base of round-bottomed (Felix) tubes, whereas, negative reaction shows a compact button-like deposit (Fig. 13.6).

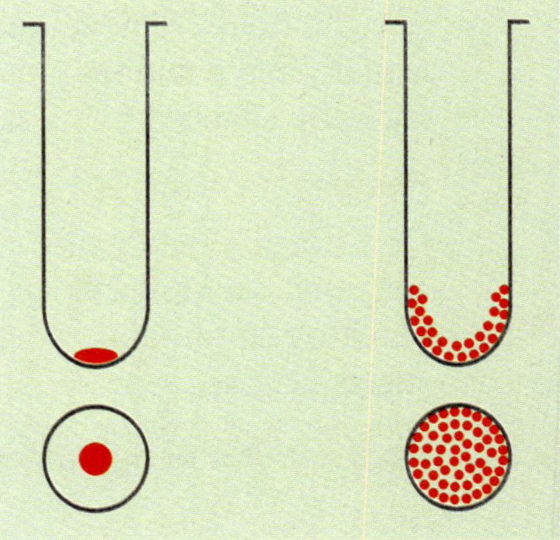

Fig. 13.6. Tube agglutination test.

Tube agglutination test for brucellosis may be complicated by prozone phenomenon and the presence of blocking antibodies. To avoid false negative results due to prozone, several dilutions of the serum should be tested. *Blocking antibodies may be detected by doing the test in hypertonic (5%) saline, albumin saline or more reliably by the antiglobulin (Coombs') test.* Rh antibodies are also incomplete antibodies.

Heterophile agglutination

Weil-Felix reaction for serodiagnosis of typhus fever and ***Streptococcus* MG agglutination** for the diagnosis of primary atypical pneumonia are the examples of **heterophile agglutination test**. Red blood cells are used as antigens in **cold agglutination** and **Paul-Bunnell test**. IgM antibodies capable of agglutinating human red cells at 0–4°C (cold agglutinins) are sometimes found in certain human diseases including primary atypical pneumonia, malaria, trypanosomiasis and acquired haemolytic anaemia. Sera of the patients suffering from infectious mononucleosis agglutinate sheep RBCs (see Chapter 10).

Antiglobulin (Coombs') test

Anti-Rh antibodies are of IgG type, but they normally do not agglutinate Rh-positive RBCs (incomplete antibodies). The inability of these antibodies to agglutinate is perhaps due to the presence of insufficient antigenic determinants on the RBCs to permit the antibody to overcome the normal electrostatic repulsion that exists among RBCs. When sera containing incomplete anti-Rh antibodies are mixed with Rh-positive red cells, the antibody coats the surface of erythrocytes but they are not agglutinated. When such antibody-coated erythrocytes are washed to free all unattached protein and are treated with anti-human gammaglobulin (**antiglobulin or Coombs' serum**), the cells are agglutinated.

Coombs' test is of two types – direct and indirect.

1. **Direct Coombs' test:** The sensitization of erythrocytes with incomplete antibodies takes place *in vivo* as in case of haemolytic disease of newborn due to Rh incompatibility. Therefore, when washed RBCs from such patient are mixed with antiglobulin or Coombs' serum, agglutination takes place.
2. **Indirect Coombs' test:** The sensitization of RBCs with incomplete antibodies is performed *in vitro*. Rh-positive RBCs are mixed with the serum to be tested for Rh-antibodies and then after a short incubation and washing, antiglobulin or Coombs' serum is added. If the test serum contained anti-Rh antibodies, agglutination will take place.

Uses of Coombs' test

- Detection of anti-Rh antibodies
- Demonstration of nonagglutinating antibodies in brucellosis

Q. 4. Describe briefly passive (indirect) agglutination giving suitable examples.

Ans. A precipitation reaction can be converted into agglutination reaction by coating soluble antigen onto the surface of carrier particles such as RBCs, latex, bentonite and gelatin particles. Such test is more convenient and more sensitive for detection of antibodies. Most polysaccharide and lipopolysaccharide antigens may be adsorbed by simple mixing with the cells. For adsorption of protein antigens, tanned red cells are used. Some of the examples of passive agglutination are given below:

- In rheumatoid arthritis, **RA factor** (an antigammaglobulin autoantibody) appears in the serum of the patient. It acts as an antibody to human IgG. Latex polystyrene beads coated with denatured human IgG when mixed with patient serum leads to agglutination of latex polystyrene beads.
- Latex particles coated with antibodies to meningococci, *Haemophilus influenzae* type b and pneumococci can be used to detect corresponding antigens in cases of **pyogenic meningitis**.
- Latex agglutination tests are also widely used for detection of hepatitis B, antistreptolysin O, C-reactive protein, human chorionic gonadotropin hormone and many other antigens.
- One of the most widely used passive agglutination tests employing erythrocytes is ***Treponema pallidum* haemagglutination (TPHA)** for serological diagnosis of treponemal infection.
- For the detection of **anti-HIV antibodies**, gelatin particles can be sensitized (coated) with inactivated HIV antigen. When these sensitized particles are mixed with the patient serum or plasma these particles are agglutinated if the anti-HIV antibodies are present in the sample. The test procedure is extremely simple using a microtitre technique and is particularly suitable for mass screening of specimens. The test is time-saving and results are readable by the naked eye after about two hours.

When, instead of antigen, antibody is adsorbed on the carrier particles in tests for estimation of antigens, the technique is known as **reversed passive agglutination**.

Q. 5. Describe principle and clinical applications of coagglutination.

Ans. This is based upon the principle that most strains of *Staphylococcus aureus* (especially Cowan strain I) possess protein A on their surface. Protein A binds IgG molecules, non-specifically, through Fc region leaving specific Fab sites free to combine with specific antigen. When suspension of such sensitized staphylococcal cells is treated with homologous (test) antigen, the antigen combines with free Fab sites of IgG attached to staphylococcal cells leading to visible clumping of staphylococci within two minutes. This is known as coagglutination (COA).

COA test can be used for detecting the presence of bacterial antigens in serum, urine and CSF. For example, typhoid bacillus antigen is consistently present in the blood in the early phase of disease, and also in the urine of the patients. This antigen can be detected by COA test. Similarly, meningococcal, pneumococcal and *Haemophilus* antigens can be detected by COA test in the CSF. Identification of *Neisseria gonorrhoeae* and serogrouping of β-haemolytic streptococci A, B, C, D and G can also be carried out by COA test.

Q. 6. Describe briefly complement fixation test and other tests employing complement.

Ans. The ability of antigen-antibody complexes to fix complement is made use of in complement fixation test (CFT). This is a very versatile and sensitive test. This can detect as little as 0.04 μg of antibody nitrogen and 0.1 μg of antigen. CFTs include **Wassermann reaction** and **Reiter protein complement fixation test (RPCFT)** for the serodiagnosis of syphilis. Similarly, CFTs for the identification of various viral antigens are also available.

In most of the cases fixation of complement with antigen-antibody complex causes in itself no visible effect. Therefore, it is necessary to use an indicator system consisting of sheep red cells coated with anti-sheep red cell antibody. Complement lyses antibody coated red cells. CFT, therefore, is performed in two stages.

Stage 1: Test serum (for the detection of antibody) and the antigen are mixed in the presence of carefully measured amount of complement and then incubated at 37°C for 1 hour. If the test serum contains antibody then antigen-antibody complexes are formed and complement gets fixed on it.

Stage 2: Indicator system, antibody-coated sheep red cells, is added to determine whether the complement has been fixed in stage 1 reaction or not. If the complement has been taken up during stage 1 reaction then it will not be available to lyse the red cells. Therefore, a positive CFT is indicated by absence of lysis of red cells whilst a negative test, with unused complement, is shown by lysis of the red cells (Fig. 13.7).

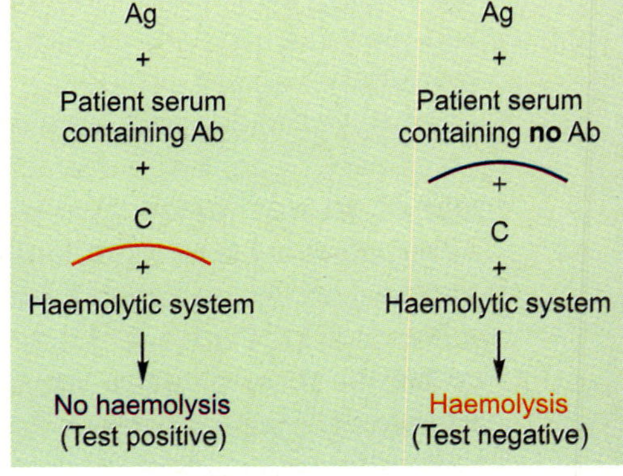

Fig. 13.7. Complement fixation test.

The antigen in this test may be soluble or particulate. Prior to commencement of test the serum should be inactivated by heating it at 56°C for 30 minutes to destroy any complement activity serum may have and also to remove some non-specific inhibitors of complement. The source of complement for laboratory use is guinea-pig serum. Guinea-pig serum is first titrated for complement activity. One unit or **minimum haemolytic dose (MHD) of complement** is the highest dilution of guinea-pig serum that lyses one unit volume of washed sheep RBCs in the presence of excess of haemolysin (amboceptor) within a fixed time (usually 30–60 minutes) at 37°C. Similarly, amboceptor should also be titrated. **One MHD of haemolysin** may be defined as highest dilution of the serum that lyses one unit volume of washed sheep RBCs in the presence of excess complement within a fixed time (usually 30–60 minutes) at 37°C.

Anti-complementary effect

Non-specific adsorption of complement may give false positive results. Some sera may develop anti-complementary properties on ageing, and after bacterial contamination. Haemolysed blood serum also has anti-complementary effect.

Other tests employing complement

Immune adherence

Some bacteria, like *Vibrio cholerae* and *Treponema pallidum*, react with specific antibody in the presence of complement and particulate material such as erythrocytes or platelets; the bacteria are aggregated and adhere to the cells. This is known as immune adherence. **Adherence occurs through the activated C3b component of complement.**

Treponema pallidum immobilization test

The test serum is incubated anaerobically with a suspension of live treponemes and complement. If antibodies are present, the treponemes will be found to be immobilized.

Cytolytic or cytocidal tests

When *V. cholerae* is mixed with its antibody in the presence of complement, the bacterium is killed and lysed.

Q. 7. Describe neutralization tests and their *in vivo* and *in vitro* applications.

Ans. These are of two types – virus neutralization tests and toxin neutralization tests.

Virus neutralization tests

Neutralization of viruses by their antibodies in a patient serum may be quantitated by their ability to reduce the infectivity of a stock virus preparation. The test serum is diluted serially, incubated with a known amount of virus and the mixture is then added to indicator systems – animals, embryonated hen's egg and tissue culture. The highest dilution of serum ablating infectivity in 50% of virus-serum mixtures tested is taken as the titre. Neutralization of bacteriophages can be demonstrated by plaque inhibition test. When bacteriophages are seeded in appropriate dilution on lawn cultures, plaques of lysis are produced. Specific antiphage serum inhibits plaque formation.

Toxin neutralization

Bacterial exotoxins are highly antigenic and their activity may be completely neutralized by appropriate concentrations of specific antibody. Antibody to bacterial exotoxin is usually referred to as antitoxin. Bacterial endotoxins are poorly antigenic and their toxicity is not neutralized by antisera.

The neutralizing capacity of an antitoxin can be assayed by neutralization test in which mixture of toxin and antitoxin is injected into a susceptible animal and the least amount of antitoxin that prevents death or disease in the animal is estimated. In case of diphtheria toxin, which in small doses causes cutaneous reaction, neutralization test can be carried out on the human skin. The Schick test is based on the ability of circulating antitoxin to neutralize the diphtheria toxin given intradermally. Neutralization (no reaction) indicates immunity, and erythema and induration indicates susceptibility to diphtheria.

If a toxin has a demonstrable *in vitro* effect, this effect can be neutralized by specific antitoxin. For example, **antistreptolysin O**, present in the serum of the patient suffering from *Streptococcus pyogenes* infection, neutralizes the haemolytic activity of the streptococcal O haemolysin. Another example of *in vitro* toxin-antitoxin neutralization is **Nagler's reaction**. *Clostridium perfringens* produces α-toxin which is a phospholipase (lecithinase-C). This produces opalescence in serum or egg yolk media. This reaction is specifically neutralized by the antitoxin.

Q. 8. Write briefly about immune and nonimmune opsonization.

Ans. A substance, such as complement or antibody, that can bind to the surface of a cell or a particle, making it more readily phagocytosed is known as opsonin. Enhanced complement-mediated phagocytosis can occur either in the presence or absence of antibody. Phagocytes such as macrophages, monocytes and neutrophils possess surface receptors (CR1) for C3b and Fc receptors for antibody. If immune complexes have activated the complement system then Fc and CR1 receptors, present on the phagocyte, bind Fc region of antibody and C3b bound on immune complexes respectively thus facilitating their phagocytosis. This facilitated phagocytosis by antibody and complement is known as **immune opsonization** (Fig. 13.8).

In contrast, **nonimmune opsonization** requires only C3b (opsonin) for opsonization. Bacteria in the blood stream can activate the alternative pathway and generate C3b, which coats the bacteria. C3b binds to CR1 receptors present on the phagocytes thus facilitating their phagocytosis. Viruses, soluble immune complexes and tumour cells are also opsonized and removed by the same mechanism (Fig. 13.8).

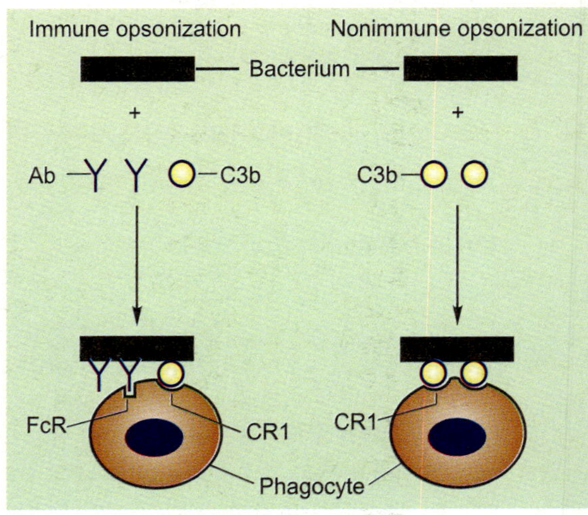

Fig. 13.8. Opsonization.

Q. 9. Describe immunofluorescence. Highlight the features of direct and indirect immunofluorescence with merits and demerits of both.

Ans. Fluorescent dyes absorb invisible UV light between 290–495 nm and emit visible longer wavelength (525 nm) green light. Therefore, if microorganisms or tissue cells are stained with a fluorescent dye and examined under the microscope with UV light instead of visible light they are seen as bright objects against a dark background. This principle is used in fluorescence microscopy. Coons and his colleagues (1942) showed that fluorescent dyes, such as fluorescein isothiocyanate (FITC), can be conjugated to antibodies (without affecting their specificity) permitting their ready detection, when attached to an antigen associated with a cell. Immunofluorescence (IF) is now used extensively to detect:

- Tissue antigens.
- Antibodies to tissues including autoantibodies.
- The antigens of infecting organisms in the body.
- Antigen-antibody complexes.

It is more sensitive than precipitation and complement fixation test. Fluorescence can be observed under a fluorescence microscope (FM), which contains a high intensity UV light source (mercury lamp) instead of visible light. Two types of filters are fitted in the FM:

1. *Primary filter:* It is fitted close to the lamp. This ensures the maximum emission of radiation (UV light) of the required wavelengths.
2. *Secondary filter:* It is placed in the eyepiece to cut out UV rays which might damage the observer's eye.

Fluorescence-staining techniques are of two types – direct and indirect (Fig. 13.9).

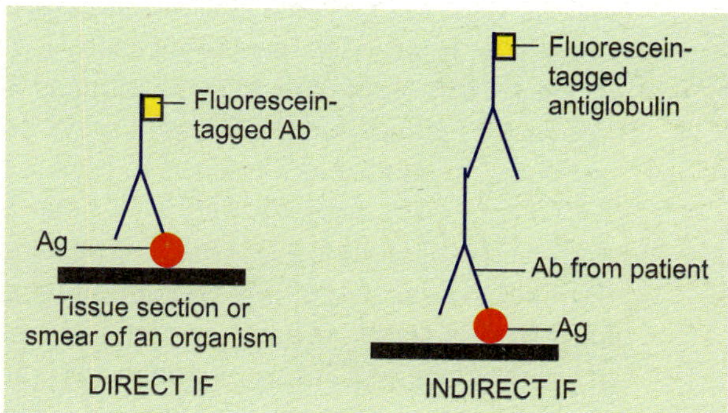

Fig. 13.9. Immunofluorescence.

Direct IF

This consists of bringing fluorescein-tagged antibodies in contact with antigens (bacteria, viruses and other antigens) fixed on a slide (e.g., in the form of a tissue section or a smear of an organism), allowing them to react, washing off excess antibody and examining under FM. The site of union of the labelled antibody with its antigen can be seen by the apple-green fluorescent areas on the slide. Direct IF is routinely used as a sensitive method of diagnosing rabies, by detection of **rabies virus antigens** in brain smears. **A disadvantage of this method is that separate fluorescent conjugates have to be prepared against each antigen to be tested.**

Indirect IF

This method can be used for detection of specific antibodies in sera or other body fluids and also for identifying antigens. The disadvantage of direct IF, mentioned above, is overcome by this method. An example of this method is the **fluorescent treponemal antibody test**

for the diagnosis of syphilis. Here a drop of the patient serum is placed on a smear of *T. pallidum* on a slide and after incubation, the slide is washed well to remove all free serum, leaving behind only antibody, if present, coated on the surface of the treponemes. Whether or not the patient serum contains antibodies to *T. pallidum* is shown by means of a fluorescein-tagged antihuman gammaglobulin (antiglobulin).

If patient serum contains anti-treponemal antibodies fluorescein-tagged antiglobulin will react with it. After washing away all the unbound fluorescent conjugate, when the slide is examined under FM the treponemes will be seen as bright objects against a dark background. If the patient serum is negative for anti-treponemal antibodies, there will be no antibody coating on the treponemes and, therefore, they will not take up the fluorescent conjugate. Therefore, they will not fluoresce. **The advantage of this technique is that a single antihuman gammaglobulin fluorescent conjugate can be employed for detecting human antibody to any antigen.** Indirect IF is also a convenient method for detecting autoantibodies that have bound to membrane antigens, *in vivo*.

The direct method is simple and rapid to perform with fewer nonspecific reactions, however, it is less sensitive. The indirect method is more sensitive and gives brighter fluorescence, however, due to increased cross-reactivity it is less specific.

Q. 10. Explain the procedure and uses of radioimmunoassay.

Ans. RIA is a very sensitive and specific method. It involves the use of either antiserum or more usually antigen labelled with ^{125}I. The amount of radioactive label bound to antigen-antibody complex can be measured, and hence the concentration of antigen or antibody in a specimen can be determined. RIA permits measurement of analytes up to picogram (10^{-12} gram) quantities. It has been used to measure a variety of serum proteins including Igs, hormones, drugs, tumour markers and viral antigens. RIA is based on the competition of radiolabelled, known antigen and unlabelled, unknown antigen for limited binding sites on known specific antibody in solution or attached to a plate or tube (solid phase).

To establish an assay, antibody must be produced against the known antigen and the antigen radiolabelled, e.g., with ^{125}I. A standard curve is established by adding fixed amounts of radiolabelled antigen, specific antibody and increasing concentrations of known unlabelled antigen to a series of tubes or wells in a plastic microtitre plate. Following incubation, the amount of labelled antigen bound to antibody is determined after separation from free labelled antigen in a gamma spectrometer. If a test serum contains antigen for the antibody, then there is competition with labelled antigen. This appears as reduction in the amount of labelled antigen bound in the complex. The concentration of the antigen in the sample can be determined from the standard curve.

Q. 11. Explain the principle of enzyme immunoassay. Discuss methods and uses of various types of enzyme-linked immunosorbent assay.

Ans. Enzyme immunoassay is an important immunological method for detecting and measuring antigens or antibodies. It is based on the same principle as that of radioimmunoassay. The key difference is that for enzyme immunoassays the antigen or antibody is conjugated to an enzyme rather than a radioactive isotope. The enzyme is then detected by its ability to convert a colourless substance to a coloured one. Obviously the method requires that, in the enzyme immunoglobulin conjugate, the enzyme retains its enzymatic activity and the antigen or antibody its immunological activity.

Enzyme immunoassays have become very popular in view of their high sensitivity, safety, economy and the simple instrumentation requirements. Solid-phase immunoassays are more widely used. Such systems are called enzyme-linked immunosorbent assays (ELISAs). The ELISA can be used to detect and determine concentrations of antigen or antibody. The test may be done in polystyrene well (microtitre plate) or tube. Different types of ELISA have been developed (Fig. 13.10).

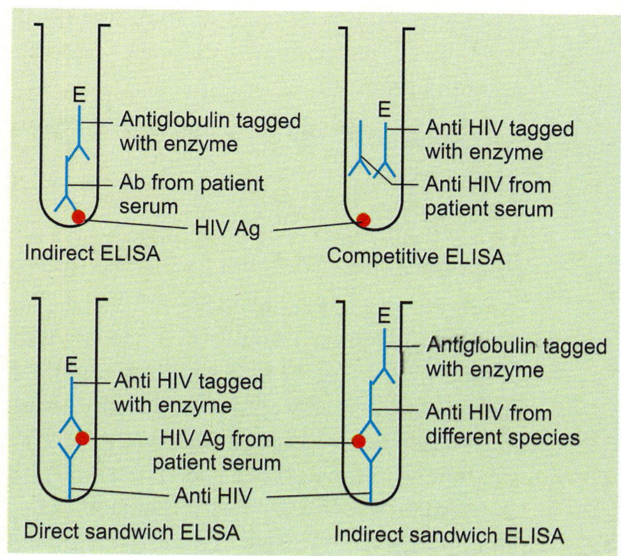

Fig. 13.10. ELISA.

1. Indirect ELISA

The principle of this test can be illustrated by outlining its application for detection of anti-HIV-1 and anti-HIV-2 antibodies in the patient serum. The wells of the polystyrene microtitre plate are coated with purified HIV-1 and HIV-2 antigens or synthetic peptides representing immunodominant epitopes of HIV-1 and HIV-2, which constitutes the solid-phase antigen. Diluted test serum or plasma sample is added to such a well and incubated. If antibodies specific for HIV-1 and/or HIV-2 are present in the test sample they will form stable complexes with antigens coated on the well. Well is then washed and a conjugate of goat antihuman immunoglobulin, which has been labelled with the enzyme horseradish peroxidase, is added. If the antigen-antibody complex is present, the peroxidase conjugate will bind to the complex and remains in the well. The conjugate fraction remaining free in the well is removed by washing and the presence of enzyme immobilized on the complexes is shown by incubation in the presence of a colourless enzyme substrate (ortho-phenylene-diamine dihydrochloride solution). Incubation with enzyme substrate produces a yellow-orange colour in the test well. If the sample contains no anti-HIV-1 and/or anti-HIV-2, then the labelled antibody cannot be found and no colour develops. The absorbance value of each well is read by an ELISA plate reader at wavelength of 492 ± 2 nm.

2. Competitive ELISA

The principle of this test too can be illustrated by outlining its application for detection of anti-HIV antibodies in the patient serum. The wells of the polystyrene microtitre plate are coated with HIV antigens which constitutes the solid-phase antigen. The test sample and human anti-HIV, which has been labelled with the enzyme horseradish peroxidase, are incubated in such a well. When the sample contains no anti-HIV, solid-phase antigen/labelled antibody complex will be formed. The incubation with enzyme substrate produces a yellow-orange colour in the test well. If anti-HIV is present in the test sample, it competes with the labelled antibody for the available solid-phase antigen and no colour or reduced colour develops. Competitive ELISA takes less time than indirect ELISA and no predilution of test serum is required.

3. Sandwich ELISA

The most frequently used ELISA for detecting microbial antigen is the sandwich solid-phase ELISA. It is of two types:

1. Single antibody or direct sandwich ELISA

Antibody is attached to the solid-phase. The test sample is then exposed to the solid-phase antibody, to which the antigen, if present, will bind. The solid-phase antibody-antigen complex is then rinsed free of unbound test sample and exposed again to antibodies reactive against the test antigen and conjugated with the enzyme. The conjugated antibody will react with the antigen held to the solid-phase by the first antibody, forming an antibody-antigen-antibody sandwich on the solid-phase. The solid-phase sandwich is again separated from unreacted test sample by rinsing. The second antibody (conjugated to an enzyme) can be detected with an appropriate substrate. This is a single antibody or direct sandwich ELISA.

2. Double antibody or indirect sandwich ELISA

In the double antibody ELISA the second antibody as above is not conjugated with the enzyme. The second antibody can be detected by treating it with an antiimmunoglobulin-enzyme conjugate. In the double antibody ELISA, the second antibody of the sandwich must be from a different species than the solid-phase antibody, otherwise, the antiimmunoglobulin conjugate reacts with the solid-phase antibody, producing high background activity.

ELISA is a simple and versatile technique. It needs only microlitre quantities of reactants. ELISA kits are commercially available for the detection of anti-HIV, hepatitis B surface antigen and rotavirus. ELISA kits have also been developed for detecting:

- *Entamoeba histolytica* antigens in faeces.
- *Toxoplasma* antigens in the patient serum.
- *Haemophilus influenzae* antigens in spinal fluid.
- β-haemolytic streptococcal antigens in spinal fluid.
- Hepatitis A virus in stools.
- Respiratory syncytial virus in pharyngeal secretions.
- Adenovirus antigens in nasopharyngeal specimens.
- Labile enterotoxin of *Escherichia coli* in stools.

14

Architecture of the Immune System

Q. 1. Describe structure, functions and classification of T and B lymphocytes.

Ans. Of the many cells involved in specific response to antigen, lymphocytes are the most important effector cells. They are small, round, 5–15 μm in diameter and are found in peripheral blood, lymph, lymphoid organs and in many other tissues. In peripheral blood, they constitute 20–40% of the leucocyte population, while in lymph and lymphoid organs they form the predominant cell type. They may be small (5–8 μm), medium (8–12 μm) and large (12–15 μm). The small lymphocytes are most numerous. They may be short-lived (life-span about two weeks) or long-lived (life-span three years or more or even for life). Short-lived cells are effector cells in immune response, while long-lived cells act as memory cells. Long-lived cells are mainly thymus-derived. Lymphopoiesis takes place in the bone marrow, central lymphoid organs and peripheral lymphoid organs.

Lymphocytes possess antigen recognition mechanism on their surface, enabling each cell to recognize only one or a small number of antigens. Two major classes of lymphocytes are recognized which are designated **T cells** and **B cells**. T and B cells are indistinguishable by conventional light microscopy.

Classification of lymphocytes on the basis of surface markers makes use of two important characteristics:

1. Cluster of differentiation or cluster determinant (CD).
2. Antigen recognition receptors.

1. Cluster of differentiation or cluster determinant

CDs represent families of surface glycoprotein antigens that can be recognized by specific antibodies produced against them. Thus a cell displaying CD1 is identified by the binding of antibodies against CD1. Each class of leucocyte displays a diagnostic pattern of CDs, for example:

- CD3 is expressed only by T cells.

- CD19 is expressed only by B cells.
- CD64 is expressed only by monocytes.
- CD66 is expressed only by granulocytes.
- CD68 is expressed only by macrophages.
- On the other hand, CD18 and CD45 are expressed by a variety of leucocyte types.
- A total of more than 150 CDs are known.

2. Antigen recognition receptors

These include membrane-bound (surface) immunoglobulins (mIgs or sIgs) in B cells, and T cell receptors (TCRs) in T cells. In contrast to CDs, which can serve as diagnostic feature for all leucocytes, antigen recognition receptors are limited to B and T lymphocytes only. These receptors are required for B and T cells to be antigen reactive. Both mIgs and TCRs serve as specific surface receptors, recognizing and interacting with only single antigenic determinant on the antigen. Reaction of antigens with mIgs and TCRs activates B cells and T cells respectively, leading to proliferation and differentiation. Thus the antigen specificity of the mIgs in B cells and TCRs in T cells is predetermined, and the sole effect of antigen is to select out a cell with appropriate surface receptor and induce it to clonally expand and differentiate into a cell that will produce the antibody it has been predetermined to make or produce specific clones of effector T cells respectively.

B lymphocytes

Lymphocytes possessing mIgs are termed B cells. They arise from pleuripotent stem cells in bone marrow, they mature in bone marrow itself and then emigrate to the peripheral lymphoid organs where, upon contact with antigen, they can differentiate into antibody-producing **plasma cells**. Antibodies are formed by clonal selection. Each individual has a large pool of different B lymphocytes (about 10^9) that have life-span of days or weeks and are formed in the bone marrow, lymph nodes, and gut-associated lymphoid tissue (e.g., tonsils or appendix). Each B cell possesses about 10^5 mIg molecules, primarily of IgM and IgD classes. Following activation, immunoglobulins of other classes might also reside on B lymphocyte membranes. Immature B cells do not possess mIg receptors.

A single B cell or a clone of B cells possess mIg receptors specific for only one (monospecific) antigenic determinant. Thus billions of B cells display a diversity of receptors capable of reacting with any antigenic determinant that might be encountered. Receptor immunoglobulin and secreted immunoglobulin of a single cell or clone of cells are identical in the variable regions of the antibody molecule.

Most B cells and macrophages, and certain activated T cells express class II major histocompatibility gene products or immune associated (Ia) antigens in the mouse, and HLA-DR antigens in humans. Receptors for the Fc portion of IgG (FcR) are found on all B cells, macrophages and certain subsets of T cells. Some cells express receptors for other classes of immunoglobulin as well. These receptors bind antigen-antibody complexes. Receptors for C3 component of complement are found on most B cells. These are known as complement receptors (CRs). These receptors are thought to play a role in the regulation of the B cell response to antigen. Because of the presence of CRs on the surface of B cells they bind to sheep RBCs which have been coated with antibody and complement forming EAC rosettes. They undergo blast transformation on treatment with bacterial endotoxins.

T lymphocytes

Pleuripotent stem cells in the bone marrow give rise to precursor T cells, which migrate to the thymus (Fig. 14.1). Once they enter the cortex of the thymus they are known as **thymocytes**. As T cells mature, their surface antigens including CDs and TCRs change. Monoclonal antibodies are used to identify the antigenic subsets of T cells. Approximately 65% of mature T cells that leave the thymus display CD2+CD3+CD4+CD8–TCR+ phenotype (CD4+ cells), while approximately 35% display CD2+ CD3+CD4–CD8+TCR+ phenotype

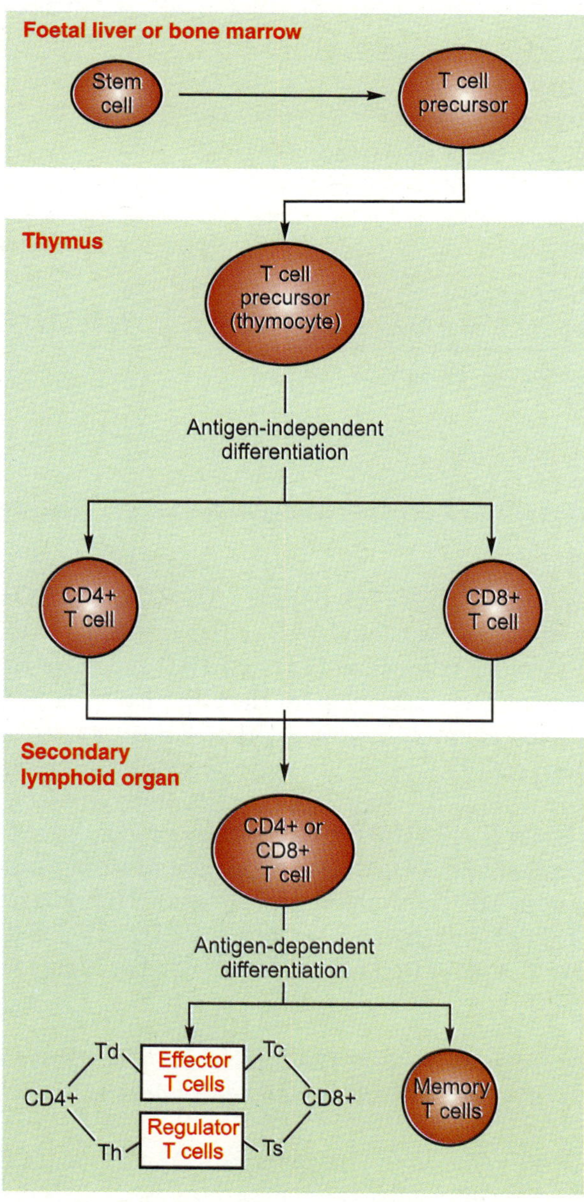

Fig. 14.1. T cell differentiation.

(CD8+ cells). A very small number express neither CD4 nor CD8 and consequently have a phenotype of CD2+CD3+ CD4–CD8–TCR+ (CD4–CD8– cells).

Q. 2. Tabulate differences between T and B cells.

Ans. Differences between T and B cells are given in Table 14.1.

Table 14.1. Differences between T and B lymphocytes

Property	T cell	B cell
Antigen recognition receptors	TCRs	mIgs
Surface glycoprotein antigens	CD3	CD19
Receptors for Fc piece of immunoglobulins (FcR)	–*	+
Receptors for C3 component of complement (CRs)	–	+
EAC rosette	–	+
E rosette	+	–
Thymus specific antigens	+	–
Blast transformation on treatment with	PHA and Con A	Bacterial endotoxins

*Certain subsets of T cells possess FcR

Q. 3. Describe briefly T cell subsets.

Ans. Four distinct subsets of T cells are known. Two each of these are regulator and effector cells.

Regulator cells

1. *Helper T cells (Th cells):* They possess CD2, CD3 and CD4 surface antigens. They help in the antigen-specific activation of B cells and effector T cells. Th cells have two different profiles of cytokine production (Th1 and Th2) and these patterns select between the two basic types of response mediated by Th cells. Th1 cytokines include interferon-γ (IFN-γ), IFN-β, and interleukin-2 (IL-2) and Th1 cells are involved in cell-mediated inflammatory reactions. Several Th1 cytokines activate cytotoxic inflammatory and delayed hypersensitivity reactions. By contrast, Th2 cells are typified by the production of IL-4 to 6, IL-9, IL-10 and IL-13. Th2 cells encourage production of antibody especially IgE, and Th2 cytokines are associated with regulation of strong antibody and allergic responses. Cytokines from Th1 cells inhibit the actions of Th2 cells and vice versa.
2. *Suppressor T cells (Ts cells):* They possess CD2, CD3 and CD8 surface antigens. They suppress expression of immune response by other lymphocytes.

Effector cells

1. *Delayed-type-hypersensitivity T cells (Td cells):* They possess CD2, CD3 and CD4 surface antigens. They are involved in delayed hypersensitivity and cell-mediated immune responses.
2. *Cytotoxic T cells (Tc cells):* They possess CD2, CD3 and CD8 surface antigens. They are also involved in cell-mediated immune responses and lyse target cells by direct cell-cell contact.

Immune response is regulated by mutually opposing influence of Th and Ts cells. **Overactivity of Th or decreased activity of Ts causes abnormal immune responses as seen in autoimmunity. Diminished Th function or increased activity of Ts leads to immunodeficiency.**

During maturation and differentiation in thymus, T cells also learn to recognize self-major histocompatibility (MHC) antigens. CD4+ cells recognize class II MHC antigens and CD8+ cells recognize class I MHC antigens.

T cells bind to sheep RBCs at 37°C forming SRBC or E rosettes while B cells do not. They undergo blast transformation, evidenced by enhanced DNA synthesis, on treatment with mitogens such as phytohaemagglutinin (PHA) and concanavalin A (Con A).

Q. 4. What are null cells? Describe briefly various types of null cells.

Ans. Null cells

A small proportion (5%) of lymphocytes that lack distinguishing phenotypic markers characteristic of T or B lymphocytes are known as null cells or non-T and non-B lymphocytes. They do not possess TCRs or mIgs. A few null cells in the circulation might be immature T or B cells.

Types

Killer cells or K cells

A subpopulation of null cells possess surface receptors for Fc part of IgG. They are capable of lysing or killing target cells sensitized by IgG antibody. They are known as killer or K cells. **They are responsible for antibody-dependent cell-mediated cytotoxicity (ADCC) in contrast to the action of cytotoxic T lymphocytes which are independent of antibody.**

Natural killer or NK cells

Another subpopulation of null cells is natural killer or NK cells. These are large lymphocytes containing azurophilic granules in the cytoplasm. They are, therefore, known as large granular lymphocytes (LGL). **NK cells are capable of non-specific killing of virus-transformed target cells and are involved in allograft and tumour rejection.** They differ from K cells in being independent of antibody.

15

Immune Response

Q. 1. Discuss primary and secondary immune responses.

Ans. **Primary humoral response**

Phases

Antibody production follows characteristic phases (Fig. 15.1):

1. **Lag phase:** After first injection of the antigen there is a long lag phase of several days before antibody appears. The lag phase depends upon the kind and amount of antigen given, the route of administration, species of animal and its health.
2. **Log phase:** As the lag period ends, the titre of antibody gradually increases over a period of a few days to a few weeks.
3. **Plateau or steady state:** There is equilibrium between antibody production and catabolism.
4. **Phase of decline:** Catabolism exceeds the production of antibody and the titre falls.

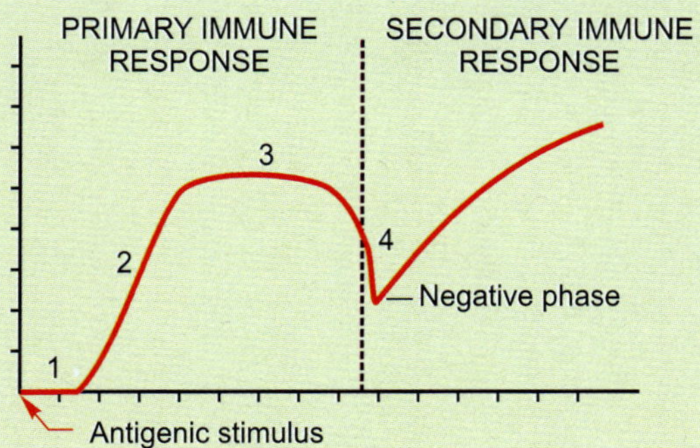

Fig. 15.1. Immune response.

Secondary humoral response

If the same animal is subsequently exposed to the same antigen there occurs a temporary fall in the level of antibodies due to the combination of the antigen with pre-existing antibody. This is known as **negative phase**. After two to three days a marked increase in antibody level becomes evident. This goes on increasing for several days thus exceeding the initial level. This is also known as **booster response**. The booster response is attributed to the persistence of antigen sensitive 'memory cells' following the primary response.

The antibody formed in primary response is predominantly IgM and in secondary response IgG. The first dose is known as **priming dose** and subsequent injection as **booster dose**. Both these doses are particularly essential in case of killed vaccines. *With live vaccines a single dose is usually sufficient as multiplication of organisms in the body provides a continuing antigenic stimulus that acts both as priming and booster doses.*

Q. 2. Comment on fate of antigen in tissues.

Ans. Antigens introduced subcutaneously are mainly localized in the draining lymph nodes, only a small amount being found in the spleen. On the other hand, antigens introduced intravenously are rapidly localized in the spleen, liver, bone marrow, kidneys and lungs. 70–80% of these are broken down by reticuloendothelial (R.E.) cells and excreted in the urine.

Q. 3. Describe production of antibodies, and T and B cell activation.

Ans. *Antigen processing and presentation*

Antigens are presented to **immunocompetent cells (ICCs)** by antigen-presenting cells (APCs) (macrophages and dendritic cells). With many antigens (T cell dependent antigens such as proteins and erythrocytes), processing by macrophages is prerequisite for antibody formation. But for T cell independent antigens, such as polysaccharides, antibody production does not require T cell participation. APC can ingest antigen, degrade it and present it to T cell. T cell is able to recognize only when the processed antigen is presented on the surface of APC, in association with MHC molecules to the T cell carrying the T cell receptor (TCR) for the epitope.

The antigen has to be presented complexed with MHC class II in case of CD4 (helper T/Th) cells and for CD8 (cytotoxic T/Tc) cells with MHC class I molecules.

T and B cell activation

The activation of Th cell requires two signals for activation. The first signal is a combination of the TCR with the MHC class II-complexed antigen. The second signal is interleukin-1 (IL-1) which is produced by the APC. The activated Th cell produces IL-2 and other cytokines required for B cell stimulation. These include IL-4, IL-5 and IL-6 which act as B cell growth factor (BCGF) and B cell differentiation factor (BCDF). They activate B cells which have combined with their respective antigens to clonally proliferate and differentiate into antibody secreting plasma cells. A small proportion of B cells, instead of being transformed into plasma cells, become long-lived memory cells producing a secondary type of response to subsequent contact with the antigen. B cells carry surface receptors which consist of IgM or other immunoglobulin classes. A plasma cell secretes an antibody of a single specificity of a single antibody class (IgM, IgG or any other single class). However, in primary humoral response, plasma cells secrete IgM and later switch over to form IgG.

CD8 (cytotoxic T/Tc) cells are activated when they come into contact with antigens presented along with MHC class I molecules. They also need a second signal IL-2, which is secreted by activated Th cells. On contact with a target cell carrying the antigen on its surface, the activated Tc cells release cytokines that destroy the target, which may be virus infected or tumour cells. Some T cells also become memory cells.

Q. 4. Describe briefly clonal selection theory of antibody production.

Ans. This theory was proposed by Burnet (1957). This theory states that during immunological development a large number of lymphocytes capable of reacting with different antigens are formed. Cells with immunological reactivity with self-antigens are eliminated during embryonic life. Such clones are known as **forbidden clones**. *Their persistence or development in the later life leads to autoimmunity*. Each ICC is capable of reacting with one antigen. Contact with specific antigen leads to cellular proliferation to form clones which synthesize antibodies. This theory is more widely accepted than other theories.

Q. 5. Discuss principle, technique and applications of monoclonal antibodies.

Ans. *Principle*

If an antigen is injected into an animal, the latter produces different types of antibodies against various epitopes of the antigen. The antibodies thus generated are polyclonal in nature. This means different clones of antibody secreting cells are simultaneously synthesizing the antibody. Different molecules will have different specificities and affinities. In all microbial infections, body reacts with polyclonal antibody production. When these polyclonal antisera are used in bacterial test systems, **cross-reactivity** often occurs.

A single antibody-forming cell or clone produces antibodies directed against specific epitope of the antigen. Such antibodies produced by a single clone and directed against a single antigenic determinant are called **monoclonal antibodies (MCA)**. In nature, MCA are produced in multiple myeloma where only one clone secretes a particular type of antibody. MCA can be generated in the laboratory. The theory of MCA production is based on clonal selection hypothesis of Burnet (1959) and the method for production of MCA was described by Kohler and Milstein in 1975, for which they were awarded Nobel Prize for Medicine in 1984.

The main breakthrough was not that a single line of monoclonal antibody producing cells could be isolated, but rather that the mouse splenic lymphocytes could be fused with mouse myeloma cells to produce **hybrid cells (hybridoma)**. Among the two cell types chosen for fusion, one provides the hybrid cell immortality (**myeloma cell**) while the other (**splenic plasma cell**) provides the antibody producing capacity. Such hybridomas can be maintained indefinitely in culture and continue to form MCA.

Technique

- Lymphocytes from the spleen of a mouse immunized with desired antigen are fused with mouse myeloma cells grown in culture which is deficient in the enzyme hypoxanthine phosphoribosyl transferase (HPRT) (Fig. 15.2).

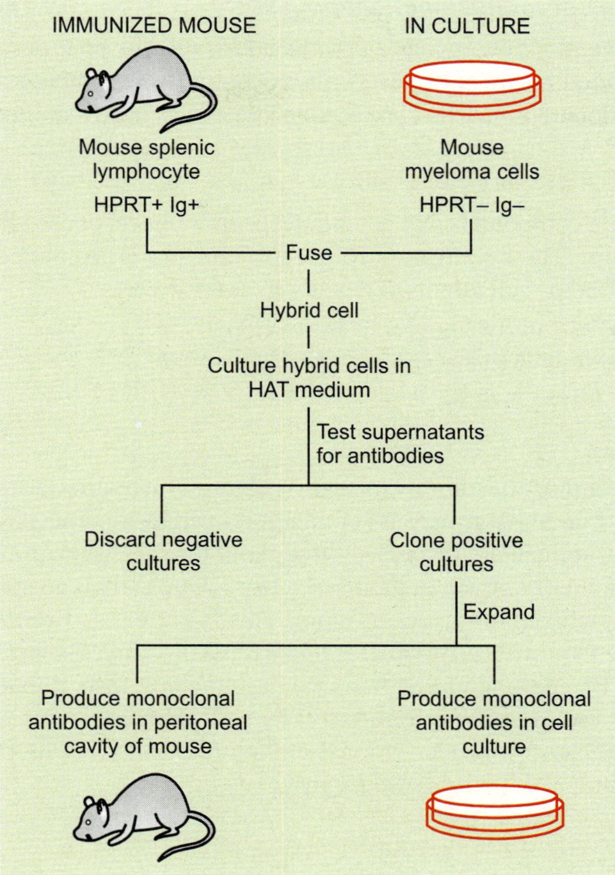

Fig. 15.2. Production of monoclonal antibodies.

- The fused cells are placed in a basal culture medium containing hypoxanthine, aminopterin and thymidine (HAT medium).
- Only hybrid cells possessing properties of both the splenic lymphocytes (HPRT+) and myeloma cells (HPRT–) can grow in culture. Normal lymphocytes cannot replicate indefinitely and unfused myeloma cells are killed by the aminopterin in HAT medium.
- The peritoneal cavity of mice, preferably of the same strain that was used for initial immunization step, can be used to grow the selected hybrid cell clone. First the peritoneal cavity is injected with an organic irritant such as pristane to produce chemical peritonitis. Next the selected hybrid cell line is injected into the peritoneal cavity. Within days, a tumour known as hybridoma develops. This tumour produces large quantities of MCA that can be harvested by aspirating ascitic fluid from mouse's peritoneal cavity.
- A tumour-bearing mouse will survive for 4–6 weeks, during which time large quantities of antibody can be recovered.
- Hybridomas can also be grown in tissue cultures where highly purified antibodies are produced without contamination from serum, ascites proteins or the cross-reactivity of histocompatibility antibodies derived from mouse tissues.

Applications of monoclonal antibodies

Monoclonal antibodies have been produced for specific epitopes of a wide variety of viruses, bacteria (including mycobacteria), parasites and fungi. Many of the commercial systems using direct fluorescence and enzyme-linked assays utilize monoclonal antibody conjugates.

Q. 6. Write short note on adjuvants.

Ans. Adjuvants are compounds that potentiate the immune response when mixed and administered with antigens. They contribute to greater and more prolonged antibody production and increased effector cell counts. They act in several ways:

1. Sustained release of antigen from the depot.
2. Stimulate lymphocytes nonspecifically.
3. Activate macrophages.

Types of adjuvants

- **Depot:** A number of substances such as aluminium hydroxide or phosphate and an aqueous solution of an antigen may be emulsified in light mineral oil so that tiny water droplets containing antigen are dispersed throughout the oil (water-in-oil emulsion). The emulsion forms a depot of antigen in the tissues from which small quantities of antigen are released slowly sometimes for a year or more. This is known as **Freund's incomplete adjuvant**.
- **Complete Freund's adjuvant:** It possesses killed mycobacteria in addition to incomplete adjuvant. Besides increasing humoral immune response, it induces high degree of cellular immunity (delayed hypersensitivity) as well. However, this adjuvant cannot be used in humans, because it produces local granuloma, and must be replaced by other adjuvants such as alum or killed *Bordetella pertussis*.

Q. 7. Describe briefly immunosuppressive agents.

Ans. Immunosuppressive agents are those which inhibit the immune response of macrophages, and B and T lymphocytes leading to lowered capacity to phagocytosis or to produce immunoglobulins and lymphokines. Organ and bone marrow transplantation became practicable on a large-scale only after powerful immunosuppressive drugs became available. They may also be used to control autoimmune responses or to prevent allergic reactions.

A wide range of physical, chemical and biologic agents have been tried (Table 15.1). Some of these were soon dropped because the margin of safety was too small and toxic effects too pronounced.

- **X-irradiation** is more cytotoxic to replicating cells and has been used to prolong transplant survival and to control certain autoimmune conditions.
- Corticosteroids and cyclosporine impair maturation of activated cells by suppressing production of interleukins (ILs). Corticosteroids are antiinflammatory drugs that diminish the responsiveness of both B and T cell pools. They can inhibit production of IL-1 and IL-2. Prolonged use of corticosteroids may lead to hypertension, bone necrosis, cataract and mental disturbances.
- Cyclosporine has been widely used as an immunosuppressant in organ transplantation. It causes immune suppression by inhibiting the production of IL-2. It may have adverse side-effects affecting the liver and kidney.

Table 15.1. Immunosuppressive agents

A. PHYSICAL AGENTS
- X-irradiation
- Surgery

B. CHEMICAL AGENTS
- *Alkylating agents*
  - Cyclophosphamide
  - Nitrogen mustard
- *Corticosteroids*
- *Antimetabolites*
  - Folic acid antagonists (methotrexate)
  - Analogues of purine (6-mercaptopurine and azathioprine)
  - Cytosine
  - Uracil (5-fluorouracil)
- *Miscellaneous*
  - Cyclosporine

C. BIOLOGICAL AGENTS
- Antilymphocytic serum

- **Cytotoxic drugs**, such as azathioprine or cyclophosphamide, act on various stages of nucleic acid synthesis preventing replication of active lymphocytes. Azathioprine, used in renal transplant, inhibits T cells, but not B cell responses. Cyclophosphamide, used in bone marrow recipients, selectively prevents B cell replication.

T cell population can be depleted by use of antilymphocytic serum produced in horses. This destroys body's T cell pool but leaves antibody production intact. Unfortunately, it also reduces the ability of the body to fight viral infection.

Q. 8. Describe cell-mediated immune responses.

Ans. Cell-mediated immunity (CMI) normally refers to specific acquired immunity, which is accomplished by effector T cells and macrophages rather than B cells and antibodies. This includes allograft rejection, delayed hypersensitivity (DH) and cytotoxic reactions against intracellular parasites. As in case of antibody-mediated immune response, cell-mediated immune response can also be divided into primary and secondary cell-mediated immune responses.

Primary cell-mediated immune response

This is produced by initial contact with a foreign antigen. Foreign antigen is presented by antigen-presenting cells (APCs) to T cells leading to their activation. T cells possess antigen recognition receptors known as T cell receptors (TCRs) that recognize foreign antigen and a self-MHC molecule on the surface of the APC (Fig. 15.3). Because of the specificity of the TCRs only particular cells become activated. These cells proliferate and produce specific clones of effector T cells (Th, Tc, Td and Ts). Cell-mediated immune response develops after several days of antigenic challenge.

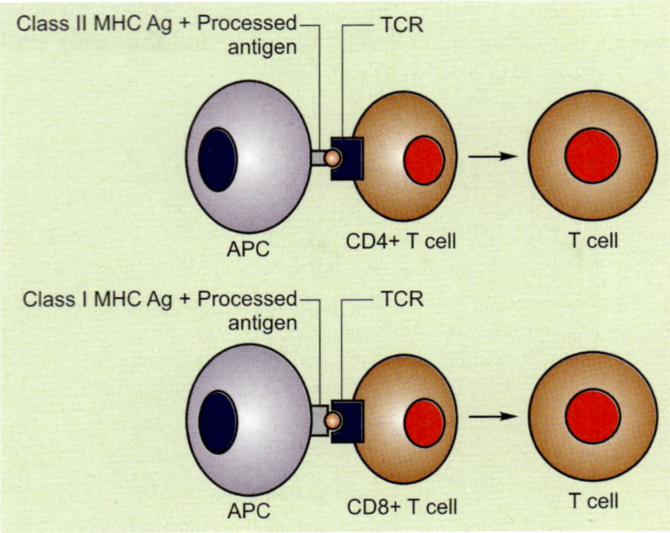

Fig. 15.3. Cell-mediated immune response.

Secondary cell-mediated immune response

If the same host is subsequently exposed to the same antigen, then the secondary cell-mediated immune response is usually more pronounced and occurs more rapidly. Because of the availability of specific memory cells, an increased number of effector cells are produced.

T cell differentiation

APCs, such as macrophages, phagocytose the antigen and degrade it. Subsequently, portions of antigen become associated with MHC antigens and are expressed on APCs surface. Two modes of processing are known (Fig. 15.3):

- One mode is seen in case of processing of phagocytosed material such as bacteria. The antigenic material dissociated from the bacteria is associated with class II MHC molecules probably within the phagosome. MHC-antigen complex then expresses on the surface of the APC.
- Second mode is seen in processing antigens derived within the cell, for example, viral antigens synthesized in infected cell. However, this antigenic determinant associates with class I MHC molecule probably in the endoplasmic reticulum. MHC-antigen complex then expresses on the surface of the APC.

CD8+ cells recognize the combination of foreign antigen and class I MHC antigen and differentiate into Tc and Ts lymphocytes while CD4+ cells recognize the combination of antigen and class II MHC antigen and differentiate into Th and Td cells.

Lysis of target cell

Tc cell recognizes foreign antigen and class I MHC antigen and gets attached to the target cell expressing these on their surface. This stimulates Tc cells to release **cytolysins**. This leads to calcium-dependent lysis of the target cell. Subsequently, the Tc cell can detach from the target cell and repeat this process with another. Recognition of target cells also stimulates Tc cells to synthesize and secrete **interferon-γ**, and thus they probably also contribute to some extent to macrophage activation.

Q. 9. What are cytokines? Name biological activities of cytokines.

Ans. These are biologically active substances produced by cells that influence other cells. They are referred to as **lymphokines** if they are derived from lymphocytes and **monokines** if they are derived from monocytes and macrophages. Interleukins are a family of cytokines that function primarily as growth and differentiation factors. Cytokines have been named based on the biological effects they produce. Various cytokines are given in Table 15.2.

Q. 10. Write short note on transfer factor.

Ans. Lawrence (1954) reported transfer of CMI in man by injection of extract from the leucocytes from immunized individual. The extract from the leucocytes contains a soluble factor called transfer factor (TF). The transferred immunity is specific in that CMI can be transferred only to those antigens to which the donor is sensitive.

TF is a nucleopeptide with a molecular weight of 2,000–4,000 daltons. It is non-antigenic. It is resistant to trypsin but gets inactivated by heating at 56°C in 30 minutes. The mode of action of TF is not known. It appears to stimulate the release of lymphokines from sensitized T lymphocytes. It does not promote antibody synthesis. TF has been used in patients with:

- T cell deficiency (Wiskott-Aldrich syndrome).
- Disseminated infections associated with deficient CMI (lepromatous leprosy, tuberculosis and mucocutaneous candidiasis).
- Malignant melanoma and other types of cancer.

Q. 11. Describe briefly immunological tolerance.

Ans. Immunological tolerance may be defined as a state of unresponsiveness to specific antigens. This unresponsiveness is specific to antigens to which the individual is tolerant. Response to other antigens is unaffected. Two forms of tolerance can be identified – natural tolerance and acquired tolerance.

Natural tolerance

It is nonresponsiveness to self-antigens. This arises during foetal development, when the immune system is being formed and maturing. If this tolerance breaks down and body responds to self molecules then an autoimmune disease will develop. Dizygotic cattle twins, which are genetically dissimilar, share the same placental circulation in utero. As adults, each twin fails to mount immune response to histocompatibility antigens on the cells of the other twin. Thus they accept transplants from each other. This could be accounted for by induction of specific immunological tolerance during foetal life. Based on this observation of Owen (1945), Burnet and Fenner (1949) suggested that the unresponsiveness of individuals to self-antigens was due to the contact of the immature immunological system with self-antigens during embryonic life.

Table 15.2. Source and activity of cytokines

Cytokine	Source	Biological activity
Macrophage stimulating factor (MSF)	Td cells	Stimulates macrophage migration to the site of action
Macrophage activating factor (MAF)	Td cells	Restricts macrophage movement and increases phagocytic activity
Migration inhibiting factor (MIF)	Td cells	Inhibits migration of macrophages
Chemotactic factor (CF)	Td cells	Stimulates chemotaxis of macrophages
Interferon-gamma (IFN-γ)	Th, Td and NK cells	Increases cytotoxicity of NK cells and macrophages
Interleukin-1 (IL-1)	NK cells, APCs, B cells and T cells	Promotes growth and expression of fibroblasts, NK cells, B cells and T cells
Interleukin-2 (IL-2)	Th cells	Promotes B cell differentiation and T cell growth
Interleukin-3 (IL-3)	Th cells	Acts as a growth factor for bone marrow stem cell
Interleukin-4 (IL-4)	Th cells	Acts as a growth factor for macrophages, mast cells, B cells and T cells
Interleukin-5 (IL-5)	Th cells	Promotes B cell growth, antibody production and maturation of eosinophils
Interleukin-6 (IL-6)	Macrophages	Promotes B cell growth
Interleukin-7 (IL-7)	Bone marrow stroma cell	Stimulates B cell and T cell proliferation
Interleukin-8 (IL-8)	Mononuclear cells, endothelial cells and skin fibroblasts.	Stimulates chemotaxis of neutrophils and T cells
Interleukin-9 (IL-9)	Activated T cells	Stimulates proliferation of IL-3 dependent myeloid cells and mast cells
Interleukin-10 (IL-10)	Th cells	Inhibits production of IFN and mononuclear cell functions
Interleukin-11 (IL-11)	Bone marrow and stromal cells	Induces acute phase proteins
Interleukin-12 (IL-12)	T cells	Activates natural killer (NK) cells
Interleukin-13 (IL-13)	T cells	Inhibits mononuclear cell functions
Interleukin-14 (IL-14)	T cells	Stimulates proliferation of activated B cells, inhibits immunoglobulin production
Interleukin-15 (IL-15)	Monocytes	Proliferation of T cells and activated B cells
Interleukin-16 (IL-16)	Eosinophils, CD8+ T cells	Chemoattraction of CD4+ T cells
Interleukin-17 (IL-17)	CD4+ T cells	Release of IL-6, IL-8
Interleukin-18 (IL-18)	Hepatocytes	Induces production of interferon-γ, enhances NK cell activity

Any antigen that comes into contact with the immunological system during its embryonic life would be recognised as a self-antigen and would not induce any immune response. They postulated that tolerance could be induced against foreign antigens if they were administered during embryonic life. Medawar and his colleagues (1953) proved it experimentally. When skin graft from one inbred strain of mice (CBA) is applied on a mouse of another strain (A), it is rejected. But if CBA cells are injected into foetal or newborn A strain mice, the latter when grow up will freely accept skin grafts from CBA mice.

Certain strains of mice that are genetically deficient in the C5 complement component make vigorous antibody response when immunized with pure C5 taken from normal animals. Normal animals (which are not deficient in C5) do not respond to similar immunization.

Acquired tolerance

It arises when a potential immunogen induces a state of unresponsiveness to itself. This has consequences for host defences since the presence of a tolerogenic epitope on a pathogen may compromise the ability of the body to resist infection. For acquired tolerance to be maintained the tolerogen must persist or be repeatedly administered. This is probably necessary because of the continuous production of new B and T cells that must be rendered tolerant.

A number of factors influence the induction of tolerance. These include species and immunocompetence of the host, physical nature, dose, and route of administration of antigen. Rabbits and mice can be rendered tolerant more rapidly than guinea-pigs and chickens. Higher the degree of immunocompetence of the host, the more difficult it is to induce tolerance. Therefore, embryos and newborns are particularly susceptible for induction of tolerance.

It is easier to induce tolerance to a soluble macromolecule than to an aggregated antigen. For example, when human gammaglobulin is heat aggregated, it is highly immunogenic in mice, but when de-aggregated it is tolerogenic. This is probably due to the fact that aggregated antigens are readily phagocytosed by macrophages, where they can be presented to antibody-forming cells thus inducing antibody synthesis. On the other hand, soluble antigens are not so easily processed and may be more effective in inducing the Ts suppressor circuit.

The induction of tolerance is dose-dependent. Generally high doses of antigen tolerize B cells, while minute doses given repeatedly tolerize T cells. A moderate dose of the same antigen might be immunogenic. The route of administration is also important. Intravenously administered antigens have faster contact with more cells at the highest concentration of tolerogen. Moreover, an intravenous injection rapidly reaches the spleen to which Ts cells migrate leading to tolerance.

Tolerance can be overcome spontaneously or by injection of cross-reacting immunogens. For example, tolerance to bovine serum albumin in rabbits can be abolished by immunization with cross-reacting human serum albumin.

16

Hypersensitivity and Autoimmunity

Q. 1. Define hypersensitivity. Classify hypersensitivity reactions. Discuss in detail type I hypersensitivity.

Ans. Hypersensitivity is an abnormal immune response which produces physiological or histo-pathological damage in the host. It may be divided into five types:

Type I	Anaphylactic
Type II	Cytotoxic
Type III	Immune complex
Type IV	Cell-mediated or delayed
Type V	Stimulatory or antireceptor

Type I, II, III and V hypersensitivity depend on the interaction of antigen with humoral antibodies and are known as immediate type reactions, although some are more immediate than others. Immediate hypersensitivity reactions develop in less than 24 hours after reexposure to an antigen. Type IV hypersensitivity or delayed hypersensitivity is mediated by T lymphocytes. Delayed hypersensitivity reactions develop in 24–48 hours.

Type I hypersensitivity: Anaphylactic

It is **mediated by IgE antibody** and is due to the powerful effects of histamine and other vasoactive amines. Hypersensitivity may be local or generalized, depending upon the amount of histamine released, the site of its release and route of stimulating antigen. Generally, small amount of antigen administered to mucous membrane or skin will induce local anaphylaxis, whereas larger amounts may induce a generalized reaction and antigen administered systemically may cause generalized anaphylaxis. Local anaphylaxis is exemplified by such conditions as hay fever and asthma. Systemic anaphylaxis is a shocklike condition that can occur in individuals who are intensely allergic to such things as bee venom, penicillin and horse serum.

Mechanism of type I hypersensitivity

In order to produce type I hypersensitivity an individual must first come in contact with an antigen and produce IgE antibodies. These antibodies bind to mast cells and basophils (Fig. 16.1). Basophils are found in the circulation while mast cells (or fixed basophils) are located in lymphoid regions of respiratory tract, gastrointestinal tract, reproductive tract, skin and lining of blood vessels including capillaries. They have large number of vesicles containing pharmacologically potent compounds like histamine and serotonin.

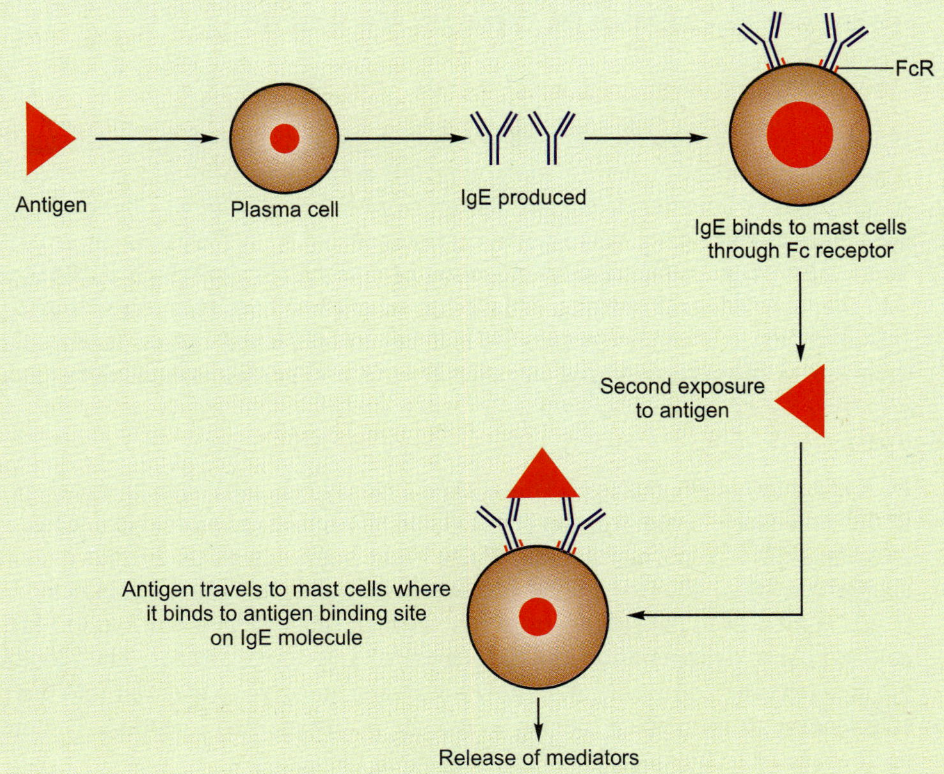

Fig. 16.1. Antigen-induced mediator release from mast cell.

Thus **after first exposure** allergen-specific IgE is fixed to the mast cells and basophils, thereby sensitizing them. The part of the IgE molecule that binds to the surface of mast cells and basophils is the Fc portion. These cells possess high affinity receptors specific for Fc portion of IgE antibodies. Thus Fab portion of IgE remains exposed. IgE antibodies can remain attached on these cells for up to six weeks. Such an individual is said to be **sensitized**.

After a second exposure the allergen travels to the mast cells and basophils, where it binds to antigen-binding site on IgE molecule. Antigen-antibody binding triggers the process of degranulation through which the mast cell explosively discharges its pharmacologically active agents. These include histamine, serotonin, bradykinin, slow-reacting substance of anaphylaxis (SRS-A), platelet-activating factors, eosinophil chemotactic factor of anaphylaxis and prostaglandins.

Q. 2. Write short note on cutaneous anaphylaxis.

Ans. If a person is suspected to be allergic to a particular substance, a **skin test** can be done. In this test a small dose of allergen is injected intradermally. In less than 30 minutes results can be read. If the individual is allergic there will be a **wheal and flare response** at the site of injection. Wheal is a pale central area of puffiness due to oedema (caused by increased capillary permeability) which is surrounded by flare (caused by hyperaemia due to vaso-dilation). Since the injection site is small, it is possible to test for hypersensitivity to hundreds of substances on a person's back. The wheal and flare response can be used to determine the specific substance to which the atopic person is sensitive.

Q. 3. Describe briefly Prausnitz–Kustner (PK) reaction.

Ans. Prausnitz and Kustner in 1921 demonstrated transmission of IgE-mediated type I hyper-sensitivity by injecting serum containing IgE antibodies from allergic person into the skin of a normal or nonallergic person. Serum from Kustner, who was hypersensitive to certain species of cooked fish, was injected intracutaneously in Prausnitz (normal) followed 24 hours later by an intracutaneous injection of cooked fish, to which Kustner was sensitive, into the same site in Prausnitz. This led to wheal and flare reaction within 20 minutes. As IgE antibody is homocytotropic, the test has to be carried out on human skin, therefore, there is risk of transmission of hepatitis B virus and human immunodeficiency virus.

Q. 4. Write short note on passive cutaneous anaphylaxis.

Ans. PCA is similar to PK reaction. This is used to assay IgE antibodies in experimental animals. In this procedure, serum from an anaphylactically sensitized animal is injected intradermally into the skin of a normal animal. Forty eight hours later this animal is challenged with allergen (to which the first animal was sensitive) and Evans blue dye, injected intravenously. If IgE is present in the serum (from first animal), the allergen will bind to IgE on the mast cell and cause degranulation and the release of vasoactive amines. The blood capillaries in the area become permeable and allow the Evans blue dye to leak out into the dermis of the skin leading to immediate blueing at the site of intradermal injection. The area of blueing can be related to the quantity of IgE present in the serum.

Q. 5. Write short note on anaphylaxis *in vitro*.

Ans. In 1910, Schultz and Dale demonstrated that sensitized strips of smooth muscle contract, *in vitro*, following exposure to antigen. Thus intestinal and uterine muscle strips from a sensitized animal (guinea-pig) held in Ringer's solution bath contract vigorously on addition of specific antigen. Smooth muscle strips can be passively sensitized by bathing them in serum from a hypersensitive animal. The actual test is done by adding the antigen and observing subsequent contractions.

Q. 6. Give detailed description of atopy.

Ans. The term atopy refers to chronic human allergic states. These include **hay fever**, **allergic asthma**, **atopic dermatitis (urticaria)** and **food allergies**. The antigens commonly involved in atopy are inhalants (pollen, house dust, animal dander or other types of fine particles suspended in air) or ingestants (milk, milk products, eggs, meat, fish or cereal). Some of them are contact allergens, to which the skin and conjunctiva may be exposed. The mechanism of development of atopy is essentially the same as that of systemic anaphylaxis. Atopy is likely to develop when allergen is localized or absorbed slowly, on the other hand systemic anaphylaxis is likely to develop if large quantities of allergen are quickly distributed throughout the body.

Hay fever (allergic rhinitis)

It is an IgE-mediated allergic reaction that affects the mucosal surfaces of upper respiratory tract. It leads to nasal congestion, headache, running nose, watery eyes, itching and sneezing. The specific stimuli that cause allergic rhinitis include antigenic components of grass, weed and tree pollens, dust, mites, animal dander, organic dusts, components of tobacco smoke, and noninfectious components of fungal and bacterial allergens. If the allergen cannot be removed, then antihistaminics are the pharmacological agents of choice for the treatment of allergic rhinitis since histamine seems to be the major mediator of this allergy.

Allergic asthma

It is a severe form of respiratory allergy. It leads to contraction of the trachea and bronchi. The specific stimuli that cause allergic asthma include airborne allergens. In addition, asthma-producing foods such as milk, milk products, eggs, meat, fish or cereal may also precipitate allergic asthma. Some patients may even be sensitive to normal microbial flora leading to endogenous asthma. The main mediators of this allergy are serotonin and SRS-A. Therefore, antihistaminics are not able to reverse the smooth muscle contraction. The drug of choice for the treatment of this allergy is adrenaline (epinephrine). It is dispensed as atomizers for quick delivery. In addition, corticosteroids and cromolyn sodium have proved beneficial in treating attacks of allergic asthma.

Atopic dermatitis (urticaria)

Allergic skin eruptions in the form of wheals (whitish swelling), hives (red lesions), or eczema (scaly sores) may develop from varied sources such as foods, drugs, chemicals and clothing materials. Avoidance of these is the treatment. If it is not possible then antihistaminics are indicated.

Food allergies

Food allergy occurs in infants and children, but is uncommon in adults. Certain foods such as eggs, milk, peanuts, seafoods, citrus fruits and chocolate are frequent causes of food allergy. Consumption of the food in a patient with food allergy leads to nausea, vomiting, diarrhoea and cramps with typical urticaria and wheezing or upper airways congestion. Best cure for food allergy is to avoid that food unless it is a common ingredient of prepared foods such as flour.

Q. 7. Describe mechanism of type II hypersensitivity. Describe briefly clinical examples of type II hypersensitivity.

Ans. This involves the combination of IgG and IgM serum antibodies with foreign antigenic components on a cell surface. Alternatively, a free foreign antigen or hapten such as a drug or microbial product may be adsorbed onto a cell membrane, which subsequently combines with antibody. Two different antibody-dependent mechanisms are involved in this type of hypersensitivity.

1. Complement-mediated cytotoxicity

Some of the cytotoxic reactions are complement dependent. After the antibodies become membrane bound, complement may be activated. Activation of classical complement pathway leads to the lysis of the cell through generation of membrane attack complex (MAC) (Fig. 12.1). Activation of complement cascade also leads to the formation of C3a and C5a fragments. These fragments are chemotactic for phagocytic cells. Fab portions of the antibodies bind to the cell bound antigens and complement gets fixed at the Fc portions of the antibody molecules. The phagocytes, which arrive at the site by the chemotactic activity of C3a and C5a possess complement receptors (CRs) and lead to the phagocytic response (Fig. 16.2).

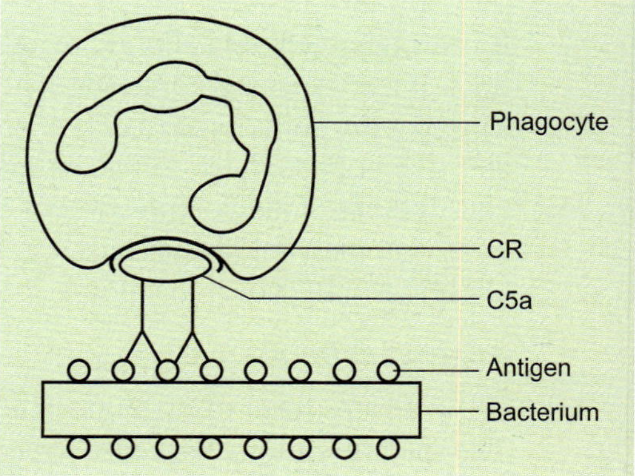

Fig. 16.2. Complement-mediated cytotoxicity.

2. Antibody-dependent cell-mediated cytotoxicity (ADCC)

This is the second possible mechanism involved in type II reactions. Fc portions of IgG or IgM absorbed onto the target cell through Fab interact with Fc receptors (FcRs) of NK cell which, in this context of ADCC, is often referred to as a K cell. Macrophages and eosinophils also indulge in this type of activity. This leads to lysis of target cells (Fig. 16.3). Lysis of target cells requires contact with K cells but does not involve phagocytosis or fixation of complement.

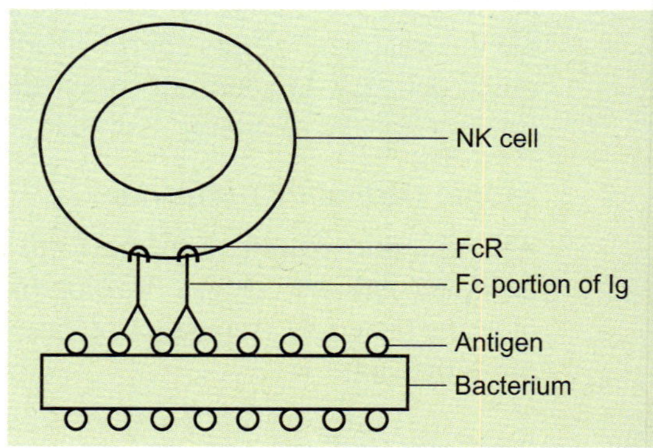

Fig. 16.3. Antibody-dependent cell-mediated cytotoxicity.

Clinically, antibody-mediated reactions occur in following situations:

1. Drug-induced immune haemolytic anaemia

A type II hypersensitivity reaction involving haemolytic anaemia may be induced by administration of certain drugs. Drugs such as antibiotic penicillin, and alpha-methyldopa for the treatment of hypertension can bind to the surface of red blood cell and form an antigenic complex with the surface of these cells. This can bring about the production of complement-fixing antibody to the drug. Reaction of this antibody with the RBC-bound drug activates the complement system, resulting in RBC lysis and anaemia.

2. Transfusion reactions

When a person receives incompatible blood transfusion, the antibodies normally present in recipient's serum agglutinate and lyse donor RBCs with the liberation of free haemoglobin into the plasma. This leads to jaundice, fever and failure of kidney function. Serum of the donor may also agglutinate and lyse recipient's RBCs. For example, transfusion of group O whole blood or plasma to group A or group B or group AB recipients may lead to haemolysis. But this reaction is mild since the donor's serum gets considerably diluted in the circulation of the recipient.

3. Rh incompatibility

Rh antibodies are major cause of **haemolytic disease of newborn (HDN)**. When an Rh-negative woman carries an Rh-positive foetus, she may be immunized against Rh antigen by passage of foetal red cells into maternal circulation. Minor transplacental leaks may occur any time during pregnancy, but it is during delivery that foetal cells enter the maternal circulation in large numbers. Therefore, the mother is usually immunized only at first delivery, and consequently, the first child escapes damage (except where the woman has been sensitized already by prior Rh incompatible blood transfusion). During subsequent pregnancy, Rh antibodies of IgG class pass from the mother to the foetus and damage its erythrocytes. The clinical features of HDN may vary from a mere accentuation of the physiological jaundice in the newborn to erythroblastosis foetalis or intrauterine death due to **hydrops foetalis**.

4. Autoimmune haemolytic anaemia, agranulocytosis and thrombocytopenia

Some persons develop antibodies against their blood elements, resulting in autoimmune haemolytic anaemia, agranulocytosis or thrombocytopenia.

5. Anaemia due to infectious diseases

A variety of infectious diseases due to *Salmonella* and mycobacteria are associated with haemolytic anaemia. Studies in *Salmonella* infections have revealed that the haemolysis is due to an immune reaction against a lipopolysaccharide bacterial endotoxin that becomes coated onto the erythrocytes of the patient.

Q. 8. Describe mechanism of type III hypersensitivity. Describe briefly clinical examples of type III hypersensitivity.

Ans. If an antigen is not cell-bound but is rather small and soluble, the body can encounter severe difficulties if it is repeatedly exposed to that antigen. Antigen-antibody complexes formed under these conditions may lead to type III or immune complex-mediated hypersensitivity. Monocytes and macrophages are very efficient at binding and removing large precipitating antigen-antibody complexes. They can also eliminate the smaller complexes made in antibody excess but are relatively inefficient at removing those formed in antigen excess. The formation of antigen-antibody complexes in serum, with subsequent deposition of the complexes in tissues, is the key event in type III hypersensitivity. Antigen-antibody complexes can then activate serum complement, platelets and phagocytes, all of which lead to tissue damage.

As a result of activation of complement, fragments C3a and C5a are created. Both these fragments are anaphylatoxic since they bind to plasma membrane receptor sites on basophils, mast cells and platelets causing histamine release leading to inflammatory response. C5a fragment also attracts polymorphonuclear leucocytes. These cells release their degradative lysosomal enzymes leading to tissue damage.

The degree and site of damage depends on the ratio of antigen to antibody. At equivalence or slight excess of either component, the complexes precipitate at the site of antigen injection and a mild local type III hypersensitivity or Arthus reaction develops. On the other hand, the complexes formed in large antigen excess become soluble and circulate, causing more serious systemic reactions, i.e., serum sickness or eventually deposit in organs, such as skin, joints, kidneys and heart.

Arthus reaction (local immune complex disease)

Arthus (1903) observed that when rabbits were repeatedly injected subcutaneously with normal horse serum, the initial injections were without any local effect, but with later injections, there occurred intense local reaction consisting of oedema, induration and haemorrhagic necrosis. This is known as Arthus reaction. The tissue damage is due to formation of local precipitating immune complexes which are deposited on the endothelial lining of the blood vessels. Antigen-antibody complexes can then trigger and activate complement leading to inflammation and tissue damage as discussed above.

Passive cutaneous form of the Arthus reaction

In this an antiserum is first injected intravenously into a nonsensitive recipient and the corresponding antigen is then injected into the skin.

Reversed passive Arthus reaction

In this the antiserum is injected into the recipient's skin and the antigen is then injected into the same dermal site or intravenously. Both injections are made at about the same time so that sufficient amount of antibody will remain near the injection site to precipitate with the antigen and cause local inflammation and necrosis.

Serum sickness (systemic immune complex disease)

This is a systemic form of type III hypersensitivity. This develops in persons who receive a single injection of a high concentration of horse antitoxin against tetanus, gas gangrene, diphtheria, etc. for prophylactic and therapeutic purposes. Seven to 12 days after the injection, patient may develop fever, lymphadenopathy, splenomegaly, arthritis, glomerulonephritis, endocarditis, vasculitis, urticarial rash, abdominal pain, nausea and vomiting. It is due to the immune response to horse antigens and it has also been encountered in allergic reactions to certain drugs. After 7–12 days, antibodies to horse antigens appear while horse antigens are still persisting because a large dose was administered. Initially they form antigen-antibody complexes in antigen excess. These soluble complexes can circulate and get deposited in various sites throughout the body particularly in skin, joints, kidneys and heart.

Antigen-antibody aggregates can fix complement leading to inflammation and tissue damage as discussed above. The plasma level of complement falls due to massive complement activation and fixation by antigen-antibody complexes. Initially, the circulating immune complexes are in antigen excess and produce inflammatory lesions, but as antibody production rises, the immune complexes increase in size as zone of equivalence is reached. These larger immune complexes are more easily phagocytosed and cleared by the cells of reticuloendothelial system of liver and spleen. Once all immune complexes are removed from the circulation, symptoms are usually resolved within a week.

Raised levels of immune complexes have been demonstrated in many infective and other conditions:

(a) **Bacterial infections**
- Endocarditis
- Poststreptococcal glomerulonephritis
- Lepromatous leprosy
- Secondary syphilis
- Infected shunts in children

(b) **Viral infections**
- Dengue haemorrhagic fever
- Hepatitis B
- Cytomegalovirus
- Infectious mononucleosis
- Subacute sclerosing panencephalitis

(c) **Parasitic infections**
- Malaria
- Toxoplasmosis
- Trypanosomiasis
- Schistosomiasis
- Filariasis

(d) **Drugs**
- Penicillin
- Sulphonamides

Q. 9. Describe type IV hypersensitivity. Describe briefly clinical examples of type IV hypersensitivity.

Ans. Type IV hypersensitivity or delayed hypersensitivity (DH) is the clinically observable outcome of cell-mediated immune reaction in the tissues of a sensitized individual. The reaction is not brought about by circulating antibodies and B lymphocytes but by sensitized T lymphocytes and macrophages. It is named delayed hypersensitivity because it appears in 24–48 hours after the presensitized host encounters the antigen, while immediate hypersensitivity reactions develop in 1/2 to 12 hours. The mechanism of delayed hypersensitivity is given in Chapter 15. Two types of DH are recognized – tuberculin (infection) type and contact dermatitis type:

1. Tuberculin (infection) type

The immune response to the tubercle bacillus, observed by Robert Koch in 1880, has served a general model for DH. When a small dose (1 to 3 units) of tuberculin or purified protein derivative (PPD) is injected intradermally in an individual sensitized to tuberculoprotein by prior infection or immunization, an indurated inflammatory reaction, 10 mm or more in diameter, develops at the site of injection within 48–72 hours. It is characterized by erythema due to increased blood flow to the damaged area and induration due to infiltration with a large number of mononuclear cells, mainly T lymphocytes and about 10–20% macrophages.

In unsensitized individuals, the tuberculin injection provokes no response. Cell-mediated hypersensitivity reactions are seen in a number of chronic infectious diseases due to mycobacteria, protozoa and fungi.

2. Contact dermatitis type

Contact dermatitis is cell-mediated allergic reaction that occurs when certain substances like metals (nickel and chromium), dyes (picryl chloride and dinitrochlorobenzene), drugs such as penicillin, and toiletries come in contact with skin. Sensitization is particularly liable to occur when contact is with an inflamed area and when chemical is applied in an oily base. Application of antibiotic ointments frequently provokes sensitization. The substances involved are not antigenic by themselves but may acquire antigenicity on combination with skin proteins. Subsequent contact with allergen in a sensitized individual leads to contact dermatitis. The lesions vary from macules and papules to vesicles which break down leaving behind raw weeping areas typical of acute eczematous dermatitis.

This hypersensitivity can be detected by **patch test**. The allergen is applied to the skin under an adherent dressing. Sensitivity is indicated by itching, appearing in 4–5 hours and local reaction which may vary from erythema to vesicle or blister formation in 24 hours.

Q. 10. Tabulate differences between type I, type II, type III and type IV hypersensitivity.

Ans. Differences between type I, type II, type III and type IV hypersensitivity are given in Table 16.1.

Table 16.1. Comparison of type I–IV hypersensitivity reactions

Characteristic	Type I	Type II	Type III	Type IV
Approximate time to develop clinical signs	1/2–8 hours	5–12 hours	3–8 hours	24–48 hours
Reaction mediators	IgE, histamine, serotonin, SRS-A, etc.	IgG, IgM and complement	IgG, IgM, complement, neutrophils, eosinophils and lysosomal enzymes	T cells, macrophages and lymphokines
Response to intradermal injection of antigen	Wheal and flare	—	Erythema and oedema	Erythema and induration
Passive transfer with	Serum	Serum	Serum	T cells
Examples	Anaphylaxis, asthma, hay fever, and food and insect allergies	Transfusion reaction, HDN and drug-induced allergy	Arthus reaction and serum sickness	Tuberculin test, contact dermatitis, graft rejection and tumour immunity

Q. 11. Write short note on type V hypersensitivity.

Ans. This is an antibody-mediated hypersensitivity. Here antibody reacts with a key surface component such as a hormone receptor and switches on or stimulates the cell. An example of this type of hypersensitivity is the thyroid hyperactivity in Graves' disease due to **thyroid stimulating autoantibody**.

Normally thyroid stimulating hormone (TSH) from pituitary gland binds to thyroid cell receptors. This activates adenyl cyclase in the membrane which converts ATP to AMP. The latter stimulates activity of thyroid cells thus secreting thyroxine. **The thyroid stimulating antibody present in the sera of thyrotoxic patients is an autoantibody directed against receptors for TSH.** This antibody, therefore, binds to these receptors and brings about the same effect as that of TSH. Type V hypersensitivity differs from type II, because instead of binding to cell surface components, the antibodies, in type V hypersensitivity, recognize and bind to the cell surface receptors and stimulate the cell.

Q. 12. Describe briefly Shwartzman reaction.

Ans. It is not an immune reaction. It is, however, traditionally described along with hypersensitivity reactions because of superficial resemblance. Shwartzman (1928) observed that when culture filtrate of Gram-negative bacteria is injected intradermally in rabbit and then after 24 hours a larger dose of the same or unrelated toxin is injected intravenously, within a few hours after second injection, the site of intradermal injection shows petechial haemorrhagic area. The absence of specificity and short interval between the two doses excludes the chances of immunological basis.

Mechanism

The first dose is called **preparatory dose** and the second dose is called **provocative dose**. The preparatory dose causes accumulation of leucocytes which release lysosomal enzymes. These enzymes damage capillary walls. Following provocative dose, there occurs intravascular clotting, the thrombi leading to necrosis of vessel walls and haemorrhage. This is called **local form of Shwartzman reaction**.

When both injections are given intravenously the animal dies 12–24 hours after the second dose. Autopsy reveals bilateral cortical necrosis of kidneys and patchy necrosis of the liver, spleen and other organs. This is known as **generalized Shwartzman reaction**. In fulminating meningococcal septicaemia (**Waterhouse-Friderichsen syndrome**), there occurs adrenal haemorrhage and profound shock. These manifestations may be due to Shwartzman-like phenomenon.

Q. 13. Define and discuss mechanism of autoimmunity.

Ans. Normally we do not form potentially destructive antibodies and T cells against our own cells because our body has developed tolerance to self-antigens. However, all mechanisms have a risk of breakdown. The self-recognition mechanisms are no exception, and a number of diseases have been identified in which there is autoimmunity, due to copious production of autoantibodies and autoreactive T cells. **Self-tolerance** refers to lack of responsiveness to an individual's own antigens, and obviously it underlines our ability to live in harmony with our own cells and tissues. **Autoimmunity may, therefore, be defined as immune response to self-antigens, which can generate autoantibodies and autoreactive T cells.**

Mechanism of autoimmunity

There are several possible mechanisms involved in the development of autoimmunity:

1. Forbidden clones

According to clonal selection theory, antibody-forming lymphocytes capable of reacting with different antigens are formed. Clones of cells that have immunological reactivity with self-antigens are eliminated during embryonic life. Such clones are called forbidden clones. Their persistence or development in later life by somatic mutations can lead to autoimmunity.

2. Hidden or sequestrated antigen

Certain self-antigens are present in closed systems and are not accessible to immune system. An example is the **lens antigen of the eye**. The lens protein is enclosed in its capsule and does not circulate in the blood. Therefore, immunological tolerance against this antigen does not develop during foetal life. When the lens protein antigen leaks out, following cataract surgery or injury to the eye, it leads to immune response and damage to the other eye.

Another example of hidden antigen is seen in case of **sperm antigens**. Since sperms develop only at puberty, therefore, the sperm antigens cannot induce tolerance during foetal life. Sperms may enter into blood stream following injury of the testes and mumps. Virus probably damages the basement membrane of seminiferous tubules leading to the leakage of sperms and initiation of an immune response resulting in orchitis.

3. Neoantigens or altered antigens

Cells or tissues may undergo antigenic alteration by physical agents such as irradiation. Photosensitivity or cold allergy may be due to altered antigens by light and cold respectively. Several chemical agents including drugs can combine with cells and tissues and alter their antigenic structure. Skin contact with a variety of chemicals may lead to contact dermatitis. Drug-induced anaemia, leucopenia and thrombocytopenia often have autoimmune basis. Viruses and other intracellular pathogens may induce alterations of cell antigens leading to autoimmunity.

4. Cross-reacting antigens

Immunological damage may result from immune response induced by cross-reacting foreign antigens. For example, **Semple rabies vaccine** consists of infected sheep brain tissue inactivated with phenol. Its injection elicits an immune response against sheep brain antigens. This may lead to damage to patient's nervous tissue due to cross-reaction between human and sheep brain leading to encephalitis.

Immunological injury may be due to cross-reacting antigens present on microorganisms causing infection. An important example of this is the **non-suppurative sequelae of *Streptococcus pyogenes*** infection which include acute rheumatic fever and acute glomerulonephritis. M protein of *S. pyogenes* and heart of man share antigenic characteristics. The immune response induced by repeated streptococcal infections can, therefore, damage the heart. Nephritogenic strains of *S. pyogenes* share antigens with renal glomeruli. Therefore, immune response following infection with such strains may lead to acute glomerulonephritis.

Escherichia coli* O14** shares antigen with human colon. This organism has, therefore, been blamed to cause ulcerative colitis. Many patients suffering from syphilis develop haemolytic anaemia. It has been suggested that antibodies raised against ***Treponema pallidum* antigens** cross-react with certain blood group antigens bringing about the anaemia. There is also an evidence that antigens common to ***Trypanosoma cruzi, causative agent of Chagas' disease, and human cardiac muscle produce the immunopathological lesions seen in this disease.

5. Mutation

Immunocompetent cells may acquire an unnatural responsiveness to self-antigens by mutation.

6. Activity of helper and suppressor T cells

Helper T (Th) cells facilitate B cell response to many antigens. Suppressor T (Ts) cells inhibit antibody production by B cells. Optimal antibody response depends on the balanced activity of Th and Ts cells. *Overactivity of Th cells or decreased activity of Ts cells may lead to autoimmunity.*

17

STAPHYLOCOCCUS

Q. 1. Describe morphology, cultural characteristics and virulence factors of *Staphylococcus aureus*.

Ans. Morphology

They are spherical cocci about 0.8–1.0 μm in diameter. They are arranged characteristically in grape-like clusters. Cluster formation is due to cell division occurring in more than one plane with daughter cells remaining close together. In smear from pus, the cocci appear singly or in pairs, clusters or short chains of three or four cells (Fig. 17.1). They are non-motile (non-flagellated), non-sporing and, with the exception of rare strains, non-capsulated. They are Gram-positive but old and phagocytosed organisms may be Gram-negative.

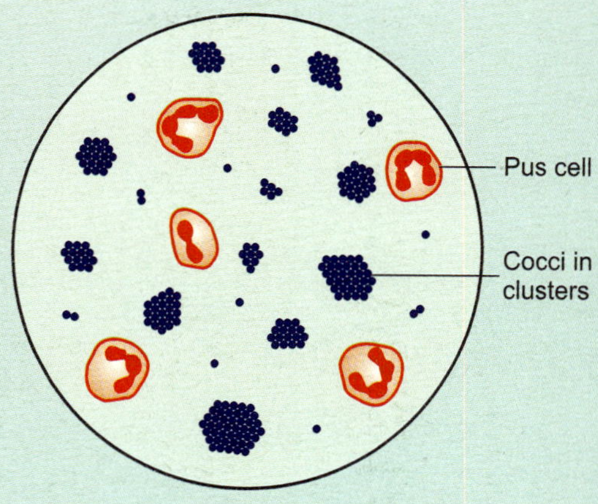

Fig. 17.1. Staphylococci and pus cells.

Cultural characteristics

They are aerobes and facultative anaerobes. Optimum temperature for growth is 37°C, range being 12–44°C. Optimum pH is 7.5. They can grow well on ordinary media.

1. Nutrient agar

After overnight incubation at 37°C, colonies are 1–2 mm in diameter with a smooth glistening surface. They are opaque and easily emulsifiable. Most strains produce golden-yellow (*aureus*) pigment, though some strains may form white (non-pigmented) colonies. Pigment production occurs optimally at 22°C and only in aerobic cultures. Pigment is not formed in liquid media.

2. Blood agar

Colonies are similar to those on nutrient agar, but may be surrounded by a zone of β-haemolysis (Fig. 17.2), especially when the medium contains sheep, ox, human or rabbit blood and it is incubated in an atmosphere of 20% CO_2. Haemolysis is weak on horse blood agar.

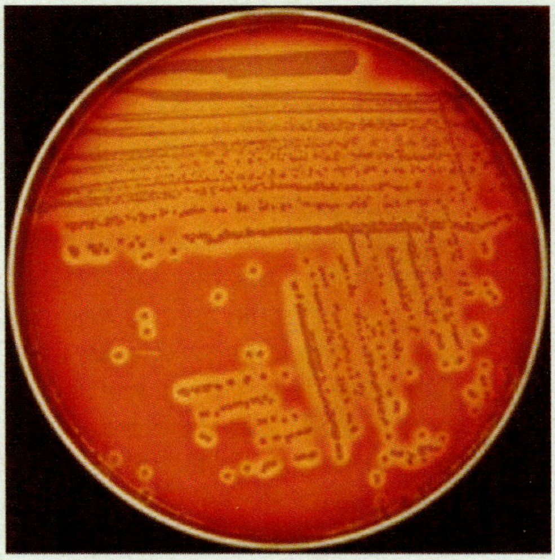

3. Mannitol salt agar

1% mannitol, 7.5% sodium chloride and 0.0025% phenol red is added to nutrient agar. This is both selective and indicator medium. Most strains of *S. aureus* ferment mannitol, therefore, due to the production of acids their colonies are surrounded by yellow zones. Otherwise the colonies resemble those seen on nutrient agar.

Fig. 17.2. Growth of *Staphylococcus aureus* on blood agar showing β-haemolysis.

Determinants of pathogenicity or virulence factors of Staphylococcus aureus

S. aureus possesses a large number of cell wall associated factors, and extracellular toxins and enzymes (Table 17.1 and Fig. 17.3), which contribute to the ability of the organism to overcome the body's defence and to invade, propagate, survive and produce disease in the host.

Table 17.1. Determinants of pathogenicity or virulence factors of *Staphylococcus aureus*

I. CELL WALL ASSOCIATED FACTORS
1. Capsular polysaccharide
2. Teichoic acid
3. Peptidoglycan
4. Protein A
5. Clumping factor

II. EXTRACELLULAR TOXINS
1. Haemolytic toxins (Haemolysins)
   - α lysin
   - β lysin
   - γ lysin
   - δ lysin
2. Leucocidin
3. Epidermolytic toxins
4. Enterotoxins
5. Toxic shock syndrome toxin-1

III. EXTRACELLULAR ENZYMES
1. Coagulase
2. Staphylokinase
3. Hyaluronidase
4. Deoxyribonuclease
5. Lipase
6. Phospholipases
7. Proteases

Cell wall associated factors

1. Capsular polysaccharide

A few strains of *S. aureus* are encapsulated and these tend to be more virulent than the non-capsulated strains. The capsule is composed of antigenic polysaccharide. It prevents ingestion of the organism by polymorphonuclear leucocytes. The capsular material may promote the adherence of the organisms to host cells and to prosthetic devices.

2. Teichoic acid

It is a major antigenic determinant of all strains

of *S. aureus*. It facilitates adhesion of cocci to host cell surface and protects them from complement-mediated opsonization.

3. Peptidoglycan

It is a polysaccharide polymer which provides rigidity to the cell wall. It stimulates both humoral and cellular immune responses in the host. In addition to their role in providing rigidity and resilience to the staphylococcal cell wall, peptidoglycan and teichoic acid also have several biologic activities that are thought to contribute to virulence.

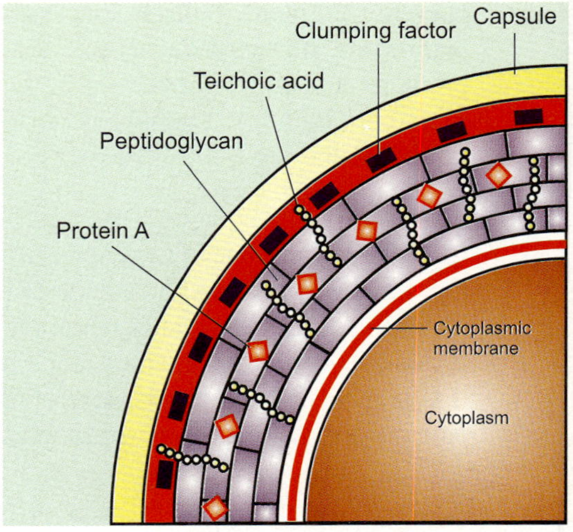

Fig. 17.3. Cell wall associated factors of *Staphylococcus aureus*.

4. Protein A

Protein A is a group-specific antigen found in the cell wall of about 90% strains of *S. aureus* (especially Cowan I strain). It has a molecular weight of 13,000 daltons. It is chemotactic, anticomplementary, antiphagocytic, mitogenic, potentiates natural killer cells, and elicits platelet injury and hypersensitivity reaction.

5. Clumping factor (bound coagulase)

It is a surface component that causes the organisms to clump when mixed with plasma. This factor reacts directly with fibrinogen in plasma, causing rapid cell agglutination. It can be detected by emulsifying a few colonies of the bacteria in a drop of normal saline on a clean glass slide and mixing it with a drop of rabbit plasma. Prompt clumping of the organisms indicates the presence of clumping factor (bound coagulase). Since this factor is detected by performing the test on a slide, therefore, the test is known as **slide coagulase test**. Almost all the clumping factor producing strains of *S. aureus* produce coagulase, whereas 12% of coagulase producing strains may not produce clumping factor. This factor is also not detectable in capsulated strains of *S. aureus*.

Extracellular toxins

S. aureus produces a variety of extracellular toxins, including haemolysins, leucocidin, epidermolytic toxins, enterotoxins and toxic shock syndrome toxin-1.

1. Haemolysins

Almost every strain of *S. aureus* produces one or more of four haemolytic, membrane-damaging exotoxins known as α, β, γ and δ lysins. They are antigenically distinct and differ from one another in their activity against the red blood cells of different animal species, lethal activity, dermonecrosis and leucocidal activity.

2. Leucocidin

Leucocidin consists of two protein components. On the basis of their migration in carboxymethylcellulose columns they are designated F (fast) and S (slow) components. These components act synergistically to damage polymorphonuclear leucocytes and macrophages, and to produce dermonecrosis.

3. Epidermolytic toxins (exfoliative toxins)

Many strains of *S. aureus*, mainly belonging to phage group II, produce two types of epidermolytic toxin (types A and B). They are proteins with a molecular weight of 30,000 and 29,500 daltons respectively. Epidermolytic toxin A is heat-stable and its production is determined by a chromosomal gene. On the other hand, epidermolytic toxin B is heat-labile and plasmid-controlled.

4. Enterotoxins

About 40% of all clinical isolates of *S. aureus* produce enterotoxins which are exotoxins that cause food poisoning in man. These have also been implicated in some cases of **pseudo-membranous enterocolitis** seen in patients after antibiotic therapy. Enterotoxins are proteins with molecular weights of 26,000–30,000 daltons. These are heat-stable, resisting boiling for 30 minutes. Therefore, once formed enterotoxins might not be destroyed even if food is heated sufficiently to kill all viable staphylococci. These are also not destroyed by gut enzymes. Nine antigenic types (A, B, C_1, C_2, C_3, D, E, H and I) of enterotoxins have been identified. Enterotoxin F is now known as toxic shock syndrome toxin-1. Type A toxin is responsible for the most cases.

5. Toxic shock syndrome toxin-1 (TSST-1)

TSST-1 is produced by certain strains of *S. aureus*. Most of the strains producing TSST-1 belong to phage group I. TSST-1 is a protein with a molecular weight of 22,000 daltons. It is antigenic and most persons over 30 years of age have circulating antibodies.

Extracellular enzymes

1. Coagulase

S. aureus produces an extracellular enzyme called coagulase. It activates a coagulase-reacting factor (CRF) normally present in plasma, causing the plasma to clot by the conversion of fibrinogen to fibrin. Clotting does not occur with plasma of certain species like guinea-pig which lack CRF. CRF is similar to prothrombin but is probably not identical with it. Coagulase is produced during the logarithmic phase of growth in a variety of media. Eight antigenic types (A–H) have been described. Most human strains produce coagulase A.

Coagulase (tube coagulase) test

0.1 ml of an overnight broth culture or broth suspension from an agar plate culture made up to the same density is mixed with 0.5 ml of a 1 in 10 dilution of human or rabbit plasma. The mixture is incubated in a water bath at 37°C for three to six hours. If positive, the plasma clots and does not flow when the tube is inverted. If clot does not appear it is left overnight at room temperature and re-examined. On continued incubation, the clot may be lysed by fibrinolysin produced by some strains. Controls with plasma alone, and known coagulase-positive and coagulase-negative cultures must be set up with each batch of tests. Human, rabbit or pig plasma which are rich in CRF can be used. Oxalate, EDTA or heparin are suitable anticoagulants. **Citrated plasma should not be used because contaminating Gram-negative bacilli may utilize the citrate and produce false positive reaction.**

For slide coagulase see clumping factor.

2. Staphylokinase (fibrinolysin)

Many strains of *S. aureus* that do not produce β lysin may produce staphylokinase. It is a protein with a molecular weight of 13,000–15,000 daltons. It has fibrinolytic activity. It is antigenically and enzymatically distinct from streptokinase produced by *Streptococcus pyogenes*. Fibrinolysin may break down fibrin clots and allow spread of infection to contiguous tissues.

3. Hyaluronidase

More than 90% strains of *S. aureus* produce hyaluronidase, but the amount varies widely. It hydrolyzes hyaluronic acid present in the intercellular ground substance of connective tissue, thus facilitating the spread of the organisms to adjacent areas.

Other extracellular enzymes produced by *S. aureus* and their activities are as under:

Extracellular enzyme	Activity
1. Deoxyribonuclease	Degrades DNA
2. Lipase	Degrades lipid
3. Phospholipases	Degrade phospholipids
4. Proteases	Cause proteolysis

Q. 2. Discuss pathogenicity and laboratory diagnosis of *Staphylococcus aureus*.

Ans. Pathogenicity

S. aureus is an **opportunistic pathogen** in that it causes infection most commonly at sites of lowered host resistance, e.g., damaged skin or mucous membranes or haematomas in the cancellous tissue of a long bone. Those with respiratory tract viral infections, such as influenza and measles, and diabetic patients are also more susceptible to staphylococcal infections.

Staphylococcal diseases may be classified as cutaneous and deep infections, exfoliative diseases, food poisoning and the toxic shock syndrome.

Cutaneous infections

These include wound and burn infection, pustules (small cutaneous abscesses), furuncles or boils (large cutaneous abscesses), carbuncles, styes, impetigo and pemphigus neonatorum.

Deep infections

These include osteomyelitis, periostitis, tonsillitis, pharyngitis, sinusitis, bronchopneumonia, empyema, septicaemia, meningitis, endocarditis, breast abscess, renal abscess and abscesses in other organs.

Exfoliative diseases

These lesions are produced by the strains of *S. aureus* which produce epidermolytic toxins. These toxins separate the outer layer of epidermis from the underlying tissues leading to blistering disease. The most dramatic manifestation of these toxins is **scalded skin syndrome** or **Ritter's disease** in which toxin spreads systemically in individuals that lack neutralizing antitoxin. Extensive areas of the skin are involved. Patient develops painful rash which sloughs off and skin surface resembles scalding.

Staphylococcal scalded skin syndrome (SSSS) occurs primarily in newborns and previously healthy young children. In adults, it occurs most commonly among patients with chronic renal failure and those with compromised immune systems. Although the mortality rate is low (0–7%) in cases seen among children, the rate in adults is as high as 50%.

Food poisoning

It is caused by staphylococcal enterotoxin. The enterotoxin is a preformed toxin already present in the contaminated food before consumption. Food is often contaminated by a food handler, who is either a carrier of *S. aureus* or is suffering from staphylococcal skin infection. Milk and milk products, and animal products like fish and meat kept at room temperature after cooking are mainly incriminated. When kept at room temperature, the contaminating staphylococci multiply and produce enterotoxin. It may also be produced in uncooked food contaminated with *S. aureus* and kept at room temperature. The enterotoxin is heat stable, resisting heat at 100°C for 10–40 minutes, therefore, it is not inactivated by cooking.

Patient develops nausea, vomiting and diarrhoea 2–6 hours after consumption of food containing preformed enterotoxin of *S. aureus*. It is a self-limiting condition.

Toxic shock syndrome (TSS)

It is a multisystem illness characterized by high fever, headache, confusion, conjunctival reddening, subcutaneous oedema, vomiting, diarrhoea, scarlatiniform rash and fine desquamation of the hands and feet. Severe cases progress to acute renal failure, disseminated intravascular coagulation, peripheral gangrene, profound hypotensive shock and death.

Laboratory diagnosis

Specimens

Specimens to be collected include pus from suppurative lesions, blood from a patient with pyrexia of unknown origin, mid-stream urine from a patient with urinary tract infection, sputum from a patient with bronchopneumonia and faeces, food remains and vomit from cases of food poisoning. Nasal and perineal swabs may be collected from suspected carriers.

Microscopy

Examine a Gram-stained smear of pus or wound exudate which may show pus cells and Gram-positive cocci in clusters (Fig. 17.4).

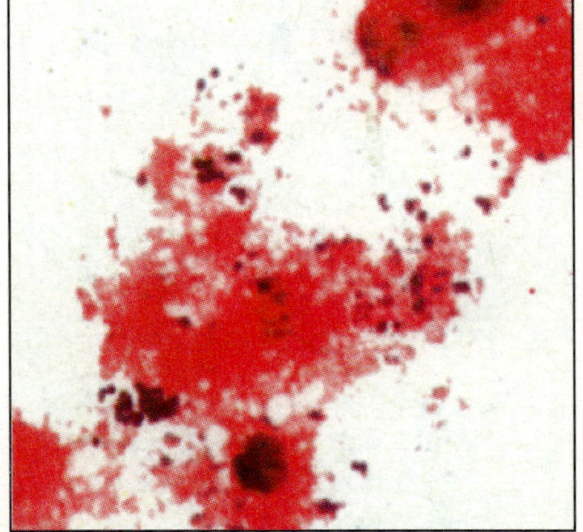

Fig. 17.4. Staphylococci in Gram-stained smear of pus.

Culture

The specimens are cultured on a blood agar plate. Specimens, where staphylococci are expected to be outnumbered by other bacteria (e.g., wound swab and faeces), are inoculated on selective media like salt agar or salt milk agar. The inoculated media are incubated at 37°C for 24 hours. Next day, the plates are inspected for golden-yellow or white colonies and are confirmed by slide coagulase test. On blood agar plate, look for haemolysis around the colonies (Fig. 17.2). Other tests which may be carried out include tube coagulase, mannitol fermentation, DNAse and phosphatase production, and gelatin liquefaction. As a guide to treatment, antibiotic sensitivity tests should be done and for epidemiological purposes bacteriophage typing may be done.

Q. 3. Write short note on methicillin-resistant staphylococci.

Ans. MRSA is any strain of *S. aureus* that has developed, through the process of natural selection, resistance to beta-lactam antibiotics, which include the penicillins (methicillin, oxacillin, dicloxacillin, nafcillin, etc.) and the cephalosporins. It is also called oxacillin-resistant *Staphylococcus aureus* (ORSA). Strains unable to resist these antibiotics are classified as methicillin-sensitive *Staphylococcus aureus* or MSSA. The evolution of such resistance does not cause the organism to be more intrinsically virulent than strains of *S. aureus* that have no antibiotic resistance, but resistance does make MRSA infection more difficult to treat with standard types of antibiotics and thus more dangerous.

MRSA is responsible for several difficult-to-treat infections in humans. It is especially troublesome in hospitals, where patients with open wounds, invasive devices, and weakened immune systems are at a greater risk of infection than general public. The main cause of concern now is the emergence of community acquired MRSA (CA MRSA) which was earlier restricted to the hospital setting hospital associated MRSA (HA MRSA).

Q. 4. Write short note on vancomycin-resistant staphylococci.

Ans. Vancomycin is the drug of choice, and sometimes the only drug available, for serious staphylococcal infections, and thus the development of vancomycin resistance has been a serious concern. In 2002, isolates of **Vancomycin-resistant *S. aureus* (VRSA)** were reported in the United States, isolated from patients undergoing long-term vancomycin treatment.

Q. 5. Write short note on coagulase-negative staphylococci.

Ans. Coagulase-negative staphylococci (CoNS) form part of the normal flora of the skin. Some species of CoNS, e.g., *S. epidermidis* and *S. saprophyticus*, can produce human infections. They are morphologically similar to *S. aureus* and the methods for isolation are the same. Their colonies are white (non-pigmented) and they can be distinguished from *S. aureus* by their failure to coagulate plasma and by their lack of clumping factor and DNAse.

Staphylococcus epidermidis

The role of *S. epidermidis* as an aetiologic agent of disease has become increasingly evident. Infections caused by *S. epidermidis* are predominantly hospital acquired. Some of the predisposing factors are instrumentation procedures such as catheterization, prosthetic heart valve implantation, and immunosuppressive therapy. Infections caused by this organism include endocarditis of native and prosthetic valves, intravenous catheter infections, CSF shunt infections, peritoneal dialysis, catheter-associated peritonitis, bacteraemia, osteomyelitis, wound infections, vascular graft infections, prosthetic joint infections and mediastinitis. *S. epidermidis* is probably the most common cause of hospital acquired urinary tract infections.

Many strains of *S. epidermidis* can adhere to plastic catheters and prosthetic devices. Adherence of CoNS to plastic prosthetics is, most likely, facilitated by nonspecific binding related to electrical charge and/or hydrophobic interactions between the bacterial surface and the surface of plastic devices. Many strains of *S. epidermidis* are capable of producing large amounts of polysaccharide glycocalyx known as **slime**. It is produced readily when the bacteria are growing on a solid surface such as a plastic catheter allowing the formation of microcolonies. Slime has been thought to play a role in the adherence of staphylococci to surfaces. Slime-producing strains also utilize this adherence factor to inhibit the action of lymphocytes and neutrophils.

Staphylococcus saprophyticus

S. saprophyticus is a well documented pathogen causing primarily acute urinary tract infections in young healthy sexually active women. In this population *S. saprophyticus* is the most common cause of cystitis after *Escherichia coli*. When present in urine cultures, it may be found in low numbers and yet considered significant. It is found to adhere more effectively to the epithelial cells lining the urogenital tract.

Patients with this infection usually present with dysuria, pyuria, and haematuria. Upper urinary tract infections (e.g., pyelonephritis) may be seen in 41–86% of patients, and occasionally *S. saprophyticus* bacteraemia may be seen as a complication of upper urinary tract infection. It may also cause urethritis in men and women, catheter-associated urinary tract infections, prostatitis in elderly men, and rarely bacteraemia, sepsis and endocarditis.

18

STREPTOCOCCUS AND ENTEROCOCCUS

Q. 1. Describe morphology, cultural characteristics, biochemical reactions and antigenic structure of *Streptococcus pyogenes*.

Ans. ***Morphology***

They are Gram-positive, spherical cocci about 0.6–1.0 μm in diameter. They occur in chains of varying lengths. Chain formation is due to the cocci dividing in one plane only and the daughter cells failing to separate completely (Fig. 18.1). They are non-motile, non-sporing and some strains produce a capsule of hyaluronic acid, which may be demonstrable during the first 2–4 hours of growth. Because many strains also produce the enzyme hyaluronidase later during the growth cycle, capsules may not be seen in older cultures. Since hyaluronic acid is a normal component of connective tissue, therefore, anticapsular antibodies are not formed.

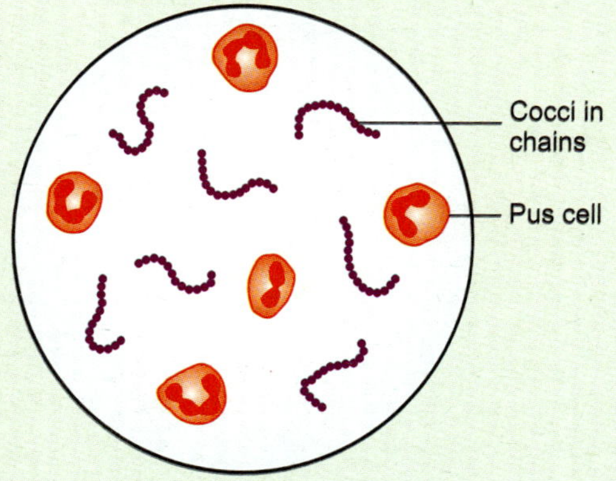

Fig. 18.1. Streptococci in Gram-stained smear of pus.

Cultural characteristics

They are aerobes and facultative anaerobes. Temperature range is 22–40°C, optimum temperature being 37°C. They can grow on blood and serum agar.

- After 24 hour incubation, colonies of *S. pyogenes* on **blood agar** are small (0.5–1 mm in diameter), semitransparent, grey-white with a matt or glossy surface. The colonies are surrounded by a wide zone of β-haemolysis. Mucoid colonies are formed by strains which produce large capsules.
- The addition of 0.0002% crystal violet to blood agar inhibits the growth of some bacteria, notably staphylococci, while permitting the growth of streptococci. **Crystal violet blood agar** is, therefore, a selective medium for isolation of *S. pyogenes*.

Biochemical reactions

It is catalase-negative and, unlike *S. pneumoniae*, insoluble in 10% bile.

Antigenic structure

Several components of bacterial cell of *S. pyogenes* (Fig. 18.2) are antigenic. These include:

1. Capsule

The hyaluronic acid of the capsule is nonantigenic, presumably because it is chemically indistinguishable from the hyaluronic acid of ground substance of animal connective tissue. Capsule has only a weak antiphagocytic effect.

2. Cell wall

Cell wall is composed of an outer layer of protein, a middle layer of group-specific carbohydrate and an inner layer of peptidoglycan.

(a) **Peptidoglycan:** Peptidoglycan is responsible for cell wall rigidity. It also has biologic properties such as pyrogenic and thrombolytic activity.

(b) **Group-specific carbohydrate:** On the basis of group-specific carbohydrate antigen contained in the cell wall, haemolytic streptococci have been divided into 21 groups (A–W

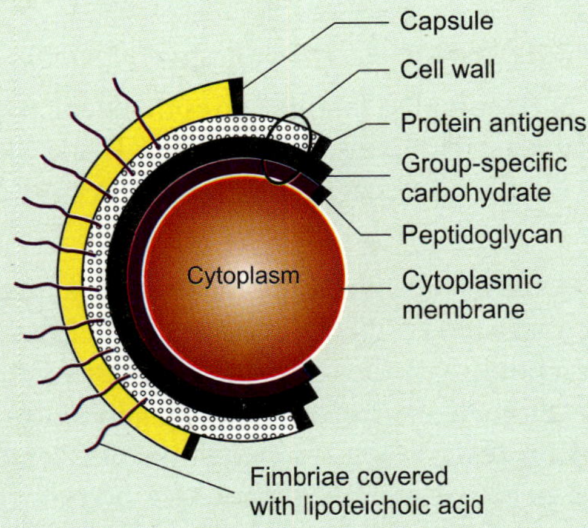

Fig. 18.2. Components of *Streptococcus pyogenes*.

except I and J). These are known as Lancefield groups. As this antigen is an integral part of the cell wall, it has to be extracted for grouping by a precipitation test with group antisera. For the test, streptococci are grown in Todd-Hewitt broth and extracted with hydrochloric acid (**Lancefield acid extraction method**) or formamide (**Fuller method**) or by an enzyme produced by *Streptomyces albus* (**Maxted method**) or by autoclaving (**Rantz and Randall method**). The extract and specific antisera are allowed to react in capillary tubes. Precipitation occurs within five minutes at the interface between the extract and the homologous antisera. *S. pyogenes* belongs to Lancefield group A. **All streptococci except the viridans group have a layer of carbohydrate.**

(c) **Proteins:** *S. pyogenes* produces three surface protein antigens (M, T and R) that are useful in serologic typing:

- **M protein:** It is the most important. It acts as a virulence factor by inhibiting phagocytosis. Specific anti-M antibody develops after infection which enhances phagocytosis. **M protein extends through the capsule as fine fimbriae.** They are covered with lipoteichoic acid. They enable the organism to attach to epithelial cells. M protein is acid- and heat-stable and trypsin-sensitive. It is antigenic and antisera can be raised against it. On the basis of antigenic differences in the M protein, *S. pyogenes* is divided into more than 80 M types. M protein can be extracted by Lancefield acid extraction method and M typing is performed by **capillary tube precipitation tests** using type-specific antisera and acid extract.
- **T protein:** It is resistant to pepsin and trypsin but is heat- and acid-stable. It is present in many serotypes of *S. pyogenes*. T typing is done by slide agglutination test using trypsin-treated whole streptococci.
- **R protein:** It is destroyed by pepsin and not by trypsin. Typing systems employing the R surface antigens are not commonly used.

Q. 2. Name and describe toxins and enzymes produced by *Streptococcus pyogenes*.

Ans. ***Toxins***

S. pyogenes produces several exotoxins and enzymes which contribute to its pathogenicity and identification.

Streptococcal pyrogenic exotoxins (Erythrogenic toxins)

There are three antigenically distinct streptococcal pyrogenic exotoxins A, B and C (streptococcal pyrogenic exotoxins – SPE A, SPE B and SPE C). **These extoxins are super-antigens** and have been associated with streptococcal toxic shock syndrome and scarlet fever.

Dick test: When 0.2 ml of suitably diluted toxin is injected intradermally in the susceptible children, it causes localized erythematous reaction at least 1 cm in diameter in 12–24 hours. This indicates susceptibility to the toxin and thus to scarlet fever. This test is known as Dick test. This toxin is antigenic. It is neutralized by antibodies found in convalescent sera.

Schultz-Charlton test: When the patient serum contains demonstrable antitoxin, the skin test becomes negative and an injection of homologous antitoxin intradermally in a patient of scarlet fever causes local blanching of the rash. This is known as Schultz-Charlton test.

Enzymes

Haemolysins (Streptolysins)

S. pyogenes produces two types of haemolysins. One of these is oxygen-labile hence designated as streptolysin O (SLO) and the other is oxygen-stable and soluble in serum hence designated as streptolysin S (SLS).

Streptolysin O: It is a heat-labile protein with a molecular weight of 50,000–75,000 daltons. It binds to the cholesterol containing erythrocyte membrane and produces large holes in it, leading to complete lysis. On blood agar, SLO activity is seen only in pour plates, and in anaerobic cultures. It is inactive in oxidised form, but may be reactivated by treatment with reducing agents. It is irreversibly inactivated by cholesterol. It is lethal on intravenous injection into animals and has particularly toxic effect on the heart and leucocytes.

SLO is strongly antigenic. It induces brisk antibody response, usually within 10–14 days. **Antistreptolysin O (ASO)** may be demonstrated, *in vitro*, by its capacity to inhibit the haemolytic action of the toxin. It provides a very important tool for determining a recent group A streptococcal infection. Such information is an important aid in the diagnosis of the late complications of streptococcal infections, which usually occur after the organisms have been eliminated from the host.

Streptolysin S: It is a small polypeptide with a molecular weight of less than 20,000 daltons. It is nonantigenic. It is oxygen-stable, so it is responsible for haemolysis around the surface colonies. In addition to causing β-haemolysis, it is able to inhibit chemotaxis and phagocytosis.

Streptokinase

Streptococci of groups A, C and G produce a substance called streptokinase which is actively fibrinolytic for human fibrin (blood clot) and can be recovered in streptococcal culture filtrates. This acts on plasminogen, a factor present in normal plasma, which is converted into plasmin, an active proteolytic enzyme that lysis fibrin. It is thought to be at least partially responsible for the rapid spread of streptococcal infection by preventing the formation of a fibrin barrier around the infected site. It is an antigenic protein and neutralizing antibodies appear in convalescent sera. Antistreptokinase antibody provides retrospective evidence of streptococcal infection. It is given intravenously for the treatment of early myocardial infarction and other thromboembolic disorders.

Deoxyribonucleases (streptodornases)

S. pyogenes also elaborates enzymes that degrade DNA. Four immunologically and electrophoretically different types (A, B, C and D) of deoxyribonucleases have been found in streptococcal culture filtrates. Of these, B is most antigenic in man and demonstration of **anti-deoxyribonuclease B** is useful in the retrospective diagnosis particularly of skin infections, where ASO titre may be low. One or more of these enzymes are produced by all strains of *S. pyogenes*. They are capable of depolymerizing the highly viscous DNA which accumulates in thick pus as a result of disintegration of polymorphonuclear leucocytes. Thus these enzymes are probably responsible for serous character of streptococcal pus. Mixtures of streptokinase and streptodornase have been used therapeutically for breaking down blood clots, thick pus and fibrinous exudates in closed spaces such as joints or pleural cavity.

Hyaluronidase (spreading factor)

It is an enzyme which splits hyaluronic acid binding tissue cells together and also that of streptococcal capsules, consequently strains which produce large amounts of hyaluronidase produce little hyaluronic acid capsule. This enzyme is expected to play a part in the virulence of *S. pyogenes* by facilitating its spread. It is antigenic and antibodies to the enzyme are formed after infection. Hyaluronidase is produced by strains of groups A, B, C and G streptococci.

Serum opacity factor (SOF)

SOF is an enzyme, lipoproteinase. It exists both as cell-bound and released from it. It produces opacity when applied to agar gel containing horse or swine serum. It is produced by group A streptococci of certain M types. It thus provides a means of classifying group A streptococci into two categories – SOF-producing and non-SOF-producing strains.

Nicotinamide adenine dinucleotidase (NADase)

This acts on the coenzyme NAD and liberates nicotinamide from the molecule. It is antigenic and is specifically neutralised by the antibody in convalescent sera. Its role in the virulence of the organisms is not known.

Q. 3. Discuss pathogenicity of *Streptococcus pyogenes*.

Ans. *S. pyogenes* is intrinsically a much more dangerous organism than *S. aureus* and has a much greater tendency to spread in the tissues, therefore, it is more likely to give rise to septicaemia. Various strains of *S. pyogenes* are carried normally in the respiratory tract, mouth and the skin of about 5% of general population. The carrier rate is generally higher in children between 1–15 years of age. Carriers and patients with acute infections are the sources of infection which is acquired by respiratory droplets or by direct or indirect contact. *S. pyogenes* causes:

I. Suppurative diseases.
II. Non-suppurative sequelae.

I. Suppurative diseases

1. ***Tonsillitis and pharyngitis:*** The main site of streptococcal infection is the throat where purulent tonsillitis is the most typical lesion. This generally develops 2–4 days after exposure to the pathogen. This condition characteristically occurs in older children and adults where it may constitute 30–40% of all cases of sore throat. In younger children, the infection is more diffuse (pharyngitis rather than tonsillitis) and less acute in character. The more acute localized lesion of older persons is believed to depend on a previous acquired allergy.

   From the throat the infection may spread locally particularly to the neighbouring lymph nodes causing cervical lymphadenitis and to the middle ear causing otitis media and mastoiditis. Occasionally, a peritonsillar or retropharyngeal abscess is produced and infrequently diffuse cellulitis of the floor of the mouth, known as **Ludwig's angina**, develops. From the throat, the organism may also involve the meninges leading to meningitis and the lungs leading to pneumonia.

2. ***Scarlet fever:*** Scarlet fever is a complication of streptococcal pharyngitis that occurs when the infecting strain is lysogenized by a bacteriophage that mediates production of a pyrogenic exotoxin. The disease consists of a combination of a streptococcal sore throat and a generalized erythema, although occasionally the rash can accompany a streptococcal wound infection. The rash consists of widespread erythema with punctate spots. The skin of the face is generally clear. Whether the rash is secondary to a direct action of the circulating toxin or to a generalized cutaneous hypersensitivity reaction is not known. In the favour of the latter possibility is the observation that infants under the age of two years rarely develop the disease and do not show positive Dick test.
3. ***Impetigo:*** This is caused predominantly by *S. pyogenes*. It may also be caused by group C and G streptococci and by *S. aureus*. Impetigo is a skin infection that occurs most often in young children, particularly those living in crowded, low socioeconomic conditions. Streptococcal impetigo is characterized by the occurrence on the skin of a superficial discrete crusted spot seldom exceeding an inch in diameter, which lasts for 1–2 weeks and heals spontaneously without leaving a scar. Lesions may also appear in groups. Group A streptococci causing impetigo are frequently nephritogenic, that is, leading to acute glomerulonephritis.
4. ***Erysipelas:*** This is an acute, spreading, intensely erythematous skin lesion with a sharply demarcated but irregular edge and sometimes with superficial vesicles and bullae. In facial erysipelas the attack may be preceded by a streptococcal sore throat and in others an infected abrasion or surgical wound may be associated but in many a primary lesion is not identifiable. The sufferers are usually adults, many of them elderly, and the Dick test is usually negative early in the disease.
5. ***Streptococcal toxic shock syndrome:*** Patients with invasive and bacteraemic *S. pyogenes* infections, and in particular necrotizing fasciitis, may develop toxic shock syndrome. The disease, which was first described in the late 1980s, is the result of the release of the streptococcal toxins to the blood stream. A striking feature of this acute fulminating disease is severe pain at the site of initial infection, usually the soft tissue. The additional clinical signs resemble those of staphylococcal toxic shock syndrome and include fever, malaise, nausea, vomiting and diarrhoea, dizziness, confusion and a flat rash over large parts of the body. If not treated, the disease progresses to shock and general organ failure (e.g., kidney, lungs, liver, heart).
6. ***Other group A streptococcal infections:*** *S. pyogenes* is the most important cause of **puerperal sepsis**. In this condition, the organisms are almost invariably derived from attendant nurses or doctors or from contaminated instruments. It may also cause wound and burn infections.

II. Non-suppurative sequelae

There is a considerable evidence that *S. pyogenes* is in some way the cause of acute rheumatic fever (ARF) involving the heart and joints, and acute glomerulonephritis (AGN) involving the kidneys. These conditions differ from suppurative infections in that:

(a) These conditions appear only between 2–3 weeks after infection with *S. pyogenes*. *S. pyogenes* is no longer detectable when the complications set in.

(b) Many cases are not preceded by overt streptococcal infection but in many of these, high titres of antibodies to streptococcal extracellular antigens, particularly to streptolysin O, are frequently demonstrable.
(c) Streptococci are not directly demonstrable in the lesions in these conditions.

- **Acute rheumatic fever (ARF):** ARF develops in a small percentage (roughly 3%) of individuals, 2–3 weeks after the onset of acute streptococcal pharyngitis caused by any type of group A streptococci. It is characterized by fever, migrating polyarthritis, and carditis, and is frequently associated with subcutaneous nodules. Recovery from ARF occurs without residual injury to the joints, but permanent damage to the heart may occur. The mechanism by which streptococci produce rheumatic fever is still obscure.

  There have been reports that a common cross-reacting antigen exists in some group A streptococci and the heart. In this case, antibodies synthesized in response to the streptococcal infection could react with antigens in the heart, causing cellular destruction and permanent damage. This theory is supported by the observation that following a streptococcal epidemic, most patients who develop ARF have higher titre of antistreptococcal antibodies in their sera than do those who escape the disease. Circulating immune complexes have also been found in serum of the patients with ARF.
- **Acute glomerulonephritis (AGN):** AGN is less frequently a consequence of streptococcal infection than is ARF. It is almost always produced by group A streptococci but group C streptococci may also be involved. In contrast to ARF which occurs only after pharyngitis, AGN may be seen after a pharyngeal or cutaneous infection. Most cases of AGN occur 2–3 weeks following skin infection or pharyngitis caused by certain pyodermal (M types 1 and 12) and pharyngeal (M types 49, 53–55 and 59–61) strains of *S. pyogenes*. These strains are known as nephritogenic strains.

  Poststreptococcal AGN probably develops because some components of glomerular basement membrane are antigenically similar to the cell membranes of nephritogenic β-haemolytic streptococci. Therefore, antibodies which are produced by the host against the latter cross-react with the former. Alternatively, streptococcal antigen-antibody complexes may lodge in the glomeruli. In either case, the activation of the C3 and C5 components of complement leads to tissue destruction. This is supported by the detection of C3 as well as γ-globulin and streptococcal antigens in the glomerular lesion.

Q. 4. Describe laboratory diagnosis of *Streptococcus pyogenes* infection.

Ans. In acute infections, diagnosis is established by identification of β-haemolytic streptococci that have been isolated from the patient, while in non-suppurative complications, diagnosis is based on the demonstration of rising titre of antibody to one or more streptococcal antigens.

Specimens

Throat and nasal swabs from cases of sore throat or from suspected carriers, high vaginal swabs from cases of puerperal sepsis, pus or pus swabs from suppurative infections and blood from cases of systemic infections are the usual specimens collected.

Gram staining

The observation of typical Gram-positive cocci arranged in chains on microscopic examination of smear of pus or CSF may indicate the likelihood of the presence of streptococci.

Fluorescent antibody technique

The examination of throat swab by the direct fluorescent antibody technique may be used for rapid identification of group A streptococci.

Culture

Inoculate pus or swab on blood agar plate immediately. Incubate it at 37°C for 24 hours and look for β-haemolytic colonies of streptococci. If there is likely to be delay, swab should be sent to the laboratory in Pike's medium (blood agar containing 1 in 1,000,000 crystal violet and 1 in 16,000 sodium azide distributed as for stab cultures in tubes). In case of bacteriological examination of skin lesions, crystal violet blood agar and PNF medium are useful selective media that inhibit many commensal organisms.

Identification

Streptococcal colonies that produce β-haemolysis are subjected to:

- **Lancefield grouping** and in case the isolate belongs to group A, it is further subjected to **M typing**.
- A rapid method for identification of group A streptococci is based on **Maxted's observation** that they are more sensitive to bacitracin than other streptococci. The plate is inoculated with a pure culture of β-haemolytic *Streptococcus*, a 0.04 units bacitracin disc is placed in the area of inoculation and the plate is incubated at 37°C for 24 hours. The inhibition of growth around the disc is seen with *S. pyogenes* but not with other streptococci. However, this test is not totally reliable as 5–15% of bacitracin-susceptible streptococci recovered from clinical sources may belong to groups other than group A. For example, 6% of group B and 7.5% of group C and G β-haemolytic streptococci are bacitracin-sensitive. About 7.5% of α-haemolytic streptococci are also bacitracin-sensitive.

Serological tests

In ARF and AGN, a retrospective diagnosis of streptococcal infection may be established by serological tests, preferably with paired sera, to detect a rise in antibody titre to one or more of the extracellular products of *S. pyogenes*.

- **Antistreptolysin O** (ASO) test is used most frequently. ASO titres higher than 200 Todd units/ml are indicative of prior streptococcal infection.
- **Anti-deoxyribonuclease B** (anti-DNase B) estimation is also commonly employed. Titres higher than 300 or 350 are taken as significant.
- Other tests, only occasionally used, are antistreptokinase, antihyaluronidase and antiNADase.
- **Streptozyme test**, which is a passive slide haemagglutination test using erythrocytes sensitized with a crude preparation of extracellular antigens of streptococci, is a convenient, sensitive and specific screening test.

Q. 5. Describe group B streptococci.

Ans. Group B streptococci (*S. agalactiae*) are the etiologic agents of bovine mastitis and their association with human disease was recognized in 1930s. In recent years, infections with group B streptococci have been reported with increasing frequency. They are now major streptococcal pathogens in neonates and young children. Infection in the neonate is divided into early-onset-type and late-onset-type.

Early-onset-type

Group B streptococci are present in the vaginal flora of about 25% of all women. Early rupture of the membranes, prolonged labour, prematurity, low birth weight and heavy colonization of mother's vagina by group B streptococci lead to early-onset-type infection. Within first five days of life the neonate develops septicaemia and pneumonia, and in spite of the intensive antibiotic therapy, such infections carry a mortality rate of 50–70%. Meningitis may also develop.

The serotype of group B streptococci isolated from the anterior nares, external auditory meatus, umbilicus and rectum of the neonate, with or without infection, in almost all the cases, is similar to that isolated from the cervicovaginal canal, urethra or rectum of the mother. The fact that some babies delivered by caesarean section become infected indicates that direct spread of the organism to the uterus may take place.

Late-onset-type

This type of infection develops between second to fourth weeks of life. Baby acquires infection from the hospital personnel during nursing procedures. Baby to baby spread may also occur. The infecting organism is rarely found in the mother's vagina. This type of infection is not as severe as early-onset-type, but has a high incidence of residual effects often of a neurological nature.

Group B streptococci may also cause adult infections, including septicaemia, endocarditis, meningitis, and local septic lesions in the female genital tract, the urinary tract, surgical wounds and skin. Occasionally, they may lead to pneumonia, empyema, arthritis and osteomyelitis.

S. agalactiae possesses the enzyme hippuricase, which hydrolyzes sodium hippurate. Another test to identify group B streptococci is the CAMP reaction (so called because it was originally described by Christie, Atkins and Munch-Petersen), which can be demonstrated as an accentuated zone of haemolysis (butterfly appearance) when *S. agalactiae* is inoculated perpendicular to a streak of *S. aureus* (NCTC 1803) on a sheep or bovine blood agar plate (Fig. 18.3). Occasional strains are bacitracin-sensitive.

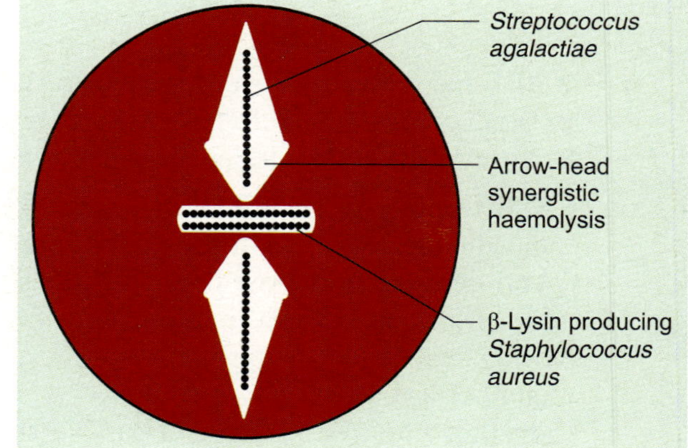

Fig. 18.3. CAMP test.

S. agalactiae produces several virulence factors, including haemolysins, capsular polysaccharide, C5a peptidase, hyaluronidase and various surface proteins that serve as adhesins. Eleven different types of capsular polysaccharide have been identified (Ia, Ia/c, Ib/c, II, IIc, III–VIII). The serotype most frequently associated with neonatal infections is type III, whereas infections in adults are more evenly distributed over the different serotypes.

Q. 6. Describe briefly group D streptococci and *Enterococcus* species.

Ans. The group D streptococci include *S. bovis* and *S. equinus*. Until the mid-1980s, the group D streptococci were divided into the enterococcal and nonenterococcal groups. Those found in the intestinal tract were part of the enterococcal group and have now been placed in a new genus, *Enterococcus*, but nonenterococcal group remains part of the group D streptococci. Both *Enterococcus* and group D streptococci can grow in the presence of 40% bile and also hydrolyze aesculin to aesculetin and glucose. One or two isolated colonies from blood agar plate are inoculated on a bile aesculin agar slant. If aesculin is hydrolyzed then aesculetin diffuses into the agar and combines with ferric citrate in the medium to give a black complex. This is known as bile **aesculin hydrolysis test**.

Group D streptococci can be differentiated from enterococci in that they fail to grow in nutrient broth with 6.5% sodium chloride, are PYRase test negative and are susceptible to penicillin. They are α-haemolytic or nonhaemolytic on sheep blood agar and do not hydrolyze hippurate. They may cause bacterial endocarditis, urinary tract infections, septicaemia, and other diseases, such as abscesses and wound infections. An association has been reported between bacteraemia resulting from *S. bovis* and the presence of gastrointestinal tumours.

Q. 7. Enlist important characteristics of enterococci.

Ans. Important characteristics of enterococci are:

1. They are normal flora of the lower intestinal tract and vagina.
2. They are non-motile, non-capsulated, Gram-positive cocci occurring in pairs or short chains.
3. These organisms may be α-, β- or non-haemolytic on sheep blood agar.
4. On MacConkey agar medium they produce tiny, deep pink colonies.
5. They can grow in the presence of 6.5% sodium chloride, at pH 9.6, and at 45°C.
6. *Enterococcus* and group D streptococci can grow in the presence of 40% bile and hydrolyze aesculin to aesculetin and glucose.
7. Enterococci are PYRase test positive.
8. They do not hydrolyze hippurate.
9. Most strains of enterococci are resistant to penicillin. They are also resistant to sulphonamides. Recently they have developed resistance to newer penicillins and cephalosporins, streptomycin and gentamicin.
10. They are relatively heat-resistant, surviving 60°C for 30 minutes.

There are currently 38 species in this genus, however, relatively few species are important human pathogens. The species most commonly associated with human disease is *E. faecalis*, but infections caused by *E. faecium*, *E. durans*, *E. avium* and other enterococci also occur. Identification of various species of *Enterococcus* is made on biochemical grounds. *E. faecalis* ferments mannitol with gas production. It is VP positive and can grow on blood tellurite agar producing black colonies.

Enterococci may cause urinary tract infection, wound infection, infective endocarditis, biliary tract infection, peritonitis, suppurative abdominal lesions and septicaemia.

Antimicrobial resistance

Enterococci are intrinsically resistant to cephalosporins and offer low level resistance to aminoglycosides. Strains resistant to penicillin and other antibiotics occur frequently.

Vancomycin is the primary alternative drug to penicillin for treating enterococcal infection. Vancomycin-resistant enterococci (VRE) have also been isolated. Resistance is most common in *E. faecalis* and *E. faecium*.

Q. 8. Tabulate differences between group D streptococci and *Enterococcus* species.

Ans. Table 18.1 shows differences between group D streptococci and *Enterococcus* species.

Table 18.1. Differences between group D streptococci and *Enterococcus* spp.

	Group D streptococci	*Enterococcus* spp.
Haemolysis type	α, none	α, β, none
Aesculin hydrolysis	+	+
Growth in presence of 40% bile	+	+
Growth in nutrient broth with 6.5% sodium chloride	–	+
Susceptibility to penicillin	+	–
Hydrolysis of hippurate	–	–*
PYRase test	–	+

*Exceptions may occur

Q. 9. Write short note on viridans streptococci.

Ans. Viridans streptococci are a heterogeneous group of α-haemolytic and non-haemolytic streptococci. Most isolates of viridans streptococci do not possess a group-specific carbohydrate; hence they cannot be classified under Lancefield classification of streptococci. They are constantly present as commensals in the mouth and oropharynx.

At least five species of viridans streptococci have been recognized. These include *S. salivarius*, *S. sanguis*, *S. mutans*, *S. mitior* (*mitis*) and *S. milleri*. Viridans streptococci, chiefly *S. mutans* and to a lesser extent *S. sanguis*, are involved in the production of **dental caries**. They break down dietary sucrose, producing acid and a tough adhesive dextran. The acid damages dentine and the dextran binds together food debris, epithelial cells, mucus and bacteria to form **dental plaques** which lead to caries.

In persons with predisposing factors, such as valvular disease of heart, they may cause **infective endocarditis (IE)**. *S. sanguis* is the most common causative agent of infective endocarditis. Tooth extraction and injury of the oral cavity in such persons is dangerous, because from oral cavity they may enter into the blood stream and cause IE. Tooth extraction in such individuals should be done under antibiotic cover. Other organisms which may also cause IE include *E. faecalis* and other enterococci, *S. aureus*, coagulase-negative staphylococci, *Coxiella burnetii* and some fungi.

Diagnosis of IE is established by repeated blood cultures. Viridans streptococci can be recognized by their α-haemolytic colonies on blood agar, their failure to grow on MacConkey medium and their sensitivity to penicillin. When isolated from mouth, throat and respiratory tract, they are regarded as harmless commensals and when isolated from blood or a closed lesion they are likely to be pathogenic. These streptococci are generally susceptible to penicillin, though some strains may be resistant. Therefore, antibiotic sensitivity of these organisms should also be carried out.

19

Streptococcus pneumoniae (Pneumococcus)

Q. 1. Describe morphology, cultural characteristics, biochemical reactions, antigenic structure, genetic variation and toxin production by *Streptococcus pneumoniae*.

Ans. ***Morphology***

The pneumococcus is a non-motile, non-sporing, Gram-positive coccus. In the material taken from the body, it occurs characteristically in pairs of **flame-shaped cocci** about 1 μm in diameter, the rounded ends of the cocci being adjacent to each other (Fig. 19.1). The cell wall of pneumococcus contains an antigen, referred to as **C substance**, that is similar to the carbohydrate antigens contained in the cell wall of β-haemolytic streptococci. In cultures they usually appear in chains like streptococci. The pneumococcus is capsulated. The capsule encloses each pair and it is best seen in the material taken directly from the exudates and may be lost on repeated cultivation. Pneumococcal capsule can be demonstrated by following methods:

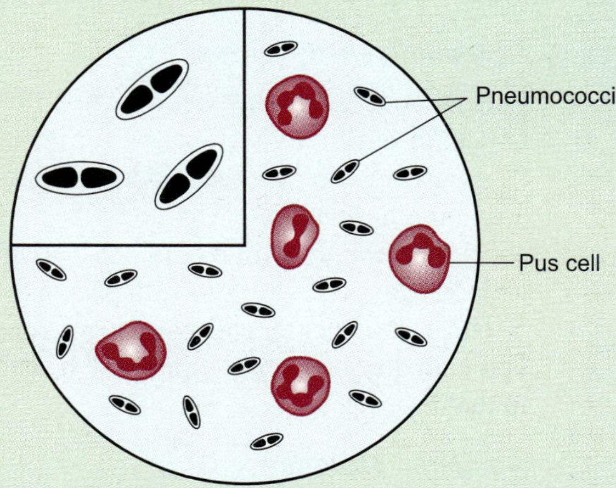

Fig. 19.1. Pneumococci in pus. Inset: enlarged view.

- As a clear halo in India ink preparation.
- By direct special staining techniques.
- It can also be seen and typed by treatment with homologous type-specific antibody which combines with the capsular polysaccharide and renders it refractile – **Quellung reaction**.

Cultural characteristics

Aerobe and facultative anaerobe, may need 5–10% CO_2 for primary isolation. Optimum temperature 37°C (range 25–40°C), pH 7.8 (range 6.5–8.3) and grows only on enriched media.

On **blood agar**, after 18–24 hour incubation at 37°C, virulent strains with abundant capsular polysaccharide produce small (0.5–1 mm in diameter), round, dome-shaped, transparent colonies. The colonies are surrounded by a 2–3 mm zone of α-haemolysis. On further incubation, the colonies develop a central depression because of autolysis with raised rim (**draughtsman colony**).

Biochemical reactions

Pneumococci ferment glucose, sucrose, lactose and inulin with the production of acid but no gas. Fermentation reactions are tested in *Hiss's serum water*. **Fermentation of inulin** by pneumococci is a useful test for differentiating them from streptococci which do not ferment it. They are catalase and oxidase negative.

Bile solubility test

Pneumococci are **bile soluble** while viridans and other streptococci are not. Bile salts, (sodium deoxycholate and sodium taurocholate) lyse pneumococci when added to actively growing cultures in an artificial culture medium. Pneumococci produce autolytic enzymes leading to autolysis in older cultures. The addition of bile salts is thought to accelerate this process.

Optochin sensitivity test

Pneumococci are highly sensitive to killing by optochin (ethyl hydrocuprein hydrochloride). Optochin sensitivity test is used for identification of pneumococci and distinguishing them from viridans streptococci, both of which produce α-haemolysis on blood agar. Optochin is a quinine derivative that inhibits the growth of pneumococci but not of viridans streptococci. For testing, a filter paper disc containing 5 μg of optochin is applied to the surface of a blood agar plate streaked with a lawn of pure culture. Plate is incubated at 37°C in air with 5–10% CO_2. Pneumococcus shows a zone of inhibition of 14 mm or more around the 6 mm optochin disc or 16 mm or more if 10 mm disc is used. Viridans streptococci grow right up to the disc.

Antigenic structure

1. Capsular antigen

The most important of pneumococcal antigens is the capsular polysaccharide on the basis of which the pneumococci are divided into more than 90 serologic types named 1, 2, 3, etc. As this polysaccharide diffuses into the culture medium or infective exudates and tissues, it is also known as **specific soluble substance (SSS)**.

The capsule of the pneumococcus is essential for virulence, its role being to protect the organism from phagocytosis. Only smooth encapsulated (S) strains are pathogenic for man and most laboratory animals. Active or passive immunization against a specific polysaccharide produces a high level of resistance to infection with pneumococci of homologous type. Laboratory strains that have lost the ability to produce a capsule are nonpathogenic.

The typing of individual isolates can be performed by:

- **Quellung reaction** in which the capsules of pneumococci are made more easily visible when acted upon by specific antisera. It is performed by mixing equal quantities of specimen (sputum, pus or sediment of CSF) or light suspension of the test organisms with type-specific pneumococcal antiserum. After waiting for 15–30 minutes, for the reaction to occur, the mixture is examined microscopically using a 100X objective. If Quellung reaction is positive, the capsule of the pneumococci will appear quite prominent as compared with those in the same specimen mixed with saline solution as a control. **The increased prominence of the capsule or swelling is apparently due to an alteration of its refractive index after reacting with the antiserum.** Pooled sera may be tested first and then in turn the individual type-specific antisera until one of them is found to give positive result.
- **Agglutination** of the cocci with the type-specific antiserum.
- **Precipitation** of SSS with the specific antiserum.

2. Somatic antigen

Pneumococcal cell wall contains a species-specific carbohydrate hapten. It is referred to as **pneumococcal C substance**. This appears to be analogous to (though antigenically different from) the group-specific C antigens of β-haemolytic streptococci.

3. M protein

Type-specific protein antigens analogous to the M protein of *Streptococcus pyogenes*, but immunologically distinct, are present in pneumococci. **Antibodies to the pneumococcal M protein do not inhibit phagocytosis and are, therefore, not protective.**

4. C-reactive protein (CRP)

CRP is an abnormal protein (β-globulin). It appears in acute phase sera of cases of pneumonia but disappears during convalescence. It also appears in some other pathological conditions. It is known as C-reactive protein because it precipitates with C antigen of pneumococci. It is not an antibody. Its production is stimulated by bacterial infection, inflammation, malignancy and tissue destruction. It disappears when inflammation subsides. It is used as an index of response to treatment in rheumatic fever and certain other conditions. It is tested by:

- Capillary precipitation of patient serum with antiserum prepared in rabbits against purified CRP; and
- Passive agglutination using latex particles coated with anti-CRP antibody.

Genetic variation

Repeated subcultures of *S. pneumoniae* may result in smooth to rough (S → R) variation. In R form, the organisms are noncapsulated, autoagglutinable, avirulent and form rough colonies. R forms arise as a result of mutation. Rough pneumococci derived from capsulated organisms of one type can be permanently transformed into capsulated organisms of a different or same type by treatment with DNA derived from different or same serotype of pneumococci. This **transformation** is of considerable historical interest since its discovery by Griffith was the first indication that the **genetic material could be transferred from one micro-organism to another**.

Toxin production

S. pneumoniae produces an oxygen-labile haemolysin (pneumolysin) and leucocidin. But both these are weak toxins and there is no conclusive evidence that they play an important role in infection.

Q. 2. Tabulate differences between *Streptococcus pneumoniae* and viridans streptococci.

Ans. Table 19.1 shows differences between *S. pneumoniae* and viridans streptococci.

Table 19.1. Differences between *Streptococcus pneumoniae* and viridans streptococci

	S. pneumoniae	Viridans streptococci
1. Morphology		
• Shape	Flame-shaped cocci	Round or oval cocci
• Arrangement	In pairs	In chains
• Capsule	Present	Absent
2. Cultural characteristics		
• On blood agar medium	After 24 hour incubation, colonies are small (0.5–1 mm), round, dome-shaped, transparent and surrounded by 2–3 mm zone of α-haemolysis. On further incubation, the colonies develop a central depression with raised rim (**draughtsman colonies**)	After 24 hour incubation, colonies are dome-shaped, opaque and surrounded by a narrow zone (1–2 mm in diameter) of α-haemolysis
• In liquid medium	Uniform turbidity	Granular turbidity, powdery deposit
3. Bile solubility	Positive	Negative
4. Inulin fermentation	Positive	Negative
5. Optochin sensitivity	Positive	Negative
6. Animal pathogenicity (Intraperitoneal inoculation in mice)	Fatal, death of mice in 1–3 days	Non-pathogenic

Q. 3. Discuss pathogenicity and laboratory diagnosis of *Streptococcus pneumoniae.*

Ans. ***Pathogenicity***

Between 5–70% of normal human adults carry one or more serological types of *S. pneumoniae* in their throats, yet epidemics of pneumococcal pneumonia are rare and morbidity low. This is due to following reasons:

- Many of the commensal pneumococci are noncapsulated and avirulent.
- Bacterial antagonism, primarily with α-haemolytic streptococci, tends to limit the growth of pneumococci in the pharynx.
- Normal epiglottal reflex, mucociliary escalator and cough reflex.

Therefore, pneumococcal pneumonia is rarely a primary infection and results only when the normal defence barriers of the respiratory tract are disturbed. Chilling, general anaesthesia, convulsions, cerebrovascular accidents, epilepsy, morphine, alcoholic intoxication and head injury predispose to pneumococcal pneumonia. These factors impair epiglottal reflex, mucociliary escalator and cough reflex, thus facilitating aspiration of pneumococci in the infected secretions from the upper respiratory tract into lower respiratory tract.

Viral infections of upper respiratory tract are a major contributory cause of pneumococcal pneumonia. Pneumococci present in the nasopharynx proliferate in the viral-modified environment and are carried down into the alveoli by the thin bronchial secretions. Aspiration of small quantities of oropharyngeal secretions can also be demonstrated in the healthy individuals during sleep. Person to person spread, by droplet infection, is uncommon.

In adults, most of the pneumococcal infections are caused by types 1–8 and 18. In children, commoner prevalent types are 6, 14, 19 and 23. The most important disease caused by *S. pneumoniae* is **pneumonia**, **either a lobar pneumonia or a bronchopneumonia**. The latter is characteristically a disease of young children and older adults over 50 years, while lobar pneumonia is almost exclusively a disease of the age group 10–50 years. Other pneumococcal lesions are **acute bronchitis**, **sinusitis**, **otitis media**, **mastoiditis**, **meningitis**, **endocarditis**, **suppurative arthritis** and **peritonitis**.

S. pneumoniae is the etiologic agent in about half of the children with otitis media. *S. pneumoniae* is a common cause of **bacterial meningitis** that affects patients of all ages. Pneumococcal meningitis is most often seen in children and the elderly. Pneumococcal meningitis may occur as a complication of otitis media or lobar pneumonia. Sometimes it is a consequence of fracture of skull with tearing of meninges. Bacteraemia may complicate pneumococcal pneumonia in about 15% of patients.

Laboratory diagnosis

The diagnosis is carried out by demonstration of pneumococci in sputum, exudate, blood and cerebrospinal fluid (CSF) by Gram staining, culture and by demonstration of pneumococcal antigen by coagglutination (COA), latex agglutination (LA) and counterimmunoelectrophoresis (CIE).

Microscopy

The sputum is homogenized by agitating the specimen for 30 minutes in a mechanical shaker with an equal quantity of distilled water and a small number of glass beads. Gram-stained smears are prepared from homogenized sputum and examined. In acute otitis media, *S. pneumoniae* may be demonstrated in fluid aspirated from the middle ear. In meningitis, the presumptive diagnosis may be made from Gram-stained films of centrifuged deposit of CSF. Gram-positive diplococci may be seen both inside the polymorphs and extracellularly (Fig. 19.2).

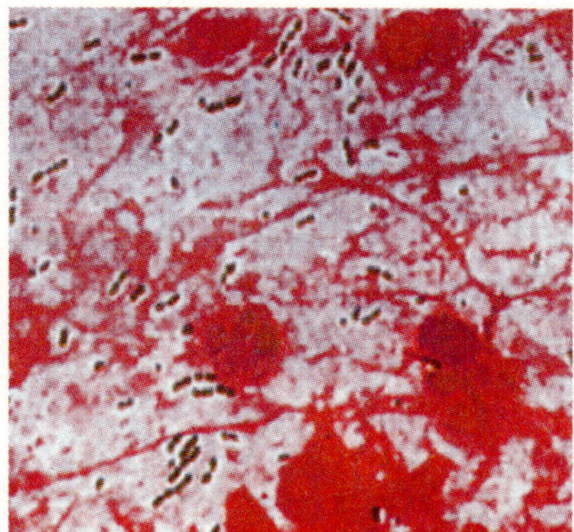

Fig. 19.2. Gram-stained sputum smear showing Gram-positive, encapsulated, extracellular diplococci from a patient of pneumococcal pneumonia.

Culture

The sputum, after homogenisation if necessary, is inoculated onto blood agar and heated blood agar media and incubated in air with 5–10% CO_2 for 18–24 hours.

If the sputum is unobtainable, as in young children, a serum-coated laryngeal swab is taken and processed. The organisms isolated are identified by their morphological and biochemical characters.

The growth of *S. pneumoniae* may be typed with appropriate antisera. Typing can also be done by Quellung reaction in wet films of sputum, pus or sediment of CSF.

- **Blood culture:** Since many healthy individuals carry pneumococci in their throats, therefore, demonstration of organisms in sputum or throat culture is not necessarily indicative of pneumococcal disease. Many pneumococcal infections are associated with a bacteraemia or septicaemia. Therefore, if pneumococci are isolated from patient's blood, the diagnosis of a severe pneumococcal infection can be made with certainty. In all cases of suspected acute bacterial pneumonia sample of blood obtained by venipuncture, prior to administration of antimicrobial drugs, should be cultured immediately in beef infusion broth and thioglycollate broth.
- **Cerebrospinal fluid:** In case of suspected meningitis, a centrifuged deposit of CSF should be examined immediately in a Gram-stained film, cultured on blood agar and heated blood agar and incubated in air with 5–10% CO_2 for 18–24 hours.

Antigen detection

In some cases, particularly if antibiotics have been given before collection of the specimen, viable cocci may not be there in the specimen and culture may be negative. In such cases, pneumococcal antigen is often detectable in CSF by COA, LA or CIE. COA test for antigen gives positive result in larger proportion of specimens than either a Gram-stained film or culture. Moreover, by COA test, result is available within a short time. In addition to CSF, capsular polysaccharide can be demonstrated in blood and urine by CIE.

Mouse inoculation

In specimens where the organisms are scanty, isolation may be obtained by intraperitoneal inoculation in mice, even if culture is negative. Inoculated mice die in 1–3 days, and *S. pneumoniae* may be demonstrated in the peritoneal exudate and heart blood.

20

NEISSERIA

Q. 1. Describe morphology, cultural characteristics, biochemical reactions, antigenic structure and determinants of pathogenicity of *Neisseria meningitidis*.

Ans. ***Morphology***

They are Gram-negative cocci, 0.6–0.8 μm in diameter. They usually occur in pairs with adjacent sides flattened or concave and long axes parallel. They are typically seen in large numbers inside polymorphonuclear leucocytes (Fig. 20.1). Fresh isolates of most *N. meningitidis* serogroups are encapsulated. They are nonsporing and non-motile.

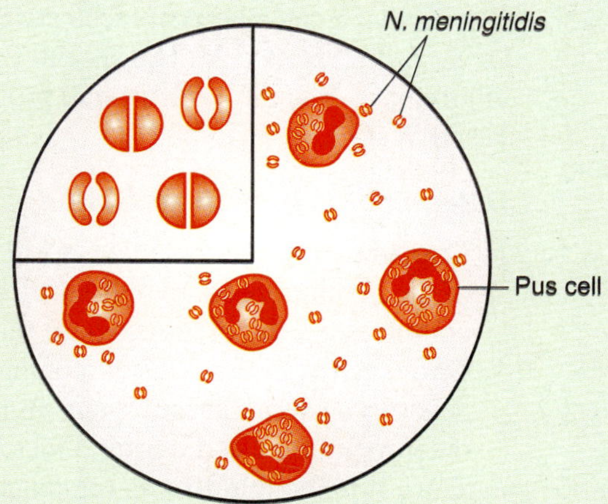

Fig. 20.1. *Neisseria meningitidis* in CSF. Inset: Enlarged view showing adjacent sides flattened or concave and long axes parallel.

Cultural characteristics

Meningococci have exacting growth requirements and do not grow on ordinary media. Growth occurs on media enriched with blood or serum. However, they grow well on trypticase-soy agar and Mueller-Hinton medium without the addition of blood or serum. They are strict aerobes, no growth occurring anaerobically. The growth is facilitated by 5–10% CO_2 and high humidity. The optimum temperature and pH for the growth of meningococci are 35–36°C and 7.0–7.4 respectively.

- On **blood agar**, after 24 hour incubation, the colonies of meningococci are small about 1 mm in diameter, round, convex, grey, non-haemolytic and translucent. After 48 hours

incubation, colonies are larger with an opaque raised centre and thin transparent margins which may be crenated.
- On **heated blood agar (chocolate agar)**, colonies of meningococci are slightly larger than those on ordinary blood agar.

Biochemical reactions

Meningococci are catalase- and oxidase-positive. It can utilise glucose and maltose with the production of acid only.

Oxidase test

When 1% solution of oxidase reagent (tetramethyl-paraphenylenediamine dihydrochloride) is poured on culture plate, *Neisseria* colonies quickly turn deep-purple. This **prompt oxidase reaction** helps in the identification of meningococci and gonococci in mixed cultures. This test may also be done by rubbing a few colonies with a glass rod on a strip of filter paper moistened with oxidase reagent. A deep-purple colour develops immediately.

Meningococci utilize glucose and maltose by oxidative method with the production of acid but no gas. They do not attack lactose or sucrose. Indole and hydrogen sulphide are not produced and nitrates are not reduced.

Antigenic structure

N. meningitidis possesses a polysaccharide capsule and on the basis of immunologic specificity of capsular polysaccharide it has been subdivided into 13 serogroups – A, B, C, D, X, Y, Z, 29E, W-135, H, I, K and L. Most meningococcal infections are caused by strains of groups A, B and C with a small proportion of infections being due to strains of serogroups Y and W-135.

Determinants of pathogenicity

1. **Capsular polysaccharide:** Capsular polysaccharide contributes to the invasive properties of the meningococci by inhibiting phagocytosis. In the presence of specific antibody and complement, the organisms are readily destroyed by phagocytic leucocytes.
2. **Endotoxins:** Endotoxins of meningococci are basically similar to those of the other Gram-negative bacteria. These organisms produce large amounts of lipopolysaccharide-containing outer membrane and during division, vesicles of this material are released extracellularly. Thus, it is thought that as organisms invade and multiply they release large quantities of lipopolysaccharide. These materials released in cells of vascular endothelium induce an inflammatory response and cause vascular necrosis. Endotoxins of meningococci are capable of producing both localized and generalized **Shwartzman reactions**. It is possible that such reactions are involved in the pathogenesis of meningococcal disease particularly **petechial haemorrhages** and **Waterhouse-Friderichsen syndrome**.
3. **IgA1 protease:** All strains of *N. meningitidis* produce an IgA1 protease that is excreted into extracellular environment. All pathogenic species have this capacity. These enzymes are neutral endopeptidases with a substrate specificity for human IgA1 immunoglobulin. IgA1 protease cleaves the subclass IgA1 molecule in the hinge region, and inactivates it. IgA2 is resistant to such cleavage because it has a shorter hinge region and lacks the proline-rich site cleaved by proteases.

4. **Transferrin-bound iron as a sole source of iron:** *N. meningitidis* can use transferrin-bound iron as a sole source of iron while non-pathogenic *Neisseria* species lack the ability to use iron from transferrin.
5. **Pili:** Meningococci possess pili on their surface which allow intimate contact with the host cell and organisms release endotoxin. Pili may also have antiphagocytic effect.
6. **Outer membrane proteins:** Outer membrane protein of meningococci can be divided into 5 classes out of which class 5 has been implicated with attachment to the host cell.

Q. 2. Discuss pathogenicity of *Neisseria meningitidis.*

Ans. Meningococci are normally carried in nasopharynx of 5–10% of healthy individuals. During epidemics the carrier rate of the epidemic strains may range from 20–90%. **An increase in carrier rate heralds the onset of an epidemic.** The carrier state may last for a few days to months. The average carriage in a nonepidemic setting is 10 months. The carrier rate is higher in the members of the household of a patient with meningococcal disease. **The meningococcal carrier is important in the transmission of meningococci and provides reservoir of infection.** Human resistance to meningococcal disease is relatively high and the incidence of healthy carriers is invariably higher than that of the cases of the disease.

Like most of the respiratory infections, meningococcal meningitis is disseminated by droplet infection, direct contact and less often by fomites. Infection is spread by patients and convalescents to a limited extent, but the healthy carriers of meningococci are of primary importance. The meningococcal disease can be divided into three stages:

1. First stage

The organisms appear in nasopharynx leading to **nasopharyngeal infection**, which is usually asymptomatic but might result in a minor inflammation. This state may last for days to months and will induce the formation of protective antibodies within a week, even though the infection remains asymptomatic. Occasionally, the infection in the nasopharynx may extend into adjacent areas, giving rise to conjunctivitis, pneumonia, etc.

2. Second stage

In a small percentage of cases, the meningococci may enter the blood stream from posterior nasopharynx, probably by way of the cervical lymph nodes. This stage is known as **meningococcaemia**. The patient develops **fever, malaise and petechial skin lesions** due to foci of infection in the capillaries. The organisms may also cause lesions in the joints and lungs and, rarely, may cause massive bilateral haemorrhages in the adrenals. This is known as **Waterhouse-Friderichsen syndrome**. Sometimes, the bacteraemia may take a chronic form causing mild symptoms of rash, arthritis or endocarditis over a long period of time.

The haemorrhagic lesions occurring in both the skin and internal organs, particularly the adrenals, are believed to be due to the release of endotoxin. Meningococci may also result in a condition known as **disseminated intravascular coagulation (DIC)**. In such situations, blood clots may block circulation to the extremities, necessitating amputation.

3. Third stage

Meningococci infect the meninges causing the major symptoms of severe headache, stiff neck and vomiting accompanied by delirium and confusion. The route of spread of meningococcus from the nasopharynx to the meninges is controversial. The organisms may spread along the perineural sheaths of the olfactory nerves, passing through the cribriform plate may reach the subarachnoid space or it may set up a preliminary sinusitis and reach the brain either via lymphatics or direct extension through the bone. Others believe that the meningococci reach the CNS via blood stream through a preliminary bacteraemia. In the favour of the latter are:

- The frequent positive blood cultures in the early stages of infection.
- The purpuric rash in many cases with the isolation of meningococci from the skin lesions.
- The occurrence, particularly during epidemics of meningococcal septicaemia with rash but no clinical meningitis.

Meningococci may occasionally cause acute urethritis, epididymitis, vulvovaginitis and cervicitis. In the absence of complete laboratory identification of the etiologic agent these conditions would be labelled as gonococcal infections.

Q. 3. Describe laboratory diagnosis of *Neisseria meningitidis* infection.

Ans. *Specimens*

CSF, blood, aspirate from skin lesions, pus from infected joint and throat, nasopharyngeal and in some cases genital swabs. Swabs should be transported in Stuart's transport medium. All specimens where meningococcal infection is suspected must be submitted to the laboratory immediately.

- **Cerebrospinal fluid:** In meningococcal meningitis, CSF is under pressure and is turbid due to a large number of polymorphonuclear leucocytes present in a typical case. For bacteriological examination, the CSF is divided into three portions.
  - **First portion** is centrifuged and Gram-stained smears are prepared from the deposit. Meningococci will be seen mainly inside polymorphs, but often extracellularly also. Strains causing meningitis are usually encapsulated and may show a distinct pink halo surrounding the cells. The capsule may also make the cells more resistant to decolorization and they may appear Gram-positive. When present in small numbers, meningococci may be detected by immunofluorescent technique. The supernatant contains meningococcal antigen, which may be demonstrated by precipitation test with polyvalent or monovalent antimeningococcal serum. Counterimmunoelectrophoresis provides a rapid and sensitive method for demonstration of meningococcal antigen.
  - **Second portion** of CSF is inoculated on blood agar or chocolate agar and incubated at 35–36°C under 5–10% CO_2. Colonies appear after 18–24 hours which may be identified by colonial morphology and biochemical reactions. The meningococcus isolated may be typed by agglutination with polyvalent or monovalent antimeningococcal serum.
  - **Third portion** of CSF is incubated for 18–24 hours, either as such or after adding an equal volume of glucose broth and then subcultured on blood agar or chocolate agar. This method may sometimes succeed where direct plating fails.
- **Blood culture:** Blood culture is often positive in meningococcaemia and in early cases of meningitis. Specimen of blood is inoculated into blood culture bottle of trypticase-soy broth. It should be incubated at 35–36°C in 5–10% CO_2 for 4–7 days, with daily subcultures on blood agar or chocolate agar. Look for oxidase-positive colonies of Gram-negative diplococci as above.

- **Pus aspiration and swabs:** In addition to blood agar and heated blood agar, **Thayer-Martin selective medium** is used for the culture of materials expected to yield a mixture of organisms. These include pus, aspirates, and throat, nasopharyngeal and genital swabs. Vancomycin, colistin and nystatin which are present in Thayer-Martin medium inhibit Gram-positive bacteria, Gram-negative bacteria and yeast contaminants respectively, while allowing the growth of pathogenic *Neisseria*. Meningococci may sometimes be demonstrated in petechial lesions by microscopy and culture.

Serological diagnosis

This may be attempted in cases of chronic meningococcal septicaemia where no organisms have been isolated. Specific antibodies to capsular polysaccharide may be demonstrated by haemagglutination test.

Polymerase chain reaction (PCR)

Meningococcal DNA in CSF or blood can be amplified and detected by PCR.

Q. 4. Describe morphology, cultural characteristics, biochemical reactions, antigenic structure and antigenic variation of *Neisseria gonorrhoeae*.

Ans. ### *Morphology*

Morphology and staining characteristics of *N. gonorrhoeae* are similar to those of *N. meningitidis*.

Cultural characteristics

Gonococci are more difficult to grow than meningococci. They are aerobes, but may grow anaerobically also. Addition of 5–10% CO_2 is essential for primary isolation. Growth occurs best at pH 7.0–7.4 and at a temperature of 35–36°C. They can be isolated on media enriched with blood either partially lysed by heat (chocolate agar) or completely lysed by saponin.

Heated blood agar may be made selective for the isolation of pathogenic neisseriae by the addition of vancomycin 3 mg/litre, colistin 7.5 mg/litre and nystatin 12,500 units/litre. This selective medium (**Thayer-Martin medium**) is valuable in isolating gonococci from heavily contaminated specimens. Trimethoprim lactate (5 mg/litre) may be added to Thayer-Martin medium to inhibit swarming *Proteus* species that are occasionally present in cervicovaginal and rectal specimens. This chocolate agar medium containing vancomycin, colistin, nystatin and trimethoprim is known as **modified Thayer-Martin medium**.

- On **heated blood agar** after 24 hour incubation, colonies are small about 1 mm in diameter, grey, convex and translucent. After 48 hour incubation, colonies are larger 1.5–2.5 mm in diameter, sometimes with an opaque raised centre and thin transparent margins which may be crenated.
- On **Thayer-Martin medium** growth is slower, although colonies are similar to those on heated blood agar.

On the basis of colonial appearance, autoagglutinability and virulence, Kellogg divided gonococci into five types (T1–T5). Type T1 and T2 form brown colonies, bear numerous pili and are designated as P^+ and P^{++} respectively. They are autoagglutinable and virulent.

Types T3, T4 and T5 form larger, granular, non-pigmented colonies, are nonpiliated (P^-), form smooth suspensions and are avirulent.

Biochemical reactions

N. gonorrhoeae resembles *N. meningitidis* with the exception that the former can utilize only glucose and the latter glucose and maltose with the production of acid only.

Antigenic structure

N. gonorrhoeae is antigenically heterogeneous. Surface structures include the following:

1. Pili

Pili are nonflagellar surface appendages. These are hair-like structures, several micrometers in length, 7 nm in diameter and are seen on the surface of gonococci of types T1 and T2. These are made up of identical protein subunits (pilin). Molecular weight of each pilin subunit ranges from 17,000–22,000 daltons. The pilins of almost all strains are antigenically different and a single strain can make several antigenically different forms of pilin. **Pili act as virulence factors.** They play an important role in attachment of gonococci to the cell. Furthermore, the pili are antiphagocytic. Removal of pili from cells by treatment with trypsin results in their phagocytosis and destruction.

2. Outer membrane proteins

Gonococci possess three major outer membrane proteins named proteins I, II and III.

(a) ***Protein I:*** This accounts for about 60% of total weight of the outer membrane. It has a molecular weight of 32,000–36,000 daltons. It forms pores in the surface.
(b) ***Protein II:*** It consists of a large, related family of proteins. They have subunit molecular weights ranging from 24,000–30,000 daltons. Because it is mostly present in the outer membrane of opaque colony variants of the same strains, therefore, it has also been referred to as opacity-associated protein. It appears to be associated with the adherence of the gonococci to the host cells.
(c) ***Protein III:*** It occurs in the outer membrane complexed with protein I to form porins. It appears to be identical in all gonococci and, as yet, it has not been associated with any specific virulence factor.
(d) ***Other proteins:*** Three other proteins named H8, iron binding protein and IgA1 protease have been described. The precise role of all these in pathogenesis of gonococci is not known. IgA1 protease splits IgA1 which is the predominant immunoglobulin involved in mucosal defence.

3. Lipooligosaccharide

It differs in its chemical structure from lipopolysaccharide (LPS) of Gram-negative bacilli. It does not have long O-antigenic side chains and is called lipooligosaccharide (LOS). Its molecular weight varies from 3,000–7,000 daltons. Toxicity in gonococcal infections is largely due to the endotoxic effect of LOS.

Antigenic variation

N. gonorrhoeae and *N. meningitidis* are among several organisms whose surface structures are known to change antigenically from generation to generation during growth of a single strain. The mechanism involved has been more extensively studied in gonococci but appears to be similar in both species. The antigenic structures of major interest are pili, protein II and LOS, for which there is evidence of antigenic variation both *in vitro* and *in vivo*.

Q. 5. Discuss pathogenicity of *Neisseria gonorrhoeae*.

Ans. *N. gonorrhoeae* causes **gonorrhoea**. It is a sexually transmitted disease that, with few exceptions, is acquired through sexual contact with an infected individual. *N. gonorrhoeae* is **exclusively a human pathogen** although chimpanzees have been infected by artificial inoculation. It is never found as a commensal although a proportion of those infected, particularly women, may remain asymptomatic. These may develop systemic or ascending infection at a later stage.

Gonococci ordinarily enter the body through the mucous membrane of the genitourinary tract, apparently penetrating between columnar epithelial cells. Stratified squamous epithelium is relatively resistant to infection. After an incubation period of 2–7 days, the organism evokes an acute inflammatory response in the subepithelial tissue giving rise to the purulent urethral or vaginal discharge, dysuria and frequency of micturition. In male, the acute urethritis may extend to the prostate, testes, seminal vesicles, epididymis and sometimes the periurethral tissue. Chronic urethritis may lead to stricture formation. The infection may spread to the periurethral tissues, causing abscesses and multiple discharging sinuses (**watercan perineum**).

In women, the endocervix is the primary site of infection. The urethra may also become infected. *In adult women, the vagina usually escapes because of the acidic pH of the vaginal secretions, but severe vulvovaginitis can occur in prepubertal girls*. The primary infection may spread from urethra, vagina and cervix to Bartholin's glands, uterus, fallopian tubes, ovaries and pelvic peritoneum causing a **pelvic inflammatory disease** resulting in sterility. Bacteraemia may occur in fulminating cases, in both men and women, and is occasionally complicated by endocarditis, acute purulent arthritis or both.

- Babies born to infected women may contract serious gonococcal infection of the eye (**ophthalmia neonatorum**) during passage through infected birth canal.
- **Anorectal infection** occurs in both sexes. In men this follows homosexual rectal intercourse. In women, it can follow rectal intercourse, but may also arise as a result of autoinoculation of rectal mucosa with infected vaginal discharge (direct contagious spread).
- **Gonococcal pharyngitis** may follow orogenital contact in either sex.
- **Conjunctivitis** may occur usually by autoinoculation with fingers.
- **Blood-borne dissemination** of *N. gonorrhoeae* occurs in less than 1% of all infections, resulting in purulent arthritis and rarely septicaemia. Fever and a rash on the extremities may also be present.

Q. 6. Describe laboratory diagnosis of gonorrhoea.

Ans. Disinfectants should not be used when preparing the patient for collection of specimen because small amounts of these may be toxic and impede the recovery of the organisms in culture. Calcium alginate and some cotton swabs have been shown to be inhibitory to *N. gonorrhoeae*, so Dacron or rayon swabs are preferred. These swabs should be either inoculated directly onto growth medium or transported to the laboratory in a transport medium such as Amies medium with charcoal and plated within 6 hours.

Specimens

I. Specimens in women

1. **Endocervical:** In women, the endocervix is the optimal site for culture. Specimen should be collected under direct visualization through a vaginal speculum because the adjacent vaginal mucosa harbours bacteria that may overgrow in cultures and may contain organisms such as *Candida* species that can inhibit the growth of gonococci. Remove excessive cervical mucous with cotton or gauze. Insert sterile specimen swab into the endocervical canal, move swab gently from side to side, leave in place for 10–30 seconds for adsorption of organisms to the swab surface.
2. **Anal canal:** Insert sterile specimen swab 4–5 cm in anal canal. Move swab from side to side to sample anal crypts, leave in place for 10–30 seconds for adsorption of organisms to the swab surface. If the swab is heavily soiled with faecal matter, a second specimen should be obtained with a fresh swab.
3. **Urethra:** Strip urethra towards orifice to express exudate and collect specimen on sterile loop or specimen swab.
4. **Vagina (in case of paediatric patients):** If hymen is intact obtain specimen from vaginal orifice and if hymen is not intact then use vaginal speculum and collect specimen from posterior vault.
5. **Bartholin's glands:** Purulent material expressed from the Bartholin's ducts should be collected on sterile sample swab.
6. **Oropharynx:** Using a tongue depressor and direct light, rub a sterile specimen swab firmly over the posterior pharynx and the tonsillar crypts.

II. Specimens in men

1. **Urethra:** Purulent discharge may be expressed at the anterior urethra and collected with a swab. If the patient is asymptomatic, the specimen is obtained by inserting a swab 2–3 cm into the anterior urethra. The swab is gently rotated as it is withdrawn to sample any exudate adhering to the urethral mucosa. Sterile bacteriological loop may also be used to collect specimen from anterior urethra by gently scraping the mucosa. Specimens from either symptomatic or asymptomatic men should not be collected until at least one hour after the patient has urinated.

   In chronic infections there may not be any urethral discharge. The morning drop of secretion may be examined or some exudate may be obtained after prostatic massage. It may also be possible to demonstrate gonococci in the centrifuged deposits of urine in cases where no urethral discharge is available.
2. **Anal canal**.
3. **Oropharynx**.

The specimens from anal canal and oropharynx of men are collected by the same method as in women.

III. Specimens in both sexes

1. **Synovial fluid:** In case of gonococcal arthritis.
2. **Blood:** In case of gonococcal septicaemia.
3. **Conjunctival swab:** In case of conjunctivitis.

Culture of blood and synovial fluid is done in trypticase-soy broth enriched with 1% isovitalex, 10% horse serum and 1% glucose.

Microscopy

Prepare smear by rolling the swab gently over the surface of a glass slide in one direction only. Do not rub swab, it may distort microscopic morphology. Do the Gram staining and see under oil-immersion lens. The observation of characteristic kidney-shaped Gram-negative diplococci lying within polymorphonuclear leucocytes with a few extracellular organisms from a symptomatic male with discharge correlates at a rate of 95% with culture and presumptive evidence of gonococcal infection.

Because women have vaginal and cervical saprophytic flora that resemble gonococci, direct Gram stain correlates in only 50% to 70% of cases with culture. If Gram-negative diplococci are seen only extracellularly, these may not be gonococci, a diagnosis should not be made on this basis. Therefore, culture must be done. If no organisms are visible on Gram staining, report the smear as negative.

Immunologic methods employing monoclonal antibodies may be used for the identification of *N. gonorrhoeae*. These methods include coagglutination and fluorescent antibody testing.

Culture

All specimens received in the laboratory for recovery of *Neisseria* species should be held at room temperature and plated as soon as possible. Media should be warmed to room temperature before inoculation, because *Neisseria* species are susceptible to cold. Roll specimen swab firmly in a 'Z' pattern onto selective medium (Thayer-Martin or modified Thayer-Martin) and then cross-streak with a sterile wire loop or needle. In case of specimen from normally sterile sites inoculate nonselective medium (heated blood agar). Incubate the cultures immediately at 35–36°C in 5–10% CO_2.

Observation

Examine plates after 18–24 hours incubation and test suspected colonies by touching with a cotton bud soaked in oxidase reagent. Oxidase-positive bacteria turn the contact area of the bud purple within 5–15 seconds. If oxidase-positive, prepare a smear from an identical colony and stain it with Gram stain. Gonococci will appear Gram-negative diplococci which can be further confirmed by biochemical reactions. Incubation of primary isolation plate is continued for 48 hours and cultures are re-examined by above procedures before any specimen can be reported negative.

Serology

From some chronic cases or from some patients with metastatic lesions such as arthritis, it may not be possible to isolate gonococci in culture media. Serological tests may be of value in such cases. Antibodies of the IgG, IgM and IgA classes are produced during gonococcal infection. Complement fixation tests with suspensions or crude extracts of gonococci have been used for many years. These are not very sensitive and may also give non-specific results. Defined gonococcal antigens including pilar and outer membrane protein antigens, have been used in radioimmunoassay, ELISA and haemagglutination tests.

Q. 7. Write short note on non-gonococcal urethritis.

Ans. Chronic urethritis where gonococci cannot be demonstrated is known as NGU. The incubation period is variable, but symptoms usually appear 7–14 days after intercourse. Patient develops urethral irritation and dysuria followed by a mucopurulent discharge. Microscopic examination of Gram-stained smears reveals more than five polymorphonuclear leucocytes (PMN) per oil-immersion field (1000X) in discharge, and more than 15 PMN per high power field (400X) in the centrifuged deposit of a first-catch urine specimen.

Causative agents

Twenty to thirty per cent cases of NGU are caused by *Chlamydia trachomatis*. *Ureaplasma urealyticum* may account for a minority of cases of NGU. Up to 10% cases of NGU are caused by *Mycoplasma genitalium*, *M. hominis* and *Bacteroides urealyticus*.

Treatment

Adequate treatment with tetracycline is effective for both *C. trachomatis* and *U. urealyticum* infections.

21

CORYNEBACTERIUM DIPHTHERIAE

Q. 1. Describe morphology, cultural characteristics and biochemical reactions of *Corynebacterium diphtheriae*.

Ans. ***Morphology***

They are thin, slender, non-sporing, non-capsulated, non-motile, non-acid-fast, Gram-positive bacilli of varying lengths with an average size of 3 × 0.3 µm. They frequently possess club-shaped swellings at one or both ends, a characteristic feature which is responsible for the name of the genus (*coryne* means club). When dividing, the bacilli snap and bend abruptly and appear as angled pairs resembling letters V or L or parallel rows of 3–4 bacilli (palisades) which resemble Chinese letters (*Chinese letter arrangement* or *cuneiform arrangement*) (Figs. 21.1 and 21.2).

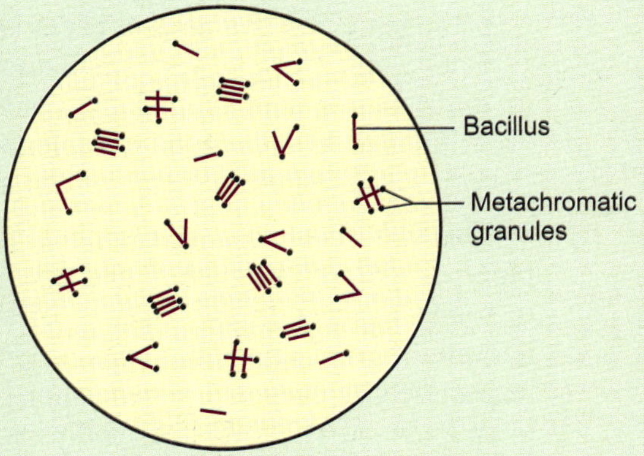

Fig. 21.1. *Corynebacterium diphtheriae* showing metachromatic granules and Chinese letter arrangement.

When stained with methylene blue or toluidine blue, the granules in the cell stain metachromatically (i.e., granules that stain a colour different from the primary dye colour) bluish black. Most cells contain 2 or 3 of these, and they tend to be on the poles. The granules consist of long-chain inorganic polyphosphates. These granules are known as *metachromatic granules* or *volutin granules* or *Babes-Ernst bodies*. In unstained wet preparations, they appear as round refractile bodies within the bacterial cytoplasm.

With Albert stain, the granules stain bluish-black and the cytoplasm green. The granules are not seen during active growth, but start to appear towards the end of the logarithmic growth period. The granule formation is best seen on Loeffler's serum slope. It appears that they represent storage depots for materials needed to form high-energy phosphate bonds. Their presence in thin slender bacilli helps to distinguish *C. diphtheriae* from short, thick, plumpy, non-pathogenic diphtheroids which lack them.

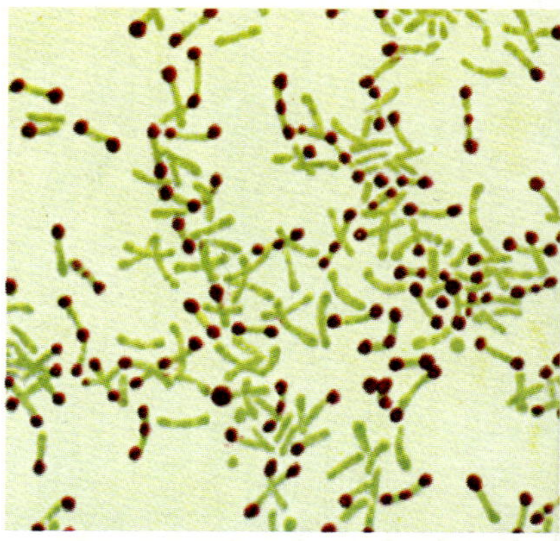

Fig. 21.2. *Corynebacterium diphtheriae* showing metachromatic granules.

Cultural characteristics

Diphtheria bacillus is an aerobe and facultative anaerobe, has an optimum temperature for growth of 37°C (range 15–40°C). It can grow on ordinary nutrient agar, but its growth is improved by the presence of animal proteins such as serum or blood. Two media are useful for this purpose:

1. **Loeffler's serum slope:** Diphtheria bacilli grow rapidly on Loeffler's serum slope, and colonies can be seen in 6–8 hours, long before other bacteria grow. The colonies are at first small, white, opaque discs, but on continued incubation increase in size and may acquire a yellow tint.
2. **Blood tellurite agar (BTA):** The addition of 0.03–0.04% potassium tellurite (K_2TeO_3) to blood agar makes the medium selective for corynebacteria by inhibiting most other pathogenic and commensal bacteria. It may retard the growth even of corynebacteria so that colonies may be very small after 24 hours, therefore, incubation should be continued for 48 hours. On this medium, colonies of *C. diphtheriae* become grey to black because tellurite or tellurous ions are able to diffuse through the cell wall and membrane and are reduced to tellurium metal, which is precipitated inside the cell.

On the basis of colonial morphology on BTA, diphtheria bacilli can be divided into three biotypes – mitis, intermedius and gravis (Table 21.1). These names were originally proposed to relate to the clinical severity of the disease produced by the three biotypes. Mitis, intermedius and gravis biotypes produce disease of mild, intermediate and severe variety respectively. However, this association is not constant. In general, biotype mitis is predominant in endemic areas, while intermedius and gravis tend to be epidemic.

Biochemical reactions

For biochemical differentiation of three biotypes of *C. diphtheriae*, starch and glycogen are used. Gravis strains ferment both but intermedius and mitis strains ferment neither.

Q. 2. Describe diphtheria toxin. What is the role of lysogeny and toxin production, and iron concentration and toxin production?

Ans. Toxigenic strains of *C. diphtheriae* produce a potent bacteriophage-encoded protein exotoxin which is an iron-free, crystalline, heat-labile protein. Its molecular weight is 61,150 daltons and is made up of two parts – A and B with molecular weights of 21,150 and 40,000 daltons respectively. Fragment B is required for transport of fragment A into the cell where it inhibits polypeptide chain elongation at the ribosome. Inhibition of protein synthesis is probably

Table 21.1. Differentiation of three biotypes of *Corynebacterium diphtheriae*

Character	Gravis	Intermedius	Mitis
1. Morphology	Uniformly stained short rods. Some degree of pleomorphism with irregularly barred tear-drop forms. Few or no granules.	Long, irregularly barred cigar-shaped rods, highly pleomorphic. Poor granulation.	Long, curved, pleomorphic, wispy rods with terminal swellings. Prominent granulation.
2. Colony characters on blood tellurite agar after 18–24 hours incubation	Dull greyish black, opaque colonies, 1.5–2.5 mm in diameter. In 2–3 days, 3–5 mm in diameter flat colony with raised dark centre, radially striated periphery and crenated edge – **'daisy-head'** colony.	Small (0.5–0.75 mm in diameter), grey colony with a darker centre and a shining surface – **'frog's egg'** colony. There is little change in size after 48 hours incubation.	Grey, opaque colonies, 1.5–2.0 mm in diameter with regular margins and glossy smooth surface. On further incubation the colony becomes flat with central elevation and regular margins – **'poached egg'** colony.
3. Haemolysis of sheep, rabbit and horse blood	Weakly haemolytic.	Non-haemolytic.	β-haemolytic.
4. Growth in broth	Surface pellicle, granular deposit and little or no turbidity.	Uniform turbidity with fine granular deposit.	Uniform turbidity with pellicle later.
5. Fermentation of starch and glycogen	+	–	–
6. Serotypes	13	4	40
7. Toxigenic strains	Almost 100%	95–99%	80–85%
8. Predominant strains in	Epidemic areas	Epidemic areas	Endemic areas

responsible for both the necrotic and neurotoxic effects of the toxin. When the toxin is treated with formalin it is converted into toxoid.

In highly susceptible species (guinea-pig, rabbit), the lethal dose of diphtheria toxin is 0.1 μg/kg or less, and in man intradermal injection of 0.1 ng will produce a visible skin reaction. Almost all strains of gravis, 95–99% of intermedius and 80–85% of mitis produce this toxin. However, toxin produced by different biotypes is antigenically similar. The classic **Park-Williams strain (PW8)** of *C. diphtheriae* isolated in 1896, is still used as a source of toxin for preparation of diphtheria toxoid (vaccine).

Lysogeny and toxin production

Only those strains of *C. diphtheriae* which are lysogenic for β phage or related temperate phages, that contain the structural gene (*tox* gene), produce diphtheria toxin. Non-toxigenic strains may be rendered toxigenic by infecting them with β phage. This is known as **lysogenic** or **phage conversion**. The toxigenicity remains only as long as the bacillus is lysogenic. When the bacillus is cured of its phage, as by growing it in the presence of antiphage serum, it loses the toxigenicity. The structural gene (*tox* gene) for diphtheria toxin resides on phage genome and is expressed under certain nutritional conditions.

Iron concentration and toxin production

Diphtheria toxin is produced most actively, *in vitro*, when iron concentration is decreased, although other factors such as osmotic pressure, amino acid concentrations and pH also have a role. Optimum iron concentration for toxin production is 0.1 mg per litre of the medium. Toxin production stops at 0.5 mg per litre of the medium. Reason for this is not known. The repressor of the *tox* gene appears to be an iron-containing protein. When sufficient iron is present repressor is formed which inhibits toxin production.

Q. 3. Describe pathogenicity of *Corynebacterium diphtheriae*.

Ans. Diphtheria remains a serious health problem within many regions of the world (e.g., the Indian subcontinent, Southeast Asia, Eastern Europe and South America). ***C. diphtheriae* causes natural infection only in man.** Experimental infection can, however, be produced in various laboratory animals. Infection spreads directly from person to person via nasopharyngeal secretions. Spread is facilitated by intimate contact. Most clinical infections are probably contracted from carriers rather than symptomatic patients. Nasal carriers are particularly dangerous because they shed large number of bacilli which may survive for many weeks in dust and on dry fomites. Children are susceptible after the age of 3–6 months when passive immunity derived from maternal antibodies has disappeared. Incidence is highest among young children, but outbreaks also occur among teenagers and young adults.

Incubation period is 3–4 days, however, it may be as short as 1 day. When toxigenic diphtheria bacilli become lodged in the throat of a susceptible individual, they first multiply rapidly on epithelial cells and produce an exotoxin (diphtheria toxin) that causes local tissue necrosis. The organisms then multiply in cell debris, produce more toxin leading to enlargement of the lesion. The combination of cell necrosis and an exudative inflammatory response of tissue leads to an accumulation of necrotic cellular material, erythrocytes, fibrin and bacteria, which forms a characteristic **diphtheritic pseudomembrane** (in Latin *diphtheria* means pseudomembrane) varying in colour from white to grey to yellow. Since epithelial cells of the mucosa are incorporated in the pseudomembrane, therefore, attempts to remove it produce bleeding.

Diphtheritic pseudomembrane usually appears first on **tonsils** or **posterior pharyngeal wall**. The infection may then spread either upwards into nasal passages or downwards into the larynx and trachea. In **laryngeal diphtheria**, mechanical obstruction may cause suffocation unless the airway is restored by intubation or tracheostomy.

Diphtheria bacilli do not, as a rule, penetrate deeply in the underlying tissues, or the blood, but they produce a powerful exotoxin. Toxin is absorbed into the blood stream from the site of infection and causes toxaemia and various systemic complications. The toxin has a **special affinity for certain tissues, notably heart muscles**, **nerve endings** and **adrenal glands**. Death often results from cardiac failure, but necrotic and often haemorrhagic lesions are usually seen in many organs at necropsy, and in laryngeal diphtheria death is due to suffocation caused by mechanical obstruction.

Although diphtheria is usually a disease of the upper respiratory tract, primary or secondary lesions may occur in other parts of body. The most common nonrespiratory site is the skin (**cutaneous diphtheria**). In cutaneous diphtheria, lesions usually appear at the site of minor abrasions as chronic, spreading, nonhealing ulcers covered by greyish membrane. Rarely, diphtherial infections of conjunctiva, cornea, vagina and ear may occur. These are almost always secondary to pharyngeal or skin infection.

The degree of toxaemia is influenced by the site of infection and the size of the local lesion. Toxin is more readily absorbed from the nasopharyngeal mucosa than from laryngo-tracheal lesions, and lesions of skin differ from those elsewhere in being associated with lower degree of toxaemia.

Q. 4. Describe laboratory diagnosis of diphtheria.

Ans. Because early administration of antitoxin is of paramount importance, specific treatment should be instituted immediately on suspicion of diphtheria, without waiting for laboratory confirmation. The disease runs a quick course and any delay may be fatal. Laboratory confirmation of diphtheria is necessary for the initiation of control measures and for epidemiological purposes. Diagnosis of diphtheria is based on isolating *C. diphtheriae* from the infected area and demonstrating its toxin-producing ability.

Specimens

Two swabs are taken from the local lesion which is usually in the throat but may also be in the nose, larynx, ear, conjunctiva, vagina and skin or from the nose and throat of contacts or suspected carriers. No antiseptics, in the form of gargles, etc., must have been applied within 12 hours. The swabs should be rubbed over the affected area and pseudomembrane, if formed, should be scraped with swab stick or where there is no definitely localized lesion the swabs should be rubbed over the mucous membrane of posterior pharyngeal wall and tonsils.

Microscopy and culture

One swab should be inoculated on Loeffler's serum slope, blood tellurite agar and a plate of ordinary blood agar, the last for differentiating streptococcal or staphylococcal pharyngitis, which may simulate diphtheria. All these media are incubated at 37°C. Loeffler's serum slope is examined after 12–18 hours. If an early result is urgently required then culture may be examined after 6–12 hours, but if it is negative the examination must be repeated after 18–24 hours.

The resultant growth is mixed by emulsifying it with a wire loop in the condensation fluid and from this smears are made and stained by Gram and Albert methods. Blood tellurite agar is examined after 24 hours, and after 48 hours if no growth is obtained after 24 hours. The growth is identified by colonial morphology, Gram staining, Albert staining and biochemical reactions (Table 21.1).

With the **second swab**, **two smears** are prepared and stained by Gram and Albert methods, but only in a small proportion of cases can positive results be obtained in this way and cultures should always be made as a routine procedure, irrespective of direct examination. Smear from Loeffler's serum slope may be the first indication of the presence of diphtheria bacillus.

Toxigenicity or virulence tests of C. diphtheriae

The identification of an isolate as *C. diphtheriae* does not mean that the patient has diphtheria. Diagnosis of diphtheria depends on showing that the isolate produces diphtheria toxin. This can be done by either *in vivo* or *in vitro* testing. *In vivo* testing is rarely done because the *in vitro* method is reliable, less expensive, and free from the need to use animal.

I. **In vivo**
   - Subcutaneous test
   - Intradermal test

II. **In vitro**
   - Elek's gel precipitation test

Subcutaneous test: Emulsify the growth from an overnight culture on Loeffler's serum slope in 2–4 ml broth and inject 0.8 ml of the emulsion subcutaneously into two guinea pigs, one of which has been protected with intramuscular injection of 500 units of diphtheria antitoxin 18–24 hours previously. If strain is virulent, the unprotected animal will die within four days.

Perform autopsy on any of the animals dying within this period. If the isolate is toxigenic then the unprotected animal shows:

- Gelatinous haemorrhagic oedema at the site of inoculation.
- Blood-stained pleural and peritoneal exudate.
- Haemorrhagic inflammation of adrenal glands.

If neither animal dies, the culture is non-toxigenic. If both animals die, the culture is virulent or toxigenic, but not *C. diphtheriae*. This method is usually not employed because the animal is sacrificed.

Intradermal test: Inoculate one colony of suspected *C. diphtheriae* isolate from BTA on a moist Loeffler's serum slope. Incubate at 37°C for 24 hours. Prepare a dense suspension of culture on this medium in 3 ml broth and inject 0.1 ml of this intradermally into the shaved side of a guinea-pig or rabbit. After four hours, the animal is injected intraperitoneally with 500 units of antitoxin. Thirty minutes later a second sample of the test suspension is injected intradermally on the opposite side.

Non-specific inflammatory reaction may occur at both sites within 24–48 hours, but if toxigenic bacilli are present, only the site injected before the antitoxin was administered will progress to form a characteristic necrotic lesion in 48–72 hours. With this test first injection acts as test and second as control and about five strains (10 injections) can be tested on each animal. Moreover, the animal does not die. Therefore, intradermal test is better than subcutaneous test.

Elek's gel precipitation test: This is a gel precipitation test. Pipette 10 ml of nutrient agar that has been cooled to 55°C in a water bath and 2 ml sterile calf serum in a petri dish and rotate 20 times to mix. Before the medium solidifies, place a 1 cm × 8 cm filter paper strip that has been soaked in the diphtheria antitoxin 500–1,000 units/ml across the middle of the plate on the surface of the agar. Allow the medium to solidify and then place the plate in the incubator with the lid ajar to allow the surface moisture to evaporate.

Inoculate the plate within 2 hours after drying by streaking a heavy inoculum of the culture to be tested across the plate at right angles to the antitoxin strip. Parallel to this streak, at a distance of about 15 mm from it, streak a known toxigenic strain of *C. diphtheriae* on one side of the test strain and streak a non-toxigenic strain on the other side. Incubate the plate at 37°C and examine after 24 and 48 hours. Look for **white lines of precipitation** a few mm from the paper strip, that extend out from the line of bacterial growth, forming an angle of about 45°.

These white precipitin lines form where the toxin from pathogenic strains of *C. diphtheriae* combines with the antitoxin in optimum concentration from the paper strip, thus identifying the strains of *C. diphtheriae* that produce the toxin. At 24 hours, the line is best seen with the help of a hand lens, at 48 hours it is more obvious. Look for continuity between the line from unknown culture and that from the known toxigenic culture (Fig. 21.3). This test is very convenient and economical.

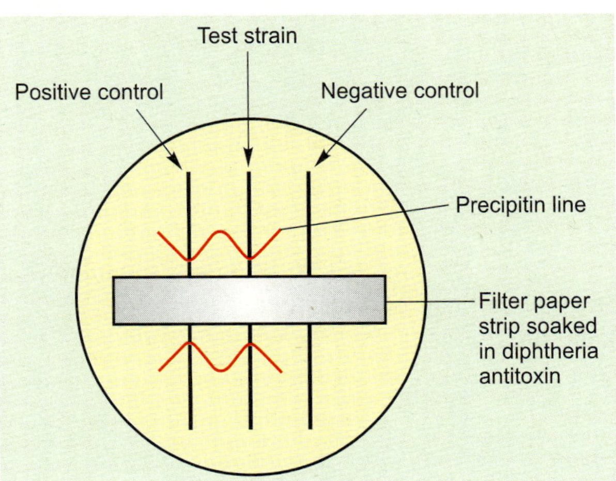

Fig. 21.3. Elek's test.

Q. 5. Describe briefly immunization against diphtheria.

Ans. *Active immunization*

This can be carried out by single and combined vaccines:

- ***Single preparations:*** These include toxin-antitoxin mixture, formol toxoid, alum-precipitated toxoid, purifed toxoid and aluminium phosphate precipitate.

- ***Combined preparations:*** These consist of diphtheria toxoid in combination with tetanus toxoid (DT) only or tetanus toxoid and killed suspension of pertussis bacilli (DPT or triple vaccine). The component antigens of DPT can be given separately also, but giving them together not only minimizes the number of injections, but also improves immune response because the **pertussis vaccine acts as an adjuvant for the toxoids**. A quadruple preparation incorporating, in addition, inactivated polio vaccine, has also been used.

  DPT and oral polio vaccines are given at the age of 6 weeks, 10 weeks, 14 weeks and 16–24 months followed by DT at the age of 5–6 years.

Diphtheria vaccine is highly effective. Fully immunized individuals may become infected with *C. diphtheriae*, because the antibodies are directed only against the toxin, but the disease is mild. Serious infection and death occur only in unimmunized or incompletely immunized individuals.

Passive immunization

This is an emergency measure, to be employed when susceptible (non-immunized) individuals are exposed to infection. It consists of subcutaneous administration of 500–1,000 units of antitoxin or antidiphtheritic serum (ADS). Contacts immunized within the previous 5 years should receive a booster dose of toxoid.

Combined immunization

Since protection conferred by passive immunization is of short duration, therefore, ADS should be administered on one arm and first dose of diphtheria toxoid on the other arm, to be continued by the full course of active immunization.

22

BACILLUS

Q. 1. Describe morphology, cultural characteristics, susceptibility to physical and chemical agents and virulence determinants of *Bacillus anthracis*.

Ans. ***Morphology***

They are large, Gram-positive, catalase-positive, non-acid-fast, non-flagellate, non-motile, spore-forming bacilli, 4–8 × 1–1.5 µm in size. In smears from infected tissues these are found singly, in pairs and in short chains, the entire chain being surrounded by a **capsule** (Fig. 22.1A). It is polypeptide in nature. It is not formed under ordinary conditions of culture but only on media containing serum or bicarbonate in the presence of excess CO_2.

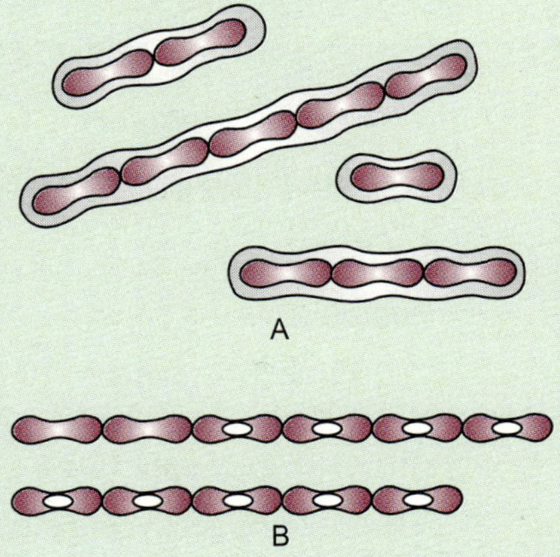

Fig. 22.1. *Bacillus anthracis.*

Spores are formed in culture or in the soil, but never in the animal body during life. Sporulation occurs under unfavourable conditions for growth and is encouraged by distilled water and 2% sodium chloride. It is inhibited by anaerobic conditions and by calcium chloride. **The spores are oval, refractile, central in position and of the same diameter as the bacilli so that they do not cause bulging of the vegetative cell.** In cultures, the bacilli are arranged end to end in long chains. The ends of the bacilli are truncated and somewhat swollen so that a chain of bacilli presents a **"bamboo-stick" appearance** (Fig. 22.1B).

Cultural characteristics

Anthrax bacilli are aerobes and facultative anaerobes. The optimum temperature for growth is 37°C but growth occurs over a wide temperature range of 12–45°C. Optimum pH for growth is 7–7.4. They can grow on ordinary media.

- On **nutrient agar**, the organisms produce large, raised, opaque, greyish-white colonies, 2–3 mm in diameter with an irregular, fringe-like edge. Under low power of the microscope, the edge of the colony is found to be composed of long, interlacing chains of bacilli, resembling curled hair-lock. This gives them the **'medusa head' appearance**. Virulent capsulated strains form rough colonies, while avirulent strains form smooth colonies. Colonies on blood agar produce very slight haemolysis.
- A selective medium (**PLET medium**) consisting of heart infusion agar with polymyxin, lysozyme, ethylenediaminetetraacetic acid (EDTA) and thallous acetate has been devised to isolate *B. anthracis* from mixtures containing other spore-bearing bacilli.
- In a **gelatin stab** culture, there is growth down the stab line with lateral spikes that are longest near the surface, giving **'inverted fir tree' appearance** with slow liquefaction commencing from the top.

Susceptibility to physical and chemical agents

Because of its ability to produce spores, *B. anthracis* is extremely resistant to adverse physical and chemical environment. In the dry state or in soil, the spores remain viable for many years and serve as a source of infection for long periods of time. With moist heat, the vegetative bacilli are killed at 60°C in 30 minutes and the spores at 100°C in 10 minutes. Spores can also be killed by dry heat at 150°C in 60 minutes and by 4% each of formaldehyde and potassium permanganate in a few minutes.

Virulence determinants

1. **Capsular polypeptide:** The capsule which is a polypeptide of D-glutamic acid inhibits phagocytosis.
2. **Anthrax toxin:** It is the plasmid-encoded toxin complex comprising of three protein components:

   (i) Protective antigen (PA),
   (ii) Lethal factor (LF), and
   (iii) Oedema factor (OF).

   The proteins act synergistically to produce the characteristic systemic effects of anthrax. PA is capable of inducing protective antibody. It has been postulated that PA binds to surface receptors on sensitive eukaryotic cells, thereby allowing translocation of OF and LF into the cell. OF is an adenyl cyclase, capable of generating high levels of cyclic adenosine monophosphate in the cytoplasm of susceptible cells leading to oedema. Entry of LF into the target cell causes cell death.

Q. 2. Discuss pathogenicity and laboratory diagnosis of *Bacillus anthracis*.

Ans. *Pathogenicity*

B. anthracis causes **anthrax**. It is a **zoonosis** – a disease of animals transmissible to man. It is primarily a disease of cattle and sheep and less often of horses and swines, but experimentally most mammals are susceptible. Bacilli are shed in large numbers from all orifices of the infected animal during the terminal stages of the disease. The organisms sporulate in the soil and remain a source of infection for a number of decades. Animals are infected by ingestion of spores present in the soil. Direct spread from animal to animal is rare.

Man acquires infection through small cuts or abrasions in the skin, by inhalation of spores and rarely by ingestion of infected meat. *Since the release of weaponized B. anthracis spores in the U.S. postal system in 2001, the potential danger associated with this organism has been re-emphasized*. Depending on the mode of infection, anthrax presents in one of the three forms – cutaneous, pulmonary and intestinal.

Cutaneous anthrax

About 95% of human cases of anthrax are cutaneous infections. It is common in farmers and veterinary surgeons handling infected animals, dock workers, factory workers, persons who handle carcasses, hides and animal hair, and those who use shaving brushes prepared from infected animal hair. The lesion starts as a small, pruritic, painless **papule** 1–5 days after contact with infected material. The papule then develops into **vesicle** containing haemorrhagic fluid. Eventually, the vesicle breaks down and is replaced by a **black eschar**, from which it derives its name. *Anthrax in Greek means coal*. Black eschar is later surrounded by a ring of vesicles containing serous fluid and an area of oedema and induration which may become extensive. This has been called a **malignant pustule**. If the lesion is not treated, the organisms may invade the regional lymph nodes and blood stream causing death.

Pulmonary anthrax

It is also known as **wool-sorter's disease** because it used to be common in workers in wool factories, due to inhalation of spores from infected wool. It may also involve workers who handle animal hides which contain spores. This is a haemorrhagic pneumonia with a high fatality rate.

Intestinal anthrax

It is extremely rare and occurs in primitive communities who eat improperly cooked carcasses of animals dying of anthrax. Patient develops haemorrhagic diarrhoea after a day or so and dies rapidly from septicaemia.

Anthrax meningitis may occur as a result of bacteraemia after pulmonary anthrax and is less common than other forms of anthrax. The cerebrospinal fluid is haemorrhagic in most cases and there is polymorphonuclear leucocytosis. Numerous bacilli are also present. Mortality is nearly 100%.

Laboratory diagnosis

Specimens

B. anthracis can be demonstrated in the material from a malignant pustule, sometimes in sputum from pulmonary anthrax, in gastric aspirates, faeces or food in intestinal anthrax and in the blood in the septicaemic stage of all forms of the disease. Specimens should be taken before antibiotic therapy has been instituted. **All procedures connected with the handling of *B. anthracis* should be carried out in microbiology laboratory that utilizes Biological Safety Level 2 (BSL2) practices. Laboratory personnel should wear protective gowns, masks and surgical gloves when processing the samples. Safety glasses or eye**

shields are recommended. After the work is over, all laboratory work benches and surfaces in the safety cabinet must be sterilized with 5% hypochlorite or 5% phenol and all the instruments used for processing the specimen must be autoclaved.

In case of malignant pustule, necessary specimens include fluid aspirated from the vesicles surrounding black eschar or material beneath the edge of the black eschar. In early cases, fluid may be obtained by scraping the lesion with a needle.

Microscopy

Prepare smears of each specimen and stain with Gram's method. Examine the stained smears under oil-immersion lens for characteristic Gram-positive anthrax bacilli.

When blood films containing anthrax bacilli are stained with **polychrome methylene blue** for a few seconds and examined under microscope, **an amorphous purplish material** is noticed around the bacilli. This represents the capsular material and is characteristic of anthrax bacillus. This is known as **McFadyean's reaction** and is employed for the presumptive diagnosis of anthrax (Fig. 22.1A). When stained with Giemsa's stain, the bacillus stains purple and capsule red.

Culture

Culture the exudate on nutrient agar, blood agar, PLET medium and nutrient broth. Incubate at 37°C for 24 hours. Examine plates for the medusa-head colonies characteristic of *B. anthracis*. Prepare a smear, stain it by Gram's method and look for tangled chains of large Gram-positive bacilli some of which have central, oval, non-bulging spores. In nutrient broth, look for a pellicle and a deposit.

Animal inoculation

Anthrax bacilli can often be isolated from contaminated tissue by applying them over shaven skin of a guinea pig. The animal dies in 48–72 hours. Autopsy reveals gelatinous, haemorrhagic oedema at the site of inoculation, petechial haemorrhages in the peritoneum and an enlarged dark red spleen. Make smears from heart blood and spleen, stain by Gram's and McFadyean's methods, and look for typical anthrax bacilli.

Serology

If the sample received is putrid so that viable bacilli are unlikely, diagnosis may be established by **Ascoli's thermoprecipitin test**. The tissue is ground up in saline, boiled for 5 minutes, filtered and layered over antianthrax serum in a narrow tube. If tissue contains anthrax antigen, a ring of precipitation will appear at the junction of the two liquids within 5 minutes at room temperature. Serological diagnosis by ELISA may be of value retrospectively.

Polymerase chain reaction (PCR)

For further confirmation PCR with specific primers may be carried out.

Q. 3. Write short note on *Bacillus cereus*.

Ans. It is widely distributed in nature and is commonly found in soil, water, milk, vegetation, and cereals such as rice and a wide variety of other foods. It is an aerobic, spore-forming, large Gram-positive bacillus resembling *B. anthracis* except that it is motile, non-capsulated, not susceptible to gamma phage and does not react with fluorescent antibody conjugate.

B. cereus produces two different toxins:

1. **Emetic toxin:** This is a heat-stable toxin. Patient develops nausea and vomiting 1–6 hours after ingestion of food that contains this toxin and recovers 6–24 hours after the onset of symptoms. Most of the outbreaks of emetic syndrome have been associated with boiled or fried rice served in oriental restaurants. The spores of certain strains of *B. cereus* found in raw rice survive boiling. When boiled rice is stored at room temperature rather than in the refrigerator (to avoid clumping of grains), the spores germinate and produce heat-stable toxin within the rice prior to preparation of fried rice. Flash frying does not always destroy heat-stable toxin.
2. **Enterotoxin:** It is heat-labile toxin formed in the intestine. Like cholera enterotoxin and labile-toxin (LT) of *Escherichia coli*, it acts on the epithelial cells of small intestine resulting in stimulation of cell-bound adenyl cyclase. This leads to increased levels of cyclic adenosine monophosphate (cAMP) in the gut epithelial cells resulting in active secretion of large volumes of fluid into the intestinal lumen.

   This toxin results in symptoms of abdominal pain and profuse diarrhoea (diarrhoeal syndrome) after an incubation period of 10–12 hours. Recovery usually occurs within 12 hours after onset. Implicated foods associated with diarrhoeal syndrome include poultry, meat, mashed potatoes and various soups. In both situations, enormous numbers of organisms (up to 10^{10} per gram) are found in contaminated food.

Laboratory diagnosis

Suspected food, faeces and vomitus are cultured on ordinary media or a special mannitol-egg yolk-phenol red-polymyxin agar (MYPA) medium. *B. cereus* is a motile bacillus, non-capsulated, not susceptible to gamma phage and does not react with fluorescent antibody conjugate. It produces lecithinase and ferments glucose but not mannitol. The inability to recover organisms from fried rice does not necessarily rule out *B. cereus* as cause of the emetic form of illness because flash frying of the fried rice can eliminate the organisms but not the heat-stable toxin.

Clostridium

Q. 1. Classify clostridia.

Ans. On the basis of biochemical reactions many clostridia can be divided into:

1. **Predominantly saccharolytic clostridia:**
   - *C. perfringens*
   - *C. septicum*
   - *C. tertium*
   - *C. fallax*

   When grown in cooked meat broth (CMB), they rapidly produce acid and gas but they do not digest the meat. The culture may have a slightly sour smell and the meat is often reddened.
2. **Predominantly proteolytic clostridia:**
   - *C. sporogenes*
   - *C. histolyticum*

   They digest protein and liquefy gelatin and coagulated serum. Culture in CMB produces blackening of meat, decomposing it and reducing it in volume with the formation of foul-smelling products.
3. **Slightly proteolytic clostridia:**
   - *C. tetani*

Q. 2. Describe morphology, cultural characteristics, biochemical reactions of and toxin production by *Clostridium perfringens*.

Ans. ***Morphology***

They are large, Gram-positive, spore-bearing bacilli, measuring 4–6 × 1 µm with parallel sides and truncated or slightly rounded ends. They occur singly, in pairs or in small bundles.

They are non-motile and form capsules in animal body. Spores are oval, subterminal or central and non-bulging (Fig. 23.1A). They are formed under natural conditions, e.g., in the bowel. They are only rarely seen in direct smears from wounds or cultures but can be demonstrated on growth in special media such as Ellner's medium.

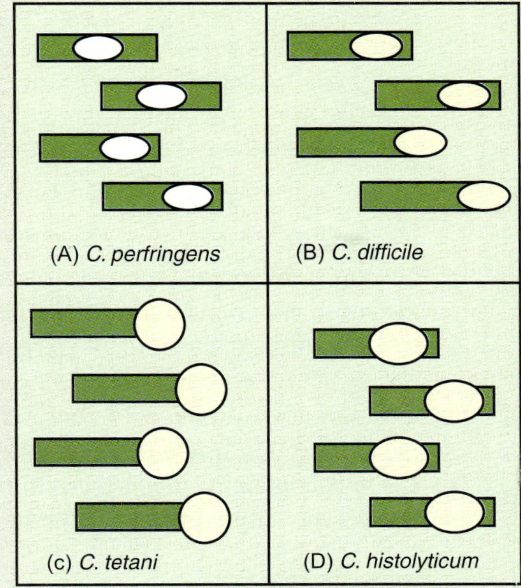

Fig. 23.1. Types of spores in different *Clostridium* species.

Cultural characteristics

It is an anaerobe, but can grow under microaerophilic conditions. Optimum temperature for growth is 37°C. It grows best on media containing carbohydrate such as **glucose blood agar** and forms two main types of colonies. One is round, 2–4 mm in diameter, smooth, regular, convex, amorphous, greyish-yellow and slightly opaque. Other is umbonate with an opaque brownish centre and a lighter, translucent, radially striated periphery with a crenated edge.

On **horse blood agar**, colonies are usually surrounded by a zone of β-haemolysis and commonly also by an outer wider zone of incomplete haemolysis owing to the action of θ and α toxins respectively (**double zone haemolysis**).

Biochemical reactions

It is actively saccharolytic and ferments glucose, maltose, sucrose, lactose and starch with the production of acid and gas.

In **litmus milk medium**, it ferments lactose and produces acid and gas. The acid clots the milk and the gas breaks up the clot resulting in **stormy clot reaction**. Production of acid is also indicated by change in the colour of the litmus from **blue to red**. The culture has sour butyric acid odour. It is indole negative, MR positive, VP negative and H_2S positive.

Gelatin is liquefied but coagulated serum is usually not liquefied. In **cooked meat broth (CMB)**, meat turns pink and is not digested. **It produces phospholipase-C** which gives opalescence around the colonies on egg yolk containing medium.

Toxins

C. perfringens produces **four major lethal, eight minor lethal or non-lethal toxins, and enterotoxin**. Major lethal toxins include α (alpha), β (beta), ε (epsilon) and ι (iota) and minor lethal toxins include γ (gamma), δ (delta), κ (kappa), λ (lambda), μ (mu), η (nu), θ (theta) and ν (eta).

On the basis of four major toxins, *C. perfringens* can be divided into **five types, A–E** (Table 23.1). Typing is done by neutralization tests with specific antitoxins by intracutaneous injection in guinea-pigs or intravenous injection in mice. Strains of *C. perfringens* type A that produce enterotoxin are associated with a mild form of food poisoning. Typical food poisoning strains (type A2) are non-haemolytic or feebly haemolytic on horse blood agar and have markedly heat-resistant spores but classical (type A1) strains are β-haemolytic and have relatively heat-sensitive spores.

Table 23.1. Typing of *Clostridium perfringens*

Type	Toxin produced			
	α	β	ε	τ
A	+	–	–	–
B	+	+	+	–
C	+	+	–	–
D	+	–	+	–
E	+	–	–	+

Alpha toxin

It is produced by all types of *C. perfringens* but most abundantly by type A strains. It is the most important toxin and is responsible for the profound toxaemia of gas gangrene. It is thermostable, lethal for mice, guinea-pigs, rabbits, pigeons and sheep, and when given intradermally, produces a necrotic lesion. It is Ca^{++} or Mg^{++} dependent phospholipase (lecithinase-C). In the presence of free Ca^{++} or Mg^{++}, it produces opalescence in serum or egg yolk containing media by splitting phospholipid complexes. This reaction can be inhibited by specific antitoxin. This is the basis of Nagler's reaction.

Nagler's reaction

A culture plate containing 6% agar, 5% peptic digest of sheep blood and 20% human serum or 5% egg yolk is prepared. The plate is dried. On one half of the plate, 2–3 drops of *C. perfringens* antitoxin are spread and allowed to dry. The plate is then inoculated with the test organisms or the exudate under study and incubated anaerobically at 37°C for 18 hours. On the section containing no antitoxin, *C. perfringens* colonies show surrounding zone of **opalescence**, i.e., Nagler's reaction whereas colonies of the remainder half of the plate show no change (Fig. 23.2). It is because of specific neutralization of the alpha toxin. Neomycin sulphate may be added to this medium to inhibit aerobic spore-forming organisms and coliforms. **Willis and Hobbs medium** also incorporates lactose and neutral red to indicate lactose-fermenting organisms, and milk to indicate proteolysis.

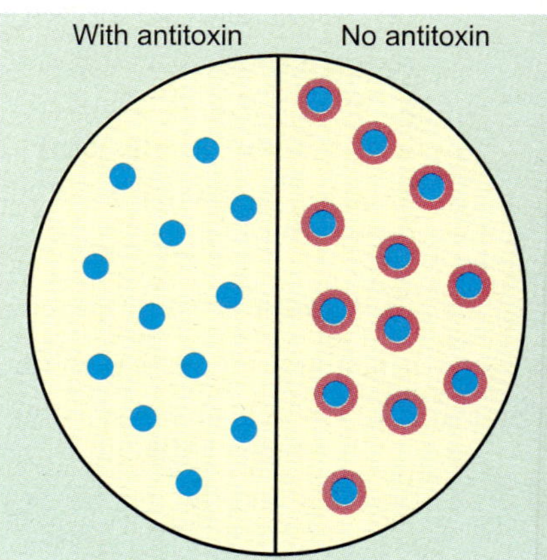

Fig. 23.2. Nagler's reaction.

Other major and minor toxins

- *Beta toxin* is not haemolytic, it is lethal to mice, and when given intradermally in guinea-pigs and rabbits it produces necrotic lesions.
- *Epsilon* and *iota toxins* are lethal and necrotizing, and non-haemolytic.
- *Gamma* and *eta* toxins are minor lethal toxins. They are neither necrotizing nor haemolytic.
- *Delta toxin* is lethal and actively haemolytic for the red cells of sheep, goat, pig and cattle.
- *Theta toxin* is oxygen-labile haemolysin antigenically related to streptolysin O. It is moderately lethal.
- *Lambda toxin* is non-lethal, non-necrotizing proteinase and gelatinase.

- *Kappa*, *mu* and *nu* toxins are collagenase, hyaluronidase and deoxyribonuclease respectively.

Enterotoxin

C. perfringens type A strains produce a potent enterotoxin. It is a heat-labile, non-diffusible protein with a polypeptide chain and a molecular weight of 34,000–35,000 daltons. *It is formed in the intestine at the time of sporulation.*

Q. 3. Discuss pathogenicity of *Clostridium perfringens*.

Ans. *C. perfringens* may lead to following infections:

1. Wound infection

C. perfringens occurs normally in the soil, particularly that of manured and cultivated land, and animal and human excreta. The infection usually results from contamination of a wound with these. Wound may get contaminated with patient's own faeces during surgery or after accident. Clostridia may also be present on the normal skin, especially on the perineum and thigh. These may also cause infection.

The presence of devitalized or dead tissue due to crushing of tissues and the severing of arteries in accidental and war injuries, blood clots, extravasated fluid, foreign bodies (bullets, shell fragments and bits of clothing) and coincident infection with aerobic organisms reduce the oxygen tension. This leads to germination of clostridial spores followed by multiplication of vegetative forms with the production of exotoxins and enzymes into the surrounding environment causing more tissue destruction and resulting in a rapid and fulminating spread of the organism in the necrotic environment. In addition, carbohydrates may be fermented, resulting in production of large quantities of gas in the tissues.

The pressure resulting from gas formation may cause still more restriction of the blood supply to adjoining tissue and hence more necrosis. Hyaluronidase produced by *C. perfringens* breaks down intercellular cement substance and promotes the spread of the infection along tissue planes. Collagenase and proteinase produced by this organism break down tissues and virtually liquefy muscles. In the absence of surgical and antitoxic treatment, severe toxaemia and death frequently ensue. Three types of clostridial wound infections are recognized:

1. ***Wound contamination:*** Here one or more clostridia are present in the traumatized tissue without evidence of infection. Up to 80–90% isolates of *C. perfringens* from hospitalized patients represent simple saprophytic wound contamination.
2. ***Clostridial cellulitis:*** In this condition, infection is confined to local fascial planes in the absence of significant toxaemia. The infecting clostridia are of low invasive power and poor toxigenicity. There is a seropurulent discharge from the wound with an offensive odour and prognosis is good.
3. ***Clostridial myonecrosis or gas gangrene:*** In this condition, there is invasion of healthy muscle tissue and striking systemic intoxication as discussed above.

The **incubation period of gas gangrene** is 2–3 days. The disease develops with increasing pain, tenderness and oedema of the affected part along with systemic signs of toxaemia. There is a thin watery discharge from the wound, which later becomes profuse and serosanguinous. Accumulation of gas (predominantly hydrogen which is less soluble than carbon dioxide) makes the tissue crepitant.

2. Food poisoning

Enterotoxin producing strains of *C. perfringens* are associated with a mild form of food poisoning. **It is third most common etiologic agent of food poisoning after *Salmonella* spp. and *S. aureus*.** Both heat-resistant (A2) and heat-sensitive (A1) strains of *C. perfringens* are capable of causing food poisoning. The incriminated food is usually meat that has been cooked hours in advance and then cooled slowly, or even allowed to stand at room temperature for several hours before being served. Before cooking, the meat may get contaminated with heat-resistant spores from the animal's intestine at the abattoir or from soil and dust during transit to shops and then from shops to houses and catering establishments.

3. Necrotizing jejunitis (Enteritis necroticans)

It is a severe and often fatal disease caused by *C. perfringens* type C. This condition is rare but sporadic cases and outbreaks have been reported from New Guinea, Germany, East Africa, Thailand and Nepal.

In addition, *C. perfringens* may also cause necrotizing colitis, gangrenous appendicitis, biliary tract infection, brain abscess and meningitis, panophthalmitis, thoracic infections, and urogenital infections.

Q. 4. Describe laboratory diagnosis of *Clostridium perfringens* infection.

Ans. The diagnosis of gas gangrene must primarily be made upon clinical grounds and initiation of treatment should not await full laboratory report. The function of laboratory is only to provide confirmation of clinical diagnosis.

Specimens

1. Edges of affected muscles,
2. Necrotic tissue, and
3. Exudate from the depth of the lesion, where infection seems to be most pronounced, to be collected with a capillary pipette.

Microscopic examination

Gram smears are prepared. If gas gangrene exists, smear shows typical Gram-positive bacilli often with other bacteria. Thick, stubby, Gram-positive rods suggest *C. perfringens*.

Culture

Aerobic and anaerobic cultures are made on fresh blood agar and heated blood agar. To prevent swarming by some anaerobes, 5–6% agar in plates is used. A plate of human serum or egg yolk agar with *C. perfringens* antitoxin spread on one half of the plate is used for Nagler's reaction.

For isolation of *C. perfringens* from faeces, inoculate CMB and heat it at 100°C for 30 minutes, cool it and incubate it at 37°C for 18 hours. Subculture on Willis and Hobbs medium, incubate anaerobically at 37°C for 18 hours. Look for colonies of Gram-positive bacilli showing Nagler's reaction.

For isolation of classical strains which are heat-sensitive, stool specimen is inoculated on Willis and Hobbs medium with neomycin 70 μg/ml. Incubate and identify as above. For isolation of *C. perfringens* from food, process it as for the isolation of classical strains from stools.

Reverse CAMP test

This test is similar to the CAMP test for identifying group B streptococci except that *C. perfringens* is inoculated over the centre of blood agar plate in place of *Staphylococcus aureus*. *Streptococcus agalactiae* is streaked at right angle to it. Positive CAMP test shows butterfly-shaped enhanced haemolysis pointing towards *C. perfringens* (Fig. 23.3).

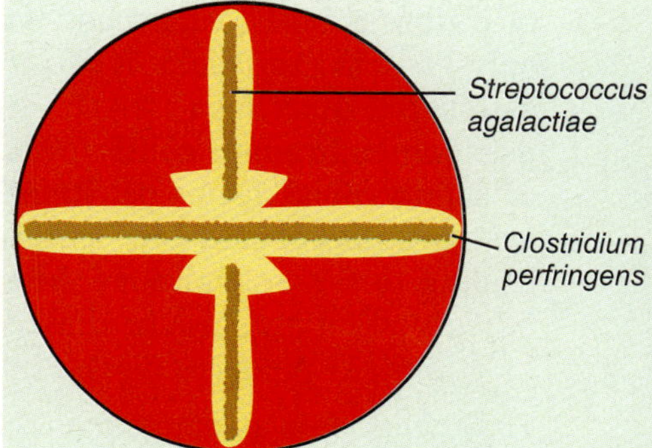

Fig. 23.3. Reverse CAMP test.

Q. 5. Describe briefly prophylaxis and treatment of gas gangrene.

Ans. *1. Toilet of the wound*

The most important preventive measure against clostridial myonecrosis is early and adequate wound debridement and irrigation of the wound to remove blood clots, necrotic tissue and foreign material. This ensures elimination of the bulk of the contaminating organisms. Wound is not sutured but is left open after thorough cleansing and loosely packed. Hyperbaric oxygen chamber, in which an infected area is placed in a chamber containing pure oxygen under pressure, has been used with some success to stop the growth of the anaerobes.

2. Chemotherapy

Surgical toilet is combined with topical and parenteral antimicrobial therapy in high doses. This should be directed against clostridial element and likely coexistence of aerobic organisms. Therefore, penicillin, metronidazole and an aminoglycoside may be given in combination. Clindamycin or a broad-spectrum β-lactam antibiotic such as cefotaxime or imipenem may also be given.

3. Antitoxic therapy

A polyvalent antiserum containing 10,000 units each of *C. perfringens* and *C. novyi* antitoxins, and 5,000 units of *C. septicum* antitoxin given intramuscular or in emergency intravenous, has been used in the prophylaxis and treatment of gas gangrene. Its efficacy has never been established and intensive antimicrobial therapy has now replaced antitoxic therapy.

Q. 6. Describe briefly morphology and pathogenesis of *Clostridium difficile*. Also describe laboratory diagnosis and treatment of *Clostridium difficile* infection.

Ans. Morphology

It is a Gram-positive bacillus, 4–8 × 0.5–1 μm in size with oval, subterminal or terminal, non-bulging spores (Fig. 23.1B). It is motile by peritrichate flagella. It is an obligate anaerobe and grows well on blood agar at 37°C. On this medium, after 24 hours incubation, colonies are non-haemolytic, glossy, greyish, low convex, and circular with irregular edges. Cefoxitin cycloserine fructose agar (CCFA) with egg yolk and neutral red, a selective medium, significantly aids in its isolation from faeces.

Pathogenesis

C. difficile is ubiquitous in nature, and has been isolated from soil, water, intestinal contents of various animals, vagina and urethra of humans, and faeces of 40–50% of neonates and only 3% of healthy adults. It has, however, been implicated as a causative agent of **antibiotic-associated diarrhoea** (AAD), **antibiotic-associated colitis** (AAC) and life-threatening **pseudomembranous colitis** (PMC). These conditions have been associated with a number of antimicrobial agents particularly clindamycin and ampicillin. Use of these antibiotics leads to killing of antibiotic-sensitive organisms and overgrowth of *C. difficile* in the intestine leading to these conditions. Most of the cases of PMC are caused by *C. difficile* but infrequently it may also be caused by *S. aureus* and *C. perfringens*.

C. difficile produces disease by the elaboration of two distinct exotoxins:

1. ***Toxin A:*** It is an enterotoxin that is primarily responsible for diarrhoea. It is capable of producing fluid accumulation in ligated rabbit ileal loop assay.
2. ***Toxin B:*** It is a potent cytotoxin capable of producing cytopathogenic effects in several tissue culture cell lines.

Laboratory diagnosis

It can be accomplished by demonstrating the toxin in the faeces of the patient by its characteristic effect on HEp2 and human diploid cell cultures or by ELISA. *C. difficile* can also be grown from the faeces of the patient.

Treatment

Discontinue the antibiotic that is presumed to have precipitated the disease, and suppress growth and toxin production of *C. difficile* by giving vancomycin or metronidazole.

Q. 7. Describe morphology, cultural characteristics, biochemical reactions and sensitivity to physical and chemical agents of *Clostridium tetani*.

Ans. ***Morphology***

C. tetani is a slender, Gram-positive bacillus, 2–5 × 0.4–0.5 μm with rounded ends. It tends to be pleomorphic and filamentous. It is non-capsulated and motile by peritrichate flagella. However, type VI strains which do not possess flagella, are non-motile. Young cultures of the organisms usually stain Gram-positive but in older cultures and in smears made from the wounds, they are Gram-variable and even frank Gram-negative. The spores are spherical, terminal and twice the diameter of vegetative cells giving them typical **'drumstick' appearance** (Fig. 23.1C). The spores do not take up the Gram stain and appear as colourless round structures.

Cultural characteristics

C. tetani is an obligate anaerobe. The optimum temperature and pH for its growth are 37°C and 7.4 respectively. It can grow well on ordinary media, but its growth is improved by the addition of blood or serum.

- **Colonies on solid media** are irregularly round, 2–5 mm in diameter with fine branching projections. Some strains form colonies with thicker, translucent, yellow brown centre and thin, translucent, colourless periphery. Isolated colonies of *C. tetani* may not be obtained because of the tendency of the organism to swarm over the surface of the medium. However, non-motile variants may produce isolated colonies.
- **On horse blood agar**, the colonies of *C. tetani* are surrounded by a zone of α-haemolysis, which subsequently develops into β-haemolysis owing to the production of an oxygen-labile haemolysin known as tetanolysin.
- **On egg yolk agar**, it does not produce opalescence or pearly layer.
- It grows well **in CMB**. The meat is not digested but shows slight blackening on prolonged incubation.

Biochemical reactions

C. tetani has slight proteolytic and no saccharolytic activity. Gelatin is slowly liquefied. Coagulated serum is rendered more transparent and softened but not liquefied. It is indole positive and MR, VP, H_2S and nitrate reduction negative.

Sensitivity to physical and chemical agents

Spores of some strains of *C. tetani* are killed by boiling for 10–15 minutes, but some resist boiling for up to 3 hours and dry heat at 160°C for 1 hour. They can, however, be killed by autoclaving at 121°C for 15 minutes. They are inactivated by exposure to iodine (1% aqueous solution), hydrogen peroxide (10 volumes) and glutaraldehyde (2%) within a few hours. In the soil, spores of *C. tetani* can survive for years.

Q. 8. Write short note on tetanus toxins.

Ans. *C. tetani* produces an oxygen-labile haemolysin (tetanolysin) but all the symptoms in tetanus are attributable to a potent neurotoxin (tetanospasmin). Different strains vary from completely non-toxigenic to very highly toxigenic.

1. Tetanospasmin

It is a heat-labile protein that may be inactivated by heating at 60°C for 20 minutes. Tetanospasmin is synthesized in the bacterium as a single polypeptide chain with a molecular weight of 150,000 daltons. On its release from the organism, a bacterial protease cleaves one peptide bond to yield 2 chains that remain linked together through a disulphide bond. The large polypeptide chain has a molecular weight of 100,000 daltons, and it possesses the specific receptors that bind the toxin to the neuronal gangliosides. The smaller polypeptide chain has a molecular weight of 50,000 daltons and is thought to exert the biologic effect of the toxin. **It is an extremely powerful toxin second in potency only to the exotoxin of *C. botulinum*.** It has a minimum lethal dose, for a mouse, of 50–75 ng. It gets toxoided spontaneously or in the presence of low concentrations of formaldehyde. It is a good antigen and is specifically neutralized by the antitoxin. The structural gene for toxin production is located on a 75-kilobase plasmid.

2. Tetanolysin

In addition to its neurotoxin, *C. tetani* produces an oxygen-labile haemolysin, antigenically related to streptolysin O and θ toxin of *C. perfringens* and *C. novyi*. There is no evidence that it plays a significant role in pathogenesis.

Q. 9. Describe pathogenesis of tetanus.

Ans. The spores of *C. tetani* are ubiquitous. They occur in the gastrointestinal tracts of man and animals. They are also present in the soil especially in manured soil. Tetanus develops following the contamination of wound with *C. tetani* spores. The source of infection may be soil, dirty clothing or faeces. Germination of spores is dependent upon the reduced tension occurring in devitalized tissue.

C. tetani remains localized at the site of initial infection and produces tetanus toxin. It is absorbed from the site of its production and ascends to the central nervous system via motor nerves. However, some toxin may be delivered from the site of infection via the blood to all nerves in the body and the subsequent transmission to the central nervous system depends upon uptake through neuromuscular nerve endings and intra-axonal transport. Therefore, the first symptoms in human tetanus appear in head and neck because of the shorter length of the cranial nerves.

Tetanospasmin resembles strychnine in its effect. It appears to act by interfering with the normal inhibition of motor impulses exercised by the upper motor neuron over the lower. This results in sustained muscle spasm and the characteristic signs of spasm of jaw muscles (**lockjaw, *trismus***) and facial muscles (***risus sardonicus***), and arching of the body (opisthotonicus).

The **incubation period** of tetanus varies from 2 days to several weeks but commonly it is 6–12 days. Tetanus is a serious disease with a high mortality rate of 80–90% without proper treatment and even with proper treatment it is 15–50%. Tetanus neonatorum and uterine tetanus have very high fatality rates (70–100%).

Q. 10. Describe laboratory diagnosis of tetanus.

Ans. The diagnosis is usually based on clinical findings alone because the isolation of the organism can occur in the absence of the disease, and it is also possible to have tetanus and never isolate the organism.

Microscopy

Collect pus or necrotic material from the wound, prepare a smear and stain it by Gram's method. Examine under microscope for typical 'drumstick' bacilli. But only a minority of specimens will show these.

Culture

Diagnosis by culture is more dependable. Pus or wound scrapings or excised bits of tissue from the necrotic depths of wound should be plated on one half of a blood agar plate and 3 bottles of CMB. Blood agar plate is incubated anaerobically at 37°C. *C. tetani* produces swarming growth which may be detected on opposite half of the plate after 1–2 days. Of the 3 inoculated CMB bottles, one should be incubated unheated, second is heated in a water bath at 80°C for 5 minutes and third for 20 minutes. The purpose of heating for different periods is to kill non-sporing bacilli, while leaving tetanus spores undamaged, which vary widely in heat-resistance. The heated bottles are also incubated anaerobically at 37°C.

Subcultures from all these bottles are made on half of a blood agar plate daily for 4 days. The plates are incubated anaerobically at 37°C and examined for the swarming edge of *C. tetani*. Incorporation of polymyxin B, to which clostridia are resistant, makes the medium selective.

In vitro toxigenicity test

A blood agar plate containing 4% agar, to minimize swarming, is divided into 2 halves. One half is smeared with tetanus antitoxin. Both halves are then inoculated with growth assumed to be *C. tetani* and incubated anaerobically for 2 days. Colonies haemolytic on the untreated half, but not on the antitoxin half, are of *C. tetani*.

In vivo toxigenicity test

The toxigenicity of the organisms is confirmed by demonstrating the production of tetanospasmin. Two mice, one unprotected and other protected, by giving 1,000 units of tetanus antitoxin intraperitoneally 1 hour before the test, are challenged with an intramuscular injection in the hind leg of 0.1 ml of a 48 hour CMB culture supernate of the isolate. The protected mouse remains well. Signs of ascending tetanus develop in the unprotected animal after several hours, they begin in the inoculated leg and extend to the tail, then the other hind limb is affected and then generalized signs appear. The animal dies within 2 days.

Q. 11. Write short note on prophylaxis of tetanus.

Ans. It is of 3 types:

1. Surgical prophylaxis

This includes prompt and adequate wound debridement, removal of foreign material, necrotic tissue and blood clots. This ensures elimination of the bulk of the contaminating organisms, and an anaerobic environment for the growth of *C. tetani* is not provided. Clean superficial wounds that receive prompt attention may not require specific protection against tetanus.

2. Antibiotic prophylaxis

This includes prompt administration of antibiotics to destroy or inhibit *C. tetani* and pyogenic bacteria in the wound, so that the production of the toxin can be prevented. A long-acting penicillin or one tablet of erythromycin 500 mg twice daily for 5 days may be given preferably before the wound toilet. However, antibiotics have no effect on the toxin, therefore, antibiotic prophylaxis does not replace immunoprophylaxis.

3. Immunoprophylaxis

It includes 3 types of immunization:

1. **Active immunization:** It is carried out with 3 spaced intramuscular injections of formol toxoid. The intervals recommended are 6–8 weeks between the first and second injections and 4–6 months between the second and third injection and booster doses every 10 years.
2. **Passive immunization:** Tetanus antitoxin often called antitetanus serum (ATS) can be obtained by immunizing horses with TT. This serum is of value if given immediately after wounding. The usual prophylactic dose is 1,500 international units given intramuscularly or subcutaneously as soon as possible after injury. The injection may be

repeated at a weekly interval till the danger of tetanus persists. Larger initial dose of 3,000–10,000 international units may be given when the wound is severe.

Disadvantages of ATS:

- *Immune elimination:* The half life of ATS in man is about 7 days, and in persons who have had prior injections of horse serum (antigenic for man) it is eliminated much quicker by combination with pre-existing antibodies to horse serum developed in response to earlier injections of ATS.
- *Hypersensitivity reactions:* Administration of ATS may lead to hypersensitivity reactions like fatal anaphylaxis and serum sickness. It is, therefore, mandatory to test for hypersensitivity before administration of ATS. The intradermal test for hypersensitivity is unreliable. A dose of 0.05 ml of ATS is given subcutaneously and patient is observed for at least half an hour for general reactions. Since even this may lead to anaphylaxis in some individuals, therefore, a syringe loaded with adrenaline (1/1,000) should invariably be kept ready.

Human tetanus immunoglobulin (HTIG) has replaced ATS for tetanus prophylaxis in many countries, because it has considerable advantage of a longer half life (3–5 weeks) and freedom from risks of hypersensitivity reactions. This is prepared by immunization of human volunteers who are free from hepatitis B, C and D, and human immunodeficiency viruses. Since HTIG is not antigenic for man, therefore, immune elimination is not seen with HTIG. The prophylactic dose of HTIG is 250–500 units by intramuscular injection.

3. **Combined immunization:** It consists of administering to a non-immune person ATS or HTIG at one site, along with the first dose of TT at another site, followed by second and third doses of TT at appropriate intervals.

Q. 12. Describe morphology, cultural characteristics, susceptibility to physical and chemical agents, antigenic types and botulinum toxin of *Clostridium botulinum*.

Ans. ***Morphology***

C. botulinum is a straight or slightly curved Gram-positive bacillus with rounded ends. It measures about 5 × 1 µm (range 3.4–8.6 × 0.5–1.3 µm) in size. It is non-capsulated and motile by peritrichate flagella. It produces heat-resistant spores that are oval, subterminal and bulging (Fig. 23.1D).

Cultural characteristics

It is an obligate anaerobe. Optimum temperature for growth is 35°C, but some strains can grow and produce toxin at 1–5°C. It can grow well on routine culture media. Surface colonies are large, irregular, smooth, semitransparent with fimbriate border. On horse blood agar, all strains except those of type G are β-haemolytic. All types except G produce opalescence and a pearly effect on egg yolk agar (EYA).

Susceptibility to physical and chemical agents

Spores of *C. botulinum* are highly resistant, surviving boiling for several hours and some strains can even survive autoclaving at 121°C for 20 minutes. However, spores of type E strains are usually much less resistant. They may be inactivated by heating at 80°C (wet heat) for 30 minutes. Insufficient heating in the process of preserving food is an important factor in the causation of botulism.

Antigenic types

On the basis of the type of toxin produced, *C. botulinum* has been divided into eight serologically distinct types, A, B, C_1, C_2, D, E, F and G. The toxins produced by different types are antigenically distinct but pharmacologically similar. Types A, B and E are the principal causes of human illness.

Properties of botulinum toxin

Botulinum toxin is probably the most toxic substance known to mankind. It is a small protein with 19 amino acids and a molecular weight of about 150,000 daltons. Minimum lethal dose, of this toxin, for a mouse, is 0.03 ng and that for humans may be 1 μg. It acts slowly taking several hours to kill. It is a neurotoxin which apparently acts by inhibiting the release of acetylcholine from the motor nerve endings of the parasympathetic system. The toxin is relatively stable being inactivated at 80°C for 30–40 minutes and at 100°C for 10 minutes. It resists digestion in the intestine and is absorbed through intestinal mucosa in an active form. It can be toxoided. It is a good antigen and is specifically neutralized by the antitoxin.

Q. 13. Describe pathogenicity of *Clostridium botulinum*.

Ans. *C. botulinum* is widely distributed in soil and decaying vegetation, thus, many foods, both vegetables and meats, may become contaminated with these organisms. It is non-invasive and its pathogenicity is entirely due to the toxin produced by it. The disease caused by this organism is known as botulism. It is of 3 types:

1. Food-borne botulism

It is due to the ingestion of preformed toxin. The causative organism, *C. botulinum*, multiplies in the food before it is consumed, and produces a powerful soluble toxin. The source of botulism is usually preserved food such as meat and meat products, fish, and vegetables. Food responsible for botulism is usually abnormal in appearance and odour. Bulging of tins and the presence of gas bubbles on opening suggest contamination with *C. botulinum*. However, at times food may look normal.

Symptoms usually begin 18–36 hours after ingestion of food and may include nausea, vomiting, thirst, constipation, double vision, difficulty in swallowing, speaking and breathing. This may be followed by muscular weakness, blurred vision, and death as a result of respiratory failure. Case fatality varies from 25–70%.

2. Wound botulism

C. botulinum has occasionally been isolated from wound in man. Toxin is produced at the site of infection and is absorbed. The symptoms are those of food-borne botulism except those of gastrointestinal system. Symptoms appear 4–14 days after injury, in persons with *C. botulinum* infection.

3. Infant botulism

This entity was recognized in 1976. Affected infants have ranged from 3 weeks to 9 months in age and both sexes have been affected equally. Older children and adults are not susceptible. The infants ingest spores, but not preformed toxin, from soil, household dust, honey, etc. About 10% of honey samples have been shown to contain type A and B spores of *C. botulinum*. **Within the intestine, *C. botulinum* multiplies and elaborates toxin.** After a period of normal development, the infant develops constipation, listlessness, difficulty in sucking and swallowing, weak or altered cry, muscle weakness, ptosis, and loss of head control. Eventually the baby appears 'floppy' (**floppy child syndrome**) and develops respiratory insufficiency or respiratory arrest. Patient excretes toxin and spores in the faeces. Management consists of supportive care and assisted feeding.

Q. 14. Describe laboratory diagnosis, treatment and prophylaxis of botulism.

Ans. ***Laboratory diagnosis***

Diagnosis may be made by demonstration of the bacillus or the toxin in suspected residual food or in faeces.

Demonstration of toxin

Botulinum toxin may be demonstrated in the food or faeces. The food is macerated in sterile saline, and the filtrate inoculated into mice or guinea pigs intraperitoneally. The test animal develops dyspnoea, flaccid paralysis and dies within 24 hours. Control animals protected by polyvalent antitoxin remain healthy. Toxin may also be demonstrated in patient serum.

Demonstration of the organism

Gram-positive sporing bacilli may be demonstrable in smears made from the residual food. For the isolation of *C. botulinum*, the specimen is inoculated on EYA, blood agar and three bottles of CMB. Hold one of these three bottles in a water bath at 80°C for 10 minutes and another for 20 minutes and third is unheated. This procedure selects heat-resistant spores and also allows heat-sensitive spores to grow in unheated CMB. The culture media are incubated anaerobically at 30°C for 3–5 days. Cultures in CMB are screened at intervals for toxin production in mice and presence of the organisms may be detected by fluorescent antibody test. Absence of toxin production up to 5 days usually rules out botulism. Subculture toxin-positive CMB culture onto EYA and blood agar. Incubate anaerobically at 30°C for 48 hours. The growth on EYA and blood agar (direct as well as subculture) is identified by Gram staining, fluorescent antibody procedure, colonial morphology and biochemical characters.

Treatment

The toxin still remaining in the stomach should be removed by lavage with 2–5% bicarbonate solution because toxin is labile in alkaline pH. Saline enemas may be given to remove toxin from the colon. Polyvalent antitoxin against common types, i.e., A, B and E or monovalent when the type of intoxication is known should be given as soon as possible. The antitoxin cannot reverse the effect of toxin already affecting the nerves but will neutralize unfixed toxin. Intensive nursing care and the use of mechanical respirator, when necessary, is of great importance.

Prophylaxis

Since botulism follows consumption of inadequately canned or preserved food, it can be prevented by proper canning and preservation of food. The food that exhibits the signs of spoilage (inflated cans, gas bubbles on opening and abnormal odour) should not be consumed. When an outbreak occurs, a prophylactic dose of polyvalent antitoxin should be given intramuscularly to all those who have consumed that food. **Those who may be exposed to the hazards of intoxication in the laboratory or of deliberate intoxication, as in biological warfare, may be protected by injecting three doses of mixed toxoid at two month intervals.**

Other question which may also be asked in the examination

Write short note on Nagler's reaction.

For answer see page 200.

24

MYCOBACTERIUM TUBERCULOSIS

Q. 1. Describe morphology, cultural characteristics, antigenic structure and pathogenicity of *Mycobacterium tuberculosis*.

Ans. ***Morphology***

Tubercle bacilli are slender, straight or slightly curved rods with rounded ends. Their average size is 3 × 0.3 µm. In sputum and other clinical specimens they may occur singly or in small clumps. They are non-motile, non-sporing, non-capsulated and acid-fast.

With Ziehl-Neelsen stain, the tubercle bacilli stain bright red, while the tissue cells and other organisms are stained blue (Fig. 24.1). Organisms in tissue and sputum smears often stain irregularly and have a beaded or barred appearance, presumably because of their vacuoles and polyphosphate content. However, *M. bovis* appear straight, stout, short uniformly stained rods.

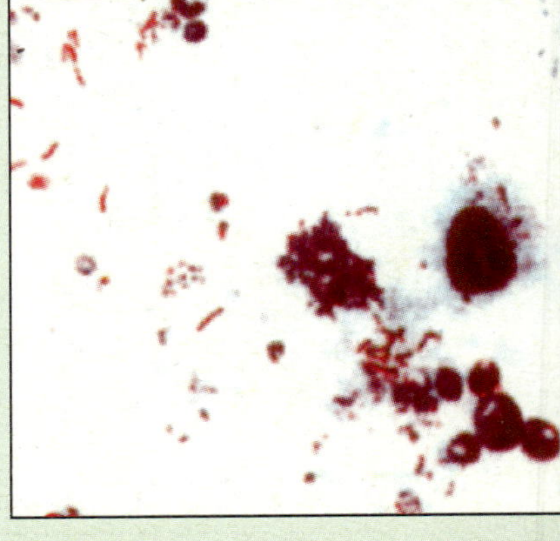

Fig. 24.1. Sputum smear showing acid-fast bacilli.

Tubercle bacilli may also be stained with auramine-rhodamine fluorescent stain and smears examined by fluorescence microscopy under low magnification. Tubercle bacilli are seen as yellow luminous organisms in a dark field. When they have been detected under low power, the morphology of the bacilli is confirmed by observation with an oil-immersion objective.

Cultural characteristics

M. tuberculosis is an obligate aerobe while *M. bovis* is microaerophilic on primary isolation, becoming aerobic on subculture. Optimum temperature for growth is 37°C (range 30–40°C) and optimum pH is 7.0 (range 6.0–7.6). Tubercle bacilli can grow on a wide range of enriched culture media but **Lowenstein-Jensen (LJ) medium** is most widely used. This medium consists of whole egg, asparagine, some mineral salts, malachite green and glycerol or sodium pyruvate, and solidified by heating (inspissation). **Malachite green inhibits the growth of organisms other than mycobacteria and provides a colour contrast against which colonies of mycobacteria can be easily seen.** The addition of glycerol improves the growth of *M. tuberculosis*, while it is without any effect or even inhibitory to *M. bovis*. Sodium pyruvate improves the growth of both *M. tuberculosis* and *M. bovis*.

The average generation time of tubercle bacilli is about 14–15 hours, prolonged incubation is, therefore, necessary. *M. tuberculosis* grows well on LJ medium (**eugonic growth**). It produces visible growth on LJ medium, incubated at 37°C, in 2–8 weeks, although on primary isolation from clinical material from patients treated with antituberculous agents, colonies may take up to 12 weeks to appear. It grows as **'rough, tough and buff'** colonies – rough due to dry, irregular growth; tough due to difficulty in lifting the colony from the surface; and buff due to the pale yellow colour. On the other hand, *M. bovis* grows poorly on LJ medium (**dysgonic growth**) forming moist, smooth, flat and white colonies which easily break up when touched.

In **glycerol broth**, the hydrophobic properties of the organisms cell surface result in a whitish wrinkled pellicle and granular deposit. Dispersed, uniform growth can, however, be obtained by subculturing them 2 or 3 times in **Dubos and Davis liquid medium** containing nonionic detergent Tween 80 (polyoxyethylene sorbitan monooleate). It wets the surface, deters aggregation of cells and permits them to grow diffusely. Virulent strains tend to grow as serpentine cords in the liquid media, while avirulent strains grow in a more dispersed fashion.

Antigenic structure

Mycobacteria possess two types of antigens – cell wall (insoluble), and cytoplasmic (soluble) antigens. Cell wall antigens include arabinomannan, arabinogalactan and lipoarabinomannan. Cytoplasmic antigens, their molecular weights and chemical nature are given in Table 24.1. These include antigen 5, antigen 6, antigen 14, antigen 19, antigen 32, antigen 38 and antigen 60.

Table 24.1. Cytoplasmic (soluble) antigens of *Mycobacterium tuberculosis*

Antigen	Molecular weight in kilodaltons	Chemical nature
5	28.5–35	Protein
6	30	Protein
14	14	Protein
19	19	Protein
32	32	Protein
38	38	Protein
60	1,000–10,000	Lipopolysaccharide protein complex

Pathogenicity

Humans become infected with *M. tuberculosis* most frequently by inhaling infective droplets coughed or sneezed into air by a patient with tuberculosis. Bovine tuberculosis is spread from animal to animal, and sometimes to human attendants, in moist cough spray. About 1% of infected cows develop lesions in the udder and bacilli are excreted in the milk which can then infect people who drink it raw. Thus, primary human tuberculosis due to *M. bovis* usually involves cervical or mesenteric lymph nodes. In developed countries, control of *M. bovis* in dairy herds and pasteurization of milk have virtually eradicated this organism. *M. avium* and closely related *M. intracellulare* (*M. avium-intracellulare*) cause lymphadenitis, pulmonary lesions and disseminated disease in 15–24% of patients with AIDS. Human tuberculosis is divisible into primary and post-primary (secondary) forms.

Primary tuberculosis

This begins with inhalation of the mycobacteria and ends with a T cell-mediated immune response that induces hypersensitivity to the organisms and controls 95% of infections. Inhaled tubercle bacilli are engulfed by alveolar macrophages in which they replicate to form the initial lesion or **Ghon focus**. It consists of a parenchymal subpleural lesion, often just above or just below the interlobar fissure between the upper and the lower lobes.

Some bacilli are transported by macrophages to the hilar lymph nodes. The Ghon focus together with the enlarged hilar lymph nodes forms the **primary complex**. In addition, the bacilli may be seeded by further lymphatic and haematogenous dissemination in many organs and tissues, including other parts of the lung. In case of *M. bovis* which enters the mouth, as in milk-borne bovine tuberculosis, the primary complexes involve the tonsil and cervical lymph nodes or the intestine, often the ileocaecal region, and the mesenteric lymph nodes.

Naive macrophages are unable to kill the mycobacteria, the latter multiply, lyse the host cell, infect other macrophages and sometimes disseminate through the blood to other parts of the lung and elsewhere in the body. Within about 10 days of infection, clones of antigen-specific T lymphocytes (CD4+ helper T cells and CD8+ suppressor T cells) are produced interacting with macrophages in two ways:

1. CD4+ helper T cells secrete interferon-gamma, which activates macrophages to kill intracellular mycobacteria. These activated macrophages are termed epithelioid cells from their microscopical resemblance to epithelial cells. These form a compact cluster or **epithelioid cell granuloma** around the foci of infection. Some of them fuse to form multinucleated giant cells.
2. CD8+ suppressor T cells kill macrophages that are infected with mycobacteria, resulting in the formation of **caseating granulomas** (delayed-type hypersensitivity reaction). Direct toxicity of the mycobacteria to the macrophages may also contribute to the necrotic centre. Activated macrophages in the granuloma are metabolically very active. They consume oxygen and the resulting anoxia and acidosis in the centre of the lesion probably kills most of the tubercle bacilli. Therefore, granuloma formation is usually sufficient to limit the primary infection.

   Surrounding fibroblasts produce dense scar tissue which may become calcified. Not all bacilli are destroyed, some remain in a dormant form as **persisters**, which when reactivated cause post-primary disease. If a focus ruptures into a blood vessel, bacilli are disseminated throughout the body with the formation of numerous granulomas. From the millet seed-like appearance of the lesions, this is known as **miliary tuberculosis**.

Post-primary (secondary) tuberculosis

It is caused by reactivation of the primary lesion (endogenous), or by exogenous reinfection. Reactivation tuberculosis is particularly likely to occur in immunocompromised individuals including the elderly, transplant recipients and those who are infected with human immunodeficiency virus (HIV). Granulomas of secondary tuberculosis most often occur in the apex of the lungs but may be widely disseminated in the lungs, kidneys, meninges, bones and other organs. The same process of granuloma formation occurs but the necrotic element of the reaction causes tissue destruction and the formation of large areas of caseation termed **tuberculomas**.

Proteases liberated by activated macrophages cause softening and liquefaction of the caseous material. Two special features of secondary tuberculosis are the presence of caseous necrosis and of cavities, which may rupture into blood vessels, spreading mycobacteria throughout the body, and break into airways, releasing infectious mycobacteria in aerosols and sputum (**open tuberculosis**).

Q. 2. Write short note on Koch's phenomenon.

Ans. The tuberculin reactivity was first demonstrated in guinea-pigs by Robert Koch (1890, 1891). The experiment that led to the demonstration of this reactivity is known as Koch's phenomenon. When a healthy guinea-pig is inoculated subcutaneously with a pure culture of tubercle bacilli, the puncture site heals quickly and there is no immediate visible reaction. But after 10–14 days a hard nodule appears which soon breaks down to form an ulcer that persists till the animal dies of progressive tuberculosis. The regional lymph nodes are enlarged and caseous.

But something totally different develops when a guinea-pig already ill with tuberculosis is inoculated. It is best to use animals that have been successfully inoculated 4–6 weeks previously. An indurated lesion appears at the site of second inoculation in a day or two which undergoes necrosis in another day to form a shallow ulcer that heals rapidly without involvement of the regional lymph nodes or other tissues. **Koch's phenomenon is a combination of hypersensitivity and immunity** and has three components:

1. A local reaction of induration and necrosis.
2. A focal response in which there occurs acute congestion and even haemorrhage around tuberculous foci in tissues.
3. A systemic response of fever which may sometimes be fatal.

Q. 3. What is the principle of tuberculin test? Describe briefly reagents, methods, uses, false negative and false positive tuberculin test.

Ans. *Principle*

Delayed, type IV or cell-mediated hypersensitivity.

Reagents

1. ***Old tuberculin (OT):*** It was originally described by Robert Koch. It is prepared by autoclaving or boiling a culture of tubercle bacilli, concentrating it 10-fold on a steam bath, filtering off the debris, and adding glycerol as preservative. OT is a crude product

and different batches vary in their activity. The active constituent in this crude product is a protein which is remarkable for its heat stability. Stock solutions retain full potency for years when stored at 5°C. It has been replaced by purified protein derivative.

2. ***Purified protein derivative (PPD):*** A slightly more refined tuberculin called purified protein derivative was prepared by Seibert (1941) by growing *M. tuberculosis* in a semisynthetic medium, autoclaving, removing debris by filtration, concentrating the filtrate by ultrafiltration and precipitating several times with 50% saturated ammonium sulphate. The product is mostly a mixture of small proteins (average molecular weight 10,000).

The dosage of PPD is expressed in Tuberculin units (TU). One large batch of PPD made by Seibert in 1939, PPD-S, was recognized by the WHO as the international standard PPD-tuberculin and arbitrarily designated it to contain 50,000 tuberculin units (TU) per mg, 1 TU equal to 0.01 ml of OT or 0.00002 mg PPD-S.

Methods

1. ***Mantoux test:*** 0.1 ml of PPD containing 5 TU is injected intracutaneously into the skin of the volar aspect of the forearm. Those suspected of having tuberculosis, and therefore likely to react strongly, may first be tested with 1 TU. The site of inoculation is palpated 72 hours later. The development of an area of palpable, firm induration 10 mm or more in diameter is recorded as positive, and those between 5 and 9 mm in diameter as doubtful. The extent of the accompanying erythema is irrelevant and should be ignored. If the reaction is completely negative, the test may be repeated by giving an injection of 100 TU.
2. ***Heaf test:*** This test is done with a multiple puncture apparatus with 6 needles that prick 1–2 mm deep into the skin. A drop of undiluted PPD is spread on the area of skin selected for inoculation. The multiple puncture apparatus is pressed against this area of skin and needles are released. The test is read after 72 hours. Erythema and induration around at least 4 of the punctures is regarded as positive. The equipment must be adequately sterilized between each use to prevent transmission of hepatitis and AIDS.

Uses of tuberculin test

1. To diagnose active infection in infants and young children.
2. To measure prevalence of infection in a community.
3. To select susceptibles for BCG vaccination.
4. Indication of successful BCG vaccination.

False negative (tuberculin anergy)

1. Early tuberculosis.
2. Advanced tuberculosis.
3. Miliary tuberculosis.
4. In patients with measles and other exanthematous reactions.
5. Occasionally after chemotherapy and removal of lung lesion.
6. Advanced age.
7. Immunosuppressive therapy and defective CMI.
8. Lymphoreticular malignancy.
9. Sarcoidosis.
10. Severe malnutrition.

False positive

False positive reactions may be seen in patients with infection by related mycobacteria (atypical mycobacteria). These are usually low grade reactions and can be differentiated by testing with tuberculin prepared from these mycobacteria.

Q. 4. Describe laboratory diagnosis of tuberculosis.

Ans. Diagnosis of tuberculosis can be established by demonstration of tubercle bacilli in clinical specimens by microscopy and cultural techniques. Only up to 50% of pulmonary and 25% of extrapulmonary tuberculosis can be diagnosed by smear examination.

Collection of specimen

- The specimen most commonly collected is **sputum** which consists of pus and mucus secretions coughed up from the lung. Patient is instructed to cough up the sputum into a clean wide-mouthed container. Disposable waxed cardboard containers are ideal. A morning specimen may be collected. If sputum is scanty, a 24 hour specimen may be collected.
- If no sputum is produced, **laryngeal swab or bronchial washings** are examined.
- In children, stomach washings may be examined as they tend to swallow sputum.
- Depending upon the site of involvement, **cerebrospinal fluid, pleural fluid, urine and aspirated fluid from bone and joint** are centrifuged and the deposits are examined.
- **Tissue biopsies** are homogenized and examined by microscopy and culture.
- In pulmonary and renal tuberculosis, three consecutive specimens of **sputum and urine** should be examined respectively.

Direct microscopy

Pour the sputum in a petri dish and examine. For preparation of smear, select **blood-tinged part** of the sputum, if it is not there then **purulent part** should be selected. The smear is stained by Ziehl-Neelsen technique and examined under oil-immersion lens. Acid-fast bacilli stain bright red against a blue background (Fig. 24.1). To be detected microscopically, there must be 50,000–100,000 bacilli per ml of sputum. A negative report should not be given till at least 300 fields have been examined, taking about 10 minutes.

Concentration of specimens

Mycobacteria in a specimen can be decontaminated and concentrated into a small volume without inactivation. Such concentrate can be used for microscopy, culture and animal inoculation. Several methods are in use:

- *Petroff's method:* It is a simple and widely used technique. Equal volumes of sputum and 4% sodium hydroxide are mixed and incubated at 37°C with frequent shaking till it gets liquefied and becomes clear. On the average, it takes 20–30 minutes. It is then centrifuged at 3,000 rpm for 30 minutes. The supernatant fluid is pipetted off and the deposit is neutralized by adding 8% hydrochloric acid in the presence of a drop of phenol red indicator.
- *Other methods:* Instead of alkali, homogenization can be carried out by treatment with dilute acids (5% oxalic acid, 3% hydrochloric acid or 6% sulphuric acid) or mucolytic agents such as N-acetyl-L-cysteine with sodium hydroxide and pancreatin.

Culture

It is very sensitive for detection of tubercle bacilli. It may be positive with as few as 10–100 bacilli per ml of sputum and it is necessary for antimicrobial drug sensitivity testing. **Concentrate of sputum** is inoculated on two slopes of LJ medium. In case of **laryngeal swab**, add enough 5% oxalic acid to the tube to cover the swab and leave it at room temperature for 30 minutes to kill non-acid-fast contaminants. Squeeze the swab against the side of the tube to remove excess fluid and rub it over the surface of two slopes of LJ medium.

In case of **gastric washings**, 15 ml of the specimen is collected in a 25 ml bottle containing 5 ml of 15% trisodium phosphate, which will neutralize the acid. Then cap and shake the bottle. In the laboratory, homogenize and decontaminate the specimen by Petroff's method. Centrifuge and examine the deposit by Ziehl-Neelsen staining and culture on LJ medium.

In case of **renal tuberculosis**, three early morning specimens of urine should be collected. Twenty four hours collection is unsatisfactory due to increased bacterial contamination and lower recovery rate as compared with a single voided specimen. Each specimen should consist of 50–100 ml. It is centrifuged at 1500 *g* for 30 minutes and treat the deposit by Petroff's method. Prepare a smear and stain by Ziehl-Neelsen staining and inoculate on two slopes of LJ medium.

Tubercle bacilli are usually scanty in **pleural and peritoneal fluids**. Therefore, at least 50–100 ml of either of these should be collected. Centrifuge these fluids and treat the deposits by Petroff's method as above. In case of **CSF**, 3–4 ml is collected and centrifuged. The deposit is used for the smear and culture. **Pus** is directly used for smear and culture.

The inoculated media are incubated at 37°C. The cultures are examined weekly for up to 12 weeks. Growth of most strains of *M. tuberculosis* may appear in 2–8 weeks. But cultures should not be discarded as negative until they have been observed for 12 weeks. Longer incubation is necessary for strains originating from patients treated with antituberculous agents.

The use of liquid medium with **radiometric growth detection**, such as BACTEC 460 TB has simplified culture method. By this method growth can be detected in 10–20 days from the time the patient specimen is brought to the laboratory. BACTEC system detects the presence of mycobacteria based on their metabolism rather than visible growth. When the ^{14}C-labelled substrate present in the medium is metabolized, $^{14}CO_2$ is produced and is measured by the BACTEC 460 TB instrument and reported in terms of growth index (GI) value.

Another method of detection of mycobacterial growth is **mycobacterial growth indicator tube** (MGIT). It is non-radiometric automated method. It consists of tubes containing liquid culture media, and a fluorescent compound is embedded on the bottom of the tube. The fluorescent compound is sensitive to dissolved oxygen in the liquid medium. Therefore, the dissolved oxygen in the uninoculated medium quenches any fluorescence from the compound. However, when the mycobacteria grow, they deplete the dissolved oxygen in the liquid medium and the compound fluoresces brightly which can be detected by observing the tube under ultraviolet light (Wood's lamp). The results are obtained in 1–2 weeks.

Animal inoculation

For many years, guinea-pig inoculation had been a popular method of diagnosis of tuberculosis, but it is now regarded as obsolete. This is due to the following reasons:

- The isolation of *M. tuberculosis* by guinea-pig inoculation is no greater than that by culture.
- Culture is simpler, safer and cheaper.
- The animals are costly to purchase and maintain, some die from intercurrent disease, and the method is time consuming. It takes 4–6 weeks for the disease to develop in the animal and it is then necessary to identify the causative agent by demonstration of acid-fast bacilli and by cultural techniques.
- The excretion of *M. tuberculosis* in the urine and faeces of infected animals creates a health hazard.

However, guinea-pig inoculation is superior to culture for the isolation of M. bovis from clinical material.

Sputum is decontaminated and concentrated by Petroff's method. 0.5 ml each of the neutralized and centrifuged deposit is inoculated intramuscularly into the thigh of two healthy, tuberculin-negative guinea-pigs. Inoculation by subcutaneous route should be avoided as it causes a local ulcer which may be infectious. The animals are weighed prior to inoculation and thereafter at weekly intervals and tuberculin test is done after 3–4 weeks. Progressive loss of weight and positive tuberculin test are indications of development of tuberculosis. As soon as the signs of disease develop, e.g., after 3–4 weeks, kill the animal. If the animals remain apparently healthy, one of them is killed at 6 weeks and other at 8 weeks. Necropsy shows:

- Caseous lesion at the site of inoculation.
- Enlarged caseous inguinal lymph nodes. The infection may spread to lumbar, portal, mediastinal and cervical lymph nodes.
- Tubercles 1–2 mm in diameter in spleen, liver, peritoneum and lungs. Kidneys are unaffected.

The identity of the bacteria is then confirmed by demonstration of acid-fast bacilli and cultural techniques from the lesions. *M. tuberculosis* is highly pathogenic for guinea-pigs and virtually non-pathogenic for rabbits, while *M. bovis* is highly pathogenic for both guinea-pigs and rabbits. Catalase-negative and INH-resistant strains and most strains isolated from South India have low virulence. The animal inoculated with strains of low virulence may have to be observed for 12 weeks or longer and sometimes the only lesion demonstrable may be an enlarged lymph node.

Molecular methods

Polymerase chain reaction (PCR) and ligase chain reaction (LCR) are used as diagnostic techniques. PCR is based on DNA amplification and has been used to detect *M. tuberculosis* in clinical specimens. The restriction fragment length polymorphism (RFLP) is used to type different strains for epidemiological purposes. The principle of this technique is that restriction endonuclease treatment yields nucleic acid fragments of different lengths, the patterns of which are strain-specific.

Serodiagnostic techniques

For the detection of antimycobacterial antibodies in patient serum, various methods such as enzyme-linked immunosorbent assay, radioimmunoassay and latex agglutination have been employed. Several antigens like glycolipids from *M. bovis* BCG, antigens 5 and 6 from *M. tuberculosis*, 64 kDa protein of *M. bovis* BCG, 32 kDa protein antigen called P32 and antigen 60 of *M. bovis* BCG have been tried for detection of antibody against them. Diagnostic utility of these tests is equivocal. WHO has recommended that these tests should not be used for the diagnosis of active tuberculosis.

Q. 5. Write short note on BCG vaccine.

Ans. It is a live attenuated vaccine introduced by Calmette and Guérin (1921). This is a strain of *M. bovis* attenuated by repeated subcultures, every 3 weeks, for 239 subcultures on slices of potato soaked in autoclaved bile containing glycerol (5%) over a period of 13 years (1908–1921). This species was selected for vaccine preparation in preference to *M. tuberculosis* because of the false assumption that it was of limited virulence in man.

BCG vaccine is available in liquid form and freeze-dried (lyophilized) form. The latter is commonly used. The lyophilized vaccine supplied by BCG vaccine laboratory, Chennai, is reconstituted by sterile physiological saline to make a final concentration of 0.1 mg (moist weight) in 0.1 ml of the vaccine. Once reconstituted, vaccine should be utilized within 3–6 hours. Following injection of 0.1 ml of vaccine intradermally, the organisms grow to a limited extent in the tissues. Immunizing capability of the vaccine depends on this. Dead vaccine or tuberculin is not effective. BCG vaccine should be administered soon after birth failing which it may be given at any time during the first year of life.

A **small nodule** develops at the site of inoculation 2–3 weeks after injection. It increases slowly in size and by about 5 weeks it attains a diameter of 4–8 mm. It then subsides or breaks into a **shallow ulcer** which heals by scarring. Such individuals become **tuberculin-positive** after 4–6 weeks. A few cases have been recorded where BCG has given rise to progressive tuberculosis.

The protective efficacy of BCG vaccine has been determined in a number of vaccine trials. The results have varied from 80% efficacy to a total absence of protection. The immunity has been reported to last for about 10 years. The consensus of opinion at present is that BCG does protect from tuberculosis. The disease runs a milder course in immunized children. It is also believed to prevent meningeal, skeletal and miliary form of tuberculosis to a large extent. BCG vaccine stimulates T lymphocytes which reportedly offer some protection against leprosy and leukaemia also.

Complications of BCG vaccination

1. *Local:*
    - Abscess
    - Indolent ulcer
    - Keloid
    - Tuberculids (small satellite BCG tubercles developing in the neighbourhood of the site of vaccination)

2. *Regional:*
   - Lymphadenitis
3. *Systemic:*
   - Fever
   - Erythema nodosum
   - Otitis media.

Contraindications of BCG

BCG vaccination is contraindicated in patients of tuberculosis, AIDS, measles, pertussis and eczema, and patients on steroids, and tuberculin positive individuals.

Q. 6. Describe briefly chemotherapy of tuberculosis.

Ans. The antituberculous drugs include rifampicin, isoniazid, pyrazinamide, streptomycin, ethambutol and thiacetazone. The first 4 of these are bactericidal and the others are bacteriostatic. Other less often used drugs include ethionamide, cycloserine, capreomycin, kanamycin and *p*-aminosalicylic acid.

In clinical practice, mutational resistance is of great importance in tuberculosis. If patient is treated with only one antituberculous drug, initially the bacilli die in large numbers but, soon resistant mutants appear and multiply unchecked. Therefore, generally three drugs are given simultaneously. Initially prolonged treatment for two or more years used to be given. But with the advent of actively bactericidal drugs like rifampicin, short course regimens of about 6 months have been found adequate in many cases.

Tubercle bacilli resistant to a number of antituberculous drugs (**multidrug-resistant tuberculosis, MDR-TB**) is a growing problem. Prevalence of MDR-TB cases is on the high in India. MDR-TB cases threaten the effectiveness of chemotherapy for both treatment and control of tuberculosis and require the use of second-line drugs that are more expensive, toxic and less effective than first-line antituberculous drugs.

Another serious condition **extensively drug-resistant tuberculosis (XDR-TB)** has emerged recently. XDR-TB is defined as MDR-TB plus resistance to fluoroquinolones and one of the second-line injectables – amikacin, capreomycin and kanamycin.

Q. 7. Write short note on Revised National Tuberculosis Control Programme (RNTCP).

Ans. RNTCP was introduced in 1993 in India. The aim was to provide standardised treatment and proper diagnostic facilities. **Directly observed treatment strategy (DOTS)** is an important component of RNTCP. Under RNTCP, any patient with cough for 2 weeks or more is included for the diagnosis of pulmonary tuberculosis. Two sputum samples are collected from the patient. One early morning and other collected on spot when the patient visits the chest clinic.

Both the sputum specimens are stained with Ziehl-Neelsen staining and examined for acid-fast bacilli (AFB). If one or both smears are positive then the patient is diagnosed as sputum positive pulmonary tuberculosis and antitubercular treatment is started. If both the sputum smears are negative for AFB, a course of antibiotics is given for 10–14 days. If cough persists after antibiotic treatment, again two sputum specimens are collected and examined for AFB. Antitubercular treatment is started if one or both smears are positive and patient is diagnosed as smear positive pulmonary tuberculosis.

If both specimens are negative, X-ray chest is done. In case X-ray chest is suggestive of tuberculosis, then the patient is diagnosed sputum negative pulmonary tuberculosis and antitubercular treatment started. In case X-ray chest is not suggestive of tuberculosis, the patient is diagnosed as not suffering from tuberculosis.

Q. 8. Tabulate differences between *Mycobacterium tuberculosis* and *Mycobacterium bovis*.

Ans. Differences between *Mycobacterium tuberculosis* and *Mycobacterium bovis* are given in Table 24.2.

Table 24.2. Distinguishing features of *Mycobacterium tuberculosis* and *M. bovis*

Character	*M. tuberculosis*	*M. bovis*
1. Microscopic morphology	Slender, straight or slightly curved rods with barred or beaded appearance	Straight, stout, short uniformly stained rods
2. Colony morphology	Dry, rough, raised, wrinkled, off-white to buff- coloured and not easily emulsifiable (rough, tough and buff)	Moist, smooth, flat, friable and white
3. Average duration of time for appearance of growth at 37°C	12–25 days. Growth is eugonic (luxuriant)	20–40 days. Growth is dysgonic
4. Susceptibility to pyrazinamide (50 µg/ml)	+	–
5. Susceptibility to thiophen-2-carboxylic acid hydrazide (10 µg/ml)	–	+
6. Biochemical reactions		
• Nitrate reduction	+	–
• Niacin production	+	–
• Tween 80 hydrolysis	Variable	–
7. Oxygen requirement	Obligate aerobe	Microaerophilic on primary isolation but becomes aerobic on subculture
8. Animal pathogenicity		
• Guinea pig	+	+
• Rabbit	–	+

25

NON-TUBERCULOUS MYCOBACTERIA

Q. 1. Describe general characters and classification of non-tuberculous mycobacteria.

Ans. Mycobacteria other than tubercle and leprosy bacilli, that normally exist as saprophytes of soil and water (environment) and occasionally cause opportunistic disease in man resembling tuberculosis are known as non-tuberculous, atypical, environmental, opportunistic, tuberculoid mycobacteria or MOTT (mycobacteria other than typical tubercle) bacilli. Infection caused by these organisms is known as **mycobacteriosis**. Atypical mycobacteria are:

- Acid-fast and alcohol-fast and may resemble or differ in morphology from tubercle bacilli.
- They may be longer and even filamentous.
- They can grow at 25°C and 37°C. Some of them (*M. xenopi*, *M. phlei* and *M. smegmatis*) can grow at 44°C.
- Some of them are rapid growers. They produce visible growth on LJ medium within one week.
- Some of them produce a bright yellow or orange pigment.
- They are resistant to antituberculous drugs such as streptomycin, isoniazid and *p*-aminosalicylic acid. All of them are resistant to at least one of these drugs. However, many strains are sensitive to rifampicin.
- They are niacin and neutral red reactions negative.
- They produce enzyme arylsulphatase.
- They are non-pathogenic for guinea-pig but pathogenic for mouse.
- They occasionally cause opportunistic disease, resembling tuberculosis in man.

Classification

On the basis of production of bright yellow or orange pigment and rate of growth, Runyon (1959) classified non-tuberculous mycobacteria into four groups (Table 25.1). These mycobacteria can grow on Lowenstein-Jensen (LJ) medium. All strains of groups I, II and III

Table 25.1. Non-tuberculous mycobacteria

Runyon group	Name	Species
I	Photochromogens	*Mycobacterium kansasii, M. marinum, M. simiae*
II	Scotochromogens	*M. scrofulaceum, M. gordonae, M. szulgai*
III	Non-chromogens	*M. avium, M. intracellulare, M. xenopi, M. ulcerans, M. malmoense, M. terrae, M. triviale, M. nonchromogenicum*
IV	Rapid growers	*M. smegmatis, M. phlei, M. chelonae, M. fortuitum*

grow slowly and form colonies in 2–8 weeks. However, group IV (rapid growers) produce colonies within one week.

Q. 2. Name and describe briefly non-tuberculous mycobacteria of group photochromogens.

Ans. They form colourless colonies when incubated in the dark, but when the young culture is exposed to light for one hour in the presence of air (cap of the culture bottle loosened) and re-incubated for 24–48 hours, they develop a bright yellow or orange pigment (beta-carotene). For testing photochromogenesis, test strain is inoculated on two LJ slopes. One of them is wrapped in aluminium foil to exclude light from it and the other is left unwrapped. Both these slopes are incubated in an incubator at 37°C with a lighted 15 watt electric bulb for 14 days. If only the unwrapped, but not wrapped culture shows a bright yellow or orange pigment, the strain is a photochromogen.

This group contains three species – *M. kansasii*, *M. marinum* and *M. simiae*.

- ***M. kansasii*** causes chronic pulmonary disease resembling tuberculosis, particularly in old persons with pre-existing lung disease. It has been isolated on several occasions from piped water supplies. It grows well at 37°C on LJ medium yielding a good growth within two weeks and reduces nitrate to nitrite. The bacterial cells are usually elongated and have a distinct beaded appearance. It is usually sensitive to rifampicin and several other antituberculous drugs.
- ***M. simiae*** was originally isolated from monkeys. Like *M. kansasii*, it grows well at 37°C and causes pulmonary disease. It synthesizes niacin in significant amounts and may thus be falsely identified as *M. tuberculosis*.
- ***M. marinum*** was originally isolated from fish. It grows poorly or not at all at 37°C. It grows well at 33°C. It causes superficial granulomatous skin disease of man known as **swimming pool granuloma** or **fish tank granuloma**. It resembles *M. kansasii* in colonial and microscopic appearance. *M. marinum* may however be distinguished from *M. kansasii* by its:
  - poor or no growth at 37°C;
  - failure to reduce nitrate to nitrite;
  - failure to produce catalase; and
  - ability to hydrolyze pyrazinamide.

Q. 3. Name and describe briefly non-tuberculous mycobacteria of group scotochromogens.

Ans. These organisms form bright yellow or orange pigment in cultures incubated in the dark, though the intensity of the colour may increase on exposure to light.

- ***M. scrofulaceum*** is an important member of this group which may cause **scrofula** (cervical lymphadenitis) in children. The bacilli may be short or long and filamentous. It is resistant to isoniazid and sensitive to cycloserine and ethionamide.
- ***M. gordonae*** is often found in water. It is a frequent contaminant of clinical specimens and a rare cause of pulmonary disease.
- ***M. szulgai*** is a scotochromogen when incubated at 37°C and photochromogen at 25°C. It may occasionally cause pulmonary disease and bursitis.

Q. 4. Name and describe briefly non-tuberculous mycobacteria of group non-chromogens.

Ans. They do not form pigment even on exposure to light. Medically important species include *M. intracellulare*, *M. avium*, *M. xenopi*, *M. ulcerans* and *M. malmoense*.

- ***M. intracellulare*** was formerly known as Battey bacillus as it was first detected in Battey State Hospital for tuberculosis in Georgia, USA. The infection with this organism is common in the Southeast USA, where the organism occurs in soil and water. It causes chronic pulmonary disease indistinguishable from tuberculosis.
- ***M. avium*** causes tuberculosis in fowls and sometimes in pigs. It can grow at 45°C. *M. avium* and *M. intracellulare* are the **commonest non-tuberculous mycobacteria** causing opportunistic infections in man. Colonies of both these species are smooth, non-pigmented and easily emulsifiable.

  Because there is no clear-cut division between *M. avium* and *M. intracellulare*, therefore, they are usually grouped together as *M. avium-intracellulare* (MAI) or *M. avium* complex (MAC). This complex possesses 28 agglutination serotypes. Types 1, 2 and 3 are regarded as *M. avium* and the others as *M. intracellulare*. In man, MAC causes pulmonary disease indistinguishable from tuberculosis, lymphadenitis and disseminated disease, particularly in patients with AIDS.

- ***M. xenopi*** was first isolated from a skin lesion in a South African toad (*Xenopus laevis*). It is a thermophile and grows well at 45°C. It may cause pulmonary lesions in man. It has a limited geographical distribution. Most of the cases of pulmonary lesions, due to *M. xenopi* have been reported from South London.
- ***M. ulcerans***, causative agent of **Buruli ulcer**, was originally isolated from ulcerative skin lesions in Australia in 1948. The name Buruli ulcer is derived from the Buruli district of Uganda where a large outbreak of the disease was extensively investigated. *M. ulcerans* grows slowly at 31–34°C but not at all at 37°C in primary culture. It produces an exotoxin which has been characterized as a high molecular weight phospholipoprotein-lipopoly-saccharide complex, which when inoculated intradermally in the guinea-pig, causes inflammation, tissue necrosis and histopathological changes similar to those seen in human lesions. Therefore, this exotoxin may be involved in the pathogenesis of the disease.
- ***M. malmoense*** causes pulmonary disease and lymphadenitis. It was first isolated from patients from Malmo in Sweden. It is a very slow-growing species. On primary isolation, colonies may not be visible until after 10 weeks incubation. It causes pulmonary disease and lymphadenitis. It is resistant to isoniazid and rifampicin and sometimes also to streptomycin and ethambutol.

- ***M. terrae*, *M. triviale* and *M. nonchromogenicum*** are rare pathogens which belong to Runyon group III (non-chromogens). They are sometimes grouped as the *Mycobacterium-terrae-trivialenonchromogenicum* group.

Q. 5. Name and describe briefly non-tuberculous mycobacteria of group rapid growers.

Ans. Rapid growers which may be photo- , scoto- or non-chromogens, produce visible growth on LJ medium within one week, usually in 2–3 days. All the chromogenic rapid growers, e.g., *M. smegmatis* and *M. phlei* are saprophytes.

- ***M. smegmatis*** forms rough colonies, white to buff in colour. The bacilli are slender rods, which may be curved and beaded. Since it is normally present in smegma, a whitish secretion around the orifice of urethra, it is a frequent contaminant of urine specimens. Some strains of *M. smegmatis* are acid-fast but not alcohol-fast, therefore, they are not seen in a Ziehl-Neelsen smear if acid-alcohol is used as decolourizer. Other strains are both acid- and alcohol-fast. In such cases, rapid growth on LJ medium and guinea-pig inoculation distinguishes it from *M. tuberculosis*. *M. smegmatis* has been implicated in rare cases of pulmonary, skin, soft tissue, and bone infections.
- ***M. phlei*** is rarely encountered and is non-pathogenic. It grows as rough colonies that at first are buff coloured and later become yellow to orange. It can be differentiated from *M. smegmatis* by its ability to grow at 52°C and survive heating at 60°C for 4 hours.
- Only two of the rapid growers, ***M. chelonae*** and ***M. fortuitum*** are human pathogens. Both these are coccoid to filamentous and form white to cream-coloured colonies. The former grows better at 25°C than at 37°C. *M. fortuitum* can further be differentiated from *M. chelonae* in reducing nitrate and assimilation of iron from ferric ammonium citrate. *M. chelonae* was originally identified as turtle and *M. fortuitum* as frog tubercle bacilli. They are found in soil and infection usually follows some injury and can lead to chronic abscess formation. They occasionally cause pulmonary or disseminated disease.

Q. 6. Describe briefly pathogenicity and laboratory diagnosis of non-tuberculous mycobacteria.

Ans. Pathogenicity

As compared to tubercle bacilli, non-tuberculous mycobacteria are of low virulence. They may occasionally cause pulmonary disease resembling tuberculosis, lymphadenopathy, skin lesions (Bruli ulcer, non-tuberculous swimming pool granuloma) and disseminated disease (Table 25.2).

Laboratory diagnosis

Specimens

Sputum, pus, exudates.

Microscopy

Ziehl-Neelsen staining of smear shows acid-fast bacilli. Repeated smear examination is necessary.

Table 25.2. Disease caused by atypical mycobacteria

Disease	Causative agents
1. Pulmonary disease	*M. kansasii, M. simiae, M. gordonae, M. szulgai, M. intracellulare, M. avium-intracellulare, M. xenopi, M. malmoense*
2. Lymphadenopathy	*M. scrofulaceum, M. avium-intracellulare, M. malmoense*
3. Skin lesions	
• Bruli ulcer	*M. ulcerans*
• Swimming pool granuloma	*M. marinum*
4. Disseminated disease	*M. avium-intracellulare*

Culture

Several LJ media should be inoculated with the specimen. These are incubated in the dark and in light at different temperatures for distinguishing various species (Table 25.3).

Biochemical reactions

Biochemical reactions are performed for distinguishing various species (Table 25.3).

Table 25.3. Differential characters of various species of non-tuberculous mycobacteria

Test	Species							
	M. kansasii	*M. marinum*	*M. scrofulaceum*	*M. avium-intracellulare*	*M. fortuitum*	*M. chelonae*	*M. phlei*	*M. smegmatis*
Growth within 7 days	–	–	–	–	+	+	+	+
Growth at								
25°C	+	+	+	±	+	+	+	+
37°C	+	–	+	+	+	+	+	+
45°C	–	–	–	±	–	–	+	+
Pigment production in dark	–	–	+	–	–	–	+	–
Pigment production in light	+	+	+	–	–	–	+	–
Urease production	+	+	+	–	+	+	+	+
Niacin production	–	–	–	–	–	–	–	–
Nitrate reduction	+	–	–	–	+	–	+	+

26

Mycobacterium leprae

Q. 1. Discuss morphology and cultivation of *Mycobacterium leprae*.

Ans. ***Morphology***

Lepra bacilli are straight or slightly curved slender bacilli about the same size as tubercle bacilli (average size: 3 × 0.3 µm). They have pointed, rounded or club-shaped ends. They are non-motile and non-sporing. They are Gram-positive and stain more readily than *M. tuberculosis*. With Ziehl-Neelsen stain, they are less acid-fast than tubercle bacilli, so 5% sulphuric acid, instead of 20%, is employed for decolorization after staining with carbol fuchsin.

The bacilli are seen singly and in groups, intracellularly and lying free outside the cell. Inside the cells they are usually present in parallel bundles of 50 or more organisms bound together by a lipid-like substance, the **glia**. These masses of bacteria are known as **globi** which are seen inside the histiocytes which have a foamy appearance. These are known as **lepra cells** (Fig. 26.1).

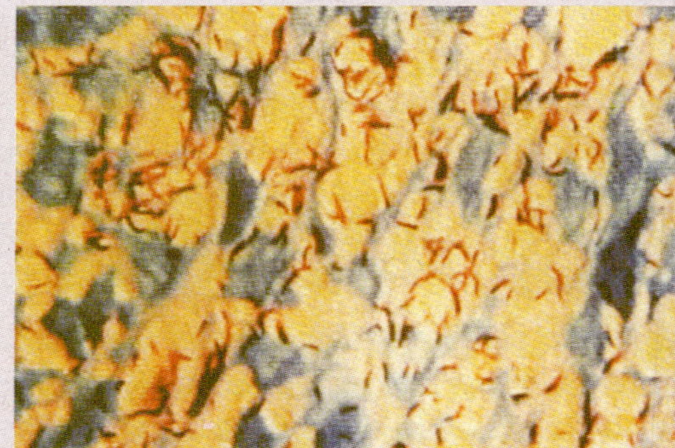

Fig. 26.1. Lepromatous leprosy showing acid-fast bacilli in macrophages (lepra cells).

Live bacilli in the smear appear solid and uniformly stained, while dead or dying forms appear fragmented, beaded and granular. The percentage of uniformly stained bacilli in the tissues is known as **morphological index** (MI). This provides a method for assessing the progress of patients on chemotherapy and is more meaningful than the old criterion, the **bacteriological index** (BI). Poorly stained bacilli are probably dead. A continuing fall in the MI is encouraging and a fall succeeded by a rise indicates development of **drug resistance** in the bacteria. Bacteriological index of a smear is the total number of acid-fast bacilli in an oil-immersion field. It can be expressed from 1+ to 6+ by Ridley's scale (Table 26.1).

Table 26.1. Bacteriological index (Ridley's scale)

Bacteriological index	Number of acid-fast bacilli
6+	More than 1000 per oil-immersion field
5+	100–1000 per oil-immersion field
4+	10–100 per oil-immersion field
3+	1–10 per oil-immersion field
2+	1–10 per 10 oil-immersion fields
1+	1–10 per 100 oil-immersion fields

Cultivation

A large number of attempts at cultivation of *M. leprae*, in artificial culture media and in tissue culture, have been made and success has been claimed from time to time, but none has been confirmed so far. One of the best known of such reports came from Indian Cancer Research Centre (ICRC), Bombay (now Mumbai) (1962), where an acid-fast bacillus was isolated from a leprosy patient, employing human foetal spinal ganglion cell culture. This is known as **ICRC bacillus**. It has been adapted for growth on Lowenstein-Jensen medium and taxonomical studies suggest that this organism is not *M. leprae* and belongs to *M. avium-intracellulare* group.

There have been many attempts to transmit leprosy to various experimental animals. But the first breakthrough was achieved by Shepard (1960) when he reported a limited localized multiplication of *M. leprae* in the **footpad of mouse** in 1–6 months. Footpad of mouse model can be used:

- for identification of *M. leprae*;
- to study the susceptibility of organisms to chemotherapeutic agents;
- to study the development of drug resistance in *M. leprae* in patients under treatment;
- to study the properties of bacilli isolated from different forms of the disease;
- to study the efficacy of various vaccines to suppress multiplication of *M. leprae*; and
- to determine viability of *M. leprae*.

The disadvantages of the footpad of mouse model are:

- Following intradermal inoculation there occurs only a limited multiplication of *M. leprae* (1×10^6 bacilli per footpad), therefore, the yield of the bacilli is not sufficient for comprehensive research on *M. leprae*.
- Mice have a short life-span and leprosy has a long incubation period and chronic course. So it is not possible to study the pathogenesis of the disease.
- The lesion produced is not of lepromatous leprosy type.

However, localized infection of Shepard model can be turned into disseminated disease, simulating human lepromatous leprosy, if immune system of mouse is knocked out by neonatal thymectomy or administration of antilymphocytic serum. Even generalized infection in immune depressed mice does not provide the quantity of bacilli required for research in various aspects of the disease and for preparation of vaccine. The minimum infective dose of *M. leprae* in mouse footpad is 10 solidly staining bacilli. The generation time of *M. leprae*, from animal experiments, has been found to be 12–13 days.

Nine-banded armadillo (*Dasypus novemcinctus*) (Fig. 26.2) is highly susceptible to leprosy. This is presumably due to low body temperature. When inoculated with *M. leprae*, about 40% armadillos develop generalized infection with extensive multiplication of *M. leprae*. Involvement of skin, nerves, lymph nodes, larynx and eye is similar to that of man. In addition, in armadillo, it involves lungs, oesophagus, meninges and cerebral cortex. In armadillo, *M. leprae* survives for about 400 days. Natural infection by a mycobacterium resembling *M. leprae* has been observed in some wild armadillos in Texas and Mexico. Wild armadillo should, therefore, be screened for mycobacterial infection and kept in quarantine for 3 months before inoculation. The advantages of armadillo are:

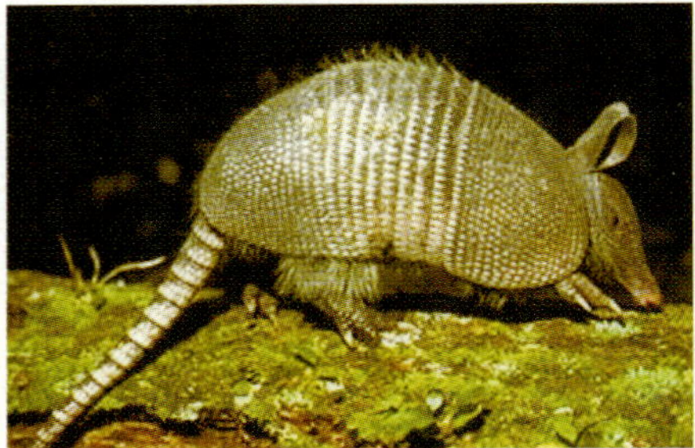

Fig. 26.2. Nine-banded armadillo.

- Relatively long life-span (12–15 years).
- Relatively low body temperature (32–35°C).
- Unique mode of reproduction by means of monozygous genetically identical quadruplets.
- *M. leprae* can be transmitted from one animal to another without any change in microbe, therefore, an abundant source of *M. leprae*, for research and the preparation of lepromin or of a vaccine, has now become available.
- The yield of *M. leprae* from armadillo skin leproma is 100–1,000 times more than that from human leproma.

The use of armadillo as an experimental model of *M. leprae* has been limited by:

- Only about 40% of the animals are susceptible to disseminated form of leprosy.
- Limits of incubation period for the development of lepromatous leprosy in armadillo are not known. It may be many years long. This is certainly the case in man. Therefore, it might be hazardous to conclude, after an arbitrarily chosen length of time, that an inoculated armadillo shall not develop disease in future.
- Some of the armadillos caught from wild life are naturally infected with mycobacteria resembling *M. leprae*.
- These animals are reported to be found only in southern parts of USA and because of their non-availability in other parts of the world their cost is very high.

Q. 2. Describe pathogenicity of *Mycobacterium leprae* and spectrum of leprosy.

Ans. ***Pathogenicity***

Leprosy is an exclusively human disease and the only source of infection is the patient. It is not considered a highly contagious disease. The exact mode of infection is not clear. Very large number of bacilli are shed in nasal secretions (over 10^8 organisms per ml) and in discharges from superficial lesions of the cases of lepromatous leprosy. Organisms may be acquired by a susceptible person by way of skin to skin contact or through respiratory tract. It has also been suggested that insect vectors may have a role in transmission of leprosy.

Once worldwide in distribution, leprosy is now confined mainly, but not exclusively, to the underdeveloped areas of tropics and the southern hemisphere. There has been a considerable decline in the number of cases, from 12 million in the 1980s to less than two million in 1996, partly as a result of control programmes. India has the maximum prevalence, with about a third of the global total. Leprosy is present in all states and territories of India, but with marked regional variations – Orissa and Bihar having the highest prevalence (> 5 per 1000 population) and Haryana the least (< 0.1 per 1000 population).

M. leprae causes **chronic granulomatous lesions** closely resembling those of tuberculosis with epithelioid cells and giant cells but **without caseation**. The organisms in the lesion are predominantly intracellular and like tubercle bacilli can proliferate in macrophages. The organism has predilection for skin, nerves and nasal mucosa though it is capable of affecting any tissue or organ.

- In **cutaneous form** of the disease, large, firm nodules are distributed widely and on the face they create a characteristic **leonine appearance**.
- In the **neural form**, segments of peripheral nerves are involved leading to **localized patches of anaesthesia**. The loss of sensations in fingers and toes increases the frequency of minor trauma, leading to secondary infection and mutilating injuries.

Both forms may be present in the same patient.

Spectrum of leprosy

On the basis of clinical, histopathologic and immunologic findings, Ridley and Joplings (1966) introduced a scale for classifying the spectrum of leprosy into 5 types with hyper-reactive tuberculoid leprosy (TT) at one pole and anergic lepromatous leprosy (LL) at the other.

- **Tuberculoid type:** It is seen in patients with high degree of resistance where cell-mediated immunity is intact. The skin lesions are few and consist of nonelevated hypo- or hyper-pigmented macular anaesthetic patches involving the face, trunk and limbs. There are very few acid-fast bacilli (AFB) so that they are generally not seen microscopically (**pauci-bacillary disease**) and numerous epithelioid cells, giant cells and lymphocytes as in tuberculosis. The local nerves are involved in the early stage and gradually the infection extends into the bigger nerve trunks which are thickened, hard and tender. In tuberculoid leprosy, lepromin test is positive due to intact CMI. Antimycobacterial and autoantibodies are rarely produced.
- **Lepromatous type:** It is the generalized form of the disease and is found in individuals where the host resistance is low. Patient develops numerous nodular skin lesions (lepromata) on face, ear lobes, hands, feet and less commonly on trunk. Skin lesions contain many macrophages, often seen as large foamy cells packed with AFB (Fig. 26.1). In advanced cases, there may be 10^9 *M. leprae*/g of skin (**multibacillary disease**). Cooler parts of the body, such as ear lobes, are particularly infiltrated by bacilli. Blood stream may be invaded, with resulting foci in the liver, spleen, adrenals, testicles and bone marrow and excretion of the organisms in milk. In addition, there is heavy infection of upper respiratory tract, particularly the nasal mucosa, from which the organisms are shed.

  There is slow and symmetric thickening of nerves and anaesthesia. Nodular skin lesions ulcerate due to repeated trauma as a result of loss of sensation. The ulcerated nodules become secondarily infected that leads to distortion and mutilation of extremities. **Lepromatous leprosy is more infectious than other types and has a poor prognosis.** Because of deficient CMI, lepromin test is negative. Humoral antibodies against mycobacterial antigens are produced in high concentrations which play no protective role. **Autoantibodies are also produced.**

• **Borderline or dimorphous type:** Many patients occupy an intermediate position on the spectrum and are classified as **borderline tuberculoid (BT), mid-borderline (BB) and borderline lepromatous (BL)**. The characteristics of these five forms are shown in Table 26.2.

Table 26.2. Characteristics of 5 types of leprosy

	TT	BT	BB	BL	LL
1. AFB in the skin	–	+/–	+	++	+++
2. AFB in nasal secretions	–	–	–	+	+++
3. Granuloma formation	+++	++	+	–	–
4. Lepromin reaction	+++	+	+/–	–	–
5. Antibodies to *M. leprae*	+/–	+/–	+	++	+++

In all types of leprosy, *M. leprae* organisms invade both sensory and motor nerves and destroy nerve fibres. **No other bacterial species has the capacity to enter nerves.** *M. leprae* invades dermal nerves and nerve trunks, but the most vulnerable sites are parts of the body that either tend to remain cool or are subject to trauma. The organisms are present in Schwann and perineural cells. The nasal bones are also involved in leprosy and their destruction may lead to **collapse of the nose**. The eye is frequently damaged by direct bacillary invasion or corneal infection secondary to paralysis of the eyelids leading to blindness.

Q. 3. Name and describe briefly lepra reactions.

Ans. Though leprosy is a chronic disease, its course is sometimes interspersed with acute exacerbations due to immune reactions. These are of two types:

1. Type 1 (Reversal reaction)
2. Type 2 (Erythema nodosum leprosum, ENL)

Type 1 (Reversal reaction)

This occurs in borderline cases (BT, BB and BL) who develop cell-mediated immunity and consequently shift towards tuberculoid part of the spectrum. Clinically there is erythema and swelling of skin lesions which may undergo ulceration. The lesions are infiltrated with lymphocytes and epithelioid cells with reduction in number of bacilli. It may rapidly cause severe and permanent nerve damage.

Type 2 (Erythema nodosum leprosum, ENL)

This is usually seen in lepromatous leprosy patients undergoing chemotherapy. Clinically crops of red nodules appear in the skin, lasting for 1 or 2 days. The lesions show intense neutrophilic infiltration and the blood vessels in the dermis show acute fibrinoid necrosis. Constitutional disturbances like fever, arthritis, iridocyclitis, orchitis and painful neuritis are common. The histological picture is that of an Arthus reaction or immune complex disease. Mycobacterial antigens are released into the circulation when the bacilli die and disintegrate during chemotherapy. The combination of these antigens with the precipitating antibodies present in the serum constitute the mechanism of ENL.

Q. 4. Write short note on immunity in leprosy.

Ans. There seems to exist a high degree of innate immunity in man, therefore, only a minority of the contacts develop clinical manifestations of disease and many others develop a localized lesion that heals spontaneously. Infection with *M. leprae* induces both antibody-mediated and cell-mediated immunity (CMI). Of these, only CMI is protective. The type of leprosy in an individual is determined by the status of CMI in him. When it is adequate, the lesions are of tuberculoid type and when it is inadequate, these are of lepromatous type. Patients with tuberculoid leprosy exhibit a strong delayed type hypersensitivity to lepromin. The macrophages phagocytose the bacilli and destroy them. Specific humoral antibodies are not prominent. There is no increase in immunoglobulin levels and the albumin globulin ratio in the serum is not altered.

Patients at the lepromatous pole of the spectrum exhibit negative lepromin test. Antibodies to *M. leprae* that cross-react with other mycobacteria may be detected in the sera of 75–95% of the patients. The albumin globulin ratio in the serum is reversed. The macrophages are able to phagocytose the bacilli, but instead of being destroyed, the bacilli proliferate in these cells. This is because of suppression of CMI in these patients. **Deficiency in cell-mediated immunity is specific to lepra bacillus antigens. Lepromatous leprosy patients are not more susceptible to viruses, parasites and other pathogens against which CMI is important.**

Q. 5. Write short note on lepromin test.

Ans. This reaction was first described by Mitsuda in Japan in 1919.

Lepromins

The lepromins used as antigen in lepromin test may be of human origin (lepromin-H) or of armadillo origin (lepromin-A) and are of two types:

1. **Integral lepromin (Mitsuda lepromin):** This was developed by Mitsuda in 1919 by boiling human lepromatous tissue rich in *M. leprae*. Standard Mitsuda lepromin contains 4.0×10^7 *M. leprae*/ml and has a shelf life of 2 years at 4°C. Mitsuda lepromin is increasingly being prepared from armadillo-derived *M. leprae* (lepromin-A).
2. **Bacillary lepromin:** This contains more of bacillary components and less of tissue. An important example of bacillary lepromin is Dharmendra antigen which is prepared by floating out the bacilli from finely ground lepromatous tissue with chloroform, evaporating it dry and removing the lipids by washing with ether. The antigen is made up in phenol saline for use.

Procedure

The test is carried out by the intradermal injection of 0.1 ml of lepromin. The response to this is biphasic:

1. **Early or Fernandez reaction:** It is characterized by an acute localized area of inflammation with congestion and oedema, more than 10 mm in diameter, appearing usually in 24–48 hours and tending to disappear in 3–4 days. Histologically, it consists of serous exudate with lymphocytic infiltration.
2. **Late or Mitsuda reaction:** It appears 1–2 weeks after the injection, reaching peak in 4 weeks. The reaction appears in the form of a nodule that may undergo central necrosis and ulceration. It takes several weeks to heal. Histologically, there is infiltration with lymphocytes, epithelioid cells and giant cells.

Fernandez reaction is like tuberculin reaction, a delayed type hypersensitivity (DTH). This reaction indicates that the patient has been infected at some time in the past. On the other hand, Mitsuda reaction is not a measure of pre-existing DTH, but is the **manifestation of cell-mediated immunity**, which the lepromin itself has induced. It thus discriminates between persons who are capable of responding to *M. leprae* and those who cannot.

Uses of lepromin reaction

1. To classify the lesions of leprosy patients. The reaction is positive in tuberculoid and negative in lepromatous leprosy patients.
2. To assess the prognosis and response to treatment. A positive reaction indicates a good prognosis and a negative one a bad prognosis. Conversion to lepromin positivity during treatment is the evidence of improvement.
3. To assess the resistance of an individual to leprosy.
4. For recruitment of persons to work in leprosy homes. Only lepromin-positive persons are recommended to be appointed.
5. To verify the identity of candidate *M. leprae*. Cultivable AFB, claimed to be *M. leprae*, should give matching results when tested in parallel with standard lepromin.

Q. 6. Describe laboratory diagnosis of leprosy.

Ans. As a routine, smears are made from affected parts of the skin and nasal mucous membrane. Material for smear is, however, sometimes taken from lymph nodes and affected nerves.

- **In lepromatous cases**, bacilli are always found in large numbers and about equally frequently in skin and nose. However, in the lepromatous cases under chemotherapy, nasal smears become negative earlier than the smears from skin lesions, consequently in cases under treatment, skin smears are more frequently positive than the nasal smears.
- **In tuberculoid cases**, as a rule, the bacilli are very few and found with great difficulty, or not at all. The characteristic histologic response in biopsy material is helpful in such cases and is essential for accurate classification of the disease within the disease spectrum.

Skin smears

The selection of site for taking smear is of great importance. Places where leprous lesions are most prominent, such as nodules, thick patches and areas of infiltration, should be selected. In case of patches, smears should be made from the thickened margins. In a patient with only diffuse infiltration, about 5–6 different areas of the skin should be sampled, including the skin over the ear lobes, buttocks, forehead, chin and cheeks. The specimen is obtained by **slit and scrape method**.

Thoroughly clean the selected portion of skin with spirit. This is necessary in order to remove any saprophytic acid-fast bacilli that may be present on the skin surface. Hold the skin pinched up and raised between the thumb and index finger of the left hand. This will squeeze out blood from the part and will minimize bleeding when the cut is made. With a small bladed-scalpel an incision, about 5 mm long and 3 mm deep, is made on the pinched skin. If any blood or lymph appears, wipe it away without releasing pressure on the held skin.

The blade of the scalpel is then turned at right angle to the cut (slit) and the bottom and sides of the slit are scraped with the point of the blade, several times in the same direction so that tissue fluid and pulp (not blood) collects on one side of the blade. This is gently smeared on glass slide.

Nasal scrapings

Smears from the nose are made by scraping a little material from the nasal septum, particularly from inferior turbinate bones, with a small-bladed knife. While examining smears from the nose, great care is needed because of the presence of weakly acid-fast diphtheroids in that site, which may be mistaken for acid-fast bacilli, especially when the smear is not properly decolourized. **Nasal smears are of great importance in deciding whether a leprosy patient is infectious or not.** They are positive in patients of leprosy of LL and BL type but are negative in all cases of BB, BT and TT. Furthermore, they disappear more rapidly from the nose as a result of chemotherapy, than they do from skin lesions.

When smears dry, these are fixed by passing the slide twice or thrice over a flame with the surface carrying the smears uppermost. The smears are then stained by the Ziehl-Neelsen technique using 5%, instead of 20%, sulphuric acid for decolourization. Bacteriological and morphological indices (as already discussed) are also determined.

Skin and nerve biopsy

Skin biopsy is collected from active edge of the patches, and nerve biopsy from thickened nerve for histological confirmation of tuberculoid leprosy when acid-fast bacilli cannot be demonstrated in direct smear. Skin biopsy is useful in the diagnosis and accurate classification of leprosy lesion but nerve biopsy is not required if a skin lesion is present.

Animal inoculation

- Injection of ground tissue from lepromatous nodules and nasal scraping from leprosy patient into the **footpad of mouse** produces typical granuloma at the site of inoculation in 1–6 months.
- **Nine-banded armadillo** is highly susceptible to leprosy. Such an animal, when inoculated with ground tissue from lepromatous nodules and nasal scrapings from leprosy patient, develops generalized infection with extensive multiplication of bacilli and the lesions produced resemble lepromatous leprosy.

The lesions which develop in the mouse and armadillo can be identified by histological examination and Ziehl-Neelsen staining.

Lepromin test or Mitsuda reaction

It is not a diagnostic test but is a guide to the resistance of the patient to *M. leprae* infection.

Serological test

Serodiagnosis of leprosy may be carried out by detection of antiphenolic glycolipid 1 antibodies by latex agglutination, *M. leprae* particle agglutination and ELISA test.

Polymerase chain reaction

PCR can be used for the diagnosis at an early stage, before appearance of clinical symptoms. It is effective even in the diagnosis of paucibacillary leprosy, as **the detection limit of PCR is as low as one bacillus**. The PCR assay can be performed on biopsy specimens, skin scrapings and nasal secretions.

27

NONSPORING ANAEROBES

Q. 1. Classify nonsporing anaerobes.

Ans. On the basis of morphology and staining characters, nonsporing anaerobes have been classified as under:

I. Cocci

A. Gram-positive
1. *Peptococcus*
2. *Peptostreptococcus*

B. Gram-negative
Veillonella

II. Bacilli

A. Gram-positive
1. *Lactobacillus*
2. *Bifidobacterium*
3. *Propionibacterium*
4. *Actinomyces*
5. *Mobiluncus*
6. *Eubacterium*

B. Gram-negative
1. *Bacteroides*
2. *Fusobacterium*
3. *Leptotrichia*
4. *Porphyromonas*
5. *Prevotella*

III. Spirochaetes
1. *Treponema*
2. *Borrelia*

Q. 2. Write short note on *Peptococcus*.

Ans. This genus has one species – *P. niger*. They are Gram-positive, non-sporing, anaerobic cocci with G + C content of DNA 50 mol %. They measure 0.4–1.2 µm in diameter and occur singly or in pairs or in clumps. They produce **black colonies on blood agar** after prolonged incubation and produce H_2S. They do not produce catalase and indole and do not reduce nitrate to nitrite.

They occur as normal flora of skin, gastrointestinal tract and genitourinary tract. However, they may cause pyogenic infections of wounds, puerperal sepsis and urinary tract infection.

Q. 3. Write short note on *Peptostreptococcus*.

Ans. This genus has 9 species – *P. anaerobius*, *P. asaccharolyticus*, *P. prevotii*, *P. magnus*, *P. indolicus*, *P. micros*, *P. productus*, *P. heliotrinreducens* and *P. tetradius* (formerly *Gafficia anaerobia*). They are Gram-positive cocci occurring in pairs, chains or irregular masses. They are **obligate anaerobes**, measure 0.5–2 μm in diameter, non-haemolytic, catalase-variable, indole production and nitrate reduction variable. Some strains ferment carbohydrates but others are asaccharolytic.

They occur as normal flora of skin, mouth, gastrointestinal tract and genitourinary tract and are the **commonest anaerobic organisms** recovered from human infections like pleuro-pulmonary disease, chronic otitis media, brain abscess, puerperal sepsis and urinary tract infections.

P. anaerobius* and *P. magnus are the commonest anaerobic Gram-positive cocci isolated from wound infections. ***P. anaerobius*** is the anaerobic coccus most commonly associated with puerperal infection.

Q. 4. Write short note on *Veillonella*.

Ans. These are Gram-negative cocci occurring in pairs, short chains and clumps. They are obligate anaerobes, oxidase-negative, catalase-negative, non-motile and measure 0.3–2.5 μm in diameter. They are present as normal flora of the mouth, gastrointestinal and genital tracts. Colonies on blood agar, after 24 hours incubation are small, round, convex, shiny, opaque, light grey and non-haemolytic. In the broth culture, abundant gas is produced. *V. parvula* is isolated from clinical specimens, but little is known of its role in the production of infection.

Q. 5. Write short note on *Lactobacillus*.

Ans. These are straight or curved rods that, like corynebacteria, frequently show bipolar bodies due to the presence of **metachromatic granules**. They are Gram-positive and non-sporing. Most strains are non-motile, while a few strains are motile by peritrichous flagella. The bacilli are of varying length and thickness with parallel sides. On an average they measure 1.5 × 1 μm in size and tend to occur singly or in chains. Occasionally, they may show filamentous forms.

Lactobacilli are normally present in mouth (*L. casei*, *L. fermentum*, *L. acidophilus* and *L. brevis*), gut (*L. acidophilus*, *L. fermentum* and *L. salivarius*) and in vagina (*L. acidophilus*, *L. fermentum*, *L. casei* and *L. cellobiosus*). In the mouth, they have been incriminated in the pathogenesis of **dental caries**. The mineral components of enamel and dentine are believed to be dissolved by the acid formed by the fermentation of sucrose and other dietary carbohydrates by lactobacilli. In the intestine, they synthesize vitamins such as biotin, vitamin B_{12} and vitamin K which may be absorbed by the host.

In the adult vagina, lactobacilli ferment glycogen which is deposited in the vaginal epithelial cells and form lactic acid, which accounts for the highly acidic pH of the vagina. This protects adult vagina from infection with gonococci. In prepubertal and postmenopausal vagina, lactobacilli are scanty. Lactobacilli occurring in vagina are collectively known as **Doderlein's bacilli**.

Lactobacilli are also found in plant materials such as silage and in food stuffs and agricultural products, particularly milk, cheese and fermented milk products and in fermented beverages such as wine and cider. In some of these products the multiplication of lactobacilli brings about desirable changes, in others it causes spoilage.

Lactobacilli grow best under microaerophilic conditions in the presence of 5% CO_2 and at pH 6. Better growth is obtained in media enriched with glucose or blood. Colonies on agar media are usually small, 1–3 mm in diameter, with entire margins. Some species form rough colonies. Selective media include Hadley's tomato juice agar (pH 5) and glucose yeast extract acetic acid agar of Rogosa et al., 1951.

Q. 6. Write short note on *Bifidobacterium*.

Ans. They are non-motile, non-sporing and pleomorphic Gram-positive rods showing true and false branching. The name is derived from the frequent bifid Y-shaped cells. Most species are obligate anaerobes, but a few species, isolated from animals and bees, can grow in the presence of 90% air and 10% CO_2. Various bifidobacteria occur as normal flora in the mouth, gastrointestinal and genitourinary tracts. *B. bifidum* is common in the faeces of breast-fed and bottle-fed infants and in the faeces of adults and of animals. Bifidobacteria are non-pathogenic to man or laboratory animals.

Q. 7. Write short note on *Propionibacterium*.

Ans. Propionibacteria are pleomorphic, Gram-positive, coryneform rods, non-acid-fast, non-motile and are often arranged in short chains or clumps. They are commonly found on the skin, conjunctiva, external ear, and in the oropharynx and female genital tract. They are aerotolerant, and growth may occasionally be obtained aerobically. Two most commonly isolated species are *Propionibacterium acnes* and *P. propionicum*. *P. acnes* is responsible for two types of infections – (1) **acne vulgaris** in teenagers and young adults, and (2) **opportunistic infections** in patients with prosthetic devices (e.g., artificial heart valves or joints) or intravascular lines (e.g., catheters, cerebrospinal fluid shunts).

Q. 8. Describe morphology, cultural characteristics, biochemical reactions, pathogenicity, laboratory diagnosis and treatment of *Mobiluncus* species.

Ans. Recent studies suggest that the genus *Mobiluncus* belongs to the order Actinomycetales and is closely related to the genus *Actinomyces*. This genus has two species: *M. curtisii* and *M. mulieris*.

Morphology

Both species are slightly curved rods and occur singly or in pairs. *M. curtisii* is short, 1.7 × 0.5 μm and Gram-variable while *M. mulieris* is long, 2.9 × 0.5 μm and Gram-negative. Both species are motile by means of multiple subpolar flagella.

Cultural characteristics

They are essentially anaerobes but can grow in an atmosphere of 5% O_2 and 95% N_2. They are fastidious and grow slowly at 33–37°C producing round, entire, low convex, smooth, translucent, colourless colonies, 2–3 mm in diameter, after anaerobic incubation on blood agar medium for five days. Addition of 10 μg/ml each of colistin and nalidixic acid to blood agar makes it selective for isolation of these organisms.

Biochemical reactions

They are oxidase- and catalase-negative. Small amounts of acetic acid and major amounts of succinic acid are produced in glycogen-containing media. Differentiating biochemical characters of both the species are given in Table 27.1.

Table 27.1. Differentiating characters of species of *Mobiluncus*

Character	*M. curtisii*	*M. mulieris*
1. Mean size of the bacterial cell	1.7 × 0.5 μm	2.9 × 0.5 μm
2. Gram staining reaction	Variable	Negative
3. Arginine hydrolysis	+	–
4. Hippurate hydrolysis	+	–
5. ONPG	+	–
6. Nitrate reduction	+	–

Pathogenicity

In association with *Bacteroides* species and *Gardnerella vaginalis*, *M. curtisii* and *M. mulieris* have been blamed to cause **bacterial vaginosis**. Of these, *Bacteroides* species constitute a major component. There is a foul-smelling (rotten fish smell) but non-purulent vaginal discharge. Rotten fish smell is accentuated when it is mixed with a drop of KOH solution. The vaginal pH is more than 4.5.

Laboratory diagnosis

Microscopic examination of fresh unstained smears of vaginal discharge show epithelial cells coated with bacteria (**'clue cells'**). *M. curtisii* and *M. mulieris* may be isolated from vaginal discharge by inoculation on blood agar and blood agar with colistin and nalidixic acid, and identified as above.

Treatment

Mobiluncus species are susceptible to benzylpenicillin, clindamycin, erythromycin and gentamicin. For the treatment of infection by *Mobiluncus* species, penicillins are appropriate drugs. *M. mulieris* is more susceptible than *M. curtisii* to metronidazole.

Q. 9. Write short note on *Bacteroides*.

Ans. *Bacteroides* occur as commensals in the mouth, gastrointestinal and female genital tracts. This genus comprises the most common anaerobes isolated from clinical specimens. They are non-sporing, non-motile, Gram-negative bacilli. They are very pleomorphic, appearing as slender rods, branching forms or coccobacilli. They occur singly, in pairs or in short chains. They grow readily in media such as brain-heart-infusion agar in an anaerobic atmosphere containing 10% CO_2. They possess capsular polysaccharide which appears to be virulence factor. The capsule confers resistance to phagocytosis and intracellular killing.

They cause peritonitis following bowel injury, pelvic inflammatory disease, abdominal and brain abscesses, and empyema. Pus is often foul smelling. *B. fragilis* is the most frequent of the non-sporing anaerobes isolated from clinical specimens. *B. melaninogenica* forms black-pigmented or brown colonies on blood-containing media. The pigment is an intracellular or cell-associated derivative of haemoglobulin (haemin). It has been isolated from lung or liver abscesses, mastoiditis, and lesions of intestine, mouth and gums.

Q. 10. Write short note on *Fusobacterium.*

Ans. Fusobacteria are Gram-negative, **strict anaerobic rods** of varied size and morphology. Some species of *Fusobacterium* produce long slender Gram-negative rods that are wide at the centre and taper towards the ends (fusiform), but others produce coccobacilli to very long and filamentous cells. They are usually non-motile and growth is often improved by 5–10% CO_2. They can be isolated on blood agar plates containing neomycin and vancomycin. After 48 hours incubation at 37°C, the colonies are striate or granular with irregular or crenated edge and a raised centre.

F. nucleatum is the most studied species. It may cause infections of head and neck region including dental and periodontal infections and cerebral abscess. *F. necrophorum* is an important animal pathogen. It may, however, sometimes cause infections in man similar to those caused by *F. nucleatum.*

Q. 11. Write short note on *Leptotrichia.*

Ans. This genus contains only one species, *L. buccalis* which is synonymous with *F. fusiforme.* They are anaerobic, non-sporing, non-motile, long, straight or slightly curved Gram-negative bacilli with considerable width and tapering ends. They measure 5–15 × 1–1.5 µm in size. They can be grown on blood agar at 37°C under anaerobic conditions with 5–10% CO_2. After 48 hours incubation, colonies are 2–3 mm in diameter, irregular and often striate. Many strains become aerotolerant after several subcultures.

L. buccalis is a normal flora of mouth and gastrointestinal tract. However, in association with *Borrelia vincentii* it is believed to cause **acute ulcerative gingivitis** or **Vincent's angina**. It is seen in patients with malnutrition, debility and poor oral hygiene. It is characterized by pain, haemorrhage, foul odour, destruction of interdental papillae, inflammation of the gums and formation of a pseudomembrane. *L. buccalis* and *B. vincentii* are present in the exudate and pseudomembrane, and diagnosis is made by direct microscopy.

Q. 12. Write short note on *Prevotella.*

Ans. *Prevotella* contains *P. melaninogenica*, *P. buccalis*, *P. denticola* and other species. *P. melaninogenica* produces black or brown colonies on anaerobic blood agar. The colour is not due to the melanin pigment but is due to hemin derivative. It causes lung or liver abscess, mastoiditis, intestinal lesions and lesions of mouth and gums. Cultures of *P. melaninogenica* and dressings from wounds infected with the bacillus produce a characteristic red fluorescence when exposed to ultraviolet light.

Q. 13. Describe laboratory diagnosis of infections caused by anaerobic bacteria.

Ans. As anaerobic bacteria form part of the normal flora of the skin and mucous surfaces, their isolation from clinical specimens has to be interpreted cautiously. The mere presence of an anaerobe does not prove its causal role.

Specimen collection and transport

Specimens should be collected in such a manner as to avoid normal resident flora. For example, the sputum is unsatisfactory for culture from a suspected case of lung abscess. In general, material for anaerobic culture is best obtained by tissue biopsy or by aspiration using a needle and syringe. Swabs are unsatisfactory specimens, but when they are to be used, they should be sent in Stuart's transport medium. Ideally, specimens should be placed in an anaerobic transport device that consists of a tube or vial containing an anaerobic gas mixture substituted for air, which protects the organisms from oxygen exposure and drying during transport to the laboratory. Specimens should be delivered within 20 minutes for culture.

Direct microscopy

Examination of a Gram-stained smear shows numerous pus cells and a variety of organisms. In case of *P. melaninogenica* infection, examination of the specimen under ultraviolet light may show the bright red fluorescence.

Culture

Freshly prepared blood agar with neomycin, yeast extract, hemin and vitamin K is inoculated and incubated at 37°C in an anaerobic jar, with 10% CO_2. Anaerobiasis can also be maintained by GasPak system. Plates are examined after 24–48 hours. Some anaerobes, such as fusobacteria, require longer period of incubation. Parallel aerobic cultures should also be set up because in most anaerobic infections aerobic bacteria are also involved. Other anaerobic media, such as cooked meat broth and thioglycollate broth, may also be used for isolation of anaerobes.

Definitive identification of the anaerobes depends on colony morphology and various biochemical tests. Gas liquid chromatography is also useful to identify anaerobes in the specimens.

28

SPIROCHAETES

Q. 1. Describe morphology, cultivation, sensitivity to physical and chemical agents and antigenic structure of *Treponema pallidum*.

Ans. ***Morphology***

It is a thin, delicate, long, motile, flexible organism which is twisted spirally round its long axis. It is 6–14 µm long. Its width is 0.13 µm in dried state, but is about 0.2 µm in the wet living state, which is just great enough for resolution with the light microscope. It has 6–12 coils which are remarkably evenly disposed at 1 µm intervals and the amplitude of spirals is 1–1.5 µm. They have tapering ends. It is actively motile exhibiting flexion and extension, translatory and corkscrew-like motility. As the spirochaete moves across the dark-field of the microscope, it often displays a **characteristic tendency to bend at right angles near its midpoint**. These secondary curves appear and disappear but its primary spirals remain unchanged.

Because of its weak refractility and slender thickness, about the limit of resolution by the light microscope, it is best seen in wet living preparation with the **dark-ground microscope**. In dried preparations, it needs to be thickened by **silver impregnation methods (Fontana's method is useful for staining films and Levaditi's for tissue sections)**. It possesses Gram-negative envelope. It cannot be stained by simple aniline dyes or by Gram's method. By prolonged **Giemsa staining** it stains pale pink. By **immunofluorescence method**, treponemes can be detected in tissues and body fluids.

Ultrastructurally, *T. pallidum* possesses usually three but occasionally four endoflagella attached subterminally at each end of the cell and extend towards the opposite pole between outer membrane and peptidoglycan layer of the cell wall. The endoflagella from the two ends are more than half the length of the organism and interdigitate over the central portion of the organism, so that in transverse section there often appear to be three or four of them in section taken from terminal regions and 4–6 in sections from the central portion.

Cultivation

Pathogenic treponemes cannot be cultivated in artificial media and are maintained by subculture in susceptible animals. **Nichol's strain** of *T. pallidum* has been maintained, in rabbit testis, for several decades by serial testicular passage since it was isolated in 1913 from CSF of a patient with neurosyphilis.

Cultivable treponemes such as *T. phagedenis* (**Reiter treponeme**) and *T. refringens* are non-pathogenic. They can be grown under strictly anaerobic conditions in Smith-Noguchi medium or in digest broth enriched with serum.

Sensitivity to physical and chemical agents

T. pallidum is a very delicate organism, therefore, syphilis is ordinarily acquired by sexual intercourse. It is readily inactivated by heating at 41.5°C for 1 hour. When infected blood is stored at 5°C in citrate anticoagulant, infectivity is lost in 5 days or less. Therefore, transfusion syphilis can be prevented by storing blood for at least 5 days in the refrigerator before transfusion.

Treponemes from rabbit syphilomas of the testis preserved in the proper suspending fluids under anaerobic conditions remain actively motile for 2 days at 37°C and 4–7 days at 25°C. Frozen in a medium containing 15% glycerol at –70°C or below, they remain viable for years and provide a reliable source of antigens for immunological tests. **Lyophilization (freeze-drying) kills the organism.**

Antigenic structure

The antigenic structure of *T. pallidum* is poorly understood. Infection with these treponemes leads to the production of three types of antibodies. On the basis of these antibodies, the treponemal antigens may be divided into specific and non-specific antigens.

Specific antigens

1. **Group-specific antigen:** It is a protein antigen present in *T. pallidum* as well as in non-pathogenic treponemes, such as Reiter treponeme. Antibody to this antigen appears in serum of syphilitic patients. The antigen used in tests to detect group-specific antibodies is derived from the Reiter treponeme.
2. **Species-specific treponemal antigen:** It appears to be polysaccharide in nature. *T. pallidum* is used as antigen for detection of species-specific antibody.

Non-specific antigen

A non-specific antibody (reagin) appears in blood of syphilitic patients that reacts with a lipid hapten extracted from beef heart. The hapten is known as **cardiolipin** and is chemically a diphosphatidyl glycerol. It is not certain whether cardiolipin is an antigen contained in *T. pallidum* itself or a product of damaged tissue caused by infection.

Q. 2. Describe pathogenicity of *Treponema pallidum*.

Ans. *T. pallidum* is a **strict parasite** and its life outside the animal body is short. It causes syphilis. Most cases of syphilis are **contracted during sexual intercourse**. The treponemes are present in the superficial genital lesions and pass from one partner to the other through **intact mucous membranes or through minor skin abrasions**. The disease may also be transmitted

congenitally, by close contact with mucous membrane lesions as in **kissing** and through **blood transfusions**. Medical personnel are occasionally infected by an **accidental finger prick** with an infected needle.

In venereal syphilis, the treponemes penetrate mucosal surfaces or abraded skin and multiply at the site of entry and after an incubation period of about a month (range 10–90 days), the clinical disease sets in. The clinical manifestations fall into four stages – primary, secondary, latent and tertiary.

1. Primary syphilis

The primary lesion of syphilis is the **chancre** which is painless, relatively avascular, circumscribed, indurated, 1–2 cm in diameter. It ulcerates in the centre. It is known as **hard chancre** to distinguish it from the non-indurated lesion (**soft sore**) caused by *Haemophilus ducreyi*. The primary lesion of syphilis is also known as **Hunterian chancre**, after John Hunter who produced the lesions on himself experimentally. Histologically, it is oedematous and infiltrated predominantly with mononuclear cells.

Most frequently chancre appears on the external genitalia – prepuce, corona of the penis (Fig. 28.1), labia and vaginal wall. It may also occur on the cervix, perianal area, anal canal or on the tongue (Fig. 28.2), and other oral mucous membranes. In some cases it may be on lips, cheeks and nipples (when it is acquired through kissing). *Chancres usually occur singly but in immunocompromised individuals, such as those infected with human immunodeficiency virus, multiple chancres may develop.*

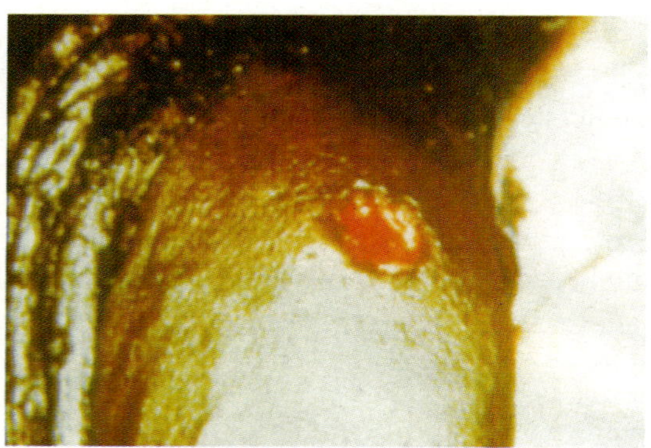

Fig. 28.1. A chancre caused by *Treponema pallidum* on the penis.

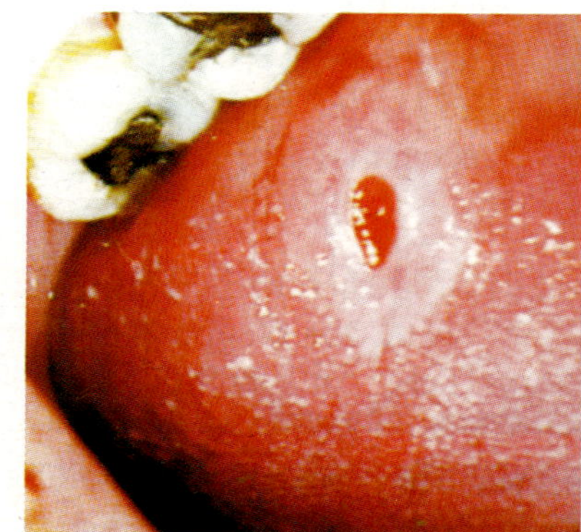

Fig. 28.2. A chancre caused by *Treponema pallidum* on the tongue.

A large number of treponemes are present in the primary lesion and in the serum that exudes from it. In the early days of infection, the spirochaetes invade the regional lymph nodes (inguinal in males and pelvic in females) and lead to **lymphadenitis**. The lymph nodes are swollen, discrete, rubbery and non-tender. From lymph nodes treponemes enter into the blood stream in large numbers. *Chancre heals spontaneously in about 3–6 weeks even without treatment leaving a thin scar.*

2. Secondary syphilis

This sets in 2–6 months after the primary lesion heals during which period the patient is asymptomatic. The secondary lesions are due to widespread multiplication of the treponemes and their dissemination through the blood. Patient develops marked constitutional symptoms, **diffuse erythematous cutaneous lesions**, particularly on the trunk and extremities, mucous patches in the oropharynx and **condylomata** at mucocutaneous junctions.

There may also be enlargement of the lymph nodes and sometimes involvement of the bones, joints, eyes and other organs. All the lesions of secondary syphilis, especially those involving mucous membranes on exposed surfaces discharge very large number of treponemes. Like the primary chancre, they constitute a very large reservoir of infection and they present a hazard to medical personnel who investigate and treat cases of syphilis. *Lesions of secondary syphilis undergo spontaneous healing in 4–5 years.*

3. Latent syphilis

After the secondary lesions disappear, the disease becomes latent and can be detected only by serological tests. In many cases, this is followed by natural cure but in others, after several years, manifestations of tertiary syphilis appear.

4. Tertiary syphilis

Decades after the primary infection, patient may develop late or tertiary syphilis. It is a slowly progressive, destructive inflammatory disease that may affect any organ. It may lead to relatively benign ulcerating lesions of the skin, mucous membranes or bones, or **gummata** of the internal organs. More serious are lesions of heart and aorta that may lead to the formation of **aneurysms**, or of the central nervous system, of which **tabes dorsalis** and **general paralysis of the insane** are the most common.

The lesions of tertiary syphilis contain very few organisms and the remarkable severity of the lesions is attributed to an intense cellular immune response to the organisms and their products. Individuals with serologic evidence of AIDS appear to be at much higher risk of developing neurosyphilis. This may be due to the immunosupression associated with AIDS.

Congenital syphilis

The treponemes can cross the placental barrier. Infection in the foetus usually occurs from primary and secondary infection of the mother. The lesions of congenital syphilis usually develop only after fourth month of gestation, the time when foetal immune competence starts appearing. This suggests that the pathogenesis of syphilis requires an immune response from the foetus. Congenital syphilis can be prevented if the mother is given adequate treatment before the fourth month of pregnancy.

Q. 3. Describe laboratory diagnosis of syphilis.

Ans. The clinical diagnosis of syphilis is confirmed in the laboratory (Table 28.1) by:

A. Demonstration of treponemes in the exudate

1. **Dark-ground microscopy:** To avoid the risk of acquiring infection, it is important to wear gloves and exercise great care in handling the lesions. The surface of the lesion is cleansed carefully with a gauze swab soaked in warm normal saline and the margins are gently scrapped so that superficial epithelium is abraded. Gentle pressure is applied to the base of the lesion until serum exudes from its surface. If it is blood stained, it should be wiped away and process repeated until a clear fluid is obtained. Wet film is now made

on a thin glass slide, covered with a thin coverslip and examined under dark-ground microscope.

T. pallidum is recognized by its slender structure, regularity of its spirals and slightly pointed ends (Fig. 28.3). Other spirochaetes are usually thicker and have rounded ends. It is motile with a to and fro drilling motion and occasional flexion of the body. Dark-ground microscopy is unsuitable for examining oral lesions because many of the non-pathogenic treponemes found there may be confused with *T. pallidum*. Numerous commensal spirochaetes that are found as the normal flora of the genital and rectal mucosal surfaces must be carefully distinguished. These may be present on the surface of the genital ulcers and are not found in the depth of the lesions. If the initial test is negative, the procedure should be repeated daily for at least 3 days. Antibiotics and local antiseptics should be withheld during this period.

2. **Direct fluorescent-antibody staining for T. pallidum (DFA-Tp):** A more definite approach to diagnosis is provided by DFA-Tp. It has the advantage that a smear of the material to be tested is made on a glass slide, fixed in acetone and sent to the laboratory. The smear is then stained with fluorescein-labelled pathogen-specific monoclonal antibody and examined under fluorescence microscope. The treponemes appear distinct, sharply outlined and have an apple-green fluorescence. The ability to scan slides quickly in search of these typical forms is a distinct advantage over dark-ground microscopy. Oral lesions which cannot be evaluated by dark-ground microscopy can be accurately examined by DFA-Tp. Non-motile *T. pallidum* can also be identified by this test. This test is 100% sensitive and specific, while dark-ground microscopy is 97% sensitive and 77% specific.

Table 28.1. Methods of laboratory diagnosis of syphilis

A. Demonstration of treponemes in the exudate
1. Dark-ground microscopy
2. Direct fluorescent-antibody staining for *Treponema pallidum* (DFA-Tp)

B. Demonstration of treponemes in tissues
- Immunofluorescence
- Silver impregnation method

C. Demonstration of treponemal antigen in the lesion
- EIA

D. Nucleic acid-based test
- PCR

E. Serological diagnosis of syphilis
1. Nontreponemal tests
   - Wassermann reaction
   - Kahn test
   - VDRL test
   - RPR test
2. Treponemal tests
   (a) Those using cultivable treponemes
   - RPCF test
   (b) Those in which pathogenic *T. pallidum* is the antigen employed
   I. Test using live *T. pallidum*
   - TPI test
   II. Tests using killed *T. pallidum*
   - TPA test
   - TPIA test
   - FTA, FTA-ABS, IgM FTA-ABS tests
   III. Tests using *T. pallidum* extract
   - TPHA
   - EIA

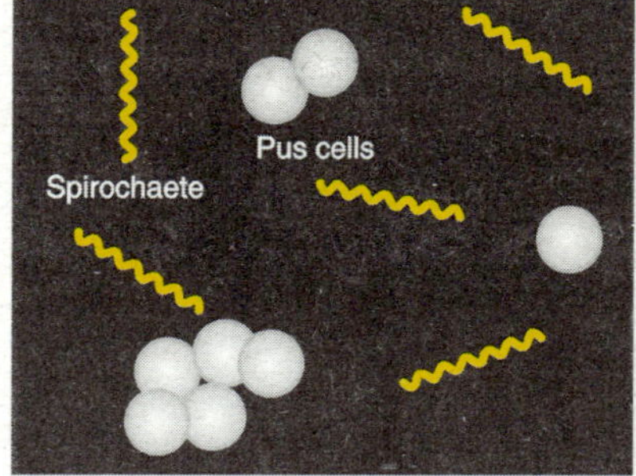

Fig. 28.3. Dark-ground illumination preparation of serous exudate from primary syphilitic chancre.

B. Demonstration of treponemes in tissues

Treponemes in the tissues can be demonstrated by immunofluorescence or silver staining.

C. Demonstration of treponemal antigen in the lesion

T. pallidum antigen in the lesion can be detected by enzyme immunoassay.

D. Nucleic acid-based test

Nucleic acid amplification test (polymerase chain reaction) has been developed for detecting *T. pallidum* in genital lesions, infant blood, and cerebrospinal fluid.

E. Serological diagnosis of syphilis

Direct detection of treponemes and treponemal antigen requires special skills or use of complex reagents with a short shelf life. Therefore, serological diagnosis of syphilis is a viable alternative. Depending upon the antigens used, serological tests for syphilis may be divided into the following:

1. **Nontreponemal tests or Standard tests for syphilis (STS)** in which cardiolipin or lipoidal antigen is used.
2. **Treponemal tests** in which treponemes are used as the antigen. These are of two types:
   (a) Those using cultivable treponemes, such as Reiter treponemes (*T. phagedenis*) as the antigen.
   (b) Those in which pathogenic *T. pallidum* is the antigen employed. These tests may further be classified according to whether the treponeme employed is live, killed or extracts of the treponemes.

Nontreponemal tests

Nontreponemal tests that can be employed are Wassermann, Kahn, Venereal Diseases Research Laboratory (VDRL) and the rapid plasma reagin (RPR) tests. The antigen used in these tests is an alcoholic extract of beef heart tissue (cardiolipin) to which lecithin and cholesterol are added. Wassermann reaction and Kahn test are complement fixation and tube flocculation tests respectively. Since Wassermann reaction offers no advantage over simple and rapid flocculation tests such as VDRL and RPR, therefore, World Health Organization (1982) recommended that its use should be discontinued. Similarly, Kahn test is rarely done these days.

VDRL test

The test is named after Venereal Disease Research Laboratory, New York, where the test was developed. It is the most widely used simple and rapid test which requires only a small quantity of serum and it is sensitive and no less specific than Wassermann reaction and Kahn test. **IgM or IgG** antibody present in the patient serum causes a suspension of cardiolipin antigen to flocculate. These antibodies are wrongly known as '**reagin**' and are different from IgE class of antibodies which carry the same name.

VDRL test is performed as a slide test in which inactivated patient serum is mixed with a freshly prepared suspension of cardiolipin-lecithin-cholesterol antigen on a glass slide. The mixture is rotated, usually mechanically, for 4 minutes after which the flocculation (aggregation of antigen-antibody complexes in suspension) can be detected under a low power objective of a microscope.

VDRL test is used as a screening test and is positive in approximately 70% of primary and 99% of secondary syphilis. Antibody becomes detectable 7–10 days after the appearance of primary chancre. The titre of antibody may rise to 8 or 16 during primary syphilis and 16–128 during secondary syphilis. It may sometimes, show false negative reaction due to prozone phenomenon when the patient serum contains high titre of antibody. Titres decline beyond the secondary stage and around 30% of patients with late syphilis are non-reactive. High titres similar to those in secondary syphilis may be found in active cardiovascular and neurosyphilis, and in patients with gummatous lesions. In some cases of neurosyphilis, reagin tests may be negative with serum but positive with the CSF. Positive result in the VDRL test usually indicates active infection, therefore, it can be used to monitor the efficacy of antibacterial therapy. *Though the majority of HIV-infected patients have a normal serologic response to treponemal infections, some demonstrate an exaggerated immune response and some a lack of immune response, resulting in a diverse serologic presentation.*

The major disadvantages of the VDRL slide test are the need to prepare fresh antigen each day and to use a microscope to read the results. Heat inactivation of sera is necessary to destroy a heat-labile inhibitory factor of IgM class which may be present in both normal and syphilitic serum. *Heat treatment inactivates HIV also thus reducing the risk of acquiring AIDS in laboratory personnel.*

RPR test

In rapid plasma reagin test, VDRL antigen is adsorbed on finely divided carbon particles and suspended in choline chloride which blocks inhibitory factors in the serum thus eliminating the need to heat the serum before testing. The antigen is also stabilized with EDTA, allowing it to be used for up to 6 months when stored at 4–10°C. This test is performed by mixing one drop of patient serum or plasma (50 µl) with a drop of this modified antigen (20 µl), on a disposable plastic card (12.5 × 7 cm in size with 10 clearly defined test areas) using a disposable stick. The card is then rocked gently to and fro for 8 minutes and observed under strong source of light. In a positive test, the flocculation of carbon particles (black aggregates) is visible with naked eye. Black aggregates may be deposited at the periphery of the liquid. In a negative test, there is a complete absence of black aggregates with a uniform greyish background. Any specimen giving a positive reaction should then be tested quantitatively using doubling dilutions of serum (1 : 2, 1 : 4, 1 : 8, 1 : 16, 1 : 32, etc.).

Most laboratories use RPR test as a screening procedure for syphilis. The sensitivity and specificity of the RPR test are essentially the same as that of the VDRL test. The RPR is quick and easy to perform and serum sample does not need to be heat-inactivated. In addition, cards can be read macroscopically, in contrast to VDRL test which requires microscopic examination for interpretation. However, only disadvantage with the RPR test is that **it cannot be used to test cerebrospinal fluid, while VDRL remains the standard test for use with cerebrospinal fluid**.

Biological false positive reactions: Antibodies against cardiolipin may be detected in the absence of *T. pallidum* infection and give what is known as biological false positive (BFP) reaction. In such cases, specific treponemal tests are negative and there is no history of present or past treponemal infection. BFP reactions may occur in 0.3–0.9% of all sera examined and are caused mainly by IgM antibody. These reactions are of two types:

- **Acute or transient BFP reactions** which may develop shortly after an acute febrile infectious disease and will disappear within a few weeks or months after the illness has subsided.
- **Chronic BFP reactions** persist longer than 6 months. These may occur in a wide variety of infectious and noninfectious conditions associated with tissue damage. These include:
  - autoimmune diseases particularly systemic lupus erythematosus,
  - leprosy particularly lepromatous leprosy,
  - malaria,
  - relapsing fever,
  - infectious mononucleosis,
  - hepatitis, and
  - tropical eosinophilia.

Treponemal tests

(a) Those using cultivable treponemes

The antigen used to detect group-specific antibody is derived from *T. phagedenis* (Reiter treponeme). It is protein in nature and the test is known as **Reiter protein complement fixation (RPCF) test**. The principle of this test is the same as that of Wassermann test, but the antigen in RPCF test is extracted from *T. phagedenis*. This is less sensitive than cardiolipin tests in early syphilis but is more sensitive in late or latent syphilis. It is much more specific than cardiolipin tests, but false reactions still occur in a few cases. With the advent of newer treponemal tests such as *Treponema pallidum* haemagglutination assay, RPCF test is rarely done now a days. New ELISA tests based on purified endoflagella of *T. phagedenis* have been developed.

(b) Those in which pathogenic T. pallidum is the antigen employed

A number of specific tests are now available for the definite diagnosis of syphilis. All require live or killed or extracts of *T. pallidum* (Nichol's strain) grown in rabbit testes.

I. Test using live *T. pallidum*

Treponema pallidum immobilization (TPI) test

This test determines the ability of patient serum to immobilize motile virulent *T. pallidum*. The test serum is incubated anaerobically with a suspension of the treponemes and complement. If antibodies are present, the treponemes will be found to be immobilized, when examined under dark-ground microscope. The test is considered reactive if more than 50% of the treponemes are immobilized, and non-reactive if less than 20% are immobilized. The test is doubtful if 20–50% treponemes are immobilized.

In the past, TPI test was the only reliable serological test for distinguishing between syphilitic and nontreponemal cardiolipin-antibody response. But it is expensive and technically difficult to perform, therefore, it has now been superseded by the widespread use of FTA-ABS test. TPI test may be negative in primary syphilis and may not become negative after treatment. Hence, **for the assessment of cure following treatment, non-treponemal tests are more useful than the TPI test**. False positive TPI reactions have been reported.

II. Tests using killed *T. pallidum*

Treponema pallidum agglutination (TPA) test

In this test, a suspension of *T. pallidum*, inactivated by formalin, is mixed with test serum and incubated. The mixture is then examined under dark-ground microscope. In the presence of antibody, treponemes are found to be agglutinated. This test is not very specific and false positive reactions are common.

Treponema pallidum immune adherence (TPIA) test

Suspension of inactivated treponemes is mixed with test serum, complement and fresh heparinised whole blood from a normal individual, and incubated. In the presence of antibodies, the treponemes will be found to adhere to the erythrocytes. In the absence of antibody, immune adherence does not take place. Both TPA and TPIA are not used in diagnostic laboratories, they serve primarily as research tools.

Fluorescent treponemal antibody (FTA) test

It is an indirect immunofluorescence test. Smears of *T. pallidum* are prepared on slides and fixed with acetone. These slides can be stored in the deep freezer for several months. The patient serum is added on the smear and incubated for the antibody to react with the treponemes. The excess serum is then washed off and the antibodies that bind to the fixed organisms are detected by treating the smear with fluorescein-labelled antihuman immunoglobulin. After incubation and washing off the unfixed conjugate, slide is examined under fluorescence microscope. In a positive test, treponemes fluoresce.

Originally patient serum was used in a dilution of 1 in 5. At this dilution, the test has high sensitivity and poor specificity. Therefore, the dilution of the serum was raised to 1 in 200. In this test, called **FTA-200**, the specificity was improved but sensitivity was decreased. Therefore, this test was further modified to **fluorescent treponemal antibody absorption (FTA-ABS) test**. Here the patient serum is first absorbed with an extract of non-pathogenic *T. phagedenis* (Reiter treponemes) to remove group-reactive antibody. FTA-ABS test has high specificity and sensitivity. It is almost as specific as the more complicated TPI test. Therefore, it is the most widely used serologic test for detection of specific treponemal antibodies. **VDRL and FTA-ABS tests can also be performed on cerebrospinal fluid.** Antibodies do not reach from the blood stream but are probably formed in the CNS in response to treponemal infection.

FTA-ABS test becomes reactive around 3rd week of infection and is positive in 80%, 100% and 95% of primary, secondary and late syphilis respectively. Unlike VDRL test, its reactivity persists after successful therapy. However, occasionally the test may become non-reactive if treatment is given early in the disease. The specificity of this test ranges from 92–99%. **False positive reactions have been observed in patients with rheumatoid arthritis, lupus erythematosus, cirrhosis and hypergammaglobulinaemia and in 1% of normal persons.**

Another modification of this test, the **IgM FTA-ABS test, can detect IgM antibodies in congenital syphilis** thus distinguishing it from seropositivity due to passively transferred maternal antibodies which are IgG in nature. In addition, in the former repeated tests will show an increase in titre, whereas in the latter titre will fall.

III. Tests using *T. pallidum* extract

Treponema pallidum haemagglutination test (TPHA)

In this test, *T. pallidum* antigen is adsorbed onto the surface of red blood cells. When these red blood cells are mixed with patient serum, specific antibody, if present, causes haemagglutination. As in FTA-ABS test patient serum is pre-absorbed with an extract of Reiter treponemes to remove group-reactive antibody. TPHA reactivity may be detectable around the 4th week of infection. It is less sensitive than FTA-ABS in primary syphilis being positive in 65% of cases, but both give similar results for secondary and late syphilis. After treatment, TPHA invariably remains positive for life. **This test can also be used to detect localised production of anti-treponemal antibodies in cerebrospinal fluid, a marker of neurosyphilis.**

TPHA is very simple to perform, therefore, it was the first of the specific tests suitable for routine screening. Because of greater convenience and lower cost, TPHA may be performed in microtitre plates. This is referred to as **microtitre haemagglutination-*T. pallidum* (MHA-TP) test**. Both these terms are used synonymously. Combination of a cardiolipin antigen test and TPHA is the most widely used screening procedure.

Enzyme immunoassay (EIA)

Ultrasonicate of *T. pallidum* antigen is coated on tubes or ferrous metal beads as a solid-phase carrier for antigen. Antibody in the patient serum is detected by enzyme immunoassay. Sensitivity and specificity of this test has been reported to be 90% and 98% respectively.

Q. 4. What is the characteristic of relapsing fever. Name causative agents and describe morphology, cultural characteristics, pathogenicity, laboratory diagnosis, and prevention and treatment of relapsing fever.

Ans. Relapsing fever is characterized by the occurrence of one or more relapses after the subsidence of primary febrile paroxysm. It occurs worldwide as epidemic or louse-borne relapsing fever, and endemic or tick-borne relapsing fever. The former is caused by *B. recurrentis* and the latter by several *Borrelia* species, including, *B. duttoni*, *B. hermsii*, *B. parkeri* and *B. turicatae*.

Morphology

Various *Borrelia* species causing relapsing fever are morphologically indistinguishable, but exhibit some antigenic differences. They are 8–20 µm long and 0.2–0.5 µm wide. They possess 15–20 endoflagella per cell end and 3–10 loose, uneven spiral coils. Spirals are coarser and more irregular than those of the treponemes or leptospires and can usually be seen with light microscopy in preparations stained with aniline dyes such as Wright or Giemsa stains. The spirochaetes may be demonstrated in the peripheral blood by direct stain. In fresh blood the organisms are actively motile, they move in forward and backward waves and in a corkscrew-like motion.

Cultural characteristics

Borrelia are microaerophilic. Optimum temperature for growth is 28–30°C. These may be grown in fluid media containing blood, serum or tissue, and on chorioallantoic membrane of chick embryo.

Pathogenicity

Relapsing fever is transmitted by infected vectors – body louse (*Pediculus corporis*) in case of *B. recurrentis*, and tick (*Ornithodoros*) in case of *B. duttoni* and others. After an infected blood meal, spirochaetes may be demonstrated in the stomach of the louse for 24 hours. Thereafter, they grow in the haemolymph of the louse but do not invade tissues. They are not found in the salivary glands, the gut or the genital organs. As a result, the excrement of the louse is non-infectious and the **bacterium is not transferred transovarially to the progeny**. However, once the louse is infected, it remains so for the rest of its life (usually about 3 weeks).

The disease is transmitted to man not by the bite of the louse, but by contamination of the wounds made by the bite itself or by scratching, with body fluids of the louse which is crushed by scratching releasing spirochaetes. The latter then enter into the tissues through damaged or intact skin or mucous membranes.

Spirochaetes causing tick-borne relapsing fever invade all the tissues of the tick, including the salivary glands, genitalia and excretory system. Infection is transmitted to man through the bite of the ticks or through their excrements. **Transovarial transmission** to the tick progeny maintains the spirochaete in the tick population.

In both forms of relapsing fever, after an incubation period of 2–14 days, the disease sets in abruptly with high fever (up to 40°C), rigors, headache, myalgia, arthralgia, photophobia and sometimes nausea and vomiting. The spleen and liver are enlarged and tender. Some patients develop jaundice, bronchitis and skin rash. During acute phase, there may be up to 10^5 spirochaetes per ml of blood. The primary illness subsides in 3–9 days. After an afebrile period of 11–15 days during which borreliae are not demonstrable in blood, a **relapse** follows which is less severe and shorter than the primary attack. The borreliae reappear in blood during the relapse of fever. The disease ultimately subsides after 3–4 relapses. In general, tick-borne relapsing fever has shorter febrile and afebrile periods than louse-borne infection.

Each episode of spirochaetaemia is terminated as a result of development of specific antibodies. The borreliae readily undergo **antigenic variation**, particularly in outer membrane protein composition, *in vivo* and this is believed to be the reason for the occurrence of relapses in the disease. As relapses continue, the borreliae tend to revert back to the antigenic types that caused the original spirochaetaemia thus clearing the infection.

Laboratory diagnosis

Wet preparation

Blood is collected during pyrexial period and a drop of it is examined as a wet film under the dark-ground or phase-contrast microscope. Borreliae can be detected by their active movements.

Staining

Thick or thin blood smears may be stained with Giemsa or Leishman stain and examined for *Borrelia*.

Animal inoculation

If direct microscopy is negative, 1–2 ml of fresh whole blood or of clot ground up in saline, is injected intraperitoneally into a newborn mouse or rat. The borreliae multiply in the animal and appear in large numbers in peripheral blood within two days. Smears are prepared from blood collected from the tail vein and examined daily for two weeks. The degree of spirochaetaemia in adult animals is much less and may not be detected for several days.

Serology

Because of the occurrence of frequent antigenic variation, serological diagnosis of relapsing fever is unreliable. Serological tests for syphilis are positive in 5–10% of cases of relapsing fever.

Prevention and treatment

Since the organisms are transmitted only by vectors, therefore, tick and louse control, and maintenance of good personal hygiene are effective measures for the control of relapsing fever. Tetracycline, chloramphenicol, penicillin and erythromycin have been used successfully for the treatment of relapsing fever. As in the treatment of syphilis, elimination of spirochaetes from the blood may result in a severe **Jarisch-Herxheimer type reaction** which is occasionally fatal.

Q. 5. Write short note on Vincent's angina.

Ans. *Borrelia vincentii* is 7–18 μm long and 0.2–0.6 μm wide, with 3–8 loose, open coils of variable size. It is actively motile. It is easily stained with dilute carbol fuchsin, methyl violet, Giemsa and Leishman stains and is Gram-negative. It is an obligate anaerobe and can be cultured in sealed tubes containing digest broth enriched with ascitic fluid. *B. vincentii* is a normal commensal of mouth but may, under predisposing conditions such as malnutrition or viral infections, give rise to **ulcerative gingivostomatitis** or **oropharyngitis (Vincent's angina)**.

In Vincent's angina, *B. vincentii* is often associated with 'fusiform bacillus' known as *Leptotrichia buccalis* (*Fusobacterium fusiforme*). This symbiotic infection is known as **fusospirochaetosis**. Vincent's angina is characterized by ulcerative lesions of mouth or tonsillar area.

For the diagnosis, smears are made from the ulcerative lesions and are stained with dilute carbol fuchsin. A clinical diagnosis of Vincent's angina is confirmed when a large number of spirochaetes and fusiform bacilli are seen together with many pus cells.

Q. 6. Name the causative agent of Lyme disease. Describe briefly morphology, cultural characteristics, pathogenicity, laboratory diagnosis and treatment of Lyme disease.

Ans. Lyme disease is caused by *Borrelia burgdorferi*. It was first identified in 1975 in Lyme, Connecticut, USA.

Morphology

It measures 4–30 μm in length and 0.2 μm in diameter. It is flexible, helical and Gram-negative.

Cultural characteristics

It is a microaerophilic spirochaete. It can be grown on BSK medium which contains N-acetyl glucosamine, yeast extract, amino acids, vitamins, nucleotides and serum. Optimum temperature for growth is 34–37°C.

Pathogenicity

B. burgdorferi causes **Lyme disease**. It is widespread in the USA, where it is most common vector-borne infection. It has been reported from other parts of the world also. Wild and domestic animals, including mice and other rodents, deer, sheep, cattle, horses and dogs are the natural hosts of *B. burgdorferi*. It is transmitted to man by ixodid ticks that become infected whilst feeding on infected animals. The organisms grow in the midgut of the tick and transmission to man occurs by regurgitation of the gut contents during the blood meal.

Patient develops a small red macule or papule at the site of bite. Three to 22 days later, redness spreads centrifugally surrounded by an induration about 2 cm wide. It is known as **erythema chronicum migrans (ECM)**. The centre of the lesion may become vesicular or necrotic. Commonly affected sites are the thigh, groin and axilla. The organism also spreads to a variety of other organs. In about one-half of the patients, multiple skin lesions develop several days after the appearance of the initial lesion. ECM is frequently accompanied with headache, fever, stiff neck, malaise and lymphadenopathy. Weeks to months later, some patients develop meningoencephalitis, myocarditis or migratory musculoskeletal pain and intermittent arthritis.

Laboratory diagnosis

The diagnosis of Lyme disease is made mainly on clinical grounds. The presence of an ECM lesion at the site of vector bite, which was followed by an expanding bright red rash would be suggestive of a positive diagnosis. However, a definitive diagnosis can be made by the isolation and identification of *B. burgdorferi* from skin lesions or blood of the infected patient. However, the culture is too slow and gives too low a yield of positive results for routine use. Microscopic detection of borreliae by dark-ground microscopy, phase-contrast microscopy, silver staining and immunofluorescence methods also lacks sensitivity. DNA probes have been developed for a gene encoding a specific outer membrane protein, however, their efficiency in detecting this in tissue samples is yet to be established.

For the **serological diagnosis**, ELISA, indirect immunofluorescence and haemagglutination tests are commonly used. However, these tests lack specificity and may give positive results in cases of relapsing fever, syphilis, yaws, pinta, leptospiral infections and collagen disorders. Lyme disease patients may give a positive FTA-ABS test, though the VDRL test is negative.

Treatment

Doxycycline, amoxycillin and cefuroxime are useful for the treatment of Lyme disease. **Jarisch-Herxheimer reactions** occur in 15% of patients following antibiotic therapy.

Q. 7. Describe morphology, cultural characteristics, pathogenicity and laboratory diagnosis of *Leptospira interrogans*.

Ans. ***Morphology***

L. interrogans are spiral bacteria, 6–20 μm long and 0.1 μm in diameter. They are actively motile and possess tightly coiled spirals and hooked ends. Because of their narrow diameter, leptospires are best observed by dark-ground, phase-contrast and electron microscopy. Leptospires rotate rapidly along their long axes and also glide across the field with either end foremost. They occasionally form secondary coils and then straighten again. They stain poorly with aniline dyes but can be demonstrated by fluorescent antibody technique, and silver impregnation techniques of Levaditi and Fontana. They possess Gram-negative cell envelope.

Cultural characteristics

L. interrogans are obligate aerobes. Optimum pH and temperature for their growth are 7.2 and 28–32°C respectively. They do not grow at 13°C and for primary isolation from infected tissues, incubation at 37°C may be advantageous. *L. interrogans* can be grown in artificial media supplemented with sterile rabbit serum or bovine serum albumin with Tween 80. A semisolid medium prepared by adding 0.2–0.5% agar to liquid medium may be used for isolation of *L. interrogans* from animal tissues. Leptospires may be grown on the chorioallantoic membrane of chick embryo. They may be demonstrated in the blood of allantoic vessels 4–5 days after inoculation.

Pathogenicity

L. interrogans causes leptospirosis. It is primarily a parasite of vertebrates other than humans, such as rodents, dogs, pigs and cattle. Leptospires localize in the kidneys, colonizing the convoluted tubules and are continuously shed in the urine of some infected animals, thereby contaminating the environment. Each serovar of *L. interrogans* appears to have its own particular animal host, for example, serovar *icterohaemorrhagiae* is normally carried by the brown rat (*Rattus norvegicus*), serovar *hebdomadis* by field mouse (*Microtus montebelloi*), serovar *canicola* by dog, serovar *pomona* by pig, serovar *hardjo* by cattle and serovars *autumnalis* and *grippotyphosa* by mice but cross-infections do occur. Most reservoir hosts remain healthy carriers.

Leptospirosis in man may be caused by any of the serovars of *Leptospira*. Man acquires infection mainly through contact with water, soil or vegetation contaminated with animal urine. The pathogenic leptospires enter the body through cuts or abrasions of the skin. They may also enter through the mucous membranes of the nose, mouth or eyes. The organisms enter the blood and invade various tissues and organs, particularly the kidney, liver, meninges and conjunctiva.

After an incubation period of 1–2 weeks, the patient develops muscular pain, headache, vomiting, photophobia, fever and chills. Jaundice occurs in about 10–20% of cases by second or third day. Purpuric haemorrhages sometimes occur on the skin and mucosa. Albuminuria is a constant feature. Leptospires can be seen in the blood during acute phase of the disease, but can seldom be demonstrated after 8–10 days. However, they persist in internal organs, particularly in the kidneys so that they may be demonstrated in the urine in the later stages of the disease.

L. interrogans serovar *icterohaemorrhagiae* produces a more severe illness. It is known as **Weil's disease** (infectious jaundice). It has a fatality rate of 25% due to renal failure and hepatic injury. Other serovars, e.g., *australis*, *bataviae* and *pyrogenes* may also cause spirochaetal jaundice.

Laboratory diagnosis

Because of the variability of signs and symptoms, leptospirosis must be considered as a possible cause of pyrexia of uncertain origin (PUO), particularly in those patients who may have been exposed to various animal hosts or have been swimming in water contaminated with animal urine. The diagnosis of leptospirosis may be established by (I) demonstration of leptospires and (II) serological diagnosis.

I. Demonstration of leptospires

Leptospires may be demonstrated in (1) the blood, and (2) the urine.

1. **Demonstration of leptospires in the blood:**
   - Leptospires can be demonstrated in the blood, by dark-ground microscopy, especially after differential centrifugation of blood. As leptospires disappear from blood after 8 days, therefore, blood examination is useful only in the early stages of the disease.
   - Inoculate a number of bijou bottles containing 3 ml of modified Korthof's medium with varying amounts of blood ranging from 1–4 drops. Incubate at 28–32°C and examine by dark-ground microscopy every 3 days up to 6 weeks before discarding it as negative. The blood from the patient is also inoculated intraperitoneally into young guinea-pigs, followed some days later by culture of the animal blood obtained by cardiac puncture.
2. **Demonstration of leptospires in the urine:** Leptospires may be present in the urine in the second week of the disease and intermittently thereafter for 4–6 weeks.
   - Centrifuged deposit of fresh urine may be examined by dark-ground microscopy and by culture on Fletcher's semisolid medium containing neomycin sulphate. Because leptospires are very sensitive to acid urine, therefore, the urine should be examined immediately after voiding.
   - For culture of urine by animal inoculation, 2 ml of fresh urine is inoculated intraperitoneally into young guinea-pigs, followed some days later by culture of the animal blood. The identification of serovar of the isolate is carried out by agglutination and agglutination absorption technique.

II. Serological diagnosis

Antibodies appear in the serum towards the end of the first week of the disease, they continue to rise for several weeks and then begin to decline. Serological tests fall into two categories:

1. Genus-specific tests.
2. Serogroup and serovar-specific tests.

1. **Genus-specific tests:** These tests detect leptospiral infection without indicating the exact infecting serovar. The antigens for these tests are prepared from nonpathogenic *L. biflexa* Patoc 1 strain. These tests include complement fixation test, sensitized erythrocyte lysis and haemagglutination test, and enzyme-linked immunosorbent assay (ELISA) which is capable of detecting IgM and IgG leptospiral antibodies.
2. **Serogroup and serovar-specific tests:** These tests identify the infecting serovar by demonstrating specific antibodies. Macroscopic and microscopic agglutination tests have been widely used.
   - In the **macroscopic agglutination test**, commercially available, formalin-killed suspensions of a number of reference strains are tested for macroscopic agglutination with serial dilutions of the test serum.
   - In the **microscopic agglutination test**, formalinized or live suspensions of well grown cultures are used and the results are read by low-power dark-ground microscopy.

29

ESCHERICHIA, KLEBSIELLA AND PROTEUS

Q. 1. Describe morphology, cultural characteristics, biochemical reactions, antigenic structure and antigenic typing of *Escherichia coli*.

Ans. ***Morphology***

It is a Gram-negative, non-sporing bacillus measuring 1–3 μm × 0.4–0.7 μm in size. Most (about 80%) strains are motile by peritrichous flagella. The fimbriae are present on 80% of the strains. A few strains, especially those from extra-intestinal infections, possess polysaccharide capsule.

Cultural characteristics

It is an aerobe and a facultative anaerobe. Optimum temperature for its growth is 37°C (range 10–40°C). It can grow on ordinary media like **nutrient agar** forming large (2–3 mm in diameter), circular, low convex, colourless, opaque or partially translucent colonies after 18 hours incubation at 37°C. Since most strains ferment lactose rapidly the colonies on **MacConkey agar** medium are red or pink in colour (Fig. 29.1). On **deoxycholate citrate agar** (DCA), the growth is partially or totally inhibited by sodium citrate and sodium thiosulphate. Colonies that form are small, pink and opaque.

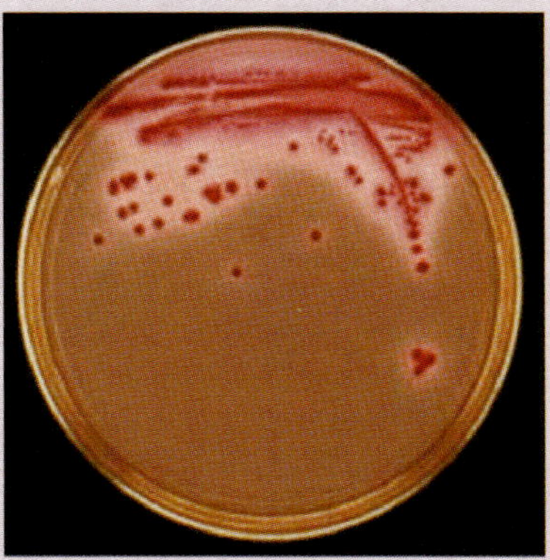

Fig. 29.1. Growth of *Escherichia coli* on MacConkey agar showing lactose fermenting colonies.

On **blood agar**, colonies of some strains of *E. coli* (especially those isolated from pathologic conditions) are surrounded by a complete zone of haemolysis. *E. coli* is not inhibited by bile salt in MacConkey medium, but is inhibited by sodium selenite, sodium tetrathionate and brilliant green in media (selenite broth, tetrathionate broth and brilliant green tetrathionate broth respectively) selective for salmonellae and shigellae. It is also inhibited by 7% sodium chloride in salt media used for isolation of staphylococci.

Biochemical reactions

E. coli is indole and methyl red (MR) reaction positive and it is negative for Voges-Proskauer (VP) reaction, citrate utilization, phenylalanine deaminase test, urease test, H_2S production, gelatin liquefaction, growth in the presence of potassium cyanide and malonate utilization. It ferments glucose, mannitol, maltose, lactose, sucrose and many other sugars with the production of acid and gas. Some strains of *E. coli* are late lactose or non-lactose-fermenters. Indole production and fermentation of sugars takes place both at 37°C and 44°C.

Antigenic structure

E. coli possesses 4 types of antigens:

1. H (flageller) antigens
2. O (somatic) antigens
3. K (capsular) antigens
4. F (fimbrial) antigens.

1. **H antigens:** So far **75 H antigens** have been recognized. These are thermolabile.
2. **O antigens:** These are heat-stable, lipopolysaccharide antigens of cell wall. **One hundred and seventy three different O antigens** have been described which are designated 1, 2, 3, 4, etc.
3. **K antigens:** This term was first used collectively for the surface or capsular antigens that cause O inagglutinability. **One hundred and three K antigens** of *E. coli* are known. K antigens act as virulence factor by protecting bacilli from the killing action of antibody and complement and also by inhibiting phagocytosis.
4. **F antigens:** These are thermolabile proteins and heating the organisms at 100°C detaches their fimbriae. *E. coli* possesses common fimbriae which are chromosomally determined, and sex pili which are determined by conjugative plasmids and appear to be organelles of conjugation.

A number of filamentous protein structures resembling fimbriae have been described in *E. coli*. These cause mannose-resistant haemagglutination. They probably play a significant role in the pathogenesis of diarrhoeal disease and in urinary tract infection. These include K88, K99 and colonization factor antigens (CFAs). K88 and K99 are heat-labile proteins and were originally placed in K antigens. By electron microscopy, they can be seen as filaments resembling fimbriae on the bacterial surface. They are encoded by transmissible plasmids. K88 causes enteritis in pigs and K99 causes enteritis in calves and lambs. CFAs are similar to K88 and K99 antigens and are also plasmid-determined. They are found in some enterotoxigenic strains that cause human diarrhoea. Till now, 4 CFAs designated as CFA I, CFA II, CFA III and CFA IV have been described. They can be detected by serological tests (agglutination and immunodiffusion) with specific antisera.

Antigenic typing

On the basis of O antigens, *E. coli* is subdivided into a number of O groups. Each O group is then divided into subgroups on the basis of K antigens. Each of these subgroups includes strains with different H antigens. Thus a strain of *E. coli* is recorded as O111:K58:H12.

Q. 2. Describe briefly toxins and haemolysin produced by *Escherichia coli.*

Ans. ***Toxins***

Some strains of *E. coli* produce enterotoxins, Verocytotoxin and haemolysin.

1. Enterotoxins

Enterotoxigenic strains of *E. coli* (ETEC) produce one or both of two different toxins, a heat-labile toxin (LT) and a heat-stable toxin (ST). Production of both LT and ST is under the genetic control of transmissible plasmids called *ent* plasmids.

(a) **Heat-labile toxin**

It is a heat-labile protein which is destroyed by heating at 65°C for 30 minutes. It is composed of one enzymatically active polypeptide A (active) subunit and five identical B (binding) subunits. The molecular weight of A subunit is 25,000 daltons and that of each B subunit is 11,500 daltons.

The B subunits of LT bind to the Gm_1 ganglioside at the brush border of epithelial cells of the small intestine. This binding facilitates the entry of subunit A into the cell, which then activates **adenylate cyclase**. This results in conversion of adenosine triphosphate (ATP) to cyclic adenosine monophosphate (cAMP). The accumulation of cAMP in the intestinal mucosa initiates the hypersecretion of electrolytes and fluids into the lumen, resulting in a watery diarrhoea.

Various strains of *E. coli* produce two types of LT toxin – LT-I and LT-II. LT-I is structurally and antigenically related to enterotoxin produced by *Vibrio cholerae* (CT). Anti-CT can neutralize LT-I. LT-II is biologically similar to LT-I, but it is not neutralized by either anti-LT-I or anti-CT. LT can be assayed by ligated rabbit ileal loop (read at 18 hours), adult rabbit skin (vascular permeability factor), steroid production in Y1 mouse adrenal cell culture, elongation of Chinese hamster ovary cells, agar gel diffusion, reversed passive latex agglutination, enzyme-linked immunosorbent assay, solid phase radioimmunoassay and DNA probes (Table 29.1).

Table 29.1. Differences between heat-labile (LT) and heat-stable (ST) enterotoxins of *Escherichia coli*

Test	LT	ST
In vivo tests		
• Ligated rabbit ileal loop		
Read at 6 hours	±	+
Read at 18 hours	+	–
• Adult rabbit skin (vascular permeability factor)	+	–
• Intragastric into 1–4 day old suckling mouse after 4 hours	–	+
In vitro tests		
• Steroid production in Y1 mouse adrenal cell culture	+	–
• Elongation of Chinese hamster ovary cells	+	–
• Agar gel diffusion	+	–
• Reversed passive latex agglutination	+	–
• Enzyme-linked immunosorbent assay	+	+*
• Solid phase radioimmunoassay	+	–
• DNA probes	+	+

* With monoclonal antibodies

(b) **Heat-stable toxin**

In contrast to LT, ST is a low molecular weight polypeptide and poorly immunogenic. Two major classes of *E. coli* ST are known. They are known as ST-I and ST-II. ST-I is not destroyed by heating at 100°C for 30 minutes. It activates **guanylate cyclase** causing the increased production of cyclic guanosine monophosphate (cGMP) and subsequent hypersecretion. ST-I has no effect on the concentration of cAMP. It can be assayed by injecting the toxin intragastrically into a 1–4 day old suckling mouse and measuring intestinal fluid accumulation (ratio of intestinal/remaining body weight) after 4 hours. It can also be assayed by ligated rabbit ileal loop (read at 6 hours). ST-I stimulates guanylate cyclase only in intestinal cells, indicating that such cells possess a unique receptor for ST-I. The activity of ST-I is rapid, whereas LT acts after a lag period.

ST-II is produced by some strains of *E. coli*. It stimulates fluid accumulation in ligated intestinal loops of piglets ranging in age from a few days to 9 weeks but not in infant mouse test. Unlike ST-I, ST-II is insoluble in methanol. The mechanism of action of ST-II is not known but it appears not to act via cAMP or cGMP.

The enterotoxin alone is not sufficient to cause diarrhoea. It must also be able to adhere to the mucosal surface of the epithelial cells of the small intestine. In humans, it is mediated by colonization factors.

2. Verocytotoxin

E. coli O157:H7 produces two cytotoxins – Verocytotoxin 1 (VT1) and Verocytotoxin 2 (VT2). VT1 is a phage encoded cytotoxin identical to the Shiga toxin (Stx) produced by *S. dysenteriae* type 1. This Verocytotoxin is cytotoxic to Vero cells (African green monkey kidney cells), hence the term Verocytotoxin. It also reacts with and is neutralized by the antibody against Shiga toxin. In contrast with VT1, VT2 is not neutralized by the antibody to Shiga toxin and is immunologically different from but biologically similar to VT1. These Verocytotoxins have also been called Shiga-like toxins but are more recently referred to as Shiga toxin 1 (Stx 1) and Shiga toxin 2 (Stx 2). *E. coli* strains that produce these toxins are known as Shiga toxigenic *E. coli* (STEC) or Verocytotoxigenic *E. coli* (VTEC). These can be detected by their cytotoxic effect on Vero and HeLa cells.

3. Haemolysin

Many strains of *E. coli* produce a haemolysin which can bring about lysis of RBCs of some species. A larger proportion of strains of *E. coli* recovered from extra-intestinal lesions of man are haemolytic than are those isolated from human faeces. In experimental animals, haemolytic strains have been found to be more virulent than non-haemolytic ones. It is likely that haemolytic strains of *E. coli* obtain iron from the lysed erythrocytes of the host.

Q. 3. Describe pathogenicity of *Escherichia coli.*

Ans. ***Pathogenicity***

E. coli forms a part of normal intestinal flora of man and animals. It can cause four main types of clinical syndrome:

1. Urinary tract infection.
2. Diarrhoea and dysentery.
3. Pyogenic infections.
4. Septicaemia.

1. Urinary tract infection

E. coli is the commonest organism causing urinary tract infection (UTI). Most frequently encountered O serotypes of *E. coli* in UTI include O1, O2, O4, O6, O7, O18 and O75. These are also known as nephritogenic strains. Special nephropathogenic potential of these strains appears to be due to:

(a) The polysaccharides of the O and K antigens protect the organism from the bactericidal effect of complement and phagocytes in the absence of specific antibodies. Strains possessing K1 or K5 antigen appear to be more virulent than those with other K antigens.
(b) Fimbriae present on the surface of *E. coli* mediate the adherence of the organism to the uroepithelial cells.

E. coli that causes UTI often originate in the gut of the patient. The bacteria may gain access to the urinary tract by the ascending or the haematogenous route. The ascending route of infection is believed to be usual one. The bacteria from the faecal flora spread to the perineum and from there they ascend into the bladder.

UTI occurs more often in females than in males. This is due to short urethra, pregnancy, infrequent voiding and sexual intercourse which may lead to **'honey-moon' cystitis**. Shorter and wider female urethra appears to be less effective in preventing access of the bacteria to the bladder. The high incidence of UTI in pregnant women can be attributed to impairment of urine flow due to pressure on the urinary tract and due to hormonal changes.

Relative infrequency of UTI in men may be due to longer male urethra and the bactericidal activity of the prostatic fluid. Causes of urinary stagnation that may predispose to UTI include enlarged prostate, urinary calculi, congenital malformations and neurological disorders. Catheterization and cystoscopy may introduce endogenous or exogenous bacteria into the bladder leading to infection.

Urinary tract infection may be defined as the presence of bacteria undergoing multiplication in urine within the urinary drainage system. Kass (1956) gave a criterion of active bacterial infection of urinary tract according to which **a count exceeding 10^5 organisms/ml denotes significant bacteriuria** and **indicates active UTI**. Contamination accounts for less than 10^4 organisms/ml and usually less than 10^3/ml. Moreover, UTI is generally caused by one species, while contaminants are generally of mixed species. **This count is, however, not applicable to tuberculosis of urinary tract because of slow rate of multiplication of mycobacteria.** Bacterial counts in urine are, however, influenced by various factors. These include a high fluid intake, use of alkalinizing or acidifying agents and inadequate chemotherapy. Therefore, a low bacterial count should be considered significant in patients with symptoms and pyuria.

2. Diarrhoea and dysentery

E. coli causing diarrhoeal diseases are divisible into six groups. They produce diarrhoea with different pathogenic mechanisms.

- ***Enteropathogenic E. coli (EPEC):*** *It is second most common cause of infantile diarrhoea after rotavirus.* It causes prolonged watery diarrhoea in babies < 1 year in developing countries. The pathogenic mechanism is not clear, however, the inflammatory reactions and epithelial degenerative changes that are observed in tissue sections may be secondary to adhesive properties of the bacteria. Common serogroups of EPEC are O26, O55, O86, O111, O114, O119, O125, O126, O127, O128 and O142.

- ***Enterotoxigenic E. coli (ETEC):*** These strains are associated with diarrhoea in infants and adults in tropical and subtropical climates, especially in developing countries, where it is one of the major causes of infantile bacterial diarrhoea. In the United States and other developed countries, ETEC diarrhoea is the most common cause of diarrhoeal disease referred to as **traveller's diarrhoea**. The diarrhoeal illness is acquired by travellers from developed countries when they visit developing countries.

  ETEC infection is commonly acquired by consuming contaminated food or water. In addition, they possess colonization factors that are specific for the host animal species. These enable the organisms to adhere to the epithelium of the small intestine. Surface attachment of the bacterial cells to the intestinal epithelial cells is a prerequisite to toxin production. Common serogroups of ETEC are O6, O8, O15, O25, O27, O63, O78, O115, O148, O153, O159 and O167.
- ***Enteroinvasive E. coli (EIEC):*** These strains invade large bowel, similar to shigellosis. It causes watery diarrhoea with excess of leucocytes, fever and abdominal pain. About 10% patients progress to dysentery. Common serogroups of EIEC are O28, O112, O124, O136, O143, O144, O152 and O164.
- ***Verocytotoxigenic E. coli (VTEC):*** In 1982, one particular serovar of *E. coli* (O157:H7) was identified as the causative agent involved in two outbreaks of a distinctive **bloody diarrhoeal syndrome**. Soon after it was recognized that some strains of other *E. coli* serovars may exhibit a similar virulence potential. The ability to cause haemorrhagic colitis has led some workers to refer to these strains as **enterohaemorrhagic *E. coli* or EHEC**.

  These strains cause **haemorrhagic colitis (HC)** and **haemolytic uraemic syndrome (HUS)**. In HC, patient develops blood-stained diarrhoea. Fever is generally absent, distinguishing it from shigellosis. It may often be preceded by abdominal pain and watery diarrhoea. HUS is characterized by acute renal failure, microangiopathic haemolytic anaemia and thrombocytopenia. It occurs in all age groups but is most common in infants and young children. It is a major cause of renal failure in childhood.
- ***Enteroaggregative E. coli (EAEC):*** Enteroaggregative *E. coli* cause acute and chronic diarrhoea in developing countries by adhering to the mucosal surface of the intestine. These strains are found to adhere to HEp-2 cells, packed in an aggregative pattern on the cells and in between the cells. These organisms produce symptoms such as watery diarrhoea, vomiting, dehydration, low-grade fever and occasionally abdominal pain. These symptoms persist for more than 2 weeks.
- ***Diffusely adherent E. coli (DAEC):*** These strains adhere to epithelial cells in a diffuse pattern and carry a gene encoding surface fimbria designated F1845. Majority of the patients with DAEC develop watery diarrhoea without blood or faecal leucocytes.

3. Pyogenic infections

E. coli may cause wound infection, peritonitis, biliary tract infection, and meningitis. *E. coli* is a common cause of meningitis in the newborn, but is much less so in older patients.

4. Septicaemia

E. coli is a very common cause of septicaemia in many hospitals. It leads to fever, hypotension and disseminated intravascular coagulation (**endotoxic shock**) with high mortality. This condition usually develops in debilitated patients.

Q. 4. Describe laboratory diagnosis of *Escherichia coli* infections.

Ans. Urinary tract infection

Collection of specimen

Normal urine is sterile, but during voiding may become contaminated with genital commensals. In order to avoid such contamination, urine used to be collected by catheterization for culture. Catheterization for this purpose is no longer considered justifiable because it carries a 2–6% risk of introducing and initiating infection. Therefore, **clean-voided midstream sample** of urine is employed for culture. The normal flora of anterior urethra must be adequately flushed out by passing some urine before the specimen is obtained.

- **In newborn infants and young children**, urine may be aspirated from the bladder into a syringe with a needle introduced aseptically through the abdominal wall just above the pubis.

Urine is an excellent culture medium, therefore, contaminating bacteria, from the anterior urethra, can readily multiply to reach significant numbers. Therefore, the urine must be processed immediately. If a delay of more than 1–2 hours is unavoidable, the specimen should be stored in a refrigerator at 4°C for upto 24 hours.

Microscopy

Microscopic examination of urine is done to detect the presence of increased number of polymorphs (pyuria) which is an indication of UTI. The deposit of the centrifuged urine can be examined under microscope to find out the presence of pus cells, red blood cells and bacteria in it. Presence of more than 3 pus cells per high power field is suggestive of infection. Red blood cells indicate damage to urinary tract hence increased susceptibility to infection.

Pyuria in addition to bacteriuria is an important factor in establishing the presence of urinary tract infection.

Culture

Measured quantity of urine (0.001 ml or 1/1000 ml) with the help of standardized loop of nichrome or platinum wire is inoculated on blood agar and MacConkey media and incubated overnight at 37°C. The number of colonies is counted and multiplied by 1000 to get the bacterial count per ml. For example, growth of 100 colonies indicates the presence of 10^5 bacteria/ml of urine (100×1000). On the basis of this result, it can be reported whether the patient has significant bacteriuria or not. The identification of the isolate is carried out by cultural characteristics and biochemical reactions.

Diarrhoea and dysentery

Faeces or rectal swab is inoculated on MacConkey agar. For detection of EPEC, *E. coli* colonies are emulsified in saline on a slide and tested by agglutination with polyvalent and monovalent O antisera against enteropathogenic serogroups. As more than one serogroup may be present in faecal cultures, it is essential to test at least 10 isolated colonies by agglutination.

EIEC can be detected by **Sereny test** in which the organism is instilled into the conjunctival sac of guinea-pig. The animal is examined after 72 hours for the production of **keratoconjunctivitis**. Simpler tests using HeLa cells or HEp-2 cells have also been described.

Monolayers of these cells are exposed to suspension of test organisms. Extracellular organisms are removed after an appropriate infection period by washing with a solution containing gentamicin and lysozyme. After a further period of intracellular growth, cells are examined microscopically for the presence of intracellular organisms.

Methods of detection of ETEC and VTEC are given in answer to Q. 2.

Pyogenic infections

For the diagnosis of pyogenic infections caused by *E. coli* pus, wound swab, blood, CSF, etc. are inoculated on MacConkey agar and blood agar followed by incubation at 37°C for 24 hours. The isolate is identified by its morphological and biochemical characters.

Septicaemia

Diagnosis of septicaemia caused by *E. coli* depends on the isolation of the organism by blood culture. Five to 10 ml of blood is inoculated into 50–100 ml glucose broth. It is incubated at 37°C for up to 7 days. After overnight incubation, subculture is made on MacConkey agar and blood agar, and processed as above. If no growth is obtained from first subculture, then subcultures should be repeated daily up to 7 days.

Q. 5. Describe morphology, cultural characteristics, biochemical reactions, antigenic structure, methods of typing, pathogenicity and laboratory diagnosis of *Klebsiella*.

Ans. ***Morphology***

Members of the genus *Klebsiella* are Gram-negative, non-sporing, non-motile bacilli, 1–2 µm long and 0.5–0.8 µm wide with parallel or bulging sides and slightly pointed or rounded ends. They occur either in end to end pairs (diplobacilli, like pneumococci) or are arranged singly.

Freshly isolated strains possess a well-defined polysaccharide capsule. It is produced in greater amounts in media rich in carbohydrates. It can be demonstrated by India ink preparation, Quellung reaction and even by Gram staining. In the Gram-stained smear, capsule appears as an empty halo around the bacterium.

The name *K. pneumoniae* is used for the species as a whole. It is further divided into 4 subspecies. The most frequently encountered, biochemically typical form of it is known as *K. pneumoniae* subsp. *aerogenes*. Other subspecies are *ozaenae*, *pneumoniae* and *rhinoscleromatis*. Indole-producing strains that are like *K. pneumoniae* subsp. *aerogenes* in other respects are classified in a separate species, *K. oxytoca*.

Another species, *K. granulomatis*, has been included in the genus *Klebsiella*. This was previously known as *Calymmatobacterium granulomatis*. It causes donovanosis.

Cultural characteristics

Klebsiellae grow well on ordinary media in a temperature range of 12–43°C with optimum growth at 37°C. On MacConkey agar, the colonies typically appear large, mucoid and red. However, some strains are not mucoid.

Biochemical reactions

Biochemical reactions of different subspecies of *K. pneumoniae* and *K. oxytoca* are given in Table 29.2.

Table 29.2. Differentiation of species and subspecies of *Klebsiella*

Property	*K. pneumoniae* subspecies				*K. oxytoca*
	aerogenes	*ozaenae*	*pneumoniae*	*rhinoscleromatis*	
Indole	–	–	–	–	+
MR	–	+	+	+	v
VP	+	–	–	–	v
Citrate	+	v	+	–	+
Urease	+	–	+	–	+
Gelatin liquefaction	–	–	–	–	v
Lactose (acid)	+	+	+	–	+
ONPG	+	+	+	–	+
Lysine decarboxylase	+	v	+	–	+
Ornithine decarboxylase	–	–	–	–	–
Growth in KCN medium	+	+	–	+	+

v, variable.

Antigenic structure

Somatic (O) antigen

Klebsiellae possess five O antigens (O1–O5). O1, O3, O4 and O5 are identical with or related to *E. coli* O antigens 19b, 9, 20 and 8 respectively. In capsulated strains, O antigens are masked by K antigens and because the latter are heat-stable at 100°C for 2.5 hours, therefore, O antigens are identifiable only in non-capsulated mutants.

Capsular (K) antigen

On the basis of capsular (K) antigens, the klebsiellae have been differentiated into 80 (1–80) serotypes, which is usually done by the microscopic demonstration of capsule swelling in wet films with capsular antiserum. Capsular type 2 is immunologically similar to type 2 pneumococcus. Human respiratory tract infection is mostly caused by capsular types 1–6.

Methods of typing

As mentioned above, klebsiellae can be typed by serotyping. Other typing methods such as phage typing, biotyping, bacteriocin (klebocin or pneumocin) typing and resistotyping have also been tried. Bacteriocin (klebocin) production in *Klebsiella* has been found to be determined by conjugative (transmissible) plasmids (Arora and Chugh, 1982).

Pathogenicity

Klebsiellae are widely distributed in nature and in the gastrointestinal tracts of humans and animals. They are found in the oropharynx of 1–6% of normal healthy individuals, however, a prevalence as high as 20% may be seen in hospitalized patients. This colonization may prove to be the source of lung infections such as severe bronchopneumonia, sometimes with chronic destructive lesions, pleuritis and multiple abscess formation in the lungs (**Friedlander's pneumonia**). Many of these patients may develop septicaemia with high mortality.

But klebsiellae, in general, are more frequently involved in hospital-associated (nosocomial) urinary tract infections, wound and burn infections and as secondary invaders in other respiratory infections. In fact, they are the most frequently encountered Gram-negative pathogens causing nosocomial infections of the lower respiratory tract and are second only to *E. coli* as a cause of primary bacteraemia by Gram-negative organisms. They may also cause meningitis and diarrhoea. The latter may be due to the production of heat-labile and heat-stable enterotoxins by these organisms (Arora et al., 1983). The strains responsible for above infections nearly always belong to *K. pneumoniae* subsp. *aerogenes*.

K. pneumoniae subsp. *ozaenae* has been associated with atrophic rhinitis, a condition known as **ozaena**, and purulent infection of nasal mucous membrane. *K. pneumoniae* subsp. *rhinoscleromatis* causes a granulomatous disease called **rhinoscleroma**. It is a chronic upper respiratory tract disease. The lesions occur in the nose, larynx, throat and to a lesser extent, in the trachea and consist of granulomatous infiltrations of the submucosa.

Laboratory diagnosis

Laboratory diagnosis is done by inoculating appropriate specimens on MacConkey agar and blood agar. The isolate is identified by colonial morphology, Gram staining, biochemical reactions and klebocin typing.

Q. 6. Name various species of genus *Proteus*. Describe morphology, cultural characteristics, Dienes phenomenon, biochemical reactions, pathogenicity and laboratory diagnosis of *Proteus*.

Ans. Genus *Proteus* has four species – *P. mirabilis*, *P. vulgaris*, *P. myxofaciens* and *P. penneri*.

Morphology

They are Gram-negative coccobacilli, 1–3 μm long and 0.6 μm wide. In young cultures, most of them are long (up to 80 μm) curved and filamentous. They may be arranged singly, in pairs or in short chains. They are actively motile by peritrichous flagella. However, non-flagellate and non-motile variants are also encountered. They also possess more than one type of fimbriae.

Cultural characteristics

They can grow on ordinary media like nutrient agar and culture emits characteristic putrefactive (fishy or seminal) odour. *P. mirabilis* and *P. vulgaris* possess the **ability to swarm** (spread) on solid media. A group of cells at the edge of a developing microcolony migrate to an uninoculated area of the medium. Swarming growth on a plate may eventually appear either as a uniform film of growth extending over the whole plate (**continuous swarming**) or as a series of concentric circles of growth around the point of inoculation (**discontinuous swarming**). Swarming of *Proteus* appears to be due to vigorous motility of the organism although the exact cause is not yet established. Swarming can be inhibited by:

- Increasing the concentration of agar in the medium from 1–2% to 6%.
- Incorporating chloral hydrate (1 in 500), sodium azide (1 in 500) or boric acid (1 in 100) in the medium. Swarming does not occur on MacConkey agar on which smooth, colourless colonies are formed. Non-motile variants do not swarm.

On **MacConkey agar** they form smooth, pale or colourless (NLF) colonies and do not swarm on this medium.

Dienes phenomenon

When two identical strains of *Proteus* are inoculated at different points of the same culture plate, without any swarming inhibiting substance, the resulting swarms of growth coalesce without signs of demarcation. When, however, two different strains of *Proteus* species are inoculated, the spreading films of growth fail to coalesce and remain separated by a narrow but easily visible furrow. This is known as Dienes phenomenon. **It has been used to determine the identity or non-identity of various strains of *Proteus*.**

Biochemical reactions

All species of *Proteus* produce acid from glucose. Lactose is not fermented. Other biochemical characters of four species of *Proteus* are given in Table 29.3.

Table 29.3. Differentiation of four species of *Proteus* and *Morganella morganii*

Property	*Proteus*				*M. morganii*
	mirabilis	*vulgaris*	*penneri*	*myxofaciens*	
Motility	+	+	+	+	+
Swarming on solid nutrient media	+	+	–	–	–
Indole	–	+	–	–	+
Methyl red	+	+	+	+	+
Voges-Proskauer	v	–	–	+	–
Citrate	v	v	–	v	–
Phenylalanine deaminase test	+	+	+	+	+
Urease	+	+	+	+	+
H_2S	+	+	–	+	–
Gelatin liquefaction	+	+	v	+	–
Lipase production	+	+	v	+	–
Ornithine decarboxylation	+	–	–	–	+
Gas from glucose	+	+	v	+	+
Acid from:					
• Mannose	–	–	–	–	+
• Maltose	–	+	+	+	–
• Xylose	+	+	+	–	–
• Trehalose	+	v	v	+	–

v, variable.

Pathogenicity

The genus *Proteus* is found in soil, water and faecally contaminated materials. *P. mirabilis* is the most important species (70–90%) recovered from humans, particularly as a causative agent of urinary tract and wound infections. **After *Escherichia coli*, *P. mirabilis* is the most**

frequently associated bacterium with urinary tract infection (UTI). It commonly involves young boys and elderly people of both sexes often with diabetes or structural abnormalities of the urinary tract. In the hospital patients, it may lead to UTI following various forms of urological instrumentation. *P. vulgaris* is more commonly recovered from infected sites in immunosuppressed hosts, particularly those receiving prolonged regimens of antibiotics.

UTI caused by *Proteus* tends to be more serious than that caused by *E. coli* and other coliforms, because these organisms are usually confined to the bladder whereas *Proteus* has a predilection for the upper urinary tract. It produces urease which liberates ammonia from urea. Ammonia inactivates complement, damages renal epithelium and makes the urine alkaline. The alkaline conditions lead to the precipitation of phosphates and the formation of calculi in the urinary tract. It may also lead to hyperammonaemic encephalopathy and coma. Occasionally, *Proteus* may cause wound infection, bed sores, osteomyelitis and in neonates it may cause infection of the umbilical stump which often leads to bacteraemia and meningitis. *P. penneri* and *P. myxofaciens* are rarely encountered in clinical laboratory.

Laboratory diagnosis

Specimens

- Clean voided midstream urine sample in case of UTI.
- Pus in case of pyogenic infections.

Collection

Specimens should be collected in sterile containers under aseptic conditions and transported immediately.

Culture

Specimens are inoculated on MacConkey agar or blood agar with 6% agar to inhibit swarming. These are incubated at 37°C for 18–24 hours. On MacConkey agar NLF colonies are seen.

Gram staining

Shows Gram-negative coccobacilli.

Hanging drop preparation

Shows actively motile bacilli.

Biochemical reactions

Proteus spp. are PPA and urease positive, and ferment glucose with the production of acid and gas. Other biochemical reactions can be used to differentiate various species of *Proteus* (Table 29.3).

30

SHIGELLA, SALMONELLA AND YERSINIA

Q. 1. Describe morphology, cultural characteristics, classification, antigenic structure and toxin production of genus *Shigella*.

Ans. ***Morphology***

Shigellae are non-motile, non-flagellate, non-sporing, non-capsulate, Gram-negative bacilli measuring 1–3 × 0.5 μm.

Cultural characteristics

They are aerobes and facultative anaerobes, growing within a temperature range of 10–40°C, with an optimum temperature of 37°C and pH of 7.4. They can grow on ordinary media.

1. On **nutrient agar** or **blood agar**, colonies are 2–3 mm in diameter, circular, convex, smooth, greyish or colourless and translucent. Colonies of *S. sonnei* are slightly larger and more opaque than those of other shigellae.
2. On **MacConkey agar**, colonies are colourless due to the absence of lactose fermentation. However, colonies of *S. sonnei*, a late lactose-fermenter, become pink when incubation is prolonged beyond 24 hours.
3. Colonies of *Shigella* on **deoxycholate citrate agar** (DCA), a selective medium for isolation of shigellae from faeces, are smaller (1–1.5 mm in diameter) and do not form a black centre. On prolonged incubation, colonies of *S. sonnei* form pink papillae due to late lactose fermentation.
4. **Xylose lysine deoxycholate** (XLD) agar is a better selective medium than DCA because it is less inhibitory to *S. dysenteriae* and *S. flexneri* than DCA. On this medium, colonies of *Shigella* are red and unlike those of most salmonellae, without black centres.
5. ***Salmonella-Shigella* (SS) agar** is a highly selective medium for the isolation of *Salmonella* and *Shigella*. The high bile salt concentration and sodium citrate, in this medium,

inhibit all Gram-positive bacteria, coliforms and many other Gram-negative organisms. This medium also contains sodium thiosulphate, a source of sulphur, and ferric citrate. Any bacteria that produce H_2S gas are detected by the black precipitate formed with ferric citrate. Presence of lactose and neutral red, in the medium, indicates lactose fermentation. Any lactose-fermenting colonies that appear are coloured red by the neutral red. Colonies of *Shigella* on this medium are colourless with no blackening, while those of *Salmonella* are colourless with black centres.

Enrichment media

Enrichment media or broths are helpful in the recovery of *Shigella* and *Salmonella*, whose number in the faeces may be as low as 200/gram while that of *E. coli* and other enteric bacilli (normal flora) may be as high as 10^9/gram. Inhibitory chemical substances in the enrichment media maintain the normal flora in a prolonged lag phase, while permitting shigellae and salmonellae to grow, therefore, these are more readily recovered from faecal samples. However, after several hours, the enrichment media no longer suppress the growth of normal flora that will ultimately overgrow the culture.

(a) **Selenite F broth:** Sodium selenite in this enrichment medium inhibits coliform bacilli while permitting salmonellae and many shigellae to grow. Therefore, it is recommended for the isolation of these organisms from faeces.

(b) **Gram-negative (GN) broth:** Because of the relatively low concentration of sodium deoxycholate, GN broth is less inhibitory to *E. coli* and other coliforms. Most strains of *Shigella* grow well. Sodium deoxycholate and sodium citrate inhibit Gram-positive bacteria. This medium also contains 0.1% glucose and 0.2% D-mannitol. The increased concentration of mannitol over glucose limits the growth of *Proteus* species and encourages growth of *Salmonella* and *Shigella* species because both these species, with the exception of *S. dysenteriae*, can ferment mannitol. Enrichment of faecal specimens in GN broth for 4–6 hours and then subculturing on DCA or XLD agar is an optimal technique for recovery of *Shigella* species in suspected cases of bacillary dysentery.

Classification

On the basis of biochemical reactions and serological specificity, shigellae are classified into four groups (A, B, C and D) or species – *S. dysenteriae*, *S. flexneri*, *S. boydii* and *S. sonnei* (Table 30.1). Shigellae are methyl red positive and negative for Voges-Proskauer reaction, citrate and malonate utilization, lysine decarboxylation, urease and H_2S production, gelatin liquefaction, phenylalanine deamination and are unable to grow in the presence of KCN. All the shigellae produce acid from glucose and with the exception of *S. dysenteriae,* from mannitol. *S. dysenteriae* serotype 1, *S. flexneri* serotype 6 and *S. sonnei* are always indole negative. Strains of other serotypes differ in their reactions.

***S. sonnei* is a late lactose-fermenter**, and colonies growing on MacConkey or DCA medium for more than 24 hours develop pink colour. Other three species are non-lactose-fermenters. Only *S. sonnei* forms ornithine decarboxylase. The general finding that enterobacteria produce catalase has important exceptions in *S. dysenteriae* serotype 1 (*S. shigae*) and many strains of *S. dysenteriae* serotypes 3, 4, 6 and 9, *S. flexneri* serotype 4a, and *S. boydii* serotype 13 which are catalase-negative. All strains of *S. sonnei* and a few strains of *S. dysenteriae* (especially serotype 1), and *S. boydii* (especially serotype 5) are ONPG positive.

Table 30.1. Differentiation of *Shigella* species

Species	Acid produced in fermentation of					Indole	Lysine decarboxy-lase	Ornithine decarboxy-lase	Number of sero-types
	Lactose	Sucrose	Mannitol	Dulcitol	Xylose				
S. dysenteriae	–	–	–	–	–	v	–	–	15
S. flexneri	–	–	+	–	–	v	–	–	6 + 2 variants
S. boydii	–	–	+	v	v	v	–	–	19
S. sonnei	–*	–*	+	–	v	–	–	+	2 phases; 26 colicin types

* negative at 24 hours, late positive at 2–8 days; v, variable.

Antigenic structure

All *Shigella* species possess somatic (O) antigens, and certain strains may possess K antigens. *Shigella* K antigens, when present, interfere with the detection of the O antigen during serologic grouping. The K antigen is heat-labile and may be removed by boiling the organism in a cell suspension. On the basis of O antigens, shigellae can be subdivided into serotypes. This is carried out by agglutination tests with absorbed specific antisera.

Group A (*S. dysenteriae*): It is subdivided into 15 serotypes of which serotypes 1 and 2 are also known as Shiga's bacillus (*S. shigae*) and Schmitz's bacillus (*S. schmitzi*) respectively. Each serotype is characterized by a different type antigen.

Group B (*S. flexneri*): Among shigellae, this group is the most complex antigenically. Based on type-specific (I–VI) and group-specific (1–8) antigens, they have been classified into 6 serotypes (1–6) and several subtypes (1a, 1b, 2a, 2b, 3a, 3b, 3c, 4a, 4b, 5a, 5b). In addition, 2 antigenic variants called X and Y are recognized which lack the type-specific antigen (Table 30.2). Serotype 6 is always indole negative and can be subdivided into three biotypes – Boyd 88, Manchester and Newcastle (Table 30.3).

Group C (*S. boydii*): Dysentery bacilli of this group resemble those of *S. flexneri* biochemically but not antigenically. This group is named after Boyd who first described these strains from India (1931).

Table 30.2. Antigens of various serotypes of *Shigella flexneri*

Serotype	Subserotype	Type antigen	Group antigens
1	1a	I	1, 2, 4
	1b	I	1, 2, 4, 6
2	2a	II	1, 3, 4
	2b	II	1, 7, 8
3	3a	III	1, 6, 7, 8
	3b	III	1, 3, 4, 6, 7, 8
	3c	III	1, 6
4	4a	IV	1, 3, 4
	4b	IV	1, 3, 4, 6
5	5a	V	1, 3, 4
	5b	V	1, 7, 8
6		VI	1, 2, 4
X variant		–	1, 7, 8
Y variant		–	1, 3, 4

Nineteen serotypes have been identified in this group. Members of this group have simpler antigenic structures than those of *S. flexneri*. *S. boydii* is isolated least frequently from cases of bacillary dysentery.

Table 30.3. Biotypes of *Shigella flexneri* serotype 6

Biotype	Indole	Fermentation of	
		Glucose	Mannitol
Boyd 88	–	⊥	⊥
Manchester	–	+	+
Newcastle	–	⊥ or +	–

⊥, acid only; +, acid and gas.

Group D (*S. sonnei*): It is antigenically homogeneous. It may, however, undergo an antigenic variation that affects the somatic antigens and has been referred to as phase or form variation. These 2 phases or forms of the culture are known as phase S or form I and phase R or form II. The former gives rise to smooth colonies while the colonies of the latter are larger, flatter and irregular. Cultures often contain a mixture of both forms, but the colonies of one form can be selected by addition of antiserum of the other form to the culture medium because form II variant is antigenically different from form I variant. By using 33 indicator strains, Horak (1980) could divide *S. sonnei* into **26 colicin types**. The ability to produce a particular colicin is a fairly stable character, therefore, the results of colicin typing are of value for epidemiological purposes.

Toxin formation

1. **Endotoxin:** All shigellae release an endotoxin after autolysis. It is thermostable lipopolysaccharide of the cell wall. It has irritating action on the intestinal wall which causes diarrhoea and subsequent ulcers.
2. **Exotoxin:** *S. dysenteriae* serotype 1, in addition to endotoxin, produces a powerful exotoxin. It is a heat-labile protein and acts as **enterotoxin** and **neurotoxin**. As enterotoxin, it acts on the intestinal mucosa causing transudation of fluid in the lumen and as neurotoxin, it damages endothelial cells of small blood vessels of the central nervous system which results in neurological complications like polyneuritis, coma and meningism.
3. **Verocytotoxin:** *S. dysenteriae* serotype 1 produces a potent toxin (shiga toxin) very similar to VT1 expressed by strains of Verocytotoxigenic *E. coli* (VTEC); however, in contrast to VTEC, the genes encoding shiga toxin are located on the chromosome. Shiga toxin is a subunit toxin comprising an A portion and five B subunits. The B subunits bind the toxin to the cells and the A subunit inhibits protein synthesis and causes cell death.

Q. 2. Describe pathogenicity, epidemiology and laboratory diagnosis of *Shigella* species.

Ans. ***Pathogenicity***

Members of the genus *Shigella* produce a serious illness known as **bacillary dysentery**. It is an acute diarrhoeal disease characterized in the more severe infections by the presence of blood and mucus in the stools. Humans appear to be the only natural hosts for shigellae and they become infected by ingestion of contaminated food or water. **The only source of infection is man – cases or carriers. The infective dose is small – 10–100 organisms.** *Shigella*, unlike *Vibrio cholerae* and most *Salmonella* serotypes, is acid-resistant and survives passage through the stomach to reach the intestine.

A patient or a carrier after contaminating his hands while cleansing himself at toilet, touches and contaminates objects like toilet seat, toilet chain, door handles, wash-basin taps, hand towels, etc. and these objects when used by other person may lead to infection. Infection may also spread via flies, fingers, food and faeces. Flies contaminate food mainly by carrying infective material on their feet (mechanical carriage) rather than in their intestines. Faeces of the patient or a carrier may also contaminate water supply.

After reaching the large intestine, the shigellae multiply in the gut lumen. Many bacteria adhere to the epithelial cells of the gut mucosa and induce these cells to ingest them. They then multiply within the epithelial cells and spread laterally into adjacent cells and deep into the lamina propria. Inflammatory reaction develops with capillary thrombosis, leading to necrosis of patches of epithelium, which slough off, leaving behind **superficial ulcers**. The cellular response is mainly by polymorphonuclear leucocytes which can be seen on microscopic examination of stool, together with red cells and sloughed epithelium.

The ulcers of the bacillary dysentery are much shallower than amoebic ulcers. The **intervening mucosa** is **inflamed and oedematous**. Thus, there is diffuse involvement, unlike the amoebic dysentery in which the mucosa in between the ulcerative lesions is healthy. Dysentery bacilli rarely invade other tissues and bacteraemia has been reported in only 2–4% of cases of bacillary dysentery particularly in malnourished children and in AIDS cases.

The incubation period is usually between 2–3 days, but may be as short as 12 hours. In the typical case there is diarrhoea, often bloody, fever, and tenesmus. The severity of disease varies widely. A considerable proportion of patients suffer from a simple diarrhoea, but in most of them there is usually some constitutional disturbance. In severe infections, toxaemia is profound and bacterial endotoxin can often be detected in the blood by means of the *Limulus* test.

The severity of the clinical illness is to some extent associated with the particular species involved. Infection with *S. dysenteriae* is usually associated with a severe illness in which there is a sudden onset of abdominal pain, tenesmus, pyrexia (due to absorption of exotoxins from gut), prostration and sometimes convulsions. The stools loose their usual faecal character, are small and frequent, and are composed mainly of **fresh blood, pus and mucus**. Exotoxin produced by *S. dysenteriae* serotype 1 appears to be much less important in pathogenesis than the ability of the pathogens to adhere, penetrate and multiply. Invasive and non-toxigenic mutants can still cause dysentery while toxigenic and non-invasive cannot do so.

Complications are most often seen in patients with *S. dysenteriae* serotype 1 infection. These include arthritis, toxic neuritis, conjunctivitis, parotitis, intussusception and haemolytic uraemic syndrome (HUS). HUS is characterized by haemolytic anaemia, thrombocytopenia and acute renal failure. It can be caused by many pathogens particularly *E. coli* O157. It is associated with complement activation and disseminated intravascular coagulation.

On the other extreme, the disease caused by *S. sonnei* is of mild type and may be associated with a few loose stools with vague abdominal discomfort. The illness caused by *S. flexneri* and *S. boydii* is more severe than that caused by *S. sonnei* and sometimes may be as severe as that caused by *S. dysenteriae*.

Epidemiology

Bacillary dysentery has a **global distribution**. It is commoner in countries with a warm than a temperate climate and in poor than in affluent countries. It is mostly associated with the overcrowding and bad hygienic conditions encountered in times of war and other disasters, and in jails and mental institutions.

The most prevalent species of *Shigella* in the United States is *S. sonnei* which can survive for many days on lavatory seats, particularly in conditions of low temperature and high humidity. It is transmitted by faecal-oral route and majority of the patients are pre-school age children, particularly those in day-care centres. In India, *S. flexneri* has always been the predominant species (50–85%) followed by *S. dysenteriae* (8–25%), *S. sonnei* (2–24%) and *S. boydii* (0–8%).

Laboratory diagnosis

Specimen

The laboratory diagnosis of bacillary dysentery can be made by the isolation of *Shigella* from faeces. It should be inoculated without delay. If this is impossible, the mucus or faeces should be transported in a buffered 30% glycerol saline solution, which prevents the dysentery bacilli from being destroyed by the acid produced during the growth of other organisms. A direct swab may be taken from the ulcer by sigmoidoscopic examination. Rectal swabs which do not allow adequate macroscopic and microscopic examination of faeces should be avoided.

Direct microscopy

Microscopic examination of the faeces or mucus shows numerous erythrocytes and polymorphonuclear leucocytes and a few macrophages. The latter must be carefully differentiated from vegetative forms of *Entamoeba histolytica* which have relatively smaller nuclei with a central karyosome.

Culture

The mucus or faeces are inoculated on MacConkey agar and DCA. SS agar and XLD medium can also be used. After overnight incubation at 37°C, the plates are inspected for pale (non-lactose-fermenting) colonies on MacConkey agar and DCA, and red and colourless colonies with no blackening on XLD and SS agar, respectively. These are tested for motility and biochemical reactions.

Enrichment media inoculation

Along with the inoculation of plating media, selenite F broth and GN broth (enrichment media) may also be inoculated. Subcultures are made on plating media after 8–12 hours and 4–6 hours respectively and processed as above.

Slide agglutination test

The colonies that give the characteristic reactions should be identified further by slide agglutination with species-specific sera and then with type-specific sera unless the strain is *S. sonnei*.

Q. 3. Describe nomenclature, morphology, cultural characteristics and biochemical reactions of salmonellae.

Ans. ***Nomenclature***

Genus *Salmonella* has been named after American microbiologist, D.E. Salmon. It consists of facultative anaerobic Gram-negative bacilli that parasitise the intestines of a large number of vertebrate species and which infect man, leading to enteric fever, gastroenteritis and septicaemia. Of all the Enterobacteriaceae, the genus *Salmonella* is the most complex, with more than 2,500 serotypes currently, described in Kauffmann-White scheme. According to this scheme, each named serotype was regarded as a separate *Salmonella* species and the convention was adopted that each new serotype should be given the name of the place where it was first isolated.

It is now generally accepted that all salmonellae belong to two species. *S. enterica* and *S. bongori*. There are six subspecies of *S. enterica*, the most important of which is *S. enterica* subsp. *enterica* (subspecies I) which includes the typhoid and paratyphoid bacilli and most other serotypes responsible for causing disease in mammals. Salmonellae are named as, for example, *S. enterica* subsp. *enterica* serotype Enteritidis. For convenience it is usual to abbreviate this to *S.* Enteritidis, or just Enteritidis for use in clinical situations. **Serotype names are capitalized and not in italics.**

Morphology

These are Gram-negative, non-sporing, non-acid-fast, non-capsulated bacilli measuring 1–3 × 0.5 μm. Most strains are motile by means of peritrichous flagella except *S.* Gallinarum and *S.* Pullorum which are non-motile. Non-motile mutants of other serotypes may sometimes be found.

Cultural characteristics

Salmonellae are aerobes and facultative anaerobes, growing within a temperature range of 15–41°C (optimum temperature 37°C). They can grow on ordinary media.

1. On **nutrient agar** or **blood agar**, colonies are 2–3 mm in diameter, greyish-white, circular, moist, convex and translucent. Rough (R) strains form opaque and granular colonies with irregular surface. They have a hydrophobic surface and tend to autoagglutinate.
2. On **MacConkey agar**, after overnight incubation at 37°C, the colonies are 1–3 mm in diameter and pale yellow or colourless due to the absence of lactose fermentation.
3. **Addition of brilliant green (0.004 g/litre) to MacConkey agar** inhibits the growth of *Escherichia coli*, *Proteus* and other commensal enterobacteria and makes it a selective medium for the isolation of salmonellae from faeces. They produce pale green translucent colonies. However, *S.* Typhi does not grow well on this medium.
4. The colonies of *Salmonella* on **deoxycholate citrate agar (DCA)**, a selective medium for isolation of shigellae and salmonellae from faeces, are similar to or slightly smaller in size than those on MacConkey agar. After 48 hours incubation, the colonies may develop a black centre.
5. On **Wilson and Blair's brilliant-green bismuth sulphite agar** medium, *S.* Typhi and *S.* Paratyphi B form small (about 1 mm in diameter) black colonies. This is due to the reduction of sulphite to sulphide. Due to the production of hydrogen sulphide, the colonies of *S.* Typhi are surrounded by a metallic sheen.
6. Most strains of salmonellae produce red colonies with black centres on XLD agar, and on SS agar salmonellae produce colourless colonies with black centres.

Enrichment media

(a) **Tetrathionate broth:** It enriches salmonellae and sometimes shigellae, but permits the growth of *Proteus*. The latter may reduce the tetrathionate, thus impairing the selectivity of this medium for salmonellae.

(b) **Brilliant green tetrathionate broth:** Brilliant green in tetrathionate broth inhibits the growth of *Proteus*, thus makes it more selective for the growth of salmonellae. But it is also inhibitory, to some extent, to *S.* Typhi and shigellae.

(c) **Selenite F broth:** Sodium selenite in this medium inhibits coliform bacilli while permitting salmonellae and many shigellae to grow. It is an excellent enrichment medium for the isolation of *S.* Typhi and *S.* Dublin, but some salmonellae, e.g., *S.* Paratyphi A and *S.* Choleraesuis and some shigellae may fail to grow in this medium.

Biochemical reactions

Salmonellae are indole negative, methyl red reaction positive, Voges-Proskauer negative and citrate positive (except *S.* Typhi and *S.* Paratyphi A which are citrate negative). Salmonellae ferment glucose, mannitol, maltose and sorbitol with the production of acid and gas. *S.* Typhi, *S.* Gallinarum and rare anaerogenic variants in other serotypes, e.g., *S.* Typhimurium form acid only. Salmonellae do not ferment lactose, sucrose, salicin and adonitol.

Q. 4. Describe antigenic structure and antigenic variation of salmonellae.

Ans. ### *Antigenic structure*

Salmonellae possess three main types of antigens (Fig. 30.1) on the basis of which they are serologically typed. These are:

- Flagellar (H) antigens.
- Somatic (O) antigens.
- Vi antigen.

In addition, several strains carry fimbriae. Fimbrial (F) antigens are not important in identification, but may cause confusion due to their nonspecific nature and widespread sharing amongst enterobacteria.

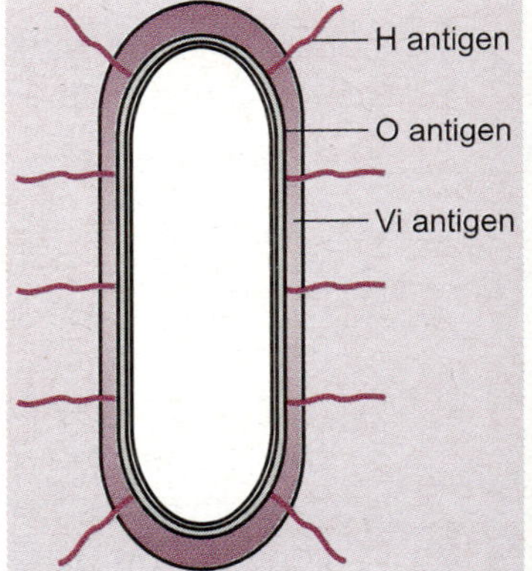

Fig. 30.1. Antigenic structure of salmonellae.

H antigens

These antigens, present on flagella, are heat-labile and alcohol-labile, but are well preserved in 0.04–0.2% formaldehyde. Heating at 100°C for 30 minutes detaches all the flagella. The H antigens of *Salmonella* are not shared by other enterobacteria. When mixed with antisera, H agglutination occurs rapidly, producing large, loose, fluffy clumps. Flagellar antigens occur in two forms called phase 1 and phase 2.

O antigens

The somatic O antigen is phospholipid-protein-polysaccharide complex which forms an integral part of the cell wall. It is identical to endotoxin. They can withstand boiling for 2.5 hours. They are also alcohol-stable, withstanding treatment with 96% ethanol at 37°C for 4 hours. They are hydrophilic and enable the bacteria to form homogeneous suspension in normal saline. When mixed with antisera, O antigen suspensions produce compact, chalky, granular clumps. O antigen is less immunogenic than H antigen. The titre of O antibody in serum after infection or immunisation is generally less than that of H antibody. O agglutination takes place more slowly and at a higher optimum temperature (50–55°C) than H agglutination (37°C). Sixty seven different O antigens have been recognized and they are designated by arabic numerals.

Vi antigen

Almost all recently isolated strains of *S.* Typhi possess surface antigen, known as Vi antigen, enveloping the O antigen. It was originally designated Vi because its presence appeared to determine virulence for mice. It is a heat-labile acidic polysaccharide. It is destroyed by boiling or heating the bacteria at 60°C for one hour. It is also destroyed by treatment with phenol, N hydrochloric acid and 0.5 N sodium hydroxide. It is unaffected by alcohol or 0.2% formaldehyde. It tends to be lost on serial subcultures. When fully expressed, it renders the bacterium inagglutinable by O antiserum but agglutinable by Vi antiserum. Vi antigen with similar antigenic specificity is also present in *S.* Paratyphi C, *S.* Dublin and some strains of *Escherichia* and *Citrobacter*.

The Vi antigen is poorly immunogenic and only low titres of antibody are produced following infection. The antibody disappears early in convalescence. Its persistence indicates the development of carrier state. It has been stated that the total absence of the Vi antibody in a proven case of typhoid fever indicates poor prognosis.

Antigenic variations

Various *Salmonella* antigens undergo phenotypic and genotypic variations:

1. H → O variation

Flagellate salmonellae (H) sometimes give rise to non-flagellate (O) strains. This kind of change is known as H → O variation. When flagellate salmonellae are cultivated on agar containing phenol (1 : 800), flagella are inhibited and O forms are produced. It is a temporary phenotypic change since flagella reappear readily when the strain is subcultured on media without phenol. Salmonellae may rarely lose flagella by mutation resulting in development of stable or irreversible mutant. For example, a stable non-motile mutant of *S.* Typhi is 901-O strain which is widely employed for the preparation of O-agglutinable bacterial suspensions.

Generally, the loss of flagella is not total and only a diminution in the number of flagella occurs. Flagellated cells are found in small numbers in such cultures. To obtain motile bacteria, rich in H antigen from such culture, selection may be carried out by use of Craigie's tube. This consists of a wide tube containing agar (0.2%) in the centre of which is embedded a short, narrow tube open at both ends in such a way that it projects above the agar. The strain is inoculated into the inner tube and after incubation, subcultures are taken from the top of agar outside the central tube. It will yield a population of motile bacteria.

Instead of Craigie's tube a U-tube of soft agar may be employed. Inoculation is made into one limb and subculture is taken from the other end.

2. Phase variation

In most salmonellae, H antigens exist in 2 alternative phases. Phase 1 antigen is either specific for a serotype or shared by a few serotypes only. Hence phase 1 is known as **specific phase**. Phase 2 antigens are widely shared and hence it is known as the '**nonspecific phase**'. A large number of flagellar antigens have been found in phase 1. These are designated by small letters of the alphabet a to z except j and then as z_1–z_{83}.

In phase 2, the bacteria form flagella with different set of H antigens. These antigens are designated by arabic numerals (1–12). The strains that possess both phases are known as **diphasic** and the strains that possess only one phase (e.g., *S.* Typhi, *S.* Paratyphi A, *S.* Enteritidis, etc.) are known as **monophasic**.

A culture contains bacterial cells with flagellar antigens of both phases, but generally one or the other phase predominates so that the culture is agglutinated only by one of the phase antisera. The definitive identification of a diphasic *Salmonella* always requires the identification of the H antigens of both phases. It is, therefore, necessary to obtain a culture in the different phase from that first isolated from the patient. This can be done by the modified Craigie's tube method in which a tube containing semisolid (0.2–0.3%) agar is used. Within the agar, containing monophasic antiserum to the original phase antigens, a small tube which is open at both the ends is placed with its upper end projecting well above the agar (Fig. 30.2). The isolated bacterium is inoculated into the inner tube and after 8–16 hours incubation, subculture is taken from the surface of the medium in the outer tube.

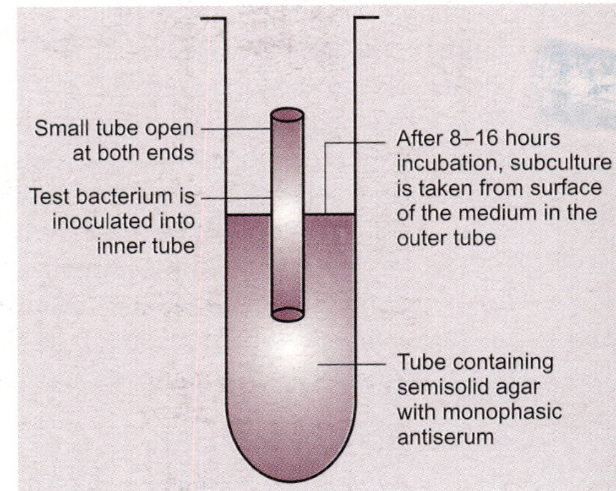

Fig. 30.2. Craigie's tube.

3. V → W variation

Almost all freshly isolated strains of *S.* Typhi carry a surface layer of Vi antigen that completely masks the O antigen. When fully expressed, such bacilli are agglutinable with Vi antiserum but not with O antiserum. This is known as V form. After several subcultures, the Vi antigen is completely lost, so that such cultures are inagglutinable with Vi antiserum but are readily agglutinable with O antiserum. This is known as W form. With partial loss of Vi antigen, the organisms are agglutinable with both O and Vi antisera and these intermediate forms are known as VW forms. Vi antigen of *S.* Paratyphi C and *S.* Dublin does not completely mask the O antigen.

4. S → R variation

Smooth-to-rough variation is associated with the change in colonial morphology from smooth to rough, and loss of O antigen and of virulence. The colonies become large, rough and are autoagglutinable in saline. The rough variants are organisms with defective capacity to synthesize polysaccharide of O antigen.

5. Variations in O antigens

A change in structural formulae of O antigen may be brought about by lysogenization with some phages resulting in the alteration of the bacterial serotype. Thus *S.* Anatum (serotype 3, 10:e, h:1, 6) is converted by phage 15 into *S.* Newington (serotype 3, 15:e, h:1, 6) and the latter into *S.* Minneapolis (serotype 3, 15, 34:e, h:1, 6) by phage 34. **It is likely that such changes occurring in nature contribute to the abundance of *Salmonella* serotypes.**

Q. 5. Write short note on Kauffmann-White scheme.

Ans. This scheme, first developed in 1934, classifies salmonellae into different O serogroups based on distinctive O antigen factors. Strains possessing factor 2 belong to serogroup A, factor 4 to serogroup B, factor 9 to serogroup D and so on. Each serogroup contains a number of serotypes. Formerly, O serogroups were designated by capital letters A–Z and those discovered later by the number 51–67. Serogroups A–Z and 51–67 represented O antigens 2–50 and 51–67 respectively.

It appears more logical to name each O serogroup by its common O antigen. These numbers are not continuous. Within each O serogroup, the different serotypes are distinguished by identification of phase 1 and 2 flagellar antigens (Table 30.4).

Table 30.4. Kauffmann-White classification of *Salmonella* showing antigenic formulae of some important serogroups and serotypes

O serogroup		Serotype	O antigens (and Vi)	H antigens	
New	Old			Phase 1	Phase 2
2	A	*S.* Paratyphi A	1, **2**, 12	a	–
4	B	*S.* Paratyphi B	1, **4**, 5, 12	b	1, 2
		S. Typhimurium	1, **4**, 5, 12	i	1, 2
7	C1	*S.* Paratyphi C	6, **7** (Vi)	c	1, 5
		S. Choleraesuis	6, **7**	c	1, 5
8	C2	*S.* Muenchen	6, **8**	d	1, 2
		S. Newport	6, **8**, 20	e, h	1, 2
9	D	*S.* Typhi	**9**, 12 (Vi)	d	–
		S. Enteritidis	4, **9**, 12	g, m	–
		S. Gallinarum	1, **9**, 12	–	–
		S. Pullorum	1, **9**, 12	–	–
3, 10	E1	*S.* Anatum	3, **10**	e, h	1, 6

Numbers in bold type are the antigens characterising the O group.

The antigenic structure of a *Salmonella* serotype is expressed as an antigenic formula which has three parts describing the O antigens, the phase 1 H antigens and phase 2 H antigens in that order. The three parts are separated by colons and the component antigens in each part by commas. More than 2,500 serotypes have so far been described in Kauffmann-White scheme.

Q. 6. Write short note on bacteriophage typing of *Salmonella* Typhi.

Ans. For epidemiological study, strains within a particular serotype may be differentiated into a number of phage types. Craigie and Yen (1937) observed that a bacteriophage acting on Vi antigen of *S.* Typhi (Vi phage II) is highly adaptable. The parent phage is known as phage A. It could be made specific for a particular strain of *S.* Typhi by serial propagation in that strain. The phage typing is done by determining the sensitivity of the culture to a series of variants of Vi phage II. Type A strains are sensitive to all adaptations of the Vi phage but most other types are sensitive to only one or a few related adaptations. As phage typing of *S.* Typhi depends on the presence of Vi antigens, a proportion of strains (Vi negative) will be untypable. At present, 97 Vi II phage types of *S.* Typhi are recognized. **Phage types E_1, O and A are the most common in India.**

Phage typing schemes have also been developed for *S.* Paratyphi A, *S.* Paratyphi B, *S.* Typhimurium, *S.* Enteritidis, *S.* Dublin, *S.* Bareilly and other serotypes in different countries.

Q. 7. Describe pathogenesis of *Salmonella* Typhi and *S.* Paratyphi.

Ans. Man acquires infection by ingestion of contaminated water or food. Water becomes polluted by the introduction of faeces from any human or animal excreting salmonellae. Infection by food usually results either from ingestion of contaminated meat or by way of the hands of the carrier. Poultry and eggs also comprise an important source of salmonellae for humans because a large percentage of chickens are routinely infected with salmonellae. Therefore, man can acquire these organisms through direct contact with uncooked chicken or by ingestion of undercooked chicken. Organisms may also be present on outer shell and in the yolk, therefore, consuming anything containing raw eggs can result in *Salmonella* infection. Slaughterhouse workers are exposed to salmonellosis, as an occupational hazard, primarily from poultry and pigs. **The infective dose of most serotypes including *S.* Typhi, varies from 10^6–10^9 organisms.**

Salmonellae cause the following clinical syndromes in man:

- Enteric fever.
- Septicaemia with or without local suppurative lesions.
- Gastroenteritis or food poisoning.

Enteric fever

Enteric fever is most usually caused by *S.* Typhi (**typhoid fever**) or *S.* Paratyphi A, B and C (**paratyphoid fever**). On reaching the gut, the bacilli attach themselves to the microvilli of the ileal mucosa by means of adhesins on the bacterial surface, which adhere specifically to mannose-containing receptors on the epithelium. They then penetrate to the lamina propria and submucosa, where they are phagocytosed by neutrophils and macrophages. They resist intracellular killing and multiply within these cells. These cells enter the mesenteric lymph nodes, where after a period of multiplication, the bacilli invade the blood stream via thoracic duct and a transient bacteraemia (**primary bacteraemia**) follows.

During this period the bacilli are seeded in the liver, gall bladder, spleen, bone marrow, lymph nodes, lungs and kidneys, where further multiplication takes place. After multiplication in these organs, bacilli pass into the blood, causing a **second and heavier bacteraemia**, heralding the onset of clinical illness.

The organisms multiply abundantly in the gall bladder and are discharged continuously into the intestine where Peyer's patches and other gut lymphoid tissues of ileum become involved. These become inflamed, undergo necrosis and slough off, leaving behind characteristic **typhoid ulcers**. Perforation and haemorrhage are occasional associated accidents.

Incubation period is usually 8–15 days, but can be as short as 5 days or as long as 50 days. The clinical course may vary from a mild undifferentiated pyrexia to a rapidly fatal fulminating disease. The onset is usually gradual with headache, malaise, anorexia, a coated tongue and abdominal discomfort with either constipation or diarrhoea. In the untreated case the temperature shows a step-ladder rise over the first week of illness, remains high for 7–10 days and then falls by lysis during third or fourth week.

Physical signs include a relative bradycardia for the height of the fever, hepatomegaly, splenomegaly and often a rash of **rose spots**. These are 2–4 mm in diameter, slightly raised discrete irregular macules. They are most often found on the front of the chest during the second or third week and fade on pressure. They are seldom noticeable in dark-skinned patients.

The most important complications are intestinal perforation, haemorrhage and circulatory collapse. Other complications include cholecystitis, arthritis, periosteitis, nephritis, haemolytic anaemia, venous thromboses, peripheral neuritis and rarely osteomyelitis. In about 5–10% cases, relapse occurs during convalescence. Mortality in untreated patients is 20%. **The development of cell-mediated immunity is probably the main means by which the infection is overcome.**

Q. 8. Describe laboratory diagnosis of enteric fever.

Ans. Laboratory diagnosis of enteric fever can be made by:

- Isolation and identification of the causative agent from the patient blood, faeces, urine, bone marrow, rose spots, etc.
- Demonstration of circulating antigen.
- Demonstration of antibodies in the patient serum.

Since the onset of symptoms is associated with bacteraemia, blood culture is positive in about 90% of cases in the first week of fever. The frequency with which causative agent can be isolated from the blood falls thereafter so that blood culture is positive in about 75% of cases in the second week, 60% in the third week and 25% after till the fever disappears.

Salmonellae are shed in the faeces throughout the course of the disease and even in convalescence, with varying frequency. During the first week of illness, organisms can be isolated from the faeces in about half the cases and they are most easily isolated between third to fifth week of illness. However, isolation from the faeces is of less certain significance, since salmonellae may be present in the faeces of carriers. Salmonellae are shed in the urine irregularly and infrequently. Urine cultures are generally positive only in the second and third weeks in about 25% of cases.

Testing of patient serum for *Salmonella* antibodies (Widal test) can afford only indirect evidence of infection, and its interpretation may be rendered difficult by past exposure to infection, previous immunization with TAB vaccine or early antibiotic treatment. Therefore, the significance of the results of the Widal test is often doubtful.

Blood culture

With all aseptic precautions, 5–10 ml of blood is collected by venipuncture and transferred into a culture bottle containing 50–100 ml of 0.5% bile broth. Before transferring blood into blood culture bottle, the cap of the bottle is thoroughly cleaned with spirit. The blood should be transferred through a hole in the cap by inserting the needle of the syringe rather than opening the bottle, thus it avoids contamination from the external environment. As far as possible, sample of blood should be collected before starting treatment. Large quantity (5–10 ml) of blood is required, since the number of organisms in the blood, particularly in mild and recovering cases, may be quite small, even as few as one/ml. As the blood's natural bactericidal or bacteriostatic action may interfere with the growth of any bacteria present, this effect is annulled by diluting (inoculating) 5–10 ml of blood in 50–100 ml of the medium (10-fold dilution). The antibacterial effect may be further prevented by the addition of liquoid (sodium polyanethol sulphonate). *Organisms causing bacteraemia in young children are usually present in sufficient concentration, therefore, small volume (1 ml) of blood is inoculated into 10 ml of the medium (10-fold dilution).*

Blood culture bottle is incubated at 37°C for up to 7 days. After overnight incubation, subculture is made onto MacConkey agar, and blood agar (for organisms other than *Salmonella*) media. These plates are incubated at 37°C for 24 hours and the isolate is identified by its morphological and biochemical characters, and slide agglutination test. If salmonellae are not obtained from first subculture from bile broth, then subcultures should be repeated every other day up to 7 days. If no growth is obtained after 7 days, then the culture is declared as negative.

For slide agglutination test, a loopful of growth from nutrient agar plate or slope is emulsified in two separate drops of saline on a clean slide. One emulsion acts as a control to show that the strain is not autoagglutinable. If the isolate is anaerogenic (i.e., *S.* Typhi is suspected) then a loopful of factor 9 antiserum is added to one drop of bacterial emulsion on the slide. The slide is rocked gently. Prompt agglutination indicates that the isolate belongs to *Salmonella* O serogroup D. Its identity as *S.* Typhi is established by agglutination with the flagellar antiserum (anti-d serum). Sometimes, fresh isolates of *S.* Typhi are in the V form and do not agglutinate with O antiserum. Such strains may be tested for agglutination with anti-Vi serum or the growth is scraped off in a small amount of saline, boiled for one hour and tested for agglutination with O antiserum. If the isolate is nontyphoid *Salmonella*, it is tested for agglutination with O and H antisera for serogroups A, B, C1, C2, etc.

Clot culture

With strict aseptic precautions, 5 ml blood is withdrawn from the patient into a sterile test tube and allowed to clot. The separated serum is removed and used for the Widal test. The clot is broken up with a sterile glass rod and added to a bottle of bile broth containing streptokinase (100 units/ml). Streptokinase causes rapid clot lysis with release of bacteria trapped in the clot. Clot culture with streptokinase yields a higher rate of isolation than whole blood culture as the bactericidal action of the serum is obviated. Another advantage is that a sample of serum also becomes available for Widal test.

Faeces culture

A spoonful of faeces should be collected in a sterile container. Rectal swab is not satisfactory. If there is likely to be a delay of some hours before specimen of faeces for culture reaches the laboratory, the faeces can be placed in a container with 5 ml of **buffered glycerol saline** transport medium. Faecal samples are plated directly on MacConkey agar, DCA and Wilson and Blair's brilliant-green bismuth sulphite agar media. The last is highly selective and should be plated heavily.

On MacConkey and DCA media salmonellae appear as pale yellow or colourless colonies after 18–24 hours incubation at 37°C. On Wilson and Blair's brilliant-green bismuth sulphite agar, *S.* Typhi forms black colonies, with a metallic sheen after 24–48 incubation at 37°C.

For enrichment, one tube each of selenite F and tetrathionate broth are also inoculated. These are also incubated at 37°C for 8–12 hours with subsequent subculture on MacConkey and DCA media.

Other materials for culture

Salmonellae may be isolated from several other sources. These include urine, bone marrow, bile obtained by duodenal aspiration, rose spots, pus from suppurative lesions, CSF and sputum. Bone marrow and bile culture are positive in most cases. The latter may be employed for detection of carriers.

Demonstration of circulating antigen

In the early phase of the disease, typhoid bacillus antigens are consistently present in the blood and urine of the patient. *Staphylococcus aureus* containing protein A (Cowan 1 strain) is stabilized with formaldehyde and then coated with *S.* Typhi antibody. When a 1% suspension of such sensitized staphylococcal cells is mixed with patient serum on a slide, typhoid antigen present in the serum combines specifically with the antibody attached to staphylococcal cells producing visible agglutination within 2 minutes. This is known as **coagglutination**. The test is rapid, sensitive and specific, but is not positive after the first week of illness.

Demonstration of antibodies in the patient serum

Widal test is used for the demonstration of antibodies in the patient serum.

Principle

It is an **agglutination test** which detects the presence of agglutinins in patient serum against H and O suspensions of the enteric bacteria likely to be encountered, e.g., *S.* Typhi and *S.* Paratyphi A in India.

Method

Two types of tubes are used for the test:

1. Dreyer's tube (narrow tube with conical bottom) for H agglutination.
2. Felix tube (short round bottomed tube) for O agglutination.

Equal volumes (0.4 ml) of serial dilutions of the patient serum (1 : 20 to 1 : 640) and H antigens of *S.* Typhi (TH) and *S.* Paratyphi A (AH); and O antigen of *S.* Typhi (TO), are mixed in Dreyer's and Felix tubes respectively and incubated in a water bath at 37°C for 4 hours and read after overnight refrigeration at 4°C. O antigen of *S.* Paratyphi A (AO) may not be employed as it cross-reacts with TO. Control tubes containing the antigen and normal saline are set to check for autoagglutination. H agglutination leads to the formation of loose and cotton-woolly clumps, while O agglutination appears as a disc-like granular deposit at the bottom of the tube (Fig. 13.7). Control (Felix) tube shows a compact deposit. **The highest dilution of the serum showing agglutination indicates the titre of the antibody.**

Interpretation

1. Agglutinins usually appear by seventh to tenth day of the illness in enteric fever, so that a negative result at an early stage is inconclusive. The titre then increases steadily till the third or fourth week, after which it declines gradually.
2. Demonstration of rising titre, e.g., four-fold or greater rise, between tests made in the first and third weeks is highly significant. However, if the first sample is taken late in the disease, a rise may not be demonstrable. Instead a fall in titre may be seen in some cases.
3. Though it is generally stated that titres of 1 : 100 or more for O agglutinins and 1 : 200 or more for H agglutinins are significant, the results in a single test by no means prove the presence of enteric fever nor negative results its absence.
4. Serum from individuals immunized with TAB vaccine may show high titres of antibodies to *S.* Typhi, *S.* Paratyphi A and *S.* Paratyphi B. However, if a marked rise of titre to one serotype is observed, the results may be regarded as diagnostically significant. H agglutinins tend to persist for many months after vaccination but O agglutinins tend to disappear sooner, i.e., within 6 months. Therefore, rise in O agglutinins indicate recent infection.
5. For determining the serotype of infecting organism, H agglutinin is more reliable than O agglutinin because the different serotypes have some O antigens in common. Moreover, O antigens are also widely distributed among other enterobacteria.
6. Persons who had past enteric infection or who have been vaccinated may develop anamnestic response during an unrelated fever like malaria, influenza, etc. The anamnestic response shows only a transient rise, while in enteric fever the rise is sustained.
7. Test suspensions of bacteria may contain nonspecific antigens such as fimbrial antigens which may produce false positive results.

Other serological tests

These include:

1. Detection of *Salmonella* O antibodies in the patient serum by indirect haemagglutination test. The results of this test appear to correspond with those of Widal test.
2. Counterimmunoelectrophoresis of the patient serum with a veronal buffer extract of *S.* Typhi, is said to be more sensitive and specific than the Widal test.
3. ELISA is a sensitive method of measuring antibody against the *Salmonella* lipopolysaccharide (LPS).
4. Solid-phase radioimmunoassay may be used to detect antibodies against LPS and a protein fraction of *S.* Typhi and to determine their immunoglobulin class.

Salmonella antibodies may also be detected in urine and faeces of the patients and the carriers.

Q. 9. Describe briefly vaccines against typhoid fever.

Ans. Following are vaccines against typhoid fever:

A. Parenteral vaccines

1. *Killed whole cell vaccine (TAB vaccine):* Heat killed, phenol preserved, whole cell vaccines containing a mixture of cultures of *S.* Typhi, 1,000 million and *S.* Paratyphi A and B, 750

million each per ml have been used for many years in countries with a high endemic level of typhoid fever.

Dose schedule: The vaccine is injected in 2 doses of 0.5 ml each at an interval of 4–6 weeks followed by a booster dose every 3 years.

2. *Vaccine of purified Vi antigen:* This vaccine contains purified Vi antigen.

   Dose schedule: It is injected intramuscularly in a dose of 25 µg.

   In the trials conducted in black South African children and in young adults in Nepal the protection conferred by the vaccine was 64% and 72% respectively. The conjugation of purified Vi polysaccharide with a protein increases its immunogenicity.

B. Oral vaccine

Because immunity to typhoid fever appears to be primarily cell-mediated, a live vaccine will undoubtedly be more effective than killed vaccines. Therefore, several live avirulent vaccines are undergoing experimental trials.

Oral administration of live avirulent mutant strain of *S.* Typhi (Ty 21a), which is a stable mutant lacking the enzyme UDP-galactose-4-epimerase, has given encouraging results in Egypt. On ingestion, it initiates infection but 'self destructs' after four or five cell divisions, therefore, it cannot induce any illness.

Dose schedule: Three doses of the vaccine are given on alternate days to children. This oral vaccine is available in enteric coated capsules or in liquid form.

Protection: It is safe and confers 65–96% protection for 3–5 years.

Q. 10. Write short note on *Salmonella* septicaemia.

Ans. All *Salmonella* species can cause bacteremia, although infections with *S.* Typhi, *S.* Paratyphi and *S.* Choleraesuis more commonly lead to a bacteremic phase. The risk for *Salmonella* bacteremia is higher in paediatric and geriatric patients and in immunocompromised patients (HIV infections, sickle-cell disease, congenital immunodeficiencies). It is characterized by suppurative lesions such as osteomyelitis, deep abscesses, endocarditis, pneumonia and meningitis. Infection occurs by oral route and the incubation period is short. Salmonellae can be isolated from blood or exudate from focal lesions but rarely from faeces.

Q. 11. Describe briefly *Salmonella* gastroenteritis.

Ans. Salmonella gastroenteritis or food poisoning is generally a **zoonotic disease.**

Source of infection

It is caused by ingestion of food like meat, egg, milk and sweets contaminated by certain species of *Salmonella* which are primarily animal pathogens. In most parts of the world, *S.* Typhimurium is the commonest (30–40%) species. Other common species include *S.* Enteritidis, *S.* Newport, *S.* Dublin, *S.* Heidelberg and *S.* Indiana. Food contamination may result from droppings of rats, lizards or other small animals. Salmonellae can enter through the shell of the egg if the eggs are left on contaminated chicken feed or faeces, and grow inside.

Pathogenesis

The incubation period is 12–24 hours and the illness is characterised by fever, vomiting, abdominal pain and diarrhoea. It may vary in severity from the passage of one or two loose stools to an acute cholera-like disease. It usually subsides in 2–7 days. There are multiple reports that *Salmonella* serotypes secrete a cholera-like enterotoxin that induces increased levels of cAMP and that some strains produce a heat-stable enterotoxin. A cytotoxin that inhibits protein synthesis in intestinal cells has been described.

Laboratory diagnosis

It is made by isolating the causative agent from faeces and food.

Prophylaxis

- Prevention of food contamination.
- Proper cooking of food.

Treatment

- For uncomplicated, non-invasive salmonellosis, the treatment is symptomatic.
- Antibiotics should not be given. They do not help recovery, on the other hand they may increase the period of faecal shedding of the bacilli.
- However, for serious invasive cases, antibiotic treatment is needed.

Q. 12. Describe morphology, cultural characteristics, biochemical reactions, antigenic structure, determinants of pathogenicity, pathogenesis and laboratory diagnosis of *Yersinia pestis*.

Ans.

Morphology

They are Gram-negative coccobacilli or rods with rounded ends and straight or convex sides, about 1.5 × 0.7 µm in size, occurring singly or in pairs or, when in fluid culture, in chains. They are non-sporing, non-acid-fast and non-motile. In exudates from lesions and in cultures grown at 37°C, rather than at the optimum temperature of 27°C, *Y. pestis* exhibits typical capsule. In smears from the tissues stained with Giemsa or methylene blue, the bacilli show characteristic bipolar staining (safety pin appearance) in which the ends of the bacilli stain darker than the central part (Fig. 30.3). In culture, the bipolar staining is less obvious.

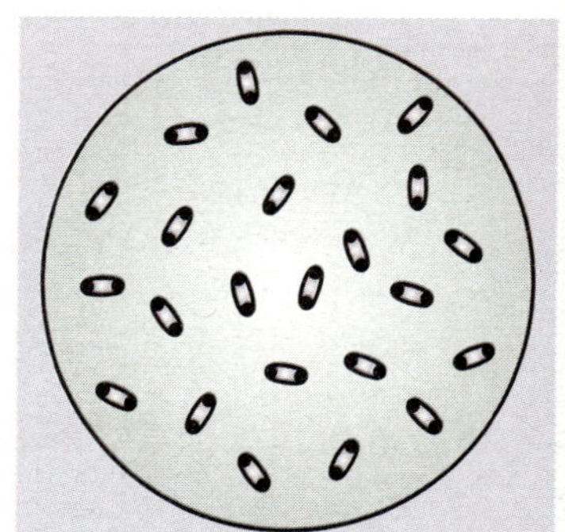

Fig. 30.3. Bipolar staining of *Yersinia pestis.*

Cultural characteristics

Plague bacilli are aerobes and facultative anaerobes. Optimum (and range) pH and temperature for the growth of these organisms are 7.2 (5.0–9.6) and 27°C (14–37°C) respectively.

It can grow on ordinary media.

- On **nutrient agar** medium, after overnight incubation, *Y. pestis* forms transparent, minute, pin-point colonies. On further incubation, they continue to increase in diameter reaching 4 mm in 5 days and become opaque.

- On **blood agar**, colonies are dark brown due to absorption of the haemin pigment.
- Colourless colonies are formed on **MacConkey agar**.
- In **broth**, it produces little turbidity but results in a granular deposit at the bottom and the sides of the tube. On prolonged incubation, a surface pellicle may appear. If a drop of sterile oil is allowed to float on the surface of an inoculated broth and provided the flask is not shaken, a characteristic growth appears which hangs down into the broth from the oil drop resembling stalactites (**stalactite growth**).

Biochemical reactions

Y. pestis is catalase-positive, indole negative, methyl red reaction positive, Voges-Proskauer and citrate negative. It is nitrate reduction positive and urease and gelatin liquefaction negative. It ferments glucose, mannitol and maltose with the production of acid but no gas. Lactose and sucrose are not fermented.

Antigenic structure

Y. pestis has a complex antigenic structure and about 20 different antigens have been identified which include:

1. A heat-labile (at 100°C) protein envelope antigen known as **fraction 1 or F1**. It is formed *in vivo* and in cultures grown at 37°C. It inhibits phagocytosis and is generally present only in virulent strains. This antigen has, therefore, been considered a virulence determinant. It plays an important role in stimulating protective immunity in mice and man. Therefore, a killed vaccine prepared from cultures grown at 37°C in which capsular material is well developed has greater immunizing properties in mice than one from cultures grown at lower temperature i.e. 25–30°C. **Production of F1 antigen is determined by a plasmid.**
2. The **V and W proteins** are also formed by virulent strains of *Y. pestis* at 37°C at low calcium concentrations. V antigen is a protein of molecular weight 90,000 and W antigen is an acidic lipoprotein of molecular weight 145,000. **Their production is also determined by a plasmid.**
3. Other antigens elaborated by *Y. pestis* include **murine and guinea-pig toxins** and some virulence associated factors such as **pesticin 1**, **fibrinolysin** and **coagulase**, **whose production is regulated by a single plasmid**.

Determinants of pathogenicity

Y. pestis possesses following determinants of pathogenicity:

1. V and W antigens.
2. F1 envelope antigen.
3. Virulence associated factors such as pesticin 1, coagulase and fibrinolysin.
4. Ability to synthesize purines.
5. Production of pigmented colonies on medium containing haemin.

Pathogenesis

Y. pestis is a natural pathogen of rodents. It causes **zoonotic disease** called **plague**. Infection is transmitted from one animal to another by the bite of rat flea. The infection normally does not pass from one animal to another unless a flea carries the organism from one to another. When a rat flea, commonly *Xenopsylla cheopsis*, bites a diseased rat, it sucks about 0.5 ml of blood per feed which contains about 5,000–50,000 bacilli. These are sufficient to infect flea. In the flea, the bacilli multiply in the stomach and block the lumen of proventriculus. In *X. cheopsis* it takes about 3 weeks (**extrinsic incubation period**). When such a flea bites another rodent blood cannot pass through. The hungry flea bites ferociously and bacteria are regurgitated into the site of bite, transmitting the infection.

When the diseased rat dies, the flea leaves the carcass and in the absence of another rat may bite man causing bubonic plague. Infection in man may also be transmitted by contamination of the wound of bite with the faeces of infected fleas. In man plague occurs in three forms – **bubonic**, **septicaemic** and **pneumonic**.

Bubonic plague

After an incubation period of 2–5 days, the lymph nodes draining the site of entry of bacillus become infected. As the plague bacillus usually enters through the bite of infected flea on the legs, the inguinal lymph nodes are involved, hence the name bubonic plague (bubo means enlarged gland in groin). The glands become enlarged and suppurate. Patient develops fever, chills, nausea and malaise. Pain may precede and accompany the bubo. The spread of disease is not stopped by the lymph nodes and hence bacteraemia occurs.

Septicaemic plague

The presence of bacteria in the blood denotes septicaemic plague. Massive involvement of blood vessels occurs resulting in haemorrhages in the skin and mucosa. This manifestation is responsible for the disease being given the name **'black death'**.

Pneumonic plague

Bacterial emboli may become trapped in the lungs causing pneumonic plague. It gives an added dimension to the disease since **it can be transmitted from man to man by droplet infection (airborne route)**. Pneumonic plague may also occur in epidemic form. Patient develops fever, 104°F or more, and cough with expectoration. The sputum at first is mucoid and blood-tinged later. It is loaded with *Y. pestis*. Patient complains of severe chest pain, difficult and rapid breathing. Towards the end, patient develops cyanosis and circulatory failure. Those who develop pneumonic plague die within 2–3 days if not treated vigorously. Death rate from bubonic plague is 50–75%, from pneumonic plague almost 100%, and with treatment it is 5–30%.

Laboratory diagnosis

The diagnosis of plague can be confirmed by demonstrating *Y. pestis* in stained films from bubos in bubonic plague or in sputum in pneumonic plague. In septicaemic plague, the bacilli may be demonstrated in blood cultures or from spleen on postmortem.

Bubonic plague

1. Puncture the bubo with a hypodermic syringe and draw the exudate for examination.
2. Prepare the films of the exudate and stain by Gram staining and methylene blue. Characteristic Gram-negative coccobacilli, and bacilli showing bipolar staining with methylene blue are suggestive of plague bacilli.

3. Culture the exudate on blood agar plate, incubate at 27°C. Pick up a single colony and subculture to obtain a pure growth. Carry out biochemical tests to confirm the diagnosis.
4. Inoculate guinea-pigs or white rats subcutaneously with exudate from bubo or with 24 hours broth culture. Infected animals die in 2–5 days. Postmortem reveals marked local inflammatory condition at the site of inoculation, with necrosis and oedema. Regional lymph nodes are enlarged and congested and may show greyish-white patches in the tissue. Prepare films from local lesions, lymph nodes, spleen and heart blood. Stain films with Gram and methylene blue stains and examine under microscope for characteristic *Y. pestis*.

Pneumonic plague

1. Prepare films from sputum and stain by Gram and methylene blue stains. Examine stained films microscopically for characteristic Gram-negative and bipolar stained coccobacilli respectively.
2. Inoculate on blood agar plate and proceed further as in case of bubonic plague.
3. Inoculate sputum into guinea-pigs or rats by applying the sputum to the nasal mucosa or to a shaved area of skin. The plague bacilli can enter through microabrasions caused by shaving while other organisms in sputum cannot. Carry out postmortem as in case of bubonic plague.

In the convalescent stage serology is most likely to be useful. Serum may be tested by complement fixation test, and the haemagglutination test with tanned sheep red cells to which the capsular F1 antigen has been absorbed. An enzyme-linked immunosorbent assay (**ELISA**) with F1 antigen is likely to become the method of choice.

A **polymerase chain reaction** (PCR), with primers based on F1 gene sequences, offers a rapid and less hazardous means of diagnosis than culture.

Other question which may also be asked in the examination

What is the principle of Widal test? Describe its method and interpretation.

For answer see pages 283–284.

31

Vibrio and Aeromonas

Q. 1. Describe morphology, cultural characteristics, special media (transport, enrichment and plating media) used for isolation and biochemical reactions of *Vibrio cholerae*.

Ans. ***Morphology***

These are short, curved or comma-shaped rods with rounded or pointed ends and 1.5 × 0.2–0.4 μm in size. S forms or spirals may be seen due to two or more cells lying end to end (Fig. 31.1). In old cultures, they are frequently highly pleomorphic. In stained films of mucous flakes from acute cholera cases, the vibrios are seen arranged in parallel rows, described by Koch as the **'fish in stream'** appearance. They show vigorous **darting motility** which is mediated by a single polar flagellum. When acute cholera stool or a young culture is examined under the microscope, the actively motile vibrios suggest a 'swarm of gnats'. They are Gram-negative, non-sporing, non-capsulated and non-acid-fast.

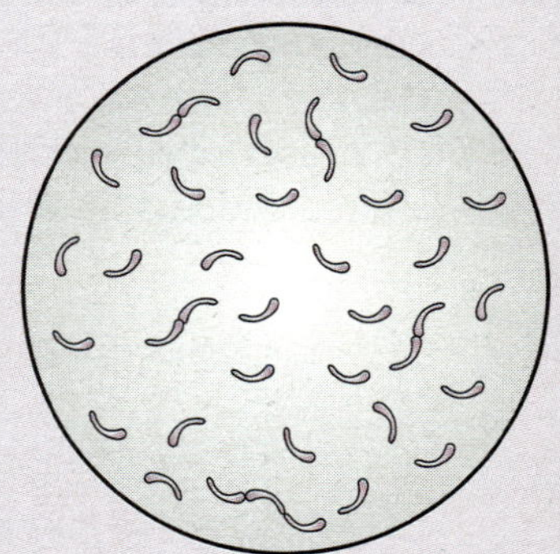

Fig. 31.1. *Vibrio cholerae.*

Cultural characteristics

V. cholerae is aerobe and facultative anaerobe, but under anaerobic conditions only scanty and slow growth is obtained. It grows within a temperature range of 16–40°C (optimum temperature 37°C). Growth occurs freely between pH 7.4 and 9.6 (optimum pH 8.2). *V. cholerae* is a non-halophilic vibrio. It cannot grow in media with a concentration of sodium chloride more than 5%. However, it can grow in the media without any sodium chloride. On the other hand, halophilic vibrios like *V. parahaemolyticus* can grow in media containing 7–10% sodium chloride and cannot grow in media lacking it.

- **Nutrient agar:** After overnight incubation at 37°C, the colonies are glistening translucent discs, 1–2 mm in diameter with bluish or greenish tinge in transmitted light.
- **MacConkey agar:** Colonies are smaller than those on nutrient agar and are colourless, but become reddish on prolonged incubation due to the late fermentation of lactose.
- **Blood agar:** Classical biotype does not produce haemolysis although some strains produce greenish discolouration around individual colonies which later becomes clear due to haemodigestion. However, colonies of El Tor biotype are haemolytic.
- **Gelatin stab:** At first a white line of growth appears along the track of the inoculating wire. Liquefaction of gelatin begins at the top which spreads downwards in a funnel-shaped form (*infundibuliform appearance*) in 3 days at 22°C.
- **Peptone water:** This organism grows as a surface pellicle because of its affinity for oxygen. The surface pellicle becomes visible in 6–9 hours.

Special media

A number of special culture media have been employed for the cultivation of *V. cholerae*. They may be classified as under:

Transport (holding) media

V. cholerae is quite sensitive to drying, exposure to sunlight and extreme changes in pH. It is also inhibited by normal intestinal flora. If the cultures cannot be put up immediately, then the stool samples should be transported in transport (holding) media:

1. **Venkatraman-Ramakrishnan (VR) medium:** About 1–3 ml of stool is added to each bottle. *V. cholerae* does not multiply in this medium but remains viable for several weeks. Moreover, it prevents overgrowth by other organisms.
2. **Cary-Blair medium:** It is a suitable transport medium for *Salmonella*, *Shigella* and *V. cholerae*.
3. If a transport medium is not available, a 5 cm × 1.5 cm strip of **thick blotting paper** can be soaked in the faecal matter, then placed in a sealed plastic bag, and sent to the laboratory.

Enrichment media

1. **Alkaline peptone water (APW):** It is particularly useful when low concentrations of organisms, in the specimen, are anticipated (e.g., in convalescent stage of the disease). High pH (8.6) of the medium suppresses the growth of many commensal intestinal bacteria while permitting uninhibited growth of *V. cholerae*. Subcultures on plating media should be done within 3–6 hours because other organisms can begin to overgrow after prolonged incubation. APW is also an excellent transport medium. About 1 g of the stool or a rectal swab should be placed into 10 ml of APW in a screw-capped tube and transported to the laboratory.
2. **Taurocholate peptone transport and enrichment medium:** Place about 1 g stool or a rectal swab in the medium and transport to the laboratory. Subculture a loopful onto a selective plating medium within 6–8 hours at ambient temperature. Also incubate it overnight at 37°C and subculture again on a plating medium next day.

Plating media

These include:

1. **Alkaline bile salt agar (BSA) pH 8.2:** This is modified nutrient agar medium containing 0.5% sodium taurocholate. The colonies on BSA are similar to those on nutrient agar medium.

2. **Monsur's gelatin taurocholate trypticase tellurite agar (GTTA) medium:** This medium is useful for the isolation of cholera and other vibrios from faeces. High (8.5) pH and potassium tellurite, in this medium, are inhibitory to most enterobacteria and Gram-positive bacteria. After 24 hours incubation, vibrios produce small (1–2 mm) translucent colonies with greyish-black centre and a turbid halo, due to hydrolysis and denaturation of gelatin. After 48 hours incubation, colonies increase in size to 3–4 mm.
3. **Thiosulphate-citrate-bile-sucrose (TCBS) agar:** This is most used selective plating medium for vibrios. This medium resembles DCA except that it has the high pH value of 8.6 and contains sucrose instead of lactose. **Sucrose-fermenting vibrios such as *V. cholerae* form yellow colonies** and non-sucrose-fermenters such as *V. parahaemolyticus* blue green ones.

Colonies of *V. cholerae* may be identified by the **string test**. Colonies of *V. cholerae* when mixed in a drop of 0.5% sodium deoxycholate, produce an extremely viscid suspension that can be drawn into a string with an inoculating loop.

Biochemical reactions

V. cholerae is strongly indole positive and reduces nitrates to nitrites. These two properties contribute to the **'cholera red reaction'**, the development of a red colour when concentrated sulphuric acid is added to a 4-day-old culture at 37°C in peptone water. It is due to the formation of **nitrosoindole** which is red in colour. It ferments glucose, sucrose, mannitol, maltose and mannose with the production of acid but no gas and ferments lactose only after several days **(late lactose fermenter)**. Arabinose and dulcitol are not fermented.

It is catalase and oxidase-positive, methyl red and urease negative and liquefies gelatin. It decarboxylates lysine and ornithine but not arginine. Voges-Proskauer reaction and haemolysis of sheep RBCs are positive in El Tor biotype and both these reactions are negative in classical biotype. The differences between classical and El Tor biotypes of *V. cholerae* are shown in Table 31.1.

Table 31.1. Differences between classical and El Tor biotypes of *Vibrio cholerae*

Property	Biotype	
	Classical	El Tor
Voges-Proskauer test	–	+
Agglutination of fowl RBCs	–	+
Haemolysis of sheep RBCs	–	+
Sensitivity to:		
• Polymyxin B	+	–
• Mukerjee's group IV phage	+	–
• Basu and Mukerjee's group V phage	–	+

Q. 2. Describe antigenic structure and phage typing of *Vibrio cholerae*.

Ans. ***Antigenic structure***

V. cholerae possesses at least 200 different O antigens on the basis of which it has been divided into corresponding number of serogroups or serovars. All strains share a common, heat-labile flagellar (H) antigen. **Epidemic cholera is caused by *V. cholerae* serogroup O1 and *V. cholerae* O139 Bengal.** Both classical and El Tor biotypes, belong to serogroup O1. They are agglutinated by *V. cholerae* O1 antiserum. The emergence of *V. cholerae* O139

Bengal as the second aetiologic agent of epidemic cholera in October 1992 in the South Indian coastal city of Chennai has shattered the long-held notion that only *V. cholerae* belonging to serogroup O1 is capable of causing epidemic (and pandemic) cholera. By mid-January 1993, similar isolates were found in Bangladesh.

Soon *V. cholerae* O139 Bengal engulfed the entire Indian subcontinent in a series of outbreaks of cholera. It also spread to several neighbouring countries in Asia. This strain does not agglutinate with O1 antiserum or with antisera to any of the other O serogroups. However, it closely resembles *V. cholerae* O1 El Tor biochemically and physiologically. Cholera caused by *V. cholerae* O139 Bengal is indistinguishable from that caused by *V. cholerae* O1.

Two recognized serogroups of *V. cholerae* which are choleragenic are serogroups O1 and O139. The serogroups O2–O200 are known as **non-O1 vibrios, non-cholera vibrios (NCV) or non-agglutinable (NAG) vibrios** because they are not agglutinated by O1 antiserum. However, they are readily agglutinated by their own antisera. From time to time, they have been associated with outbreaks of diarrhoeal or choleraic disease. Both *V. cholerae* O1 and O139 produce **enterotoxin (cholera toxin)**. Some strains of NCV also produce an enterotoxin similar to the cholera toxin.

O1 serogroup can be further subdivided into three subtypes, Ogawa, Inaba and Hikojima. This is on the basis of differences in minor O antigens (A, B and C). Antigen A is present in all the three subtypes. O antigens present in Ogawa, Inaba and Hikojima are A and B, A and C, and A, B and C respectively (Table 31.2). Ogawa and Inaba strains agglutinate with their specific absorbed antisera, while Hikojima strains which are rare are agglutinated by both Ogawa and Inaba antisera.

Table 31.2. Subtypes of *Vibrio cholerae* O1

Subtypes	Antigens
Ogawa	A and B
Inaba	A and C
Hikojima	A, B and C

Phage typing

Strains of the classical biotype of *V. cholerae* O1 can be divided into 5 types by means of 3 phages (I–III) and a fourth phage (IV) lyses all classical but not El Tor strains (Table 31.3). On the basis of lysis by 4 phages, El Tor strains can be divided into 6 types. All these strains are lysed by a fifth phage (V) (Table 31.4).

Table 31.3. Phage types of strains of classical biotype of *Vibrio cholerae* O1 (Mukerjee et al., 1957)

Phage type	Sensitivity to phage group			
	I	II	III	IV
1	+	+	+	+
2	–	+	+	+
3	+	–	+	+
4	–	–	+	+
5	+	+	–	+

Table 31.4. Phage types of strains of El Tor biotype of *Vibrio cholerae* O1 (Basu and Mukerjee, 1968)

Phage type	Sensitivity to phage group				
	I	II	III	IV	V
1	+	+	+	+	+
2	+	+	+	–	+
3	+	+	–	+	+
4	+	+	–	–	+
5	+	–	–	–	+
6	–	+	–	–	+

Q. 3. Describe pathogenesis of *Vibrio cholerae.*

Ans. *V. cholerae* O1 causes an acute diarrhoeal disease known as **cholera**. It occurs only in man. The vibrios enter orally by the ingestion of faecally contaminated food or drink. Infective dose of *V. cholerae* is 10^8 organisms. After passing the acid barrier of the stomach, they multiply in the alkaline contents of the small intestine and produce a potent toxin known as **cholera toxin (CT), cholera enterotoxin or choleragen**. It resembles heat-labile toxin (LT) of *Escherichia coli* chemically, antigenically and in its mode of action. **CT production is determined by a filamentous phage integrated in the bacterial chromosome.**

CT is a heat-labile multimeric protein, inactivated by heating at 56°C for 30 minutes. It has a molecular weight of 85,600. It consists of a single A (active) subunit of molecular weight 27,215 and five B (binding) subunits each of molecular weight 11,677. The A subunit is responsible for the activity of the toxin and is synthesized as a single inactive polypeptide which is subsequently nicked by *V. cholerae* O1 protease to yield 2 fragments A1 and A2 which remain covalently connected by a single disulphide bond. The A1 fragment is responsible for the biological activity of the toxin and A2 fragment apparently serves to link the B subunit to A.

The B subunit binds specifically to the Gm_1 ganglioside receptor on the cell lining of the villi and crypts of the small intestine. This is perhaps responsible for translocation of the A1 subunit into the cell. The A1 subunit stimulates cell bound adenylate cyclase. This, in turn, converts ATP to cyclic adenosine monophosphate (cAMP) in the gut epithelial cells (enterocytes). This causes an irreversible hypersecretion of electrolytes (Na^+, K^+, HCO_3^-) and water out of the cell and into the lumen of the intestine.

This leads to an outpouring of fluid that is isotonic and contains flakes of mucus and little protein and results in vomiting and profuse watery diarrhoea (*rice water stool*). This results in varying degrees of dehydration and electrolyte imbalance that can lead to metabolic acidosis, hypokalaemia, shock and death in extreme cases.

CT affects certain functions of other tissues that are known to be mediated by cAMP, for example, morphological changes (elongation) of Chinese hamster ovary (CHO) cells, histological changes and steroid production in adrenal tumour (Y1) cells and activation of lipolysis in rat testicular tissue. All these can be used for the assay of CT. It can also be assayed by chemical estimation of cAMP in tumour cells that have been treated with the toxin and immunologically by ELISA and RIA.

CT also increases the permeability of skin capillaries. Intradermal inoculation of rabbit or guinea-pig with CT or cell-free preparations of *V. cholerae* cultures or rice water stools of the cholera patients leads to the development of **erythema at the site of inoculation**. If Evans blue dye is injected intravenously afterwards, the skin over the site of inoculation becomes blue due to increased capillary permeability. This toxic activity is known as the **vascular permeability factor (PF)**. *In vivo*, CT can be detected by **ligated adult rabbit ileal loop** and **infant rabbit bowel assays**.

In addition to enterotoxin production, *V. cholerae* must adhere to the enterocytes. These bacteria are motile and produce mucinase and other proteolytic enzymes which help them to penetrate the protective mucin layer that coats the surface of gastroenteric mucosa. Bacterial attachment is a complex mechanism that requires the bacterial cells to recognize a surface marker on the epithelial cells to which they can bind. Several investigators have demonstrated that the flagella act as adhesins and bind the bacteria to cellular surfaces, whereas other studies indicate that the somatic antigens and slime layers may be responsible for the attachment of vibrios to host cells. Once epithelial cell attachment is accomplished, *V. cholerae* produces enterotoxin and the disease.

Q. 4. Describe laboratory diagnosis of cholera.

Ans. *Specimens*

- Watery stool
- Rectal swab
- Vomitus

Collection of specimens

- Fresh faecal material should be collected as early in the disease process as possible, before the administration of antibiotics. It is best collected by inserting a sterile soft rubber catheter (No. 24–26) and letting the liquid stool flow directly into a sterile screw-capped container.
- A rectal swab may also be collected. It is particularly useful for collecting specimen from a convalescent who no longer has watery diarrhoea. Collection of stool from a bedpan should be avoided because of the risk of contamination or the presence of disinfectants.
- Culture of vomitus may yield the growth of the organisms particularly in the early stages of disease.

Transportation and enrichment

The cultures should be put up immediately. If it is not possible, then the specimen should be preserved in a suitable transport (holding) medium such as VR medium or Cary-Blair medium for long periods. If the specimen can reach the laboratory within a few hours, it may be transported in enrichment media such as APW or Monsur's taurocholate tellurite peptone water, thus saving the time required for isolation. If transport media are not available, a 5 cm × 1.5 cm strip of thick blotting paper can be soaked in the watery stool and sent to the laboratory packed in a plastic envelope.

Culture

In the laboratory, the sample should be plated both directly and after enrichment, onto suitable solid media. Early in the choleraic infection, *V. cholerae* are present in very large numbers (10^7–10^9/ml) in the diarrhoeal stool, so direct plating on non-selective media might well be sufficient for the isolation of these organisms. At later stage of infection, and if antibiotics have been given, the number of *V. cholerae* in the stools will be relatively less, therefore, both enrichment and selective plating media should be used to prevent overgrowth by other intestinal bacteria.

1. Inoculate 2 ml faeces in 20 ml APW. Also inoculate non-selective culture media like 5% sheep blood agar and MacConkey agar and a selective medium like TCBS or GTTA. Incubate these media at 37°C.
2. After 3–6 hours incubation, subculture a loopful from the surface of the APW onto a second plate of selective medium. The inoculated plates are examined after overnight incubation at 37°C. On **MacConkey medium**, they form translucent colonies, on **GTTA medium** they form translucent colonies with greyish-black centre and a turbid halo, and

on **TCBS**, they form yellow colonies. Do the Gram staining from the suspected colonies and look for Gram-negative curved or comma-shaped rods. Perform motility and oxidase tests. Cholera vibrios show characteristic motility and are oxidase-positive.

3. Pick up oxidase-positive colonies with a straight wire and test by slide agglutination with *V. cholerae* O1 antiserum. If positive, the test is repeated using monospecific Ogawa and Inaba antisera. Hikojima strains will agglutinate well with both Ogawa and Inaba antisera. If agglutination is negative with one colony, repeat the test with at least five more colonies as O1 and non-O1 vibrios may co-exist in the same specimen. When the isolated strain is not agglutinated by *V. cholerae* O1 antiserum, it should be tested for agglutination with *V. cholerae* H antiserum. Any vibrio which is agglutinated by H antiserum and not by O1 antiserum is considered to be serogroup O2–O200, because H antigen is shared by all serogroups of *V. cholerae*. It should then be tested with other O antisera to establish their identity as belonging to one of O2–O200 serogroups.
4. For determination of the biotype of the O1 isolate, do VP test, agglutination of fowl RBCs, haemolysis of sheep RBCs, and sensitivity to polymyxin B, Mukerjee phages IV and V (Table 31.1).

Rapid diagnosis

For rapid diagnosis, the characteristic motility of the *Vibrio* and its inhibition by antiserum can be demonstrated under the dark-field or phase-contrast microscope, using stool from acute cases or more reliably after enrichment for 6 hours.

Q. 5. Write short note on oral rehydration therapy.

Ans. Death in cholera is caused by loss of fluids. Therefore, the mortality rate of cholera can be reduced to less than 1% by the adequate replacement of fluids and electrolytes. The more serious cases require immediate intravenous rehydration, but otherwise oral rehydration therapy (ORT) will suffice. The solution in ORT contains glucose, sodium chloride, potassium chloride and sodium citrate. The salts restore the electrolyte balance and reverse acidosis, and glucose promotes absorption of sodium by the small intestine. In fact, the use of any metabolizable carbohydrate in the salt solution appears to be effective for electrolyte replacement. Thus, a well-cooked and salted rice soup is recommended for diarrhoeal patients who are unable to take a glucose-salt-solution.

Q. 6. Describe briefly cholera vaccines.

Ans. Following vaccines are available:

- *Killed whole organism vaccine:* It is killed suspension containing 8,000 million *V. cholerae* per ml, composed of equal numbers of Ogawa and Inaba serotypes. In order to improve the antigenic stimulus, the number of organisms in the vaccine may be increased to 12,000 million per ml. Two injections are given at an interval of four weeks. The vaccine trials in Kolkata, Bangladesh and the Philippines showed that this vaccine offers about 60% protection for 3–6 months. A single dose of vaccine is ineffective in children below five years of age. However, it confers protection in adults due to its action as a booster because of prior natural infection.

- *Non-living oral B subunit-whole cell (BS-WC) vaccine:* This vaccine contains CT subunit B, 2.5 × 10^{10} heat killed vibrios each of Ogawa and Inaba serotypes of classical biotype and equal number of formalin killed vibrios each of Ogawa and Inaba serotypes of El Tor biotype. A field trial conducted in Bangladesh in 1985 revealed an overall protection of 85% for one year and 60% for two years.
- *Live vaccine:* Recombinant DNA vaccine with expression of *V. cholerae* O1 in attenuated strain of *S.* Typhi Ty21a as a carrier bacterium has been developed. The live salmonellae colonize the Peyer's patches of the small intestine and induce IgA response by local immune system of the gut. Live attenuated oral vaccine against *V. cholerae* O139 is also available in some countries.

Q. 7. Write short note on *Vibrio cholerae* non-O1.

Ans. *V. cholerae* serogroups O2–O200 are known as *V. cholerae* non-O1, NCV or NAG vibrios. They resemble *V. cholerae* O1 biochemically and genetically. They occur widely in aquatic environments. They may produce enterotoxins, cytotoxins, haemolysins and colonizing factors. Exposure to saline environments or consumption of seafoods may lead to infection with these organisms. They may cause mild to severe diarrhoeal disease resembling cholera. Occasionally, they may lead to bloody diarrhoea, accompanied by abdominal cramps. In addition, they may cause extraintestinal infections such as wound infections, septicaemia and meningitis.

Q. 8. Describe briefly *Vibrio parahaemolyticus.*

Ans. This organism was first isolated in 1951 in Japan as a causative agent of food poisoning due to consumption of sea fish. It was named as *V. parahaemolyticus* in 1963 by Sakazaki because of the true haemolysis produced by this organism on blood agar. It is now recognized as being responsible worldwide for outbreaks of gastroenteritis associated with the eating of crabs, prawns, shrimps and other seafoods. It has been isolated from shellfish, shrimps, crabs and molluscs in the warm coastal and estuarine waters of many countries.

Morphologically, it resembles *V. cholerae*. It is halophilic and does not grow in peptone water without sodium chloride or on cysteine-lactose electrolyte-deficient (CLED) agar but grows well in peptone water with 8% sodium chloride. However, peptone water without sodium chloride and CLED medium support the growth of non-halophilic vibrios. On MacConkey agar it forms pale, non-lactose-fermenting colonies and on sheep blood agar it produces β-haemolysis. On TCBS agar, the colonies are green (non-sucrose-fermenting). **Unlike other vibrios, it produces peritrichous flagella when grown on solid media. Polar flagella are formed in liquid cultures.**

It is oxidase, catalase, indole and citrate positive. It reduces nitrate to nitrite. It ferments glucose, maltose, mannitol, mannose and arabinose with the production of acid only. Lactose and sucrose are not fermented. It is VP positive and decarboxylates lysine and ornithine but not arginine.

Strains of *V. parahaemolyticus* associated with gastroenteritis lyse human erythrocytes in Wagatsuma's agar, a special high salt mannitol medium. This haemolysis is known as **Kanagawa phenomenon** and is due to a heat-stable haemolysin. Though a correlation has been observed in the ability of the organism to produce haemolysin and to cause disease, its role in the pathogenesis is still not clear.

A **heat-labile enterotoxin** can be separated from the heat-stable haemolysin. It causes morphological changes in tissue culture cells resembling those caused by CT, and LT of *E. coli*. Most strains isolated from seafood and environment are Kanagawa-negative although some of them are positive. It is likely that only a few Kanagawa-positive strains multiply in human intestine and produce disease.

V. parahaemolyticus causes food poisoning associated with marine food. It causes explosive diarrhoea, abdominal pain, nausea, vomiting and fever. Faeces contain cellular exudate and often also blood. Recovery usually occurs in three days.

V. parahaemolyticus has occasionally been isolated from extraintestinal sources, such as wounds, and ear and eye infections, and even a case of pneumonia. Invariably, the patient has a history of recent aquatic exposure or a water-associated traumatic injury to the infected site.

Q. 9. Name important pathogenic species of *Aeromonas*. Describe briefly morphology, cultural characteristics and pathogenesis of *A. hydrophila*.

Ans. The most important pathogens are *Aeromonas hydrophila*, *A. caviae*, and *A. veronii*. The organisms are ubiquitous in fresh and brackish water.

They are straight Gram-negative bacilli or coccobacilli with rounded ends. Motile strains usually have polar flagella but a few have lateral flagella. Some non-motile strains are found. They are catalase- and oxidase-positive. Nitrate is reduced to nitrite. They are aerobes and facultative anaerobes. Metabolism of glucose is both respiratory and fermentative. Carbohydrates are broken down to acid or acid and gas. The temperature range for growth is 4–42°C with an optimum temperature about 32°C, and the pH range 4.5–9.0.

A. hydrophila is more important. It grows well on nutrient agar, blood agar (producing wide β-haemolysis), MacConkey agar (producing pale colonies after 24 hours incubation and pink later), DCA and CLED agar, but growth is variable on TCBS agar, on which colonies are usually yellow. They ferment glucose, maltose, starch and usually arabinose and sucrose with the production of acid and gas.

The natural habitat of *A. hydrophila* (water lover) is fresh or sea waters and the soil where it commonly causes infectious diseases in cold-blooded aquatic animals. It may cause:

1. **Cellulitis and wound infections** following exposure to contaminated water, soil or food.
2. **Acute diarrhoeal disease** resembling cholera due to the production of **enterotoxin** which, like CT stimulates cAMP and produces diarrhoea. It may also cause dysenteric form of diarrhoea with blood and mucus.
3. **Septicaemia** in immunodeficient subjects and patients with hepatobiliary disease.
4. **Infections of ear, meninges** and **urinary tract**.

32

CAMPYLOBACTER, HELICOBACTER, SPIRILLUM, PSEUDOMONAS AND BURKHOLDERIA

Q. 1. Describe morphology, cultural characteristics, biochemical reactions, pathogenesis and laboratory diagnosis of *Campylobacter* species.

Ans. ***Morphology***

The campylobacters are slender, spirally curved (comma-shaped), Gram-negative rods measuring 0.5–5.0 µm in length and 0.2–0.5 µm in width. They are non-sporing and in old cultures they form coccal forms. They are motile by means of a single unsheathed polar flagellum at one or both poles. They spin rapidly around their long axes in corkscrew fashion. *C. jejuni* and *C. coli* are among the most rapidly motile bacteria encountered. The campylobacters resemble vibrios in their morphology, polar flagellation and oxidase-positive character, but differ in being microaerophilic, not fermenting sugars and having a lower G + C content of DNA (29–38 mol % as against 39–51 mol % in vibrios).

Genus *Campylobacter* possesses 32 species out of which *C. jejuni*, *C. coli*, *C. concisus*, *C. fetus*, *C. hyointestinalis*, *C. lari* and *C. sputorum* are of medical importance. Differential characteristics of these species are given in Table 32.1.

Cultural characteristics

Growth of campylobacters occurs under strict microaerophilic conditions, 5% oxygen concentration being optimal. Under ideal conditions, *C. fetus* and most other campylobacters produce visible growth after 24 hours at 37°C, but well-formed colonies are seen only after 48 hours. *C. jejuni*, *C. coli*, *C. lari* and *C. hyointestinalis* grow optimally at 42–43°C. They are, therefore, referred to as the thermophilic group. Colonies of most species are circular and convex but those of thermophilic group, particularly *C. jejuni*, are flat and tend to swarm on moist agar.

Biochemical reactions

The main biochemical activities are shown in Table 32.1. In comparison with other bacteria, campylobacters are biochemically inactive. They do not produce indole and are non-saccharo-

Table 32.1. Differential characteristics of medically important spp. of *Campylobacter* and *Helicobacter*

Property	*C. jejuni*		*C. coli*	*C. concisus*	*C. fetus**		*C. hyointestinalis*	*C. lari*	*C. sputorum*			*H. pylori*	*H. cinaedi*	*H. fennelliae*
	1	2			3	4			5	6	7			
Growth at 42–43°C	+	−	+	+	−	−	+	+	v	v	v	−	−	−
Flagellar arrangement	a	m/a	a	m	m	m	m	a	m	m	m	l	a	a
Catalase	+/w	v	+	−	+	+	+	+	+	−	−	+	+	+
Nitrate reduction	+	−	+	+	+	+	+	+	+	+	+	−	+	+
Hippurate hydrolysis	+	+	−	−	−	−	−	−	−	−	−	−	−	−
Urease	−	−	−	−	−	−	−	−	−	−	−	+	−	−
H_2S (TSI)	v	−	−	+	−	−	+	−	+	+	+	−	−	−
Susceptibility to														
• Nalidixic acid	S	S	S	R	R	R	R	R	R	R	v	R	S	S
• Cephalothin	R	S	R	R	S	S	S	R	S	S	S	S	S	S

1, *C. jejuni* subsp. *jejuni*; 2, *C. jejuni* subsp. *doylei*; 3, *C. fetus* subsp. *fetus*; 4, *C. fetus* subsp. *venerealis*; 5, *C. sputorum* biovar *faecalis*; 6, *C. sputorum* biovar *bubulus*; 7, *C. sputorum* biovar *sputorum*.

a, amphitrichate; m, monotrichate; l, lophotrichate; S, sensitive; R, resistant; v, variable; w, weak reaction.

* Subsp. *venerealis* can be distinguished from subsp. *fetus* by its failure to grow in the presence of 1% glycine or to produce H_2S from cysteine.

lytic. All species produce oxidase, most species produce catalase and with the exception of *C. jejuni* subsp. *doylei* reduce nitrate to nitrite. Of all the species of *Campylobacter*, only *C. jejuni* has the ability to hydrolyze sodium hippurate.

Pathogenesis

C. jejuni subsp. *jejuni* is the most important human pathogen among the campylobacters. This, along with enterotoxigenic *Escherichia coli* and rotaviruses, ranks as the major cause of **diarrhoeal disease** in the world, particularly in developing countries. All the campylobacters appear to be inhabitants of the gastrointestinal tract of wild and domestic animals, including house pets. Majority of chickens and turkeys are also colonized. Man acquires infection by faecal-oral route. Ingestion of raw milk, partially cooked poultry or contaminated water are common sources of human infections. The infective dose is not known but in volunteer studies, infection has been established with as few as 500–800 bacteria.

The organisms that escape killing by gastric acid colonize near neutral, microaerophilic environment of jejunum and ileum. The infection extends distally to affect the terminal ileum, colon and rectum. *C. jejuni* can produce diarrhoea by following mechanisms:

- It produces a **heat-labile enterotoxin** resembling CT that raises intracellular levels of cAMP leading to watery diarrhoea. The activity of this enterotoxin is neutralized by antiserum against *E. coli* LT, and CT.

- Like *Shigella* and *Salmonella*, it **penetrates gut epithelium** leading to oedematous exudative enteritis of jejunum, ileum and colon, with infiltration by polymorphonuclear leucocytes and ulceration of the mucosa. In well-developed infections, mesenteric lymph nodes are enlarged, fleshy and inflamed. There may be a transient bacteraemia. *Heat-labile enterotoxin along with the invasive property of this organism may contribute to the production of the damage.*

The common clinical manifestations are crampy abdominal pain, bloody diarrhoea, chills and fever. The infection is usually self-limited and resolves in 3–7 days. In cases of severe disease, the patient may be treated with oral erythromycin. The convalescing patients may continue to excrete organisms for up to one month.

Laboratory diagnosis

Gram staining

Gram-stained smear of diarrhoeal stool may show characteristic, Gram-negative, curved, S-shaped or long spiral forms and polymorphonuclear leucocytes.

Dark ground or phase contrast microscopy

Wet preparations viewed by dark-ground or phase-contrast illumination may reveal **darting motility**. Stool specimen for *Campylobacter* species may not be processed further unless polymorphonuclear leucocytes are present.

Culture

Faeces or rectal swabs are inoculated on selective media. Selective media for *Campylobacter* species are blood-based and contain antibiotics. In case of delay in inoculation on selective media, a transport medium should be employed. Campylobacters survive for 1–2 weeks at 4°C in Cary-Blair transport medium. Selective media for isolation of *C. jejuni* are Butzler's selective medium, Skirrow's *Campylobacter* selective medium, Preston *Campylobacter* selective medium and Blaser's medium.

Fresh specimens of faeces should be plated directly on the selective medium, but older specimens should first be enriched in an enrichment medium such as the Preston *Campylobacter* enrichment broth, for 24 hours, before plating on selective media. Inoculated plates are incubated at 42°C to favour growth of the thermophilic campylobacters (*C. jejuni, C. coli, C. lari* and *C. hyointestinalis*) over that of other faecal bacteria. If, however, the presence of *C. fetus* is suspected, additional plates should be incubated at 37°C to allow growth of this non-thermophile. Incubation must be done in an atmosphere of 5% O_2, 10% CO_2 and 85% N_2. Well-formed colonies are seen after 48 hours incubation. The growth is identified by Gram staining, motility, oxidase test and biochemical reactions.

Q. 2. Describe morphology, cultural characteristics, biochemical reactions, pathogenicity and laboratory diagnosis of *Helicobacter pylori.*

Ans. ***Morphology***

It is a curved, short, spiral or S-shaped Gram-negative bacterium measuring 3 µm in length and 0.5–0.9 µm in width. **It is motile by means of a tuft of up to 7 sheathed flagella at one**

pole (lophotrichate), while campylobacters have a single unsheathed flagellum. It is non-sporing and on exposure to air it transforms to coccal form.

Cultural characteristics

Like campylobacters, *H. pylori* is microaerophilic. It can grow in an atmosphere of 5% O_2, 10% CO_2 and 85% N_2. It does not grow anaerobically or in air, although many strains can also grow in humidified air with increased (10%) CO_2 content. High humidity is essential for growth, therefore, culture plates should not be dried off after pouring. The optimum temperature for its growth is 35–37°C, some grow poorly at 42°C but none grows at 25°C. It can be grown on moist freshly prepared heated blood (chocolate) agar and Skirrow's *Campylobacter* selective medium. After incubation at 35–37°C in a microaerophilic atmosphere, as above, for 3–5 days, *H. pylori* produces circular, convex and translucent colonies.

Biochemical reactions

H. pylori is biochemically inactive in most conventional tests. Notable exceptions are the production of urease, catalase and oxidase. **The urease enzyme produced by *H. pylori* is almost 100 times more active than that of *Proteus vulgaris*.**

Pathogenicity

H. pylori colonizes the surface of the gastric mucosa, especially of the antrum but any part of the stomach may be colonized. The bacteria are present in large numbers in the mucus overlying mucosa where the pH is about 7.0. Colonization extends into gastric glands. It has been isolated from gastric biopsy specimens and occasionally from gastric juices, saliva and bile. **Urease released by *H. pylori* produces ammonia ions that neutralize gastric acid in the vicinity of the organism, thus favouring bacterial multiplication.** Thus the enzyme urease is important for the colonization of the stomach by this organism.

The pathogenic role of *H. pylori* in peptic ulcer disease, both duodenal and gastric, is well recognized. Up to 95% of patients with duodenal ulcer, and 80% of patients with gastric ulcer are infected with *H. pylori*. Eradication of the organism leads to ulcer healing and a markedly lower incidence of recurrence. *H. pylori* has been classified by the International Agency for Research in Cancer as a **group I carcinogen and definite cause of gastric cancer** and **gastric lymphoma in humans**.

Laboratory diagnosis

Specimen

Biopsy of gastric mucosa is collected.

Microscopy and culture

Biopsy is subjected to Gram staining and culture on chocolate agar and Skirrow's *Campylobacter* selective medium followed by incubation as above. The organism is identified on the basis of its colonial morphology, Gram staining and biochemical characters.

Histopathology

In histological sections stained with haematoxylin and eosin, the bacteria are barely visible. However, Warthin-Starry silver staining shows the organisms most clearly.

Biopsy urease test

Since *H. pylori* produces abundant urease, therefore, it can be detected in biopsy material without having to grow the organism. Biopsy tissue is crushed into 0.5 ml urea solution with an indicator and incubated at 37°C. If *H. pylori* is present, the pH changes within a few minutes to 2 hours due to the production of ammonia.

Urea breath test

Urea tagged with an isotope of carbon is fed to the patient. If the patient's stomach is colonized with *H. pylori*, urea is converted into ammonia and tagged CO_2. The latter appears in the breath where it can be measured.

Serological test

Antibodies to *H. pylori* or its urease can be detected in the patient serum by ELISA test. The titre of antibodies falls after several months if infection is eradicated.

Faecal antigen test

Polyclonal antibodies are used to detect *H. pylori* antigen in faeces.

Polymerase chain reaction

Various DNA probes have been developed for the direct detection of *H. pylori* by PCR in gastric juice, and faeces.

Q. 3. Describe briefly morphology, cultivation, pathogenicity, laboratory diagnosis and treatment of *Spirillum minus.*

Ans. ***Morphology***

S. minus, the causative agent of rat-bite fever, is an organism of uncertain taxonomic position. It is a spiral, Gram-negative organism measuring 2–5 µm (sometimes up to 10 µm) in length and 0.2 µm in diameter. It has 2–3 rigid spirals 0.8–1.0 µm across. It is very actively motile showing **darting motility** like that of *Vibrio cholerae*. The motility is due to 1–7 flagella attached at each pole. The organisms can be demonstrated in fresh specimens, with the dark-ground microscope or by staining with Leishman or Giemsa stain.

Cultivation

S. minus has not been grown in artificial media and is best isolated by intraperitoneal inoculation of infected tissues and blood into mice, white rats and guinea-pigs.

Pathogenicity

It is a natural parasite of rats and other rodents, causing bacteraemia. In man, it causes **rat-bite fever**. Transmission is, as the name implies, by rat bite. Man to man transmission has not been documented.

One to four weeks after the animal bite patient develops chills, headache and fever. The site of bite usually heals before the onset of symptoms but it often re-ulcerates and is accompanied by regional lymphadenitis, lymphangitis and blotchy rash. The fever usually falls after one week and reappears again after a few days. The relapses of fever may occur for weeks, months or even years. Endocarditis, meningitis, hepatitis, nephritis and myocarditis are rare complications of *S. minus* infection. Rat-bite fever occurs mainly in Japan and Far East and is known as **sodoku**. It has also been reported from other parts of Asia, Europe and USA.

Laboratory diagnosis

S. minus can be isolated by intraperitoneal inoculation of blood or material from lymph node into a mouse. The animal will show no signs of illness, but after 5–14 days small number of spirilla may be demonstrated by dark ground microscopy in its blood and peritoneal fluid. Occasionally, *S. minus* may be demonstrated directly by dark ground microscopy in exudate from the local lesion, regional lymph node or blood of the patient.

Treatment

S. minus infection responds to treatment with penicillin and tetracyclines.

Q. 4. Describe morphology, cultural characteristics, pigment production, biochemical reactions, drug resistance, toxins and enzymes, and bacteriocin (pyocin) typing of *Pseudomonas aeruginosa*.

Ans.

Morphology

It is a slender, Gram-negative bacillus, 1.5–3.0 μm × 0.5 μm, actively motile by a polar flagellum. Occasional strains have two or three flagella. Clinical isolates often possess pili. It is non-capsulated but many strains have a mucoid slime layer. Mucoid strains, particularly isolated from cystic fibrosis patients, have an abundance of polysaccharide composed of alginate polymer. This forms a loose capsule in which microcolonies of the bacillus are enmeshed and protected from host defences.

Cultural characteristics

It is a strict aerobe and grows well on ordinary media. It can grow over a temperature range of 5–42°C, the optimum temperature being 37°C.

Nutrient agar

After aerobic incubation on nutrient agar at 37°C for 24 hours, the colonies are large, 2–3 mm in diameter, smooth, translucent, irregularly round and emit a characteristic fruity odour. This is due to the production of aminoacetophenone from tryptophan. Mucoid strains often produce copious amounts of an extracellular polysaccharide on agar culture. These strains are particularly common in the sputum of patients with cystic fibrosis.

MacConkey medium

It forms non-lactose fermenting colonies.

Blood agar

Many strains are haemolytic on blood agar medium.

Nutrient broth

It produces a dense turbidity and surface pellicle.

Pigment production

P. aeruginosa produces at least 4 distinct pigments:

1. Pyocyanin

It is a bluish-green phenazine pigment soluble in chloroform and water. It diffuses into the surrounding medium. This pigment is not produced by other species of this genus, therefore, its detection is diagnostic of *P. aeruginosa*.

2. Pyoverdin (fluorescein)

It is insoluble in chloroform but soluble in water. It imparts a yellowish tinge to cultures but this is sometimes not easy to detect unless cultures are examined under ultraviolet light.

3. Pyorubrin

It is a bright red water soluble pigment. It is a phenazine pigment that is insoluble in chloroform.

4. Pyomelanin

It is a brown to black pigment and its production is uncommon. It is chemically unrelated to animal melanin.

Biochemical reactions

P. aeruginosa derives energy from carbohydrates by an oxidative rather than a fermentative metabolism. **Because the amount of acid produced by oxidative pathways is less than that produced by fermentation, special media such as the O-F medium of Hugh and Leifson must be used for diagnostic tests.** It utilizes glucose oxidatively with the production of acid only. Lactose and maltose are not utilized. Indole, MR, VP and H_2S tests are negative. All strains are **oxidase-positive within 30 seconds**. This is a useful preliminary test for identification of non-pigmented strains. None of the other oxidase-positive, Gram-negative bacilli reacts as swiftly as *P. aeruginosa*. It reduces nitrates to nitrites and further to gaseous nitrogen. It is catalase, arginine dihydrolase and gelatinase positive and lysine decarboxylase and aesculin hydrolysis negative.

Drug resistance in Pseudomonas

P. aeruginosa exhibits intrinsic resistance to a variety of antimicrobials including beta-lactams. Owing to its persistence in the hospital environment, an array of multidrug resistance mechanisms are often seen in these hospital isolates as a survival strategy. Consequently, treatment options are narrowed down to only a few antibiotics. The carbapenems have been the drug of choice for the treatment of infections caused by penicillin or cephalosporin-resistant Gram-negative bacilli. However, carbapenem resistance has been observed frequently in non-fermenting Gram-negative bacilli such as *Pseudomonas aeruginosa* and *Acinetobacter* species.

Resistance to carbapenems can develop as a result of the following mechanisms:

1. Decreased outer membrane permeability via the loss of the outer membrane porin D (OprD).
2. The up-regulation of an active efflux pump system of the cytoplasmic membrane.
3. Alteration of penicillin-binding proteins.
4. The production of metallo-β-lactamases, i.e., carbapenem hydrolyzing enzymes known as carbapenemases.

Toxins and enzymes

1. Extracellular products

Pyocyanin, produced by *P. aeruginosa*, inhibits mitochondrial enzymes in mammalian tissue and causes disruption and cessation of ciliary beat on ciliated nasal epithelium. This favours colonization of the organism in the nasal mucosa by avoiding clearance from respiratory mucosa by primary host defences.

2. Extracellular enzymes and haemolysins

P. aeruginosa produces proteases (general protease, alkaline protease and elastase), haemolysins (phospholipase C and heat-stable rhamnolipid) and lipase. These play a key role in the formation of local lesions.

3. Exotoxins

P. aeruginosa produces two exotoxins, A and S. Exotoxin A has been extensively studied. It is a polypeptide of molecular weight 66,000–72,000 that inhibits protein synthesis. Although the mechanism of action of exotoxin A is identical to that of diphtheria toxin, yet the two toxins are otherwise unrelated. Antisera to either toxin will neutralize only the homologous product.

4. Endotoxin

It is a lipopolysaccharide (LPS) exhibiting many biological properties of enterobacterial LPS including pyrogenic action, Shwartzman reaction and lethality for mouse.

Bacteriocin (pyocin) typing

Typing of *P. aeruginosa* based on pyocin production is the most popular method for typing *P. aeruginosa*. The most widely used method is the one described by Gillies and Govan (1966) and later modified by Govan and Gillies (1969). The test strain is inoculated as a one cm wide band across the tryptone soya blood agar plate, incubated overnight at 32°C for pyocin production. The resultant growth is removed by scraping with a sterile glass slide. The residual growth is killed by exposure to chloroform vapours and eight indicator strains (nos. 1–8) are cross-streaked in parallel lines at right angles to the original inoculum followed by incubation at 37°C for 24 hours.

The pattern of inhibition of the indicator strains determines the type of the strain. Further discrimination among the members of the more frequent types (1, 3, 5, 10 and untypable) can be obtained by subtyping with five additional indicator (A–E) strains. Pyocin typing is easy to perform, results are available by the third day and has a reasonable reproducibility and good discrimination.

Q. 5. Describe pathogenicity and laboratory diagnosis of *Pseudomonas aeruginosa*.

Ans. ***Pathogenicity***

P. aeruginosa is widely distributed in soil, water and sewage, and in the mammalian gut. Four to twelve per cent of humans carry it as part of normal faecal flora. Its ability to persist and multiply in moist environment of the hospital wards, bath rooms, kitchens, equipment and antiseptic or disinfectant solutions is of particular importance in cross-infection. In spite of its lack of invasiveness, *P. aeruginosa* does cause infections and severe disease. It accounts for 5–15% of nosocomial infections. The commonest infections caused by it are:

- Urinary tract infection when it is mechanically placed into the urinary tract during catheterization.
- Acute purulent meningitis when it is mechanically placed into the meninges during a lumbar puncture or after cranial injury.
- It is able to multiply on respiratory ventilators and deliver large numbers of organisms directly into the lungs of an already debilitated person leading to respiratory infections like necrotizing pneumonia.
- Septicaemia may develop in persons with leukaemia or persons receiving immunosuppressive drugs and in newborn babies and old debilitated persons.
- In drug addicts, it may cause endocarditis and septic arthritis.
- In addition, it may cause wound and burn infection, chronic otitis media and otitis externa, eye infection and acute necrotizing vasculitis which leads to haemorrhagic infarction of skin and internal organs.

Laboratory diagnosis

Specimens

Specimens to be collected include pus, wound swab, urine, sputum, CSF or blood.

Culture

The specimens may be inoculated on MacConkey agar and blood agar. It may be necessary to use selective media such as cetrimide agar for isolation of *P. aeruginosa* from faeces or other samples with mixed flora such as wound swab. The isolates are identified by their colonial morphology and biochemical characters. The typing of the organisms may be carried out by serotyping and pyocin typing.

Q. 6. Write short note on *Burkholderia mallei.*

Ans. This bacillus was isolated by Loeffler and Schutz (1882) from a horse dying of glanders.

Morphology

It is a small, 2.5 µm × 0.5 µm, non-motile, Gram-negative rod.

Cultural characteristics

It is an aerobe and facultative anaerobe and can grow on ordinary culture media under a wide range of temperature. Colonies are small and translucent initially but become yellowish and opaque on ageing.

Pathogenicity

It is an obligate animal parasite occasionally transmitted to man. In susceptible animals like horses, mules and asses, *B. mallei* produces two types of lesions:

1. ***Glanders:*** In glanders, respiratory system is affected. The infected animal develops profuse catarrhal discharge from the nose, and the nasal septum shows nodule formation. Later the nodules break down with the production of irregular ulcers.

2. ***Farcy:*** This follows infection through skin with involvement of superficial lymph vessels and lymph nodes. The lymph vessels are thickened and stand out as hard cords under the skin which are called **'farcy pipes'**.

Guinea-pigs are susceptible. Intraperitoneal inoculation of small amounts of a pure culture in male guinea-pig causes testicular swelling in 2–3 days due to bacillary invasion of the tunica vaginalis. This is known as **Strauss reaction**. This may be followed by death of the animal.

Humans may become infected via skin abrasions or wounds which come into contact with the discharges of a sick animal. Human disease may take the form of an acute fulminant febrile illness or a chronic indolent infection producing abscesses in respiratory tract or skin.

Q. 7. Write short note on *Burkholderia pseudomallei*.

Ans. ***Morphology and biochemical reactions***

B. pseudomallei resembles *B. mallei* but differs in being motile, hydrolyzing aesculin and oxidizing lactose oxidatively.

Pathogenesis

It is found in soil and water particularly in Southeast Asia, the Philippines, Northern Australia, parts of Africa and Central America. Melioidosis occurs in rats, guinea-pigs and rabbits. **Human** infection may occur through inhalation, inoculation or perhaps even by ingestion of foodstuffs contaminated with excreta of infected animals. It may also get transmitted from the animals by the bite of haematophagous insects. Agriculture workers, especially those who work in moist soil (e.g., paddy fields), are particularly prone to infection.

In humans, the clinical manifestations consist of:

- A subclinical infection diagnosed by the presence of specific antibodies.
- Benign pulmonary infection that may resemble tuberculosis.
- Multiple abscesses in various organs and tissues such as lung, liver, spleen, bones, joints, muscles and subcutaneous tissues.
- A fulminating septicaemia with a mortality rate of 80–90%.

B. pseudomallei can survive intracellularly within the elements of the reticuloendothelial system and this ability may account for latency and the emergence of symptoms.

In India, cases of melioidosis have been reported from Maharashtra, Kerala, Tamil Nadu, Orissa, West Bengal and Tripura.

Laboratory diagnosis

The organisms may be detected in very small numbers, as small, bipolar stained, Gram-negative bacilli in exudates and may be isolated from sputum, urine, pus or blood. **IgG and IgM antibody** to *B. pseudomallei* may be detected in patient serum by **ELISA and indirect haemagglutination test**. A **PCR** test has also been developed to detect *B. pseudomallei* genome in pus, sputum and other specimens.

33

HAEMOPHILUS, BORDETELLA AND LEGIONELLA

Q. 1. Describe morphology, cultural characteristics, antigenic structure and virulence factors of *Haemophilus influenzae*.

Ans. ***Morphology***

H. influenzae is a slender, short (1.5 µm × 0.3 µm), non-motile, non-sporing, Gram-negative rod or coccobacillus. It exhibits considerable pleomorphism. In sputum it usually occurs as clusters of coccobacillary forms, while in the CSF from meningitis cases, long bacillary and filamentous forms predominate. Cells from young cultures are usually coccobacillary, while older cultures are distinctly pleomorphic. The organisms are somewhat difficult to stain. Staining for 5–15 minutes with dilute carbol fuchsin or Loeffler's methylene blue often gives satisfactory results. Strains isolated from acute infections are often capsulated. Capsule can be demonstrated by **India ink wet films** and by **Quellung reaction** with type-specific antiserum. In Gram-stained direct smear the capsule appears as clear, **nonstaining area (halo) surrounding the organism** in purulent secretions.

Cultural characteristics

H. influenzae has fastidious growth requirements. Accessory growth factors known as X and V, present in blood, are essential for its growth. Therefore, it can grow on blood agar or chocolate agar and not on nutrient agar which lacks sufficient amount of them. It grows better in aerobic than in anaerobic conditions. Some strains require extra (5–10%) CO_2. The temperature range for growth is 20–42°C, the optimum temperature being 35–37°C.

X factor

It is a heat-stable protoporphyrin IX, haemin or other iron-containing porphyrin. It is necessary for the synthesis of cytochrome and other haem enzymes such as catalase and peroxidase involved in aerobic respiration.

V factor

V factor is a heat-labile (destroyed at 121°C for 30 minutes) factor present in red blood cells and in many other animal and plant cells. It is synthesized by most bacterial species other than *H. influenzae*. It is either nicotinamide adenine dinucleotide (NAD, coenzyme I) or NAD phosphate (NADP, coenzyme II). It is essential for the oxidation-reduction processes in the growing bacterial cell.

Both X and V factors are found within red blood cells including the sheep erythrocytes in sheep blood agar used in clinical laboratories. Sheep blood also contains NADase activity that slowly hydrolyzes V factor. Therefore, ordinary blood agar is not suitable for the growth of *H. influenzae* where it forms only pin-point colonies. Heating blood agar at 80–90°C until it acquires a chocolate colour, results in lysis of erythrocytes, liberation of both X and V factors and inactivation of NADase enzyme that hydrolyzes V factor. Most laboratories rely on chocolate agar for the recovery of *Haemophilus* species from clinical specimens.

When an organism, such as *Staphylococcus aureus* is streaked across a plate of blood agar on which a specimen containing *H. influenzae* has been inoculated, after overnight incubation, the colonies of *H. influenzae* will be large and well developed alongside the streak of *S. aureus*, and smaller farther away (Fig. 33.1). This phenomenon is known as **satellitism**. The lysed erythrocytes in the agar surrounding the *S. aureus* streak provide X factor, and staphylococcal cells themselves secrete V factor during logarithmic growth. The '*Staphylococcus* streak' technique can be used to recover *Haemophilus* species from clinical specimens.

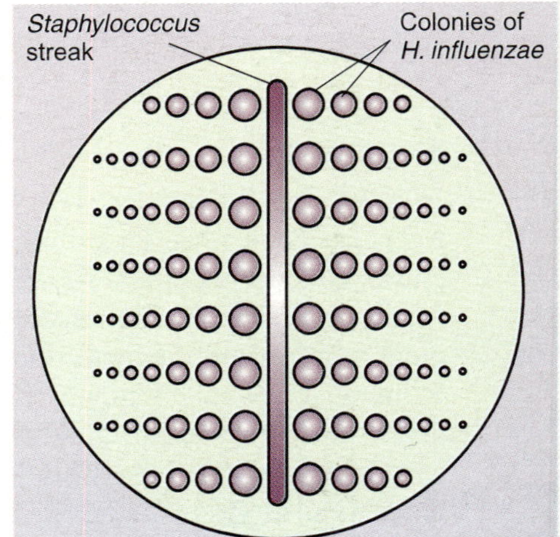

Fig. 33.1. Satellite growth of *Haemophilus influenzae*.

After 24 hour incubation at 35–37°C on chocolate agar, the colonies of non-capsulate strains are usually 0.5–1 mm in diameter, circular, low convex, smooth, pale grey and transparent. They have a characteristic fishy, seminal smell. The colonies of capsulate strains are larger (1–3 mm in diameter), high convex in shape and mucoid.

Good growth is also obtained on certain transparent media where red blood cells have been disrupted and NADase enzyme inactivated either by peptic digest (Fildes agar) or heat (Levinthal's agar). These media are useful for demonstrating capsulate strains, colonies of which are iridescent when viewed obliquely with transmitted light. Type b capsulate strains can also be detected by the presence of precipitin haloes on transparent media containing hyperimmune *H. influenzae* type b antiserum.

Antigenic structure

Three major surface antigens are present in *H. influenzae* – capsular polysaccharide, outer membrane protein (OMP) and lipooligosaccharide (LOS). Capsular polysaccharide antigen is the major antigenic determinant of capsulated *H. influenzae*, on the basis of which strains of *H. influenzae* have been classified by Pittman into six capsular types – a to f. *Most infections are caused by H. influenzae strains belonging to capsular serotype b* (Hib). These strains are associated with rapidly progressive and even life-threatening infections.

The type b capsular serotype is a polymer of ribose, ribitol and phosphate, or polyribosyl-ribitol-phosphate (PRP). Type b is the only one of the six capsular types that contains a pentose (i.e., ribose), rather than a hexose, a property that may be related to virulence. The capsular PRP antigen of Hib induces IgG, IgM and IgA antibodies which are bactericidal, opsonic and protective.

The OMP antigen shows considerable variation. These antigens of Hib have been classified into at least 13 subtypes. *H. influenzae* lipooligosaccharides are antigenically complex.

Serotyping of *H. influenzae* is done by **agglutination** or **Quellung reaction** (swelling of the capsule) with type-specific antisera. Non-capsulated strains of *H. influenzae* are antigenically heterogeneous.

Virulence factors

The virulence of *H. influenzae* is determined by the following factors:

1. **Capsular polysaccharide:** This confers on the bacterium ability to resist phagocytosis. Loss of capsule is associated with the loss of virulence.
2. **Adherence:** Most non-capsulate strains are adherent to human epithelial cells, whereas most serotype b strains are not. The lack of this adherent capability in type b organisms may explain the tendency for type b strains to cause systemic infections. The presence of adherent capability by non-capsulate strains may explain the tendency of these strains to cause more localized infections.
3. **Outer membrane proteins:** They also contribute in adhesion and invasion of host tissues.
4. **IgA1 protease:** *H. influenzae* produces enzyme IgA1 protease that splits IgA1 and inactivates its antibody activity. In addition to *H. influenzae*, IgA1 protease is an important virulence factor of *Neisseria gonorrhoeae*, *N meningitidis*, *S. pneumoniae*, *Prevotella melaninogenica* and some streptococci associated with dental disease. Production of IgA1 protease allows pathogens to inactivate the primary antibody found on mucosal surfaces and thereby eliminate protection of the host by the antibody.

Q. 2. Describe pathogenicity and laboratory diagnosis of *Haemophilus influenzae*.

Ans. *Pathogenicity*

H. influenzae is an **obligate human parasite**. Twenty five to eighty per cent of healthy adults harbour non-capsulate organisms in the nasopharynx and oropharynx. Colonization by capsulate strains is seen in 5–10%, of which capsular type b strains are found in 1–5%. *H. influenzae* causes invasive and non-invasive infections. The former are caused by capsulate strains, **type b accounting for 95% cases**, and the latter by non-capsulate strains.

I. Invasive infections

Meningitis is the most common invasive infection, followed by epiglottitis, bacteraemia, pneumonia, septic arthritis and cellulitis. These infections occur in children of 2 months to 2 years of age but epiglottitis tends to occur in slightly older children, having a peak incidence between 2 and 4 years of age. Immunity in the neonate is probably acquired by transplacental antibodies that are lost within the first few months of life. Therefore, these infections are unusual in the first 2 months of life and common thereafter up to 2–4 years of age. Antibodies generally reappear later, following exposure to type b and other organisms and these infections become less common.

Meningitis: Hib is a common cause of paediatric meningitis with case fatality rate of about 90% in the untreated. Prior nasopharyngeal colonization in a susceptible host leads to invasion of the blood stream and subsequent seeding of the meninges. Onset of meningeal symptoms may be abrupt or more commonly insidious.

Epiglottitis: Hib is the most common cause of epiglottitis. In this case, an apparently healthy child develops acute obstructive laryngeal oedema which may need immediate tracheostomy and vigorous administration of antimicrobial and supportive therapy. The epiglottis is usually markedly swollen, red and oedematous. This condition is always associated with bacteraemia and Hib can be recovered from blood cultures in more than 97% of cases.

Pneumonia: *Haemophilus* pneumonia typically occurs in infants and is accompanied by empyema and sometimes meningitis. It is caused by capsulate strains. On the other hand, bronchopneumonia may occur as a secondary infection with non-capsulate strains.

Septic arthritis: The bacteraemic spread of Hib is the most common cause of arthritis seen in children younger than 2 years of age.

II. Non-invasive infections

H. influenzae produces a number of local infections which are usually associated with some underlying anatomical or physiological abnormality. These include otitis media, sinusitis, chronic bronchitis and bronchiectasis. Acute sinusitis and otitis media are usually initiated by viral infections. These predispose to secondary infection with potential pathogenic resident microbial flora. Non-invasive infections are caused by non-capsulate strains of *H. influenzae*.

Laboratory diagnosis

Specimen collection and transportation

Depending upon the type of lesion, *H. influenzae* can be detected in cerebrospinal fluid (CSF), blood, throat swab, sputum, pus, and aspirates from joints, middle ears or sinuses, etc. In cases with epiglottitis, otitis media and pneumonia, it is often difficult to obtain a specimen from the local site of infection. In such cases blood culture should always be done and type b capsular antigen may be detected in body fluids. *As haemophili are poorly viable in clinical specimens particularly at 4°C, therefore, the specimens should never be refrigerated. For optimal yield, specimens should be transported to the laboratory and seeded onto appropriate culture media without delay.*

Direct examination

1. **Gram-stained smear** of clinical material showing poorly stained Gram-negative coccobacilli and occasionally slender filamentous forms should arouse the suspicion of *H. influenzae* infection.
2. **Immunofluorescence** and **Quellung reaction** can be employed for direct demonstration of *H. influenzae* after mixing with specific rabbit antiserum type b.
3. **Type b capsular antigen** can be detected in patient serum, urine, CSF or pus by:

- **Agglutination of latex particles** (LA) coated with rabbit antibody to type b antigen.
- **Coagglutination (COA) of *S. aureus* coated with antibody** to type b antigen.
- **Counterimmunoelectrophoresis** (CIE) with specific antiserum.

Culture

- **CSF culture:** CSF should be promptly plated on blood agar or chocolate agar. A strain of *S. aureus* should be streaked across the plate. It is then incubated at 35–37°C in air with 5–10% CO_2, overnight. The isolate is identified by its colonial morphology, phenomenon of satellitism, Gram staining, biochemical reactions and serotyping. Culture may also be done on Levinthal's medium and Fildes' agar.
- **Blood culture:** Blood culture is usually positive in cases of epiglottitis and pneumonia. Culture may be done in nutrient broth, as it will be enriched with X and V factors from the blood sample itself. For early results culture may be examined after 4–5 hours by Quellung reaction. After overnight incubation, subculture is made on chocolate agar and processed further as above.
- **Throat swab and sputum culture:** For the isolation of *H. influenzae* from throat swab and sputum, antibiotics like penicillin, bacitracin and cloxacillin may be added to the medium to inhibit the growth of normal respiratory tract flora. Sputum should be homogenized by treatment with pancreatin or by shaking with sterile water and glass beads for 10–15 minutes.

Q. 3. Describe briefly morphology, cultural characteristics, pathogenicity and laboratory diagnosis of *Haemophilus ducreyi*.

Ans. *H. ducreyi* was first reported in 1889 by Ducrey in stained smears prepared from the exudates of soft sore (chancroid) and Bezancon et al. (1900) succeeded in isolating the organisms on 30% rabbit-blood agar.

Morphology

In the purulent discharge from the ulcerated surface of chancroid or in the pus from lymph node aspirate, *H. ducreyi* appear as bipolar or evenly stained Gram-negative coccobacilli, 1–1.5 × 0.6 μm often arranged in groups, whorls or in parallel chains. They may be found inside and outside polymorphonuclear leucocytes. It is not found as a commensal in healthy persons.

Cultural characteristics

H. ducreyi grows poorly on most media. It requires X but not V factor for growth. Several other media have been devised to improve the isolation of *H. ducreyi*. These include 30% rabbit-blood agar, fresh clotted rabbit blood, heated blood agar with 1% IsoVitalex and vancomycin 3 mg/l. The latter is added to inhibit Gram-positive organisms (e.g., staphylococci and streptococci) that may be present as contaminants or superinfecting bacteria in the chancroid lesion. A humid atmosphere and increased CO_2 concentration improve the growth of *H. ducreyi* on primary isolation. Laboratory strains do not require CO_2 for growth. Optimum temperature for growth is 33–36°C. It may also be grown on chorioallantoic membrane of the chick embryo.

After 24 hours incubation, the colonies of *H. ducreyi* are small, pin-point to 0.5 mm in diameter, nonmucoid, grey, yellow or tan, translucent or semiopaque. After 48–72 hours, the colonies are 1–2 mm in diameter and semiopaque.

Pathogenicity

H. ducreyi is the aetiologic agent of **chancroid, a highly communicable sexually transmitted disease**. It is most prevalent in Africa and Southeast Asia. After incubation period of approximately 4–14 days, a nonindurated, painful lesion with an irregular edge develops, generally on the genitalia or perianal area. Inguinal lymphadenitis, either unilateral or bilateral, is common and unless treated, often results in inguinal abscess called **bubo**. Genital lesions caused by this organism are also known as **soft chancres** or **soft sores** because they are characterized by non-indurated irregular ulcers whereas primary lesion of syphilis (chancre) is sharply demarcated and indurated. In males, the lesions are generally on the penis (Fig. 33.2) and in females they may be present on the labia and within the vagina. **It is likely that the lesions of chancroid facilitate the transmission of human immunodeficiency viruses (HIV-1 and HIV-2).** Chancroid may also spread to other anatomical sites by auto-inoculation.

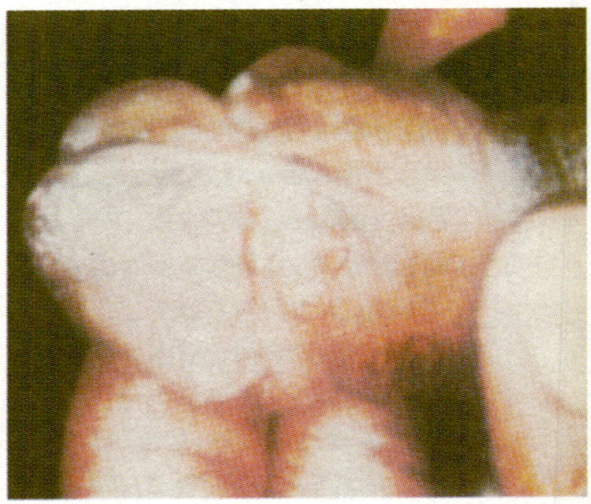

Fig. 33.2. Chancroid caused by *Haemophilus ducreyi* on the penis.

Laboratory diagnosis

1. Scrape edge of the ulcer or aspirate material from bubo.
2. Prepare the smear, do the Gram staining and look for characteristic Gram-negative coccobacilli.
3. Inoculate heated blood agar with 1% IsoVitalex. To make the medium selective, vancomycin 3 mg/l may be added. Incubate the medium at 33–36°C in a humid atmosphere and 5–10% CO_2 for 2–3 days and look for characteristic colonies.

Q. 4. Describe morphology, cultural characteristics, antigenic constituents and virulence factors of *Bordetella pertussis.*

Ans. *Morphology*

B. pertussis is a small, Gram-negative, coccobacillus, measuring 0.5–2.0 μm × 0.3–0.5 μm, arranged singly, in pairs or in small groups. On subculture, it tends to become pleomorphic. It is non-motile and non-sporing. When freshly isolated it may possess a poorly defined capsule. Fimbriae may be present in freshly isolated strains of *B. pertussis*.

Cultural characteristics

It is an **obligate aerobe**. No growth occurs anaerobically. The optimum temperature for growth is 35–36°C. It **does not require X and V factors** for its growth. However, primary isolation of *B. pertussis* requires the addition of charcoal, ion exchange resins, or 15–20% blood to neutralize growth-inhibiting effects of such substances as unsaturated fatty acids, sulphides and peroxides.

The preferred medium used for the isolation of *B. pertussis* is **charcoal blood agar** to which cephalexin has been added; the antibiotic inhibits other organisms commonly found in specimens and only minimally restricts the growth of *Bordetella* species. This medium is superior to Bordet-Gengou medium in that it supports a heavier growth of the organism on primary isolation, and the colonies are larger. The inoculated medium is incubated at 35–36°C in a humidified incubator. If it is not available, a bowl of water should be placed on the floor of the incubator to provide humidity by evaporation.

Growth of *B. pertussis* is slow. After 3–5 days incubation at 35–36°C, the colonies are small (0.5 mm in diameter), dome-shaped, smooth, opaque, greyish-white with a shiny surface resembling **'bisected pearls'** or **'mercury drops'**.

Antigenic constituents and virulence factors

Antigenic constituents and virulence factors of *B. pertussis* include:

1. Heat-labile toxin.
2. Tracheal cytotoxin.
3. Lipopolysaccharide endotoxin.
4. Pertussis toxin.
5. Adenylate cyclase.
6. Filamentous haemagglutinin.
7. Agglutinogens.

1. Heat-labile toxin (HLT)

It is a cytoplasmic protein, inactivated by heating at 56°C for 30 minutes. Mechanism of action of HLT is not known. However, it is believed that HLT-induced vasoconstriction in the respiratory tract may be responsible for inflammatory reaction. HLT in conjunction with endotoxin may be responsible for rhinorrhoea, sneezing and mild cough in the catarrhal stage of whooping cough.

2. Tracheal cytotoxin (TCT)

It is a low molecular weight toxin. It appears to be derived from the peptidoglycan of the bacterial cell wall. This toxin is probably responsible for the destruction of the ciliated respiratory epithelial cells, resulting in accumulation in the lungs of mucus, bacteria and inflammatory debris leading to severe cough from which the respiratory disease derives its name. The disruption of ciliary function may also contribute to the secondary bacterial infections which frequently complicate pertussis.

3. Lipopolysaccharide (LPS) endotoxin

It is produced by all species of *Bordetella* and comprises around 2% of the dry weight of the bacterial cell. Like other Gram-negative bacterial endotoxins, it exhibits properties like heat-stability, adjuvant activity, pyrogenicity and Shwartzman reactivity. LPS is generally considered not to be a protective antigen. However, high levels of anti-LPS antibodies of the IgG, IgA and IgM classes have been found in sera from children with pertussis.

4. Pertussis toxin (PT)

PT, also known as lymphocytosis-promoting factor, pertussigen, histamine-sensitizing factor and islet-activating factor, has a wide spectrum of biologic activity, as indicated by the variety of descriptive names attached to it. It is apparently responsible for many of the clinical signs and symptoms of pertussis, as well as the relative and absolute lymphocytosis observed during the clinical illness. Antibody against PT is protective in animal models of pertussis.

PT has a molecular weight of 117,000 and is made up of 6 polypeptide chains (S1–S5, with 2 copies of S4). PT has got two units, A (enzymatically active moiety) and B (binding component). A unit is made up of S1 polypeptide chain. It is enzymatically active. B unit consists of the remaining 5 polypeptide chains. It binds the toxin to the target cells and helps A unit to cross the membrane. Within the target cell, PT results in increased adenylate cyclase activity which in turn leads to an elevation of cyclic adenosine monophosphate (cAMP), with consequent disturbance to normal cell function.

5. Adenylate cyclase (AC)

B. pertussis produces an adenylate cyclase which can be activated by eukaryotic calcium-dependent regulatory protein, calmodulin. AC produced by the bacterium has the capacity to enter a variety of mammalian cells. Inside the cell, after activation by calmodulin, this enzyme synthesizes cAMP which is responsible for the biological effects of AC:

- Inhibition of chemotaxis, phagocytosis, phagosome-lysosome fusion, superoxide generation, and bactericidal activity of neutrophils, monocytes and macrophages.
- Chinese hamster ovary cell elongation.
- Stimulation of rat pituitary cells leading to secretion of growth hormone and adrenocorticotrophic hormone.

AC is also produced by *B. parapertussis* and *B. bronchiseptica* but not by *B. avium*.

6. Filamentous haemagglutinin (FHA)

It is a protein that exists as filamentous rods, (measuring 2 nm in diameter and 40 nm in length) extending from the cell surface of the bacterium. It mediates the initial attachment of the bacterium to the ciliated epithelial cells of the upper respiratory tract. Antibodies directed against FHA are protective, presumably by inhibiting attachment.

7. Agglutinogens (AGGs)

Mammalian bordetellae possess 14 AGGs located on the fimbriae. AGGs 1–6 are specific for *B. pertussis* and AGG 7 is common to all the three mammalian bordetellae. AGGs 14 and 12 are specific for *B. parapertussis* and *B. bronchiseptica* respectively. Agglutinogens promote virulence by helping bacteria to attach to respiratory epithelial cells. They are useful in serotyping strains and in epidemiological studies.

Q. 5. Describe pathogenicity and laboratory diagnosis of *Bordetella pertussis*.

Ans. ***Pathogenicity***

B. pertussis causes the syndrome called **pertussis** or **'whooping cough'**. All age groups are susceptible but 80% of clinical cases occur in children under the age of ten. ***B. pertussis*** is

an obligate human parasite involving primarily the ciliated epithelial cells of bronchi and trachea. They cause damage to cilia and consequently initiate the irritation that induces increased secretion of mucus which acts as a stimulus for **paroxysmal cough and bronchospasm**. The source of infection is the patient in the early stage. There is no healthy carrier. The organism is acquired through **droplet infection and is highly contagious**, with an attack rate of more than 90% in nonimmunized individuals. The clinical illness can be divided into three stages:

1. Prodromal or catarrhal stage

Infection is initiated 7–10 days after infectious aerosols are inhaled and the bacteria become attached to and proliferate on ciliated epithelial cells. It is characterized by sneezing, mild but irritating cough and little fever. The disease is **highly communicable** at this stage since a large number of organisms are present in the upper respiratory tract. Cultures collected at this time are more likely to be positive.

2. Paroxysmal stage

After 1–2 weeks, the disease enters the paroxysmal stage, in which the cough becomes very violent. During the paroxysm, the patient gets **violent spasms of continuous coughing, followed by a long inrush of air into the almost empty lungs** with a characteristic **'whoop'** that gives the disease its name. The paroxysms of coughing may be so severe that cyanosis, vomiting and convulsions follow, completely exhausting the patient. This stage usually lasts 6–8 weeks, though in some cases it may be very protracted.

3. Convalescent stage

Paroxysmal stage is followed by a convalescent stage that lasts an additional 2–4 weeks. During this period, there is a decrease in the frequency and severity of coughing spells.

The infection is limited to the respiratory tract and the organisms do not invade the blood stream. Complications that may occur during the course of the disease include:

- Secondary infection.
- Otitis media.
- High fever.
- Convulsions.
- Due to pressure effects during coughing, patient may develop subconjunctival haemorrhages, inguinal hernia or rectal prolapse.

Laboratory diagnosis

The bacilli are present in the upper respiratory tract most abundantly in the early stage of the disease. In the paroxysmal stage, the bacilli are scanty and during convalescence they are not demonstrable. Antibodies develop late and help only in retrospective diagnosis. Nasopharyngeal aspirate, cough plate, pernasal swab and post-nasal swab may be collected.

Nasopharyngeal aspirate

Nasopharyngeal aspirate collected through a soft catheter is the optimal diagnostic specimen.

Cough plate method

A culture plate is held about 10–15 cm in front of the patient's mouth during a bout of spontaneous or induced coughing. During the process of coughing, droplets of respiratory exudates are directly deposited on the medium.

Pernasal swab

B. pertussis can be recovered readily from the nasopharynx by pernasal swab. A calcium alginate swab on a flexible nichrome wire is passed gently along the floor of the nasal cavity until stopped by the posterior wall of the nasopharynx. The swab is left in place for 30 seconds to one minute to allow organisms to adsorb onto the swab. Cotton-tipped swab should not be used because cotton is inhibitory to the organisms. Pernasal swab has replaced 'cough plates' and postnasal swabs because of overgrowth by commensal bacteria. A pernasal swab acquires fewer commensals which can be suppressed by incorporation of methicillin or cephalexin in the medium.

Postnasal swab

A calcium alginate swab on a bent wire is employed to collect posterior pharyngeal wall secretions through oral cavity. West's postnatal swab may be conveniently employed. Contamination with saliva should be avoided for better results.

The specimen is inoculated immediately on charcoal blood agar to which cephalexin has been added and incubated in high humidity at 35–36°C for at least seven days before being discarded as negative. If cough plate has been collected, it should also be incubated in high humidity at 35–36°C. The colonies are identified by microscopy, biochemical characters and slide agglutination. If delay in transport is unavoidable, then the specimen may be transported in Regan-Lowe transport medium. The use of transport medium reduces the isolation rate. *B. pertussis* in nasopharyngeal secretions and organisms growing on culture plates may be identified by **direct fluorescent antibody test**.

Polymerase chain reaction (PCR)

PCR is the preferred method for the direct detection of *B. pertussis* and *B. parapertussis* from a nasopharyngeal swab or a nasopharyngeal aspirate.

Serology

Bordetella antibody can be detected in the patient serum by direct agglutination, indirect haemagglutination, complement fixation test and ELISA. However, a negative result does not exclude pertussis because the serological response is often slow and weak especially in very young children. False positive results may occur because of serological cross-reactions with organisms such as staphylococci, haemophili, moraxellae and yeasts. For accurate results paired sera should be examined.

Q. 6. Describe morphology, cultural characteristics, serogrouping, pathogenicity and laboratory diagnosis of *Legionella pneumophila*.

Ans. ***Morphology***

L. pneumophila is a Gram-negative, pleomorphic rod. In infected lung or animal tissues, it appears as short rods or coccobacilli measuring 2–5 µm × 0.3–0.9 µm with pointed ends and a tendency to filament formation on solid culture medium. It is non-sporing, non-acid-fast motile with one or more polar or subpolar flagella, pilated and non-capsulated.

It is Gram-negative but stains less well than most other Gram-negative genera. It may be demonstrated in the tissues by silver impregnation method, immunofluorescence, immuno-electron microscopy or immunoperoxidase staining.

Culture characteristics

L. pneumophila is a strict aerobe with optimum pH and temperature of 6.9 and 35°C respectively. However, it can grow in a temperature range of 29–40°C. It does not grow on ordinary nutrient media but requires the presence of cysteine and iron for primary isolation. It can be grown on buffered charcoal yeast extract agar (BCYE) and Mueller-Hinton medium containing 1% haemoglobin (source of iron) and 1% Isovitalex (source of cysteine).

On BCYE agar, colonies of *L. pneumophila* appear in 2–3 days at 35°C in the presence of 5% CO_2 but with some species primary culture may take up to 10 days and with agar-adapted strains, growth occurs more rapidly. On primary isolation, colonies of *L. pneumophila* reach 1–2 mm in diameter after 2–3 days incubation. They are circular, grey or grey-blue and low convex with a slightly irregular edge. Under the plate microscope, the colonies show 'cut glass' appearance.

Serogrouping

L. pneumophila possesses both flagellar and somatic antigens. On the basis of direct or indirect immunofluorescence with specific antisera and by slide agglutination, it can be divided into 15 (1–15) serogroups. All these serogroups have been associated with human disease but most infections are due to serogroup 1.

Pathogenicity

The natural habitat of *L. pneumophila* is water. The organisms have been isolated from a number of air-conditioning cooling towers, cooling water systems, domestic hot-water systems in hotels and hospitals, whirlpool spa baths and showers, shower heads, industrial coolants and respiratory ventilators. Contaminated water is believed to be a source of infection for those inhaling mist from such sources. Following entry into the alveoli through aerosols, legionellae multiply inside the monocytes and macrophages. Dissemination occurs by endobronchial, haematogenous, lymphatic and contiguous spread.

Outbreaks have also occurred in areas where excavation has taken place. It is, therefore, believed that the organisms may reside in soil and may be transmitted to man by contaminated dust. It has also been shown that *L. pneumophila* may be engulfed by, and survive within, free-living amoebae. When these amoebae form cysts, then the organisms are protected from drying and disinfectants. Person to person spread has not been demonstrated.

Virtually, no data exists on the prevalence of *Legionella* in India. In one report from India 9% of clinical samples and 76% of the environmental samples were positive for *Legionella*.

Legionella infection may occur in two main forms:

1. **Legionnaires' disease:** It is a pneumonia which may also progress to involve virtually every system of the body including the kidney, heart and central nervous system. After an incubation period of 2–10 days, patient develops malaise, fever, myalgia, headache, confusion, respiratory distress and non-productive cough. Reported death rate varies from 20% to more than 50% in immunologically deficient patients.

Incidence of Legionnaires' disease is more in diabetics, alcoholics, smokers, patients with pre-existing lung disease and patients receiving steroid or immunosuppressive therapy. **Pneumonia is the predominant manifestation of *Legionella* disease and places the organism among the top four causes of community-acquired bacterial pneumonia (along with *Streptococcus pneumoniae*, *Mycoplasma pneumoniae*, and *Chlamydia pneumoniae*).**

2. **Pontiac fever:** It is a self limiting, brief febrile influenza-like illness. The disease affects previously healthy people.

Rarely, *L. pneumophila* may be associated with other infections such as prosthetic valve endocarditis or wound infection. These are usually nosocomial infections. Because of their intracellular location, humoral antibodies are ineffective. Cell-mediated immunity plays an important role in the host immunity by preventing intracellular growth of the organisms.

Laboratory diagnosis

The tests employed in diagnosis of *Legionella* infection include the following:

1. Microscopy

Legionellae can be detected in the clinical specimens such as sputum, bronchial aspirate or washings, pleural fluid and lung biopsy or autopsy material, by fluorescent antibody technique, with labelled specific monoclonal or polyclonal antisera. Gram-stained films are of little value because legionellae stain poorly. However, the presence of poorly staining Gram-negative rods in a normally sterile site may suggest the presence of legionellae.

2. Culture

The clinical specimen is inoculated on BCYE agar and BCYE agar containing selective agents – vancomycin, polymyxin B and an antifungal agent such as anisomycin. Contaminated materials such as sputum or postmortem material may be heated at 50°C for 30 minutes in order to diminish growth of other less heat-stable respiratory tract organisms which may inhibit the growth of legionellae. The culture plates are incubated at 35°C in the presence of 5% CO_2 for up to 10 days. The cultures are identified by colonial morphology and by fluorescent antibody technique as above.

3. Detection of Legionella antigen

Legionella antigen in the urine can be detected by enzyme-linked immunosorbent assay (ELISA). This is a rapid and specific test for the identification of *L. pneumophila* as the likely cause of pneumonia. This antigen can also be detected by latex agglutination test.

4. Detection of Legionella antibodies

Antibodies of *L. pneumophila* develop 6–8 days after the clinical onset of the illness, and can be detected by ELISA and indirect fluorescent antibody test with heat-fixed or formalin-fixed antigens. A four-fold or greater rise in antibody titre or a high titre (>256) of antibody in a sample taken late in the illness may be considered diagnostic.

34

Brucella, Mycoplasma and Ureaplasma

Q. 1. Name important *Brucella* species and their hosts.

Ans. The following are the important *Brucella* species and their hosts:

1. *B. melitensis* is the classical species of the genus and is usually pathogenic for sheep and goats but other animals like cattle may also be infected. Man is also susceptible to infection with this organism.
2. *B. abortus* infects cattle, usually causing abortions. It may also infect other animals including sheep, goats, horses and dogs. It can also cause brucellosis in man.
3. *B. suis* is a natural parasite of pigs but other animals and man may also be infected.
4. *B. canis* causes abortion in dogs. Occasional cases of infection, with mild pyrexial illness, have also been reported in man.
5. *B. ovis* causes sexually transmitted epididymitis in rams.
6. *B. neotomae* causes infection of wood rats.

B. ovis and *B. neotomae* do not cause disease in man.

Q. 2. Describe morphology, cultural characteristics, biochemical reactions, antigenic structure, classification and pathogenicity of *Brucella* species.

Ans. ***Morphology***

Brucellae are small, Gram-negative, coccobacilli measuring 0.6–1.5 µm in length and 0.5–0.7 µm in width. They are arranged singly, sometimes in end to end pairs, small clusters or short chains of 4–6 bacteria. They are non-motile, non-sporing, non-capsulated and non-acid-fast.

Cultural characteristics

Brucellae are strict aerobes and **many strains of *B. abortus* and nearly all of *B. ovis* are**

capnophilic, requiring 5–10% CO_2 for growth. The optimum temperature for growth is 37°C (range 20–40°C). The optimum pH for growth is 6.6–7.4. They may grow on nutrient agar, though the growth tends to be slow and colony size small. Growth is improved by the addition of blood, serum and tissue extracts. Trypticase soy agar, serum dextrose agar, serum potato infusion agar and tryptose agar are employed for cultivation of brucellae. **Addition of bacitracin, polymyxin and cycloheximide to the above media makes them selective.** These can be used for isolation of brucellae from contaminated material. **Erythritol has a stimulatory effect on the growth of brucellae.**

On solid media, after incubation at 37°C for 48 hours, they produce small, low convex, circular, smooth, transparent colonies 0.5–1 mm in diameter. Less fastidious strains, especially of *B. melitensis* and *B. suis* can grow on bile salt media producing non-lactose-fermenting colonies. In liquid media, growth is uniform. A powdery or viscous deposit is formed in old cultures.

Biochemical reactions

Brucellae are catalase-positive, urease positive (variable in *B. melitensis*) and usually oxidase-positive but *B. neotomae*, *B. ovis* and some strains of *B. abortus* are oxidase-negative. Most *Brucella* strains reduce nitrates to nitrites. *B. ovis* and occasionally strains of the other species do not reduce nitrate. *B. neotomae*, many strains of *B. abortus* and some strains of *B. suis* produce H_2S from sulphur-containing amino acids. Other species produce it in small quantities or not at all. Citrate is not utilized, indole is not produced and MR and VP are negative.

Antigenic structure

Three major species of *Brucella* contain two main somatic antigenic determinants, A and M. These are present in different amounts. Antigen A is dominant (about 20 times as much as M antigen) in *B. abortus* and antigen M is dominant in *B. melitensis* (about 20 times as much as A antigen). *B. suis* has an intermediate antigenic pattern. Absorption of the minor antigenic components from an antiserum leaves most of the major antibody component. Such absorbed A and M monospecific sera are useful for species identification by agglutination test. However, species identification of *Brucella* strains is not so straightforward and strains are often seen that behave biochemically as *abortus* and serologically as *melitensis* and vice versa. Besides antigenic structure, species and biotype identification depends on a variety of other factors (Table 34.1).

Classification

On the basis of CO_2 requirement, H_2S production, urease production, growth in the presence of 20 μg/ml of basic fuchsin and thionin, and agglutination by monospecific sera, brucellae can be divided into six species (Table 34.1).

Pathogenicity

Brucellae show distinct host preferences. However, they are capable of causing infection in a wide range of host species, including man. *B. melitensis* is the most pathogenic species for man followed by *B. suis*, *B. abortus* and *B. canis*.

Brucellosis is a **zoonosis**. Man acquires infection by:

1. Direct contact with animal tissues. Therefore, farmers, dairy workers, abattoir workers, butchers, live stock producers and veterinarians are particularly at risk.

Table 34.1. Differential characteristics of *Brucella* species and biotypes

Species		CO_2 requirement	H_2S production	Urease production	Growth in the presence of 20 µg/ml of		Agglutination by monospecific sera against			Common reservoir hosts
					Basic fuchsin	Thionin	A	M	R	
B. melitensis	1	–	–	Variable	+	+	–	+	–	Sheep, goat
	2	–	–	Variable	+	+	+	–	–	Sheep, goat
	3	–	–	Variable	+	+	+	+	–	Sheep, goat
B. abortus	1	+(–)	+	1–2 h	+	+	+	–	–	Cattle
	2	+(–)	+	1–2 h	–	–	+	–	–	Cattle
	3	+(–)	+	1–2 h	+	+	+	–	–	Cattle
	4	+(–)	+	1–2 h	–(+)	+	–	+	–	Cattle
	5	–	–	1–2 h	+	+	–	+	–	Cattle
	6	–	+(–)	1–2 h	+	+	+	–	–	Cattle
	9	–	+	1–2 h	+	+	–	+	–	Cattle
B. suis	1	–	+	0–30 min	–(+)	+	+	–	–	Pig
	2	–	–	0–30 min	–	+	+	–	–	Pig, hare
	3	–	–	0–30 min	+	+	+	–	–	Pig
	4	–	–	0–30 min	–(+)	+	+	+	–	Reindeer
	5	–	–	0–30 min	–	+	–	+	–	Rodents
B. canis		–	–	0–30 min	–	+	–	–	+	Dog
B. ovis		+	–	–	–(+)	+	–	–	+	Sheep
B. neotomae		–	+	0–30 min	–	–	+	–	–	Wood rat

+(–), variable but most strains positive; –(+), variable but most strains negative; h, hours; min, minutes; A, *B. abortus*; M, *B. melitensis*; R, rough *Brucella*.

2. Ingestion of contaminated meat, raw infected milk or milk products.
3. Inhalation of aerosolized organisms.
4. In the laboratory, brucellae may be acquired as a result of accidental ingestion, inhalation, injection, and mucosal and skin contamination.
5. Rarely, the disease may be transmitted from person to person by sexual contact and by the transfer of tissues including blood and bone marrow.

After entering into the body, brucellae enter into the lymphatics and lymph nodes, leading to **lymphadenopathy** and subsequent blood stream invasion. From the blood, the organisms are localized in the reticuloendothelial system particularly in liver sinusoids, spleen and bone marrow. However, they may also localize in many other sites like joints, heart, kidneys, central nervous system and genital tract. Intracellular organisms are protected from antibodies and antibiotics. Cellular immune defence mechanisms are required to contain the intracellular bacteria. Infected tissues may have granulomas, microabscesses and unusually caseation.

Following an **incubation period of about three weeks** (with a range from one week to six months), the onset of symptoms may be acute or insidious.

Acute brucellosis

It is characterized by an intermittent fever with a maximum temperature varying from 38–41°C and sometimes higher. The body temperature is usually near normal during the early part of the day but rises sharply during evening. This is accompanied by chills, shivering, malaise, night sweats, severe headache, myalgias and arthralgias. After reaching its peak the temperature shows a rapid fall, accompanied by profuse sweating.

The name '**undulant fever**' has been given to brucellosis because of the periodic noctural fever that may occur over weeks, months or years particularly in untreated cases. Lymphadenopathy, splenomegaly and hepatomegaly may also be present.

Chronic brucellosis

When the disease persists for 6 months or more it is regarded as chronic. It is usually non-bacteraemic low-grade infection with periodic exacerbations. The symptoms are generally related to a state of hypersensitivity. The common manifestations are sweating, lassitude and joint pain, with minimal or no pyrexia. The illness lasts for years.

Q. 3. Describe laboratory diagnosis of brucellosis.

Ans. *I. Culture of brucellae*

Blood culture is the most definitive method for the diagnosis of brucellosis. Chances of getting positive blood culture are more if the blood is collected during the pyrexial phase, preferably when the temperature is rising. Because the organisms may be scanty, at least 5–10 ml should be inoculated into a bottle of **trypticase soy broth or serum dextrose broth** and incubated at 37°C in an atmosphere containing 5–10% carbon dioxide. Other materials such as **bone marrow, solid tissue samples or exudates** are also suitable for culture. Bone marrow cultures yield a higher rate of isolation and remain positive long after the blood culture has become negative.

The intracellular localization of *Brucella* within reticuloendothelial cells may account for the positive cultures from bone marrow aspirates at a time when blood culture from the same patient is negative. Blood culture should be repeated on three successive days. **Subcultures are made every 3–5 days for eight weeks on trypticase soy agar or serum dextrose agar before being discarded as negative.** *B. melitensis* and *B. suis* are more frequently isolated from blood than are *B. abortus* or *B. canis*.

The need for frequent subculture can be avoided by use of a two-phase system or **Castaneda method** of blood culture. In this method, both liquid and solid media are contained within the same bottle (Fig. 34.1). The blood is inoculated into the broth and the bottle incubated in the upright position. For subculture, the bottle is tilted so that the broth flows over the surface of the agar slant. It is again incubated in upright position. In positive cases, colonies appear on the slant. This technique reduces the chances of contamination and risk of infection to laboratory personnel.

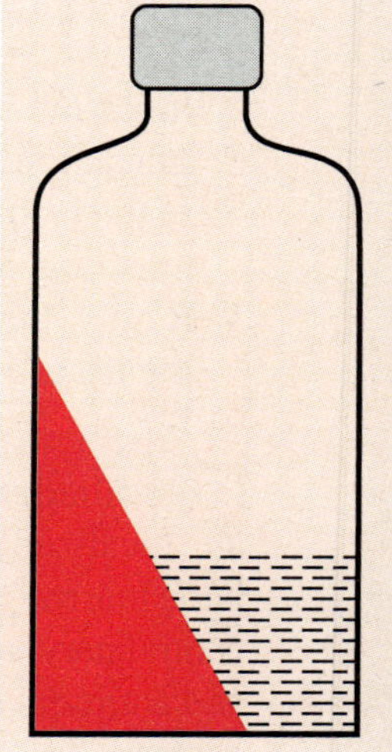

Fig. 34.1. Castaneda blood culture medium.

II. Serological tests

Blood cultures are positive only in about 30–50% of cases, even when repeated samples are tested. Therefore, serological investigation of the patient is of paramount importance for the diagnosis of the disease. Antibodies appear within 7–10 days of onset of the disease. IgM antibodies appear first. They are rapidly followed and superseded by IgG and to a lesser extent IgA antibodies. These antibodies reach their maximum titres in the third or fourth week of disease and then slowly decline, but they usually persist throughout the active phase of the disease and in some cases long thereafter.

Agglutination test identifies mainly the IgM antibody, while both IgM and IgG can fix complement. During the acute phase of illness when IgM agglutinating antibodies predominate, it is easy to detect agglutination. However, as IgG and IgA antibodies are formed during the course of the infection some of them bind with antigen, thus preventing its agglutination by larger IgM molecule. These IgG and IgA antibodies are known as **blocking** or **non-agglutinating antibodies**.

Brucella antibodies can be detected by a variety of serological tests. The most useful are:

- standard tube agglutination test (SAT),
- 2-mercaptoethanol (2ME) agglutination test,
- Rose Bengal plate test,
- complement fixation test,
- anti-human globulin (Coombs') test,
- enzyme-linked immunosorbent assay (ELISA), and
- radioimmunoassay (RIA).

Standard tube agglutination test (SAT)

The most widely used procedure is SAT. This is a tube agglutination test in which equal volumes of serial two-fold dilutions of (uninactivated) patient serum from 1 in 20 to 1 in 640 and the standardised antigen (heat-killed smooth *Brucella* cells in saline containing phenol 0.5%) are mixed, and incubated at 37°C for 24 hours.

Most patients with acute brucellosis develop agglutinin titres of 640 or more by the end of the third or fourth week of illness. Thereafter the titre falls. In normal individuals agglutinin titres vary with geographic location and exposure to the organisms but it is usually less than 1 in 100. A single titre greater than 1 in 160 by SAT is presumptive evidence of recent *Brucella* infection.

Prozone phenomenon is sometimes observed in the agglutination test. This may be due to the antibody excess (therefore, a range of serial dilutions of patient serum should be tested) or due to the presence of blocking or non-agglutinating antibodies. **Blocking antibodies can be detected by anti-human globulin (Coombs') test.** Organisms are exposed to patient serum, incubated for half an hour and then centrifuged, washed and resuspended in normal saline. Washed cells are treated with anti-human globulin which will cause agglutination if blocking antibodies are present in the patient serum.

Agglutination test is usually positive in acute infection as it mainly detects IgM antibodies, but may only be weakly positive or even be negative in chronic cases. The complement fixation test is more useful in chronic cases as it detects both IgG and IgM. 2ME agglutination test has been reliably used to demonstrate IgG (2ME-resistant) agglutinins. 2ME reduces the disulphide bonds that link IgM molecules to release the subunits.

ELISA and RIA

These tests are very sensitive tests and can distinguish IgM, IgG and IgA *Brucella* antibodies. Therefore, these tests are helpful to distinguish acute and chronic brucellosis.

Rose Bengal plate test

It is a rapid slide agglutination test with a buffered stained antigen. It is widely used as a screening test in farm animals, but also gives good results in human brucellosis. It is not affected by prozones or immunoglobulin switching.

Immunofluorescence

Brucellae may be demonstrated microscopically in pathological specimens by immunofluorescence.

III. Polymerase chain reaction

Polymerase chain reaction with primers specific for the *omp 2*, *omp 25* and *rss-rrl* genes can detect *Brucella* specifically and also give an indication of species and biovar. Promising results have been obtained in clinical studies.

IV. Brucellin test (skin test)

This test, similar to tuberculin test, is no longer recommended as it does not differentiate active from past or subclinical infection. Moreover intradermal antigen preparations are not readily available and some interfere with serological response to infection.

Q. 4. Describe briefly morphology and general characters of *Mycoplasma* and *Ureaplasma*.

Ans.

1. Mycoplasmas and ureaplasmas are smallest free-living bacteria. They measure 0.2–0.3 μm in diameter. Therefore, they can pass through the bacterial filters.
2. Mycoplasma cell contains minimum set of organelles essential for growth and replication – a plasma membrane, ribosomes, and a genome consisting of a double-stranded circular DNA molecule.
3. They differ from other bacteria in that they **lack a rigid cell wall** and their cell membrane contains sterols. In contrast, other cell wall-deficient bacteria (called **L forms**) do not have sterols in their cell membrane and can form cell walls under appropriate growth conditions.
4. *Mycoplasma*, *Ureaplasma*, *Spiroplasma* and *Anaeroplasma* **cannot synthesize their own cholesterol** and require it as a growth factor in the culture medium. However, *Acholeplasma* synthesizes carotenol as a substitute for cholesterol, but will incorporate cholesterol if it is provided.
5. Because they lack a rigid cell wall, they are **extremely pleomorphic** varying in shape from coccoid to filamentous and other bizarre forms.
6. Also because of the lack of bacterial cell wall containing peptidoglycan, these organisms are **insensitive to cell wall-active antibiotics** such as penicillins and cephalosporins. The mycoplasmas are susceptible to antibiotics, such as tetracyclines and chloramphenicol, that inhibit protein synthesis on prokaryotic ribosomes.

7. They possess a **small genome** (molecular weight 5–10 × 10^8 daltons). Therefore, these organisms have limited biosynthetic capabilities. Hence for their cultivation, media enriched with precursors for nucleic acid, protein and lipid biosynthesis, and with the exception of *Acholeplasma*, a sterol component are required.
8. They **multiply by binary fission** (typical of all bacteria), grow on artificial cell-free media and contain both RNA and DNA. Cytoplasmic division may lag behind genome replication. This results in the formation of multinucleate filaments and other shapes.
9. They **do not possess flagella or pili**, but some mycoplasmas including *M. pneumoniae*, exhibit gliding motility on liquid-covered surfaces. This is attributed to specialized tip structures that also help the organisms in the attachment to the host cell.
10. They stain poorly by Gram stain and are Gram-negative. They stain well with Giemsa and Dienes' stain.
11. The organisms of the genus *Ureaplasma* can hydrolyze urea while other genera cannot do so.
12. Most species, on solid media, form characteristic small **'fried egg'** colonies.

Q. 5. Describe cultural characteristics of *Mycoplasma* and *Ureaplasma*.

Ans. With the exception of *Anaeroplasma*, the organisms of the order Mycoplasmatales are aerobes and facultative anaerobes. However, for primary isolation, an atmosphere of 95% N_2 and 5% CO_2 is preferred. They can grow within a temperature range of 22–41°C, the parasitic species growing optimally at 35–37°C. For fermentative organisms, the initial pH of the medium should be adjusted to 7.3–7.8, for arginine-metabolizing organisms it should be about 7 and for ureaplasmas, range of pH should be 6.0–6.5.

A medium widely used for the isolation of mycoplasmas consists of bovine heart infusion broth (PPLO broth) to which are added 20% horse serum and 10% fresh yeast extract along with glucose and phenol red as a pH indicator. High concentration of serum is necessary as a source of cholesterol and other lipids. Growth of *M. pneumoniae* is detected by turbidity and colour change (red to yellow) of phenol red indicator due to fermentation of glucose.

Ureaplasma and other mycoplasmas which do not ferment glucose show only turbidity. This medium can be solidified by the addition of agar. Penicillin and polymyxin B may be added to the medium to inhibit contaminating bacteria and amphotericin B to inhibit contaminating fungi. Since thallium acetate is inhibitory for *U. urealyticum* and *M. genitalium*, and highly poisonous for humans, therefore, it should not be added to the medium. A diphasic medium in screw-capped bottle containing an agar phase that is overlain with broth medium of similar composition may also be used.

Colonies usually appear after incubation for 2–3 days. However, media for isolation of genital mycoplasmas and *M. pneumoniae* should be incubated for 1 and 4 weeks respectively, before a final culture report is made. Initially, the mycoplasma cells multiply within the agar to form an opaque ball-shaped colony that grows up to the surface of the agar and spreads around it forming a translucent peripheral zone. Such a colony presents a **'fried egg'** appearance (Fig. 34.2). Colony size varies from 200–500 μm for 'large colony' mycoplasmas to 15–60 μm for the ureaplasmas. The small colonies of the latter usually lack the peripheral zone.

Colonies may be seen with a hand lens. However, visualization of colonial morphology is facilitated by application of **Dienes' stain** directly to the agar surface. For this a block of agar containing the colony is cut and placed on a slide. It is covered with a cover slip on which an alcoholic solution of methylene blue azure has been dried.

Mycoplasmas with the fried egg colony morphology appear highly granular and stain with a dark blue centre and a light blue periphery. The agar background appears clear or slightly violet. Mycoplasmas other than *M. pneumoniae* remain stained, but *M. pneumoniae* reduces the methylene blue after a period of time and becomes colourless.

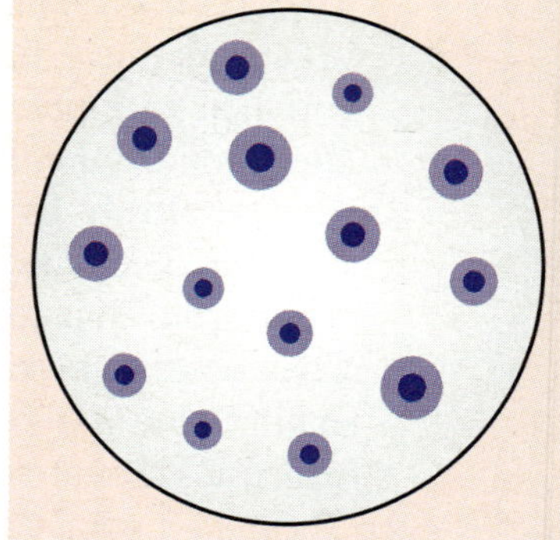

Fig. 34.2. Colonies of *Mycoplasma* on agar, showing 'fried egg' appearance.

Q. 6. Describe briefly pathogenicity of *Mycoplasma pneumoniae, Ureaplasma urealyticum, Mycoplasma hominis* and *Mycoplasma genitalium*.

Ans. Mycoplasmas are **opportunistic infectious agents**. Therefore, the infections caused by these organisms occur more frequently in patients with hypogammaglobulinaemia, Hodgkin's disease, lymphoma, leukaemia, organ transplant and AIDS.

Mycoplasma pneumoniae

1. *M. pneumoniae* (also called **Eaton agent** after the investigator who originally isolated it) commonly causes tracheobronchitis, pharyngitis, sinusitis and **primary atypical pneumonia (PAP)** accompanied by formation of (i) cold haemagglutinins that agglutinate human red cells in cold, (ii) *Streptococcus* MG agglutinins, and (iii) antibodies giving biological false positive Wasserman reaction. Penicillin has no effect on PAP which has served to differentiate PAP from typical pneumonias.
2. *M. pneumoniae* has been shown to produce an exotoxin that is believed to play a major role in the damage to the respiratory epithelium that occurs during acute infection. This toxin, named the **community acquired respiratory disease (CARD) toxin**, is an ADP-ribosylating and vacuolating cytotoxin similar to pertussis toxin. The organism also has the ability to exist and possibly replicate intracellularly, which may contribute to chronicity of illness and difficult eradication.
3. In addition, *M. pneumoniae* may also cause extrapulmonary lesions such as arthritis, hepatitis, meningoencephalitis, cerebral ataxia, transverse myelitis, Guillain-Barré syndrome, haemolytic anaemia, myocarditis and pericarditis.

M. pneumoniae is transmitted from person to person through airborne transfer of droplets containing the organisms. They attach to epithelial cells in the respiratory tract and multiply. *M. pneumoniae* possesses a membrane-associated 169 kDa protein called PI, which is known to mediate the adherence of this organism to the host cell. **It is a surface parasite. It does not penetrate the epithelial cells of the respiratory tract but remains localized and invasion of blood stream is very rare.**

Incubation period is 1–3 weeks. The onset is gradual. Patient develops fever with chills, malaise, headache, sore throat, nasal congestion and nonproductive cough. The disease is self-limited, recovery occurring in 3–10 days without antimicrobial therapy.

Ureaplasma urealyticum

1. *U. urealyticum* may cause nonchlamydial, non-gonococcal urethritis (NGU), epididymitis, vaginitis and cervicitis. However, *Chlamydia trachomatis* appears to be responsible for 30–50% cases of NGU and cervicitis.
2. Ureaplasmas may cause prematurity, postpartum endometritis, chronic lung disease of the premature infant and infection of wounds and soft tissues.
3. Ureaplasmas are the commonest organisms isolated from the CNS or lower respiratory tract of sick premature or newborn infants.
4. Ureaplasmas have also been blamed to cause male and female infertility and low birth weight but there are conflicting reports.

Mycoplasma hominis

1. *M. hominis* may cause salpingitis, tubo-ovarian abscess, pelvic abscess, septic abortion, puerperal infection, septic arthritis, septic thrombophlebitis, peritonitis and brain abscess.
2. It may cause PAP similar to that caused by *M. pneumoniae* and meningitis in newborn.

Mycoplasma genitalium

M. genitalium has been associated with some cases of non-gonococcal urethritis and pelvic inflammatory disease. Its prevalence is not known, but it may be primarily a resident of the gastrointestinal tract that occurs secondarily in the genitourinary or respiratory tract. It is very difficult to recover from culture and may require 2–3 months of incubation.

Q. 7. Describe laboratory diagnosis of *Mycoplasma* and *Ureaplasma*.

Ans. Laboratory diagnosis of *Mycoplasma* and *Ureaplasma* infections may be carried out by (i) culture and (ii) serological tests.

I. Culture

M. pneumoniae may be recovered from throat swabs, nasopharyngeal swabs, sputum, throat washings, bronchoalveolar lavage, tracheal aspirate and lung tissue specimens. Genital mycoplasmas may be isolated from urethral, vaginal and cervical swabs, semen, prostatic secretions, urine, blood, CSF, amniotic fluid, respiratory tract secretions, synovial fluid, pericardial fluid, and biopsy specimens from endometrium, fallopian tubes, placenta and aborted foetus.

Because of the fastidious nature of these bacteria, the culture media should be inoculated as soon after collection as possible. Standard *Mycoplasma* broth medium dispensed into small vials may be used for transport of swab specimens, while other specimens may be transported in sterile screw-capped containers. In the laboratory, if inoculation is not possible immediately, then the specimen may be held up to 24 hours at 4°C. If delay more than 24 hours is expected, then the specimen should be frozen at –70°C. Urine specimen should be centrifuged and deposit inoculated into the culture medium. If inoculation is not immediately possible, then urine deposit should be diluted with equal volume of transport medium and frozen.

Mycoplasma broth medium, containing penicillin, polymyxin B, amphotericin B, glucose and phenol red as a pH indicator is inoculated with the specimen and incubated at 37°C preferably in an atmosphere of 95% N_2 and 5% CO_2. If specimen contains *M. pneumoniae*, its growth is revealed by turbidity and a colour change (red to yellow) of phenol red, due to fermentation of glucose. It usually occurs in 4–28 days. Ureaplasmas and other mycoplasmas which do not ferment glucose will show only turbidity. It is then subcultured on agar medium and incubated in air for 5–7 days. *M. pneumoniae* form large (200–500 μm) colonies with a characteristic 'fried egg' appearance, while colonies of ureaplasmas are small, 15–60 μm in diameter and usually lack peripheral zone. Colonies of *M. pneumoniae* may be identified by:

1. ***Haemadsorption test:*** Colonies growing on the surface of the agar are flooded with 2 ml of 0.2–0.4% suspension of washed guinea-pig erythrocytes suspended in *Mycoplasma* broth medium. The plate is then incubated at 35°C for 30 minutes. It is occasionally rotated during this time. It is then washed with 3 ml of *Mycoplasma* broth medium by gently rotating the plate. Wash fluid is removed by aspiration with a pipette and colonies examined under 50× to 100× magnification. Colonies of *M. pneumoniae* adsorb the erythrocytes to their surface. This is due to binding of the *Mycoplasma* to sialic acid-containing oligosaccharides present on the surface of erythrocytes. However, colonies of *M. genitalium* also share this property.
2. ***Tetrazolium reduction test:*** Colonies of *M. pneumoniae* appear red when these are flooded with solution of tetrazolium compound which is colourless. *M. pneumoniae* reduces tetrazolium (colourless) to red-coloured compound.
3. ***Serological techniques:*** These include inhibition of colony development around discs impregnated with specific antiserum, or the fluorescence of colonies treated with such antiserum labelled with a fluorochrome.

II. Serological tests

These are of three types: (a) detection of antigen; (b) detection of specific DNA; and (c) detection of antibody.

(a) ***Detection of antigen:*** Detection of antigen in respiratory exudates by direct immunofluorescence and counterimmunoelectrophoresis techniques, immunoblotting with monoclonal antibodies and enzyme immunoassay.

(b) ***Detection of specific DNA:*** Detection of specific DNA by dot blot hybridization and PCR in respiratory exudate.

(c) ***Detection of antibody:***

1. **Cold agglutinins:** Cold agglutinins (IgM antibodies that bind the I antigen on the surface of human erythrocytes at 4°C) can be detected by agglutination of O Rh-negative erythrocytes at 4°C. Cold agglutinins appear about one week after infection with a peak at 4–5 weeks. Thereafter, titre declines rapidly and the test becomes negative after about 5 months. A four-fold rise in cold agglutinin titres or a single titre of 64 or more is suggestive of *M. pneumoniae* infection. However, demonstrable cold agglutinin titres develop in 50% of patients only. Moreover, cold agglutinins are occasionally induced in other diseases such as infectious mononucleosis, rubella, adenovirus infections, psittacosis, tropical eosinophilia, trypanosomiasis, cirrhosis of liver, paroxysmal haemoglobinuria and haemolytic anaemia.

2. ***Streptococcus* MG agglutination test:** In this test, a heat-killed suspension of *Streptococcus* MG is mixed with serial dilutions of patient's unheated serum. The agglutination is observed after overnight incubation at 37°C. An antibody titre of 1 : 20 or more is suggestive of *M. pneumoniae* infection.
3. **Complement fixation test:** This is the most widely used serological test for diagnosis of *M. pneumoniae* infection. The antigen used is a glycolipid from the organism that is extracted by chloroform-methanol. A recent infection is indicated by four-fold or more rise in antibody titre or a single titre of 64 or more. Complement fixing antibodies appear 7–10 days after infection with the organism and reach peak titre after 4–6 weeks. Such results are obtained in about 80% of cases.
4. **Enzyme immunoassay:** This is more sensitive test than complement fixation test. It can be used to detect specific IgM, IgG and IgA antibodies against *M. pneumoniae*.

Q. 8. Write short note on atypical pneumonia.

Ans. In the past, any patient who presented with a sudden onset of fever with shaking chills, pleuritic pain and the production of rust-coloured sputum was thought to have typical pneumonia attributable to *Streptococcus pneumoniae*. All other patients who did not show this characteristic picture were referred to as patients with 'atypical pneumonia'. *M. pneumoniae*, *Legionella pneumophila* and *Chlamydophila pneumoniae* are three atypical pathogens responsible for community acquired pneumonia (CAP). The only thing 'atypical' about these pathogens is that they are not recovered on routine sputum cultures.

Atypical pathogens do not respond to β-lactam antibiotics and their presence is often overlooked untill patients fail to respond to standard penicillin or cephalosporin therapy. β-lactam antibiotics act by inhibiting cell wall synthesis. This makes them ineffective against *Mycoplasma*. Neither penicillin nor cephalosporins have good intracellular penetration. Hence they are also ineffective against *Chlamydia* and *Legionella*.

35

Rickettsia, Orientia, Ehrlichia, Anaplasma, Neorickettsia, Coxiella and Bartonella

Q. 1. Describe morphology and general characters of *Rickettsia* and *Orientia*.

Ans. 1. The organisms of these genera are small (0.3–0.5 × 0.8–1.0 μm) Gram-negative bacilli. They are non-motile and non-capsulated. The stains commonly used for staining these organisms are Gimenez, Macchiavello and Giemsa. They appear deep red with Gimenez and Macchiavello, and purple with Giemsa stain.

2. They are **obligate intracellular parasites**.
3. They require an arthropod vector as part of their natural cycle and are **transmitted to man by blood sucking arthropods**. They are found in the alimentary canal of arthropods. The species that are pathogenic for humans parasitize endothelial cells almost exclusively.
4. They multiply by binary fission.
5. They possess a trilaminar cytoplasmic membrane and cell wall of bacterial type.
6. They are sensitive to lysozyme and antibiotics.
7. They possess both RNA and DNA.
8. They are large enough to be seen under the light microscope and are held back by bacterial filters.
9. Scrub typhus rickettsiae appear to be fundamentally different and have been placed in a separate genus as *Orientia tsutsugamushi*.

Q. 2. Describe cultural characteristics, antigenic structure and pathogenicity of *Rickettsia* species.

Ans. ***Cultural characteristics***

Rickettsiae are **unable to grow on cell free media**. Growth generally takes place in the cytoplasm of infected cells, but in the case of spotted fever rickettsiae, growth may take place in the nucleus as well. **Embryonated hens' eggs, inoculated in the yolk sac** during the 5th or 6th day of development, are highly susceptible to infection. Rickettsiae grow in the cells of the membrane surrounding the yolk.

The inoculated eggs are incubated for eight days. Optimum temperature of incubation for most rickettsiae is 35°C and for those of the spotted fever group is 33°C. After incubation, the eggs are harvested and the yolk sac membrane is removed. It serves as an excellent source of organisms for diagnostic antigens and vaccines. Limited growth occurs on the chorioallantoic membrane also.

They can also grow on **mouse fibroblasts, HeLa, HEp-2, Detroit 6 and other continuous cell lines**, but tissue cultures are not satisfactory for primary isolation of rickettsiae from the patient. They may also be propagated in **arthropods**. **Guinea pig and mice** are commonly used laboratory animals for isolation of *Rickettsia* from patients.

Antigenic structure

Rickettsiae possess at least three types of antigens:

1. A **group-specific soluble antigen** present on the surface of the organisms. This can be separated from the organisms by repeated washing and centrifugation.
2. A **species-specific**, and in case of scrub typhus **strain-specific** antigen associated with the cell wall of the organisms.
3. An **alkali-stable polysaccharide** found in some rickettsiae and in some strains of *Proteus* (OX19, OX2 and OXK). This sharing of antigen between rickettsiae and *Proteus* is the basis of **Weil-Felix reaction** used for the diagnosis of rickettsial infections, by demonstration of agglutinins to the above *Proteus* strains.

Pathogenicity

Rickettsiae are transmitted to man by the bite or faeces of an infected arthropod vector. On entry into human body, they multiply locally and enter the blood stream followed by multiplication of the organisms in the endothelial cells lining the small blood vessels. This leads to endothelial proliferation and perivascular infiltration which results in thrombosis of the vessel leading to rupture and necrosis.

Rickettsiae exhibit two types of toxicity. They possess an endotoxin that kills mice following intravenous injection. Endotoxin activity is specifically neutralized by antiserum. The second toxic activity is haemolysis of sheep and rabbit erythrocytes. However, the role of endotoxin and haemolytic activity in human rickettsial disease remains conjectural.

Diseases caused by various species of *Rickettsia* include typhus fevers, spotted fevers and scrub typhus (Table 35.1).

Q. 3. Describe typhus fevers. How will you differentiate *Rickettsia typhi* from *Rickettsia prowazekii*?

Ans. This group consists of epidemic (classical) typhus and its recrudescent infection (Brill-Zinsser disease), and endemic (murine) typhus.

Epidemic (classical) typhus

It has been **one of the great scourges of the world**, appearing during periods of crowding, war, poverty, famine and starvation. The disease has been reported from all parts of the world, but has been particularly common in Russia and Eastern Europe and was a major factor in Napoleon's defeat in Russia in 1812. Epidemic typhus, relapsing fever and dysentery were responsible for ruin and misery during the Irish famine of 1845–50.

Table 35.1. Rickettsial diseases of man

Group	Disease	Causative agent	Insect vector	Mode of transmission
1. Typhus fevers	• Epidemic typhus	*R. prowazekii*	Human body louse	Louse faeces scratched into skin
	• Recrudescent typhus (Brill-Zinsser disease)	*R. prowazekii*	—	—
	• Murine typhus (syn. *R. mooseri*)	*R. typhi*	Rat flea	Rat flea faeces scratched into skin
2. Spotted fevers	• Rocky mountain spotted fever	*R. rickettsii*	Ixodid ticks	Tick bite
	• Boutonneuse fever	*R. conorii*	Ixodid ticks	Tick bite
	• Australian tick typhus	*R. australis*	Ixodid ticks	Tick bite
	• Siberian tick typhus	*R. sibirica*	Ixodid ticks	Tick bite
	• Rickettsialpox	*R. akari*	Mites	Mite bite
3. Scrub typhus	• Scrub typhus	*O. tsutsugamushi*	Trombiculid mites	Mite bite

R. prowazekii, the causative agent of epidemic typhus, is named after von Prowazek who died of typhus fever while investigating the disease. It can infect both the human body louse (*Pediculus humanus corporis*) and the head louse (*Pediculus humanus capitis*). However, the former is a more significant vector and pubic louse is not infected by *R. prowazekii*. Lice become infected by ingesting the blood from a rickettsiaemic human. The rickettsiae multiply in the gut of lice and appear in the faeces after about a week. Lice do not transmit *R. prowazekii* to their progeny but succumb to the infection within 2–4 weeks, remaining infective till they die. Lice are sensitive to temperature. They abandon a host with a body temperature of 40°C or more or the cooling carcass and parasitize other persons.

Lice defaecate while feeding. The feeding process is irritating and scratching by the host produces minute abrasions that function as portal of entry for the rickettsiae in the louse faeces. Occasionally, infection may also be transmitted by inhalation of dried louse faeces containing viable rickettsiae or through the conjunctiva. *R. prowazekii* has been demonstrated in flying squirrels in the United States and a small number of associated human infections have occurred. Therefore, flying squirrels may act as a non-human reservoir of *R. prowazekii*.

After an **incubation period of 10–14 days**, patient develops severe headache, chills, generalized myalgia, high fever (39–41°C) and vomiting. Four to seven days after the onset of illness, a macular rash appears first on the trunk and then spreads to the limbs but sparing face, palms and soles. In the second and third weeks, the patient may become comatosed or delirious. Patient may also develop patchy pneumonia and gangrene of toes, feet, tips of fingers, ear lobes, nose, penis, scrotum or vulva. Mortality rate varies from 10–40% and increases with age.

Brill-Zinsser disease (Recrudescent typhus)

In some individuals who recover from epidemic typhus, **the rickettsiae may remain latent in the lymphoid tissues or organs for years**. Such latent infection may be reactivated, many years later, leading to recrudescent typhus. Lice that feed on a patient with recrudescent typhus can become infected and if conditions are favourable for louse-human-louse transmission, an outbreak of epidemic typhus may result. Therefore, latent human infections, act as a reservoir of *R. prowazekii*.

Brill-Zinsser disease is a milder illness. The duration of disease is shorter (less than two weeks), skin rash is rare, fever is erratic and case fatality rate is lower. Patient develops severe headache, malaise and myalgia. The disease was first noticed by Brill (1898), and Zinsser (1934) isolated *R. prowazekii* from such cases. Hence the disease is called Brill-Zinsser's disease.

Endemic (murine) typhus

It is a milder disease than epidemic typhus. It is caused by *R. typhi* (syn. *R. mooseri*). Rat acts as a reservoir and the rickettsiae are passed from rat to rat by two of its ectoparasites, the rat flea (*Xenopsylla cheopis*) and the rat louse (*Polypax spinulosa*), the former is also the vector for man. Rat flea acquires infection by feeding upon a rickettsiaemic rat. The rickettsiae multiply in the gut of the flea. It may infect other susceptible rats and thus a natural cycle of flea-rat-flea infection may become established. The flea is not incapacitated and goes on excreting rickettsiae in its faeces for long periods. Infection in flea is not transmitted trans-ovarially.

Man acquires the infection usually through the bite of infected fleas. When infected flea takes a blood meal, it defaecates on the host. The latter rubs the infected faeces into minute abrasions (produced by scratching) that function as portal of entry for rickettsiae in the infected faeces. Infection may also be transmitted by:

1. ingestion of food contaminated with infected rat urine or flea faeces,
2. inhalation of dried flea faeces, and
3. contamination of respiratory tract or conjunctiva, with infective flea faeces.

Man-to-man transmission does not occur. ***R. typhi*** **can be differentiated from *R. prowazekii* by the following tests:**

1. *Neil-Mooser or tunica reaction:* When a male guinea-pig is inoculated intraperitoneally with blood from a case of endemic typhus or with a culture of *R. typhi*, it develops fever and a characteristic scrotal inflammation. The scrotum becomes enlarged and the testes cannot be pushed back into the abdomen because of inflammatory adhesions between the layers of the tunica vaginalis. This is known as Neil-Mooser or tunica reaction. This reaction is negative with *R. prowazekii*.
2. Partial sequence homology with *R. prowazekii*.
3. The two rickettsiae can also be differentiated by IFA, ELISA and PCR-based DNA tests.

Clinically, endemic typhus resembles epidemic typhus but it is usually a mild illness of shorter duration, has fewer complications and has a case fatality rate of less than 1%. Patient develops fever, headache, malaise and myalgia. Macular rash appears on third to fifth day on trunk and spreads to the extremities. As in epidemic typhus, the involvement of palms, soles and face is rare. Untreated, the illness may last up to two weeks.

Q. 4. Describe spotted fevers.

Ans. Rickettsiae of spotted fevers possess a common soluble group antigen and grow in both the nucleus and the cytoplasm of infected cells. These diseases include Rocky Mountain spotted fever (RMSF), boutonneuse fever, Australian tick typhus, Siberian tick typhus and rickettsialpox. The infection is transmitted by ticks except in case of rickettsialpox, in which mite is the vector (Table 35.1). *Rickettsiae are transmitted transovarially in ticks and mites which act both as vectors and reservoirs*. Human infection occurs by the bite of an infected tick or mite or by ingestion of food contaminated with their faeces. Rickettsiae do not harm ticks and mites. An eschar frequently develops at the site of tick bite in spotted fevers except RMSF.

Rocky Mountain spotted fever

RMSF is the most serious type of spotted fevers. It is caused by *R. rickettsii*. After an incubation period of about one week, the patient develops fever (39.4–40°C), severe headache, myalgia, anorexia, vomiting, abdominal pain, diarrhoea, photophobia and cough. The rash usually appears on the fourth day of fever, initially on wrists, ankles, palms and soles and then becomes generalized. The rash is maculopapular early in the disease but may later become petechial, and in grave cases, haemorrhagic. In addition to haemorrhagic rash, vascular damage may lead to hypovolaemia, hypotensive shock, hemiplegia and other neurological signs and symptoms, and the patient may die within five days of onset of symptoms. Average mortality in untreated cases of RMSF varies from 6–70%.

Other tick-borne diseases

Other tick-borne diseases, i.e., Boutonneuse fever, Australian tick typhus (North Queensland tick typhus) and Siberian tick typhus (North Asian tick-borne spotted fever) caused by *R. conorii*, *R. australis* and *R. sibirica* respectively (Table 35.1), resemble RMSF in many respects. All these three rickettsiae are maintained in nature in ixodid ticks and wild animals. Humans only accidentally enter their natural cycle of infection. Diseases produced by these rickettsiae resemble RMSF but are milder. A black spot having a necrotic centre (eschar) is normally present at the site of tick bite in the early stage of disease.

Rickettsialpox

This is a benign febrile disease with a papulovesicular rash resembling that of chickenpox. It is caused by *R. akari* (*akari* means mite). Common house mouse (*Mus musculus*) acts as a reservoir and the rickettsiae are passed from mouse to mouse by its ectoparasite, the mite (*Liponyssoides sanguineus*). **The mite infects its progeny transovarially.** As in case of several other rickettsial diseases, humans enter this cycle of infection only accidentally. When murine hosts are scarce, the mite readily attacks humans.

Clinically, patient develops a papulovesicular lesion at the site of bite and the enlargement of regional lymph nodes. This is followed in 3–10 days by fever, chills, headache, malaise and myalgia. About 3–4 days after the appearance of fever, a generalized papulovesicular rash, not unlike the rash in chickenpox appears. The illness lasts for 10–14 days, after which recovery occurs.

Q. 5. Write short note on scrub typhus.

Ans. It is caused by *O. tsutsugamushi*. Scrub typhus normally occurs in a range of mammals, particularly field mice and rats and also birds including migratory birds, all of which can act as host reservoirs. Migratory birds may act as transporters of the disease agent over long distances. The rickettsiae are transmitted from animal to animal by trombiculid mites.

In scrub typhus, as in rickettsialpox, RMSF and murine typhus, humans only accidentally enter a natural cycle of rickettsial infection. Trombiculid mites have four-stage life cycles (egg, larva, nymph and adult). The larva (chigger) is the only stage that feeds on vertebrates. Mites lay their eggs in the soil and the larvae hatch later and feed on animals, including humans. After feeding, larvae drop off and metamorphose into nymphs and subsequently into adults. The latter two stages are free living in the soil. However, transmission of *O. tsutsugamushi* occurs from larva to nymph to adult and transovarially from adult to egg. Thus, the mite can act both as a vector and as a reservoir for scrub typhus.

After 1–3 weeks of chigger bite, patient abruptly develops severe headache, chills, fever, conjunctivitis, deafness and a characteristic eschar at the site of chigger bite. Spleen, and lymph nodes proximal to eschar enlarge. About one week after the onset of fever, a maculopapular rash appears on the trunk which later becomes generalized. This may be accompanied by stupor and prostration. Case fatality rate varies from 10–60%.

Q. 6. Describe laboratory diagnosis of rickettsial infections.

Ans. It may be carried out by:

1. Isolation of rickettsiae in laboratory animals, embryonated hen's eggs and cell cultures.
2. Direct detection of the organisms and their antigens in clinical specimens.
3. Serology.

1. Isolation of rickettsiae

As rickettsiae are highly infectious, **isolation should be attempted only in laboratories equipped with appropriate safety provisions.** Blood clot ground in skimmed milk or brain-heart infusion broth is inoculated intraperitoneally in male guinea-pigs or mice. The inoculated animals are observed for 3–4 weeks. The response of animals to different rickettsial infections vary:

- In RMSF, guinea-pigs develop fever, scrotal necrosis and may even die due to overwhelming infection of *R. rickettsii*.
- In *R. typhi*, *R. conorii* and *R. akari* infection, guinea-pigs develop fever and tunica reaction.
- In *R. prowazekii* infection, the animals develop fever without any testicular inflammation.
- For isolation of *O. tsutsugamushi*, mice are preferred over guinea-pigs. The infected animals become ill and develop ascites.
- Smears from peritoneum, tunica and spleen of infected animals may be stained by Giemsa or Gimenez methods to demonstrate the rickettsiae.
- Rickettsiae can also be grown in the yolk sac of embryonated hens' eggs and cell cultures.

2. Direct detection of the organisms and their antigens

Biopsy specimens from the rash of spotted fever, and chronic hepatitis, impression smears from the organs of infected animals, and endolymph from ticks may be stained with Giemsa, Macchiavello or Gimenez stains and with direct and indirect immunofluorescence techniques. In tissue smears, rickettsiae are usually seen as bipolar rods occurring near cells or free in the cytoplasm. *R. rickettsii* may also be seen within the nuclei of infected cells.

Immunofluorescence technique has the benefits of greater sensitivity and specificity as compared with classical staining methods. The sensitivity of the procedure in the detection of antigens of *R. rickettsii* is approximately 70% and the specificity approaches 100%. By immunofluorescence technique, antigens can also be demonstrated in paraffin-embedded, formalin fixed specimens if the section is treated first with trypsin to unmask antigens.

Molecular methods

Primers and probes for unique sequences in the genome of the rickettsiae or its plasmids have been synthesized and the sequences amplified by PCR.

3. Serological diagnosis of rickettsial diseases

Serological diagnosis of rickettsial diseases may be done by Weil-Felix (WF) reaction or by specific tests using rickettsial antigens. The latter include:

- Complement fixation test with purified antigens.
- Immunofluorescence on microdots of purified rickettsiae.
- Enzyme immunoassay with particulate or extracted antigens.
- Latex agglutination test.

Complement fixation test is very specific but relatively insensitive for the diagnosis of rickettsial infections. Latex agglutination test is commercially available for the diagnosis of RMSF. It is positive only during an acute infection, so a single positive test is diagnostic.

Weil-Felix reaction

It is an agglutination test which detects anti-rickettsial antibodies that cross-react with certain strains of *Proteus*. The basis of this test is the sharing of an **alkali-stable carbohydrate antigen** of some rickettsiae with O antigen of certain non-motile strains of *Proteus* – *P. vulgaris* OX19 and OX2, and *P. mirabilis* OXK. The test may be performed as a micro-agglutination reaction in microtitre plates with round bottomed wells with haematoxylin-stained antigen or as a tube agglutination test.

Sera from patients with epidemic and endemic typhus strongly agglutinate OX19 and weakly agglutinate OX2. In Brill-Zinsser disease, the test is negative or weakly reactive. In spotted fevers both OX19 and OX2 are agglutinated. OXK agglutinins are present only in scrub typhus (Table 35.2). However, this test is both insensitive and nonspecific. The agglutinins usually appear as early as 5–7 days and reach peak titres of up to 1 : 1,000 or 1 : 5,000 by the end of second week and decline rapidly during convalescence.

Table 35.2. Weil-Felix reaction in rickettsial disease

Disease	Agglutination with		
	OX19	OX2	OXK
Epidemic typhus	+++	+	–
Brill-Zinsser disease	±/–	–	–
Endemic typhus	+++	±	–
Spotted typhus	++	++	–
Scrub typhus	–	–	+++

Q. 7. Describe briefly species of *Ehrlichia*, *Neorickettsia* and *Anaplasma*, and their laboratory diagnosis.

Ans. 1. ***Ehrlichia chaffeensis:*** It infects human monocytic cells and causes **human monocytic ehrlichiosis**. It produces febrile illness with leucopenia, thrombocytopenia, perivascular

lymphohistiocytic infiltrates in many organs and non-necrotizing granulomata in bone marrow and liver. It is transmitted to humans by ticks (*Amblyomma americanum*). It occurs in the USA, Europe and Africa.
2. ***E. ewingii:*** It was found in the blood of patients with human monocytic ehrlichiosis like disease.
3. ***Neorickettsia sennetsu:*** It produces **sennetsu neorickettsiosis**, an illness resembling glandular fever (*sennetsu* means glandular fever). Patient develops lymphoid hyperplasia and atypical lymphocytosis. It is suspected to be ingested with raw fish. It occurs in Japan and Malaysia.
4. ***Anaplasma phagocytophilum:*** It infects human granulocytic cells and causes **human granulocytic anaplasmosis**. It produces febrile illness with leucopenia and thrombocytopenia. Like, *E. chaffeensis* it is also transmitted to humans by *Ixodes ricinus*-like ticks. It occurs in the USA and Europe.

Laboratory diagnosis

1. Human granulocytic anaplasmosis may be diagnosed by demonstration of **bluish intracytoplasmic inclusion (morula)** in Giemsa-stained peripheral blood neutrophils. Inclusions in monocytic ehrlichiosis are less common.
2. Diagnosis may be established by demonstration of specific antibodies by indirect immunofluorescent methods using cell culture-propagated organisms.
3. *E. chaffeensis* and *Anaplasma phagocytophilum* infections have also been diagnosed by PCR.

Q. 8. Describe morphology, resistance to physical and chemical agents, pathogenicity, laboratory diagnosis and prophylaxis of *Coxiella burnetii*.

Ans. ***Morphology***

Coxiella burnetii is also an obligate intracellular pathogen. It is a pleomorphic, coccobacillary bacterium measuring 0.4–1.0 × 0.2–0.4 μm in size. It has a Gram-negative cell wall but it does not stain well. It grows within the phagolysosome of macrophages of the vertebrate host.

Resistance to physical and chemical agents

It is more resistant to heat and drying than many non-sporing microorganisms. **It survives holder method (63°C for 30 minutes) of pasteurization of milk** and is at borderline of inactivation by the flash method (72°C for 15–20 seconds) of pasteurization. It can remain infectious for months in milk, tap water, soil, dried blood and on wool. Therefore, it can survive in dust and aerosols and can be transmitted as an airborne infection. It can be inactivated by 2% formaldehyde, 1% lysol and 5% hydrogen peroxide.

Pathogenicity

C. burnetii causes **Q fever** which has a worldwide distribution. In nature, there are two cycles of infection with this organism, one in wild animals with ixodid ticks and the other in domestic animals (cattle, sheep and goats). The latter cycle is not dependent on arthropod transmission, but is maintained primarily through airborne transmission. Infected domestic animals do not appear ill, but shed large numbers of infectious organisms in their milk, urine, faeces and particularly in their placental product. Infectious organisms in placental products become aerosolized after parturition which contaminate the surrounding area. Dust in sheep or cattle sheds may become heavily contaminated and function as a source of infection for susceptible animals and man.

Human infections have been traced to:

1. consumption of infected milk,
2. handling of infected wool or hides,
3. soil contaminated with faeces of infected animals,
4. infected straw, and
5. contaminated clothing.

Man to man transmission of Q fever can also occur. Ticks do not play any significant role in transmitting the infection to man. After an incubation period of 2–4 weeks, patient develops fever, chills, headache, malaise, myalgia, pneumonia, hepatitis, endocarditis and meningoencephalitis. Unlike most rickettsial diseases, no skin rash occurs in Q fever. The organisms may remain latent in the tissues of patients for months or years and latent infection may become activated naturally or by use of X-ray treatment or multiple cortisone injections.

Laboratory diagnosis

C. burnetii can be isolated from clinical specimens by intraperitoneal inoculation of guinea-pigs and mice, and yolk sac of embryonated hen's eggs. However, **unless special facilities are available, isolations should not be attempted**. Therefore, diagnosis mainly relies on the demonstration of specific antibodies by complement fixation test and indirect immunofluorescence assay. Weil-Felix test is negative in Q fever.

Prophylaxis

Measures for control of Q fever include:

- Separate facilities for animal parturition.
- Destruction of suspected placentas.
- Heat treatment of milk at 74°C for 15 seconds.
- Abattoir workers should take care like wearing of gloves, glasses, mask, etc. while handling carcasses and animal hides.

Q. 9. Describe morphology, cultural characteristics, pathogenicity, laboratory diagnosis, and treatment and prophylaxis of *Bartonella bacilliformis*.

Ans.

Morphology

B. bacilliformis is small, Gram-negative coccobacillus (0.3–1.5 × 0.2–0.5 μm). The organisms occur singly, in pairs, chains or clumps. They are motile by means of 10 flagella situated at one end of the bacterium.

Cultural characteristics

They are strict aerobes, optimum pH and temperature for growth are 7.8 and 25–28°C respectively. They can grow in semisolid nutrient agar containing rabbit serum and haemoglobin. Growth is slow and becomes visible after 10 days incubation.

Pathogenicity

B. bacilliformis causes **Oroya fever**, spread by sandflies. After the bite, the bacteria reach blood circulation, multiply and invade RBCs. This causes an increase in the fragility of the RBCs, thereby facilitating their removal by the reticuloendothelial cells of the spleen, thus leading to severe anaemia. After an incubation period of 3 weeks to 3 months patient develops fever, severe headache and chills, followed by severe anaemia. Patient may also develop enlargement of spleen and liver, and haemorrhages into the lymph nodes. Case fatality rate may be up to 40%.

Several weeks after recovery, or even without the initial attack of Oroya fever, patient may develop nodular lesions on skin usually of exposed parts of the body, on mucous membranes or in internal organs. These may become secondarily infected producing ulcers and haemorrhagic lesions. This condition is known as **verruga peruana**.

Laboratory diagnosis

1. *B. bacilliformis* can be demonstrated in blood smears stained by Giemsa. Organisms are seen in the cytoplasm of erythrocytes as well as adhering to the cell surfaces.
2. Organisms may be isolated from the blood, in semi-solid medium containing rabbit serum and haemoglobin.
3. Guinea pig inoculation leads to verruga peruana but not Oroya fever

Treatment and prophylaxis

1. *B. bacilliformis* is susceptible to penicillin, streptomycin, tetracycline and chloramphenicol. These may be used for the treatment of Oroya fever and verruga peruana.
2. Insecticides such as DDT should be used to eliminate the sandfly inside and outside the houses.

Q. 10. Describe morphology, cultural characteristics, pathogenicity and laboratory diagnosis of *Bartonella quintana*.

Ans.

Morphology

B. quintana (formerly *Rochalimaea quintana*) is a small, Gram-negative bacillus measuring 0.3–0.5 × 1.0–1.7 μm. It does not possess flagella, although it may exhibit twitching movement caused by fimbriae.

Cultural characteristics

It grows slowly on rabbit or sheep blood agar at 35°C in 5% CO_2 in air. Colonies appear after two weeks in primary culture and 3–5 days in subsequent passages. It proliferates in an extracellular environment in the arthropod host, in the lumen of the gut rather than within the intestinal epithelial cells. It is not possible to transmit these organisms to common laboratory animals such as mice, rats, guinea-pigs and hamsters, chick embryos and tissue culture. Besides man and louse, only rhesus monkeys can be infected. No animal reservoir other than humans has been identified.

Pathogenicity

B. quintana causes **trench fever** which was first recognized in the First World War as a **five-day fever** in men engaged in trench warfare in Europe. It is an exclusively human disease.

The disease is spread from human to human by the body louse in a human-louse-human cycle of infection. The faeces of the lice become infectious 5–9 days after feeding on a trench fever patient. Infection is acquired when infected lice faeces are scratched into the skin. The lice are unharmed and remain infectious for life. Vertical transmission does not occur in lice.

Clinically, after an incubation period of 14–30 days patient develops headache, malaise, fever, chills, severe pain in the back and legs and a roseolar rash on the chest, abdomen or back. Recovery is frequently followed by relapses occurring at five day intervals (hence the species name, quintana). The infection is mild, recovery is slow and fatalities are rare.

Laboratory diagnosis

B. quintana does not grow in mice or guinea-pigs. However, it can be isolated by allowing healthy lice to feed upon the patient and the bartonellae may be detected in the gut of these lice. It can also be cultivated from patient's blood on rabbit or sheep blood agar. *B. quintana* has been detected in the tissues by PCR. **Weil-Felix reaction, in trench fever, is negative.**

Q. 11. Describe briefly morphology, cultural characteristics, pathogenicity and laboratory diagnosis of *Bartonella henselae*.

Ans. ### *Morphology*

B. henselae is a small, slightly curved Gram-negative bacillus measuring about 2.0–2.5 × 0.5–0.6 μm. It displays twitching motility.

Cultural characteristics

It can be grown on chocolate agar, columbia agar with 5% sheep or rabbit blood and blood-supplemented brain-heart-infusion agar. Growth appears after 5–15 days incubation at 35–37°C in 5% CO_2. Colonies of *B. henselae* are white, dry, adherent, cauliflower-like and embedded in the agar.

Pathogenicity

B. henselae causes **cat-scratch disease**, a severe condition of regional lymphadenopathy and fever resulting from contact, scratch or bite of an infected cat. It occurs throughout the world. It most frequently involves cervical and axillary lymph nodes, although other sites may be involved as well. Single-node involvement occurs in about half of the patients. *B. henselae* may also cause endocarditis. In AIDS patients, as a result of immunosuppression, *B. henselae* may lead to **bacillary angiomatosis**, a condition resembling Kaposi's sarcoma.

Laboratory diagnosis

1. Diagnosis can be established by demonstration of clusters of bacillary organisms in sections of lymph node biopsies stained with the Warthin-Starry silver impregnation stain.
2. *B. henselae* can be isolated by inoculation of clinical specimens on chocolate agar or columbia agar with 5% sheep or rabbit blood.
3. ELISA, with various protein antigens, is the most useful serological test.
4. Most *Bartonella* species can be detected and differentiated by PCR methods.

Cat-scratch disease is usually self-limiting requiring no therapy.

36

CHLAMYDIA, CHLAMYDOPHILA, ACTINOMYCETES, GARDNERELLA VAGINALIS AND KLEBSIELLA GRANULOMATIS

Q. 1. Describe classification and general characters of Chlamydiaceae.

Ans. ***Classification***

Family Chlamydiaceae consists of two genera – *Chlamydia* and *Chlamydophila*. The genus *Chlamydia* has one species – *C. trachomatis* and the genus *Chlamydophila* has three species – *C. psittaci*, *C. pneumoniae* and *C. picorum* (Table 36.1).

Table 36.1. Classification of Chlamydiaceae

Order	Family	Genera	Species
Chlamydiales	Chlamydiaceae	*Chlamydia*	*C. trachomatis*
		Chlamydophila	*C. psittaci*
			C. pneumoniae
			C. picorum

General characters

1. They are small, **obligate intracellular**, **Gram-negative bacteria**.
2. They possess both RNA and DNA, ribosomes and cell wall similar to that of Gram-negative bacteria. However, they differ from most true bacteria in that they do not have peptidoglycan.
3. They lack the ability to produce their own ATP, therefore, they use host's ATP (**energy parasites**).
4. They multiply by binary fission.
5. They are non-motile and stain poorly with Gram, but readily with Giemsa, Castaneda, Gimenez and Macchiavello methods. They stain blue by Castaneda, and red by Macchiavello and Gimenez techniques. Giemsa staining is preferable for staining

inclusions in cell culture. Inclusion bodies of Chlamydiaceae are basophilic in nature. Mature inclusions of *C. trachomatis* possess glycogen matrix, therefore, iodine stains them coppery brown. Inclusions of *C. psittaci* do not possess glycogen matrix, therefore, they do not stain with iodine.

6. They can also be demonstrated by direct immunofluorescence staining.
7. They multiply in the cytoplasm of the host cell forming microcolonies or inclusion bodies which drape around the nucleus like a cloak or mantle (*chlamys* means mantle).
8. Most strains of *C. trachomatis* and *C. psittaci* possess plasmid DNA of 7.3 and 6.2 kilobase pairs respectively. However, *C. pneumoniae* does not appear to have plasmid DNA.
9. Like Gram-negative bacteria, the outer membrane of various Chlamydiaceae possess several proteins of which major outer membrane protein (MOMP) has species-specific epitopes.
10. They possess a genus-specific lipopolysaccharide-protein complex antigen.
11. They infect a wide spectrum of vertebrate hosts including birds, mammals and humans.
12. They are susceptible to a wide range of antibiotics such as tetracyclines, erythromycin, macrolides and rifampicin. *C. trachomatis* is sensitive to sulphonamides, but *C. psittaci* and *C. pneumoniae* are not.

Q. 2. Describe morphology and developmental cycle of Chlamydiaceae.

Ans. ***Morphology***

There are two morphologically distinct forms of Chlamydiaceae, namely **elementary body (EB)** and **reticulate body (RB)**.

- The EB is the extracellular infectious particle. It is a small (200–300 nm in diameter), spherical body in case of *C. trachomatis* and *C. psittaci* and pear-shaped in case of *C. pneumoniae*. It has an irregular electron-dense central nucleoid and a rigid trilaminar cell wall similar to the cell walls of Gram-negative bacteria.
- The RB is the intracellular, metabolically active form that divides by binary fission to form EBs. It is 500–1000 nm in diameter and its cell wall is fragile and pliable, leading to pleomorphism.

Developmental cycle

1. Infection is initiated by the attachment of infectious EB to the susceptible host cell (Fig. 36.1). The type and range of susceptible host cells vary with the species and biovar. For example, biovars trachoma and lymphogranuloma venereum (LGV) of *C. trachomatis* infect squamocolumnar epithelial cells and lymphoid cells respectively, while *C. psittaci* infects a wide range of host cells. Specific adhesin and receptors have yet to be identified. It is presumed that epitopes in variable domains of MOMP on the surface of the EB may act as adhesin and a trypsin-sensitive protein on the surface of the susceptible host cell as a specific cell receptor.
2. After attachment, organism enters the host cell within a vesicle. Chlamydiaceae-dependent modification of the endocytic membrane prevents lysosomal fusion and thus escapes degradation.

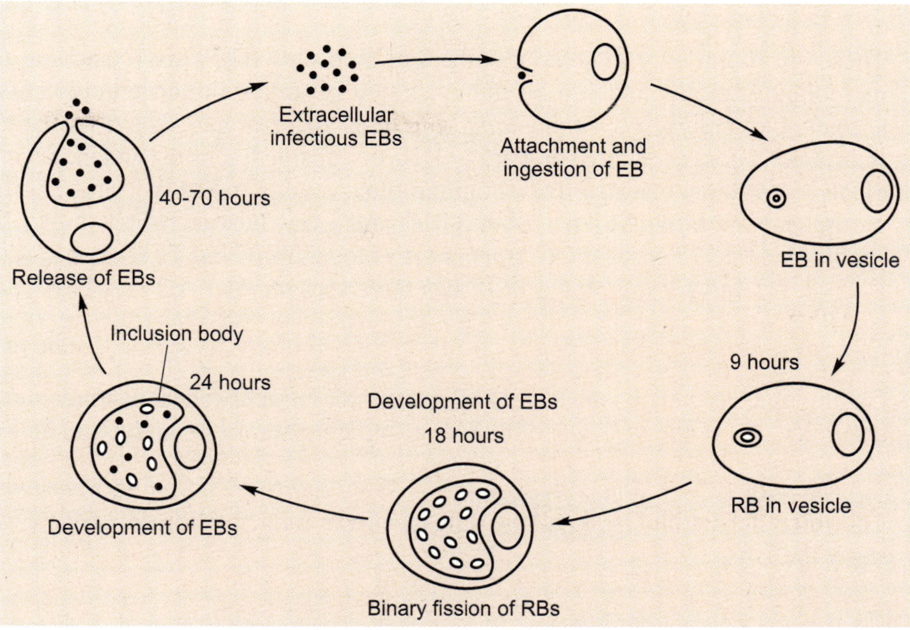

Fig. 36.1. The developmental cycle of Chlamydiaceae.

3. By 9 hours after infection, the EB within the vesicle loses its dense DNA core, its cell wall becomes less rigid due to breaking of the disulphide bonds, increases in size and differentiates into RB. It does not possess cytochrome and lacks the ability to produce ATP, therefore, they use host's ATP.
4. By 18 hours, within the enlarging vesicle, the RB divides by binary fission to yield pleomorphic organisms, and genus-specific antigens become associated with the host cell surface.
5. By 24 hours, there is condensation of DNA within the RB, disulphide bonds are formed in the outer membrane proteins and new EBs develop within the vesicle. The developing chlamydiaceal microcolony, within the vesicle, is termed as **inclusion body** which is typically perinuclear and may contain 100–500 EBs.
6. By 40–70 hours, infectious EBs are released from the cell by rupture of the inclusion which may infect new cells.

Q. 3. Describe antigenic structure of Chlamydiaceae.

Ans. Chlamydiaceae possess the following antigens:

1. Genus-specific antigen

It is heat-stable, complement fixing, genus-specific antigen common to all Chlamydiaceae. It is a lipopolysaccharide resembling the LPS of enteric Gram-negative bacilli.

2. Species-specific protein antigens

These are present at the envelope surface. They help in classifying Chlamydiaceae into different species.

3. Serotype-specific antigens

These are found only in some members of a species. They are located on the major outer membrane proteins and can be demonstrated by microimmunofluorescence. Within each species, particularly *C. trachomatis*, a number of serotypes (serovars) can be defined. *C. trachomatis* possesses three biovars – (1) those causing trachoma and inclusion conjunctivitis (TRIC), (2) those causing lymphogranuloma venereum (LGV), and (3) the one causing mouse pneumonitis (MoPn). Both TRIC and LGV biovars which infect humans can be subdivided into 15 serovars. *C. trachomatis* biovar TRIC has 12 serovars (A, B, Ba, C, D, E, F, G, H, I, J and K) and biovar LGV has three serovars (L1, L2 and L3).

Q. 4. Describe cultural characteristics of Chlamydiaceae.

Ans. Chlamydiaceae can be isolated (1) by intranasal, intraperitoneal or intracerebral inoculation into mice, (2) in the yolk sac of 6–8-days-old chick embryo, and (3) in cell cultures.

1. Mice

The mice die within 10 days and smears of the lung, peritoneal exudate, spleen or brain show the EBs.

2. Yolk sac

In the yolk sac, the organisms multiply in the endothelial cells and can be detected in impression smears stained by the Giemsa, Macchiavello or Gimenez methods. For the growth of *C. trachomatis* and *C. psittaci*, the inoculated embryonated eggs should be incubated at 35°C and 39°C respectively.

3. Cell culture

Cells that have been irradiated or treated with a metabolic inhibitor are used for isolation of Chlamydiaceae. Cycloheximide-treated McCoy cells are the most commonly used cell line although *C. pneumoniae* grows better in HeLa or monkey kidney cells. Mouse fibroblast cell lines can also be used for isolation of Chlamydiaceae. *C. psittaci* can even be propagated in fish and lizard cells. The presence of the organism, in the cell culture, is detected by staining for inclusions or elementary bodies.

Q. 5. Describe pathogenicity of chlamydiaceal infections.

Ans. Chlamydiaceae produces infections of eye, and genital and respiratory tracts of man (Table 36.2).

Infections of eye

Trachoma

It is a communicable chronic keratoconjunctivitis characterized by follicles, papillary hyperplasia, pannus formation and in late stages, cicatrization. It occurs only in humans. It is endemic in the Middle East, Africa, India and the Far East. In endemic areas, the prevalence of trachoma is maximum in children below 9 years of age. It is caused by *C. trachomatis* biovar TRIC and serovars A, B, Ba and C. The infection is transmitted from eye to eye by direct contact with fingers or contaminated towels and clothing. Flies may also transmit the infection mechanically. Incubation period of the disease appears to be 7–14 days.

Table 36.2. Chlamydiaceal infections of man

Site of infection	Disease	Organism	Biovar	Serovar
Eye	• Trachoma	*C. trachomatis*	TRIC	A, B, Ba, C
	• Inclusion conjunctivitis	*C. trachomatis*	TRIC	D–K
	• Ophthalmia neonatorum	*C. trachomatis*	TRIC	D–K
Genital tract				
Male	• Urethritis, epididymitis, proctitis	*C. trachomatis*	TRIC	D–K
Female	• Urethritis, cervicitis, salpingitis, infertility, perihepatitis, peri-appendicitis, proctitis	*C. trachomatis*	TRIC	D–K
	• Abortion, stillbirth (ovine strains)	*C. psittaci*	—	—
Male and female	• Lymphogranuloma venereum	*C. trachomatis*	LGV	L1–L3
Respiratory tract	• Pneumonitis of infant	*C. trachomatis*	TRIC	D–K
	• Pharyngitis, pneumonia	*C. pneumoniae*	—	—
	• Psittacosis	*C. psittaci*	—	—

Inclusion conjunctivitis

It is caused by *C. trachomatis* biovar TRIC serovars D–K, natural habitat of which is genital tract of both sexes. It is most prevalent in sexually active young people and is spread from genitalia to eye. The incubation period is 1–2 weeks. The onset is acute, with intense hyperaemia, mucopurulent discharge and follicular hyperplasia. Unlike trachoma, lesions are most pronounced in the lower than in the upper lid. Some patients may develop scarring, corneal lesions or pannus formation. Genital symptoms are minimal or absent particularly in women. Disease is usually self-limiting and does not lead to blindness.

Ophthalmia neonatorum (Inclusion blennorrhoea)

It is the neonatal form of inclusion conjunctivitis. It develops when the infant acquires infection from the birth canal. About 5–12% of all pregnant women have a chlamydiaceal infection of the cervix and 50% of infants born to such mothers develop conjunctivitis. Five to 12 days after birth the neonate develops swelling of the eyelids, hyperaemia and a purulent infiltration of the conjunctiva. A proportion of untreated neonates develop pneumonia.

Genital infections

Genital infection due to *C. trachomatis* is the most prevalent among the bacterial sexually transmitted diseases. *C. trachomatis* infection, if undiagnosed and untreated, can result in pelvic inflammatory disease, epidydimitis, etc., finally damaging the human reproductive tract irreversibly. Further to this, growing evidence indicates that active *C. trachomatis* infection is an important risk factor facilitating sexual transmission of HIV infection. Thus, early diagnosis and treatment of chlamydial infection is important to prevent HIV risk and devastating clinical consequences.

Males

C. trachomatis biovar TRIC serovars D–K account for at least 30% of cases of non-gonococcal urethritis (NGU). This condition develops 7–14 days after sexual intercourse. A minority of cases of NGU are caused by *Ureaplasma urealyticum*. *C. trachomatis* is also responsible for

50% cases of epididymitis in men under 35 years and 15% in men above this age. It may also cause proctitis in homosexual males.

Females

C. trachomatis biovar TRIC serovars D–K may cause urethritis, mucopurulent cervicitis, vaginitis and vaginal discharge, endometritis, salpingitis, infertility, perihepatitis and periappendicitis. Endometritis and salpingitis, singly or together may be referred to as **pelvic inflammatory disease**. Ovine strains of *C. psittaci* can cause abortion and stillbirth.

Lymphogranuloma venereum

C. trachomatis biovar TRIC serovars L1–L3 can cause lymphogranuloma venereum in both males and females. Usually 1–3 weeks after sexual contact, male patient develops a small (5–8 mm) painless papule or ulcer on the penis. Rectal infections occur in homosexuals. In women, the commonest site is the fourchette. In both sexes, the primary lesions may pass unnoticed. Primary lesions may occasionally occur on extra-genital sites such as fingers or tongue. The primary lesion soon heals but after 1–2 months, the regional lymph nodes (inguinal in males and intrapelvic and pararectal in females) become enlarged and tender, and may break open with the formation of sinuses. These enlarged lymph nodes are called **bubos**.

Respiratory tract

Chlamydophila pneumoniae was first isolated in 1965 from a Taiwanese (TW) child thought to have trachoma and later from a case of acute respiratory (AR) infection. It was originally named TWAR and thought to be a variant of *C. psittaci* but later classified as a separate species – *C. pneumoniae*. It appears to be the **third most common cause of pneumonia** following *Streptococcus pneumoniae* and *Haemophilus influenzae*. It causes an acute infection of lower respiratory tract in man. Infection seems to spread from person to person without the intervention of an avian host.

Psittacosis is a disease of the birds of the psittacine (parrot) family, transmissible to man. Similar organisms are also present in a great variety of non-psittacine birds including pigeons, ducks and domestic fowl. The disease acquired by contact with non-psittacine birds is known as **ornithosis**. Infection in birds exists as an asymptomatic, latent infection that can become overt following stresses such as caging and overcrowding leading to diarrhoea, mucopurulent respiratory discharge and emaciation. Faecal excretions and nasal discharge contain many organisms and provide the source of infection for other birds and humans.

C. pneumoniae has been implicated as an important factor in **asthma and cardiovascular disease**, where it has been isolated from atherosclerotic tissue. Infection with *C. pneumoniae* has also been established as a risk factor for **Guillain-Barré syndrome**.

Man acquires infection by the inhalation of dried infected faeces of birds. After an incubation period of 1–2 weeks, patient develops clinical disease which may vary from a mild 'influenza-like' syndrome with general malaise, fever, anorexia, rigors, sore throat, headache and photophobia to severe illness with pneumonia, septicaemia, meningo-encephalitis, pericarditis, myocarditis, endocarditis, arthritis or a typhoid-like syndrome with enlarged liver and spleen, and a rash.

Q. 6. Describe laboratory diagnosis of chlamydiaceal infections.

Ans. *Collection of specimens*

For the diagnosis of chlamydiceal infections ocular, urethral, vaginal and cervical specimens are best collected by scraping the mucosa. In addition, depending upon the site of involvement, blood, respiratory secretions, sputum, lung and other tissues can be collected. In case of LGV, pus from the bubo should be collected. These specimens are processed as under:

I. **Direct detection of chlamydiaceal antigens:**

1. ***Light microscopy:*** *C. trachomatis* infections of conjunctiva, urethra and cervix may be diagnosed by demonstrating typical **reniform inclusion bodies** surrounding the nucleus (Fig. 36.2), in the conjunctival, urethral and cervical smears stained with Giemsa, Castaneda or Macchiavello methods and seen under light microscope. Because the inclusion bodies possess a glycogen matrix, therefore, they may be stained with iodine solution also. This method has a low sensitivity.
2. ***Immunofluorescence (IF):*** Staining of smears is done with FITC-labelled antibodies (usually monoclonal) against either the species-specific or genus-specific antigen of *C. trachomatis*. The use of the latter will also detect *C. psittaci* and *C. pneumoniae* (Fig. 36.3). It has a sensitivity and specificity of 90% and 95% respectively and it can be done rapidly in less than one hour.

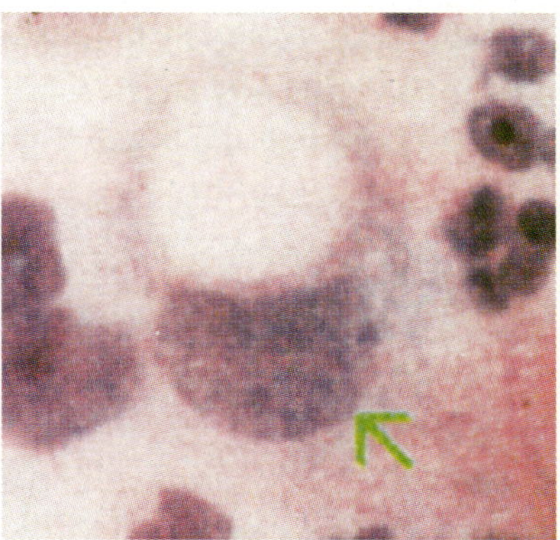

Fig. 36.2. Perinuclear inclusion body of *Chlamydia trachomatis*.

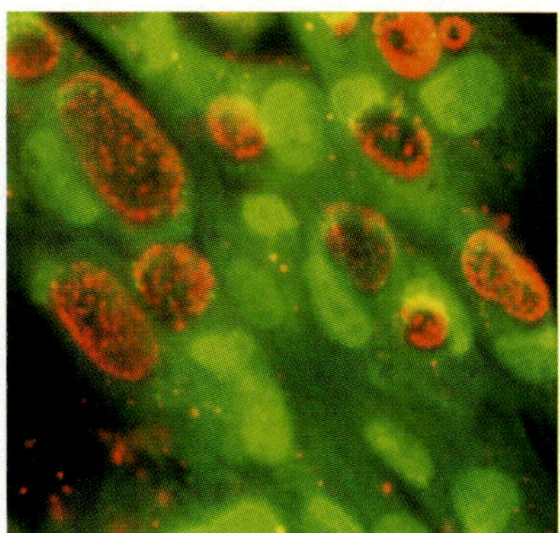

Fig. 36.3. Inclusion body of *Chlamydia trachomatis* under fluorescence microscope.

3. ***ELISA for detection of chlamydiaceal antigens:*** This test is based on detection of soluble genus-specific antigen captured by antibody attached to a solid surface such as plastic bead or microtitre well and then detected with an enzyme-labelled detector system and a chromogenic substrate. The sensitivity and specificity of ELISA is similar to that of IF.
4. ***DNA probes:*** DNA hybridization can be used for detection of *C. trachomatis* DNA in conjunctival and cervical smears.
5. ***Chemiluminescence assay:*** It uses an acridium-ester-labelled single stranded DNA probe, which is complementary to RNA of *C. trachomatis*. The labelled DNA-RNA hybrid is detected in a luminometer which measures light emitted by the acridium ester label. Sensitivity and specificity of this method are 95% each.

6. ***Polymerase chain reaction (PCR):*** Common endogenous plasmid DNA, the *omp1* gene which codes for MOMP and the 16S rRNA gene can be amplified and detected by PCR. This method is more sensitive than culture.

II. **Isolation of Chlamydiaceae:** Chlamydiaceae may be isolated in mice, yolk sac of 6–8 days old chick embryo and in cell cultures.

III. **Detection of chlamydiaceal antibody:**

1. Antibodies against *C. psittaci* and serovars L1–L3 of *C. trachomatis* can be detected by complement fixation test.
2. Antibodies against *C. trachomatis* and *C. pneumoniae* can be detected by micro-immunofluorescence, using elementary bodies of standard serovars, immuno-peroxidase and ELISA test.

A high level (> 64) of IgM and a rising titre of IgG are taken as diagnostic. In neonatal chlamydiaceal pneumonia, detection of IgM is diagnostic. Detection of IgG cannot distinguish maternal from neonatal infection. High titres of antibodies against *C. trachomatis* may be seen in acute salpingitis and infertility.

IV. **Skin test:** A skin test (**Frei's test**) is available for the diagnosis of LGV. A heat-inactivated *C. trachomatis* biovar LGV (0.1 ml) grown in yolk sac of embryonated egg is injected intradermally on the forearm and a control prepared from uninfected yolk sac on the other forearm. A positive reaction is indicated by an inflammatory nodule appearing on the test arm in 2 days and reaching a maximum in 4–5 days, measuring at least 7 mm in diameter. This test becomes positive 2–6 weeks after infection and remains positive for several years. Because of the availability of sensitive and rapid tests, it is now discarded.

Q. 7. Describe morphology, cultural characteristics, pathogenicity and laboratory diagnosis of *Actinomyces israelii*.

Ans. ***Morphology***

Actinomyces are Gram-positive, non-motile, non-sporing, non-acid-fast, 0.5–1 µm in diameter. They often grow in mycelial forms and break up into coccoid and bacillary forms. Most show true branching.

Cultural characteristics

They are facultative anaerobes. They grow best under anaerobic or micro-aerophilic conditions with the addition of 5–10% CO_2. The optimum temperature for growth is 35–37°C. They can be grown on brain-heart-infusion agar, heart-infusion agar supplemented with 5% defibrinated horse, rabbit or sheep blood. Suitable liquid media include brain-heart-infusion broth and thioglycollate broth which may be supplemented with 0.1–0.2% sterile rabbit serum. Most species show good growth after 3–4 days' incubation, however, *A. israelii* may take 7–14 days.

Pathogenicity

The *Actinomyces* causes the disease known as actinomycosis. In man, it is usually caused by *A. israelii*. It is a chronic suppurative disease characterized by peripheral spread to contiguous tissues, rare haematogenous spread, formation of sinus tracts which drain suppurative lesions and presence in the pus of colonies of *Actinomyces*. These colonies are 0.25–2 mm in diameter, white to yellowish and are known as **'sulphur granules'**. There are four important sites of primary infection in actinomycosis.

1. Cervicofacial

About two-thirds of cases of actinomycosis, in man, occur in the cervicofacial region. The primary lesion is usually in the mandible or maxilla and probably occurs by direct extension from a periodontal abscess, a traumatic lesion resulting from neglected carious or broken teeth, dental extraction or accidental fracture of jaw. Maxillary lesions may extend to the orbit, the cranial bones, the meninges and brain.

2. Thoracic

Thoracic actinomycosis commences in the lung probably as a result of aspiration of hyphal fragments of *Actinomyces* from tooth surfaces or dental caries or of *Actinomyces*-containing granules which commonly grow in tonsillar crypts without invading tonsillar tissue. The lesions in the lung may involve pleura and pericardium and spread outwards through the chest wall producing multiple draining sinuses.

3. Abdominal

Abdominal actinomycosis begins most often in appendix or rarely as a complication of perforating gastric ulcer or penetration of the mucosa of the colon by an object such as fish bone.

4. Pelvic

Pelvic actinomycosis occasionally occurs in women fitted with plastic intra-uterine contraceptive devices.

Actinomycotic cholecystitis and actinomycosis of breast have also been reported by the author.

Laboratory diagnosis

Specimens

Pus, sinus discharge, bronchial secretions, sputum or infected tissues are collected aseptically. These specimens may contain innumerable 'sulphur granules'. The granules may also be present on dressings removed from a draining sinus tract.

A. Microscopy

Pus from suspected cases is shaken with sterile water in a tube. **'Sulphur granules'** settle to the bottom. These are removed with a pasteur pipette. Granules are crushed between two slides and stained with Gram, and Ziehl-Neelsen staining using 1% sulphuric acid for decolourization. The granules are seen to consist of **Gram-positive hyphal fragments** 0.5–1 μm in diameter, sometimes remaining as intact hyphae several micrometers long and rarely with branches, surrounded by a peripheral zone of swollen radiating club-shaped structures presenting a **sun ray appearance**. These clubs are Gram-negative, and are believed to be antigen-antibody complexes. Acid-fast staining shows central part as non-acid-fast and acid-fast clubs.

'Sulphur granules' and mycelia in tissue sections can also be identified by direct **fluorescence microscopy**.

B. Culture

'Sulphur granules' are washed thoroughly in sterile normal saline in a petri dish or tube and crushed in a drop of saline with a glass rod. It is then inoculated on brain-heart-infusion agar, blood agar and in thioglycollate broth, and incubated both anaerobically and aerobically with 5–10% CO_2 at 35–37°C for up to 14 days. The colonies of *A. israelii* are 0.5–2 mm in diameter, white to grey-white, smooth, entire or lobulated resembling molar teeth (Fig. 36.4). The identity of the isolate may be confirmed by direct fluorescence microscopy and biochemical tests.

C. Biopsy

In haematoxylin and eosin stained sections, the 'sulphur granules' are deeply stained with haematoxylin except in the periphery which is stained with eosin, which shows short, radiate, club-like structures (Fig. 36.5). On Gram staining, the filaments are Gram-positive and periphery Gram-negative. The tissue reaction is a chronic suppurative, fibrosing, inflammatory process.

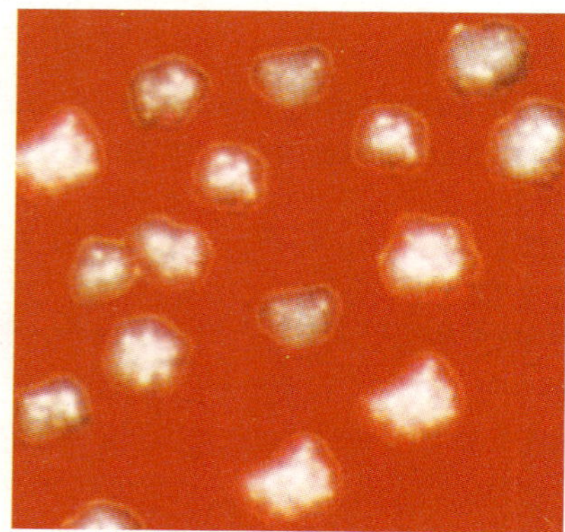

Fig. 36.4. Colonies of *Actinomyces israelii* on blood agar medium. These resemble molar teeth.

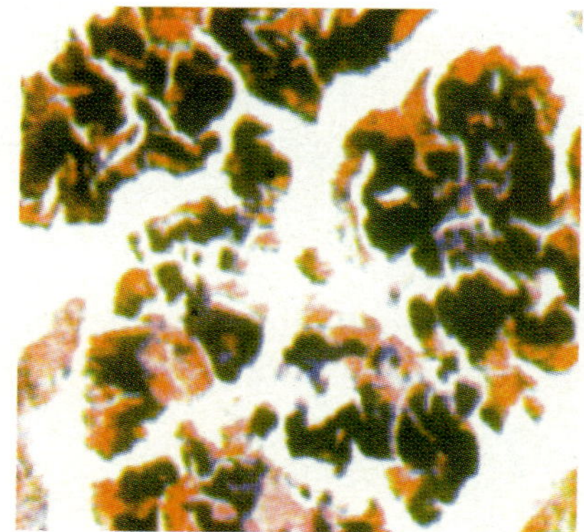

Fig. 36.5. Actinomycosis showing a grain of *Actinomyces israelii.* It is deeply stained with haematoxylin except in the periphery which is stained with eosin.

Q. 8. Describe morphology, cultural characteristics, pathogenicity and laboratory diagnosis of *Nocardia asteroides.*

Ans. ***Morphology***

Nocardiae are strictly aerobic, non-motile, Gram-positive bacteria (Fig. 36.6). They form hyphae that often fragment in situ or on mechanical disruption into rod-shaped or coccoid elements. They are acid-fast when decolourized with 1% sulphuric acid (Fig. 36.7).

Cultural characteristics

Nocardiae readily grow on nutrient agar, Sabouraud dextrose agar, brain-heart-infusion agar and yeast extract-malt extract agar. The inoculated plates should be incubated at 36°C for up to 3 weeks and examined both macroscopically and microscopically for growth every few days. Nocardiae form white, yellow, pink or brown colonies.

Fig. 36.6. Gram-stained sputum smear showing Gram-positive branched mycelia from a patient suffering from pulmonary nocardiosis.

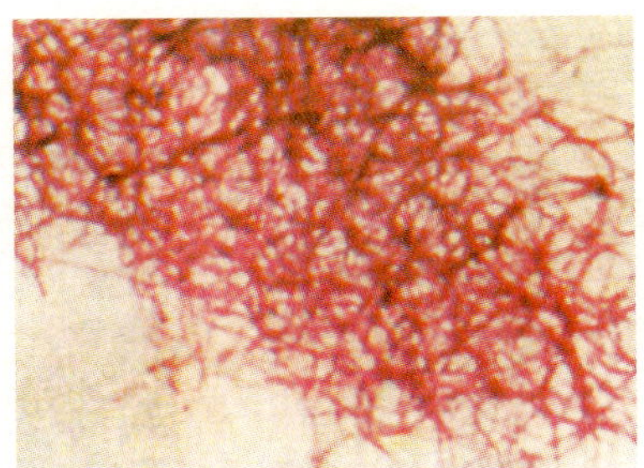

Fig. 36.7. Modified Ziehl-Neelsen staining showing acid-fast filaments of *Nocardia*.

Pathogenicity

N. asteroides produces opportunistic pulmonary disease known as nocardiosis in usually, but not always, immunocompromised individuals including those receiving immunosuppressive therapy and those with AIDS. Soil and composting matter is known to be the natural habitat of *Nocardia*. It is, therefore, believed that man and animals acquire infection by inhalation of the organism from environmental sources.

Nocardiosis is a systemic bacterial disease. It generally originates as a pulmonary infection, varying in its course from mild and slowly progressive to fulminant and fatal. It may be characterized by single or multiple nodules, miliary pattern, scattered infiltrations, bronchopneumonia, abscesses, masses with central cavitation, pleural effusions and empyema. Dissemination from the primary focus of infection may occur through pleural extension, lymphohaematogenous spread or invasion of blood vessels with bacteraemia.

Although every organ of the body may be affected, involvement of brain, meninges and spinal cord is said to be commoner than that of other parts such as skin, subcutaneous tissues, eye, liver, lymph node, etc. Infection with *Nocardia* oraganisms is serious. Approximately 40% of the diagnoses are made at autopsy. The mortality rate is high, and those who survive often suffer significant tissue damage.

Localized cutaneous and subcutaneous nocardiosis is encountered less frequently. Infection may occur through contaminated wound and by traumatic implantation. It usually involves feet and hands. The infection begins as a localized subcutaneous abscess that is invasive and quite destructive of the tissues and underlying bone. This lesion is known as **mycetoma**. It is characterized by swelling, draining sinuses, and granules. About half of the mycetomas are caused by actinomycetes and the remaining half are caused by fungi. As the infection progresses, burrowing sinuses open to the skin surface and drain pus. The pus may contain 'sulphur granules' which are masses of filamentous organisms bound together by calcium phosphate. The granules of *Nocardia* species are soft, white to cream coloured, and 0.5–1.0 mm in size.

Laboratory diagnosis

Microscopy

Pus or purulent blood-flecked sputum is spread on a slide by crushing between two slides. The smears are stained by Gram and Ziehl-Neelsen techniques and examined under oil-immersion lens. Granules may be seen in specimens from cutaneous infection. Sampled tissue and pus from the draining sinuses are the specimens of choice for direct examination. The granules may be visualized by separating them from the pus with an inoculating needle and then washing in sterile saline. These may be crushed between two glass slides which are then used for Gram and Ziehl-Neelsen staining.

Culture

Pus, sputum or the granules are inoculated on nutrient agar, Sabouraud dextrose agar and brain-heart-infusion agar, and incubated at 36°C for 3 weeks. Culture media are examined both macroscopically and microscopically every few days for identification of the isolate.

Nocardia can be isolated from sputum by **paraffin bait technique** by incubating paraffin coated glass rod in sputum for one to six weeks and subculturing the actinomycete from the rod.

Q. 9. Describe morphology, cultural characteristics, pathogenicity and laboratory diagnosis of *Gardnerella vaginalis*.

Ans. ***Morphology***

G. vaginalis is small (1.5–2.5 μm × 0.5 μm), non-motile, non-sporing coccobacillus. It is Gram-variable, but because the cell wall contains lipopolysaccharide it appears to be Gram-negative. The G+C content of the DNA is 42–44 mol%. Clusters of cells may palisade, giving the appearance of Chinese letters as is seen in case of *Corynebacterium diphtheriae*. Metachromatic granules are produced when the organism is grown in the presence of a fermentable compound or sodium phosphate. The granules appear positive by Gram stain or metachromatic with alkaline methylene blue stain. It is non-motile, non-capsulated and non-sporing.

Cultural characteristics

It is facultative anaerobe; growth occurs in air but is stimulated by 5–10% CO_2. Optimum temperature and pH for its growth are 35–37°C and 6.0–6.5 respectively. It grows on enriched media such as blood agar or chocolate agar. Colonies are β-haemolytic on human and rabbit but not on sheep blood agar.

Pathogenicity

G. vaginalis is a member of the endogenous vaginal flora in up to 69% of women. However, it is present in large numbers in the vaginal secretions of the majority of women with bacterial vaginosis. This condition presents with an increased vaginal discharge with a characteristic 'rotten fish' odour. This becomes more pronounced on alkalization, and can be evoked by placing a drop of potassium hydroxide solution on the fresh exudate on a slide or the speculum used for the vaginal examination. The discharge adheres to the vaginal wall in a thin film that varies from white to grey in colour.

The pH of the vaginal secretions is over 4.5 (normal pH is <4.5). It contains many anaerobes in addition to *G. vaginalis*. There is an absence of other common causes of vaginitis such as *Trichomonas vaginalis* or yeasts. Bacterial vaginosis is associated with a mixed bacterial flora consisting of *G. vaginalis*, *Mobiluncus mulieris*, *M. curtisii*, *Bacteroides bivius*,

B. disiens, *Porphyromonas* spp., *Prevotella* spp. and *Mycoplasma hominis*. *Mobiluncus* spp. have been found in the vaginal secretions of over 80% of women with vaginosis but rarely in women without vaginosis. It appears that both the combination of species and their relative numbers are of importance in the development of the syndrome.

Laboratory diagnosis

In wet smears bacterial vaginosis yields **'clue cells'** which are vaginal epithelial cells with their surface studded with numerous small bacteria.

Q. 10. Describe briefly morphology, cultural characteristics and pathogenicity of *Klebsiella granulomatis*.

Ans. ***Morphology***

It is a small, capsulate, Gram-negative, coccobacillus 1–2 × 0.5–1.5 μm in size. It often shows bipolar staining giving rise to **'safety pin' appearance**. In the infected tissues, it can be best stained by Wright-Giemsa method, which stains the body of the bacillus blue and the capsule pink. They are contained within the cytoplasmic vacuoles (phagosomes) of large macrophages and are known as **Donovan bodies**. These are sometimes seen inside polymorphonuclear leucocytes or lying free outside the cells. Vacuoles may contain up to 30 bacteria before these are liberated by cell rupture. It is non-flagellate, non-sporing and non-acid-fast.

Cultural characteristics

It can be cultured readily in the yolk sac of embryonated hen's eggs and with great difficulty on media containing fresh egg-yolk.

Pathogenicity

K. granulomatis causes a chronic granulomatous disease known as **granuloma inguinale**, **granuloma venereum** or **donovanosis**. The initial lesion is commonly on the genitals, indicating transmission by sexual contact. Anal lesions occur after anal intercourse. The incubation period is not known. It may vary between a few days to 3 months. The initial subcutaneous nodule breaks down to give ulcers that unlike those of chancroid are **painless**.

37

General Properties of Viruses, and Bacteriophage

Q. 1. Describe general properties, structure and shape of viruses.

Ans. ***General properties***

Viruses are the **smallest infective agents**. They are **obligate intracellular parasites**. Three main properties distinguish viruses from other microorganisms:

1. Small size

Viruses are smaller than other organisms. **They vary in size from 10–300 nm.** Therefore, they can pass through bacterial filters and they cannot be seen by light microscope. However, the poxviruses which are the largest members of the virus family and are very similar in size to the smallest bacteria, are close to the resolution of light microscope. For visualization of all other viruses an electron microscope is necessary. Virus particles can be measured by:

- **Passage through membrane filter:** Membranes are available with pores of different sizes. If the viral preparation is passed through a series of membranes of known pore size, the approximate size of any virus can be measured by determining which membranes allow the infective unit to pass and which hold it back.
- **Ultracentrifugation:** If particles are suspended in a liquid, they will settle at the bottom at a rate that is proportionate to their size. In an ultracentrifuge, forces of more than 100,000 times gravity may be used to drive the particles to the bottom of the tube and the rate of sedimentation permits determination of particle size.
- **Electron microscopy:** By this method, both size and shape of the viruses can be studied. Latex particles of known size can be included in the suspension and the size of the virus compared and calculated.

2. Genome

A virus carries its own genetic information in the form of either RNA or DNA, but not both. The genome may be single-stranded or double-stranded, circular or linear, and segmented or unsegmented. The type of nucleic acid, its strandedness, and its size are major characteristics used for classifying viruses into families.

3. Metabolically inert

Viruses have no metabolic activity outside susceptible host cells. They do not possess ribosomes or protein-synthesizing apparatus although some viruses contain one or more enzymes within their particles. Viruses, therefore, cannot multiply in inanimate media but only inside living cells. Inside the living cells the virus genome is capable of replicating new virus particles.

Structure

Viruses consist of nucleic acid core surrounded by a protein coat called **capsid**. The capsid is composed of repeating protein units called **capsomers**. The capsid with the enclosed nucleic acid is known as **nucleocapsid**.

Functions of capsid

- It protects the viral genome from physical destruction and enzymatic inactivation by nucleases in biological material.
- It serves as a vehicle of transmission from one host to another.
- It provides binding sites that enable the virus to attach to specific receptor sites on the host cell.
- It facilitates the assembly and packaging of viral genetic information.
- It is antigenic and specific for each virus type.
- It provides the structural symmetry to the virus particle.

Virus symmetry

Capsid of the virus particles shows three types of symmetry. It is determined by the arrangement of the capsomers around the nucleic acid.

1. ***Icosahedral symmetry:*** The capsomers are arranged as if they lay on the faces of an icosahedron which has 20 equilateral triangular faces and 12 corners or apices (Fig. 37.1).
2. ***Helical symmetry:*** The nucleic acid and the capsomers are wound together in the form of a helix or spiral.
3. ***Complex symmetry:*** Viruses (e.g., poxviruses) which do not show either icosahedral or helical symmetry due to complexity of their structure are referred to have complex symmetry.

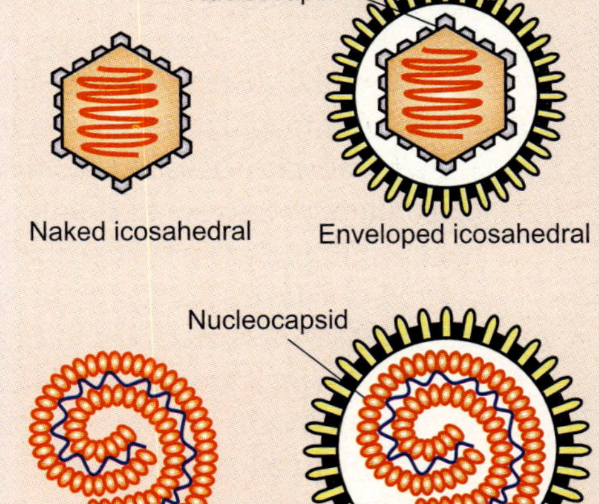

Fig. 37.1. Symmetry of viruses.

Envelope

Generally, DNA viruses replicate and are assembled in the nucleus, and RNA viruses are assembled in the cytoplasm. The final assembly of some viruses occurs at the nuclear or cytoplasmic membrane. As the virus particle moves from the nucleus to the cytoplasm or passes from the cytoplasm to the extracellular space, an external lipid-containing envelope (host origin) with virus-coded polypeptides or virus-specified glycoproteins is added to the nucleocapsid. In mature virus particle the glycoproteins often appear as projecting spikes on the outer surface of the envelope. These are known as **peplomers**. A virus may have more than one type of peplomers, e.g., the influenza virus carries two kinds of peplomers, the **haemagglutinin** which is a triangular spike and the **neuraminidase** which is a mushroom-shaped structure.

Functions of peplomers

- Many peplomers mediate attachment of the virus to the host cell receptors to initiate the entrance of the virion into the cell.
- Some viral glycoproteins attach to receptors on red blood cells, leading to haemagglutination.
- Other glycoproteins possess enzymatic activity like neuraminidase which cleave neuraminic acid from host cell glycoproteins.

Shape

The overall shape of the virus particle varies in different groups of viruses. Most of the animal viruses are roughly spherical, some are irregular and pleomorphic. Poxviruses are *brick-shaped*, rabies virus is *bullet-shaped*, tobacco mosaic virus is *rod-shaped* and bacteriophages have a *complex morphology*. The extracellular infectious virus particle is known as **virion**.

Q. 2. Describe briefly viral haemagglutination and elution.

Ans. Viral haemagglutination

A large number of viruses contain haemagglutinin spikes (peplomers) on the capsid or envelope which can agglutinate red cells of different species. *Haemagglutinin* of influenza virus has been studied extensively. The viral haemagglutinin (glycoprotein) has got a special affinity for another but different glycoprotein located in the receptor area on the surface of RBC. When RBCs are added to serial dilutions of viral suspension, the RBCs and the viruses collide in the suspension and adhere to each other resulting in haemagglutination.

The haemagglutination reaction is important in laboratory work because it provides a simple and rapid method for detection of viruses in egg or tissue culture fluid. When red cells are added to serial dilutions of a viral suspension, the highest dilution that produces haemagglutination provides the haemagglutination titre. The haemagglutination test can be carried out in test tubes or in special plastic trays. As inactivated virus can also haemagglutinate, the test serves to titrate killed influenza vaccine.

RBCs which are not agglutinated settle at the bottom in the form of a button while the agglutinated cells are seen spread into a shield-like pattern or irregular ragged pattern. As haemagglutination is specifically inhibited by the antibody to the virus, **haemagglutination inhibition** provides a convenient test for the antiviral antibody.

Elution

Some viruses, particularly influenza and parainfluenza viruses, also carry on their surface another peplomer, the enzyme *neuraminidase*, which acts on the receptors on RBCs and destroys them. It is, therefore, known as **receptor destroying enzyme** (RDE). It is also produced by many bacteria including *Vibrio cholerae* and is also present in many vertebrate cells. Destruction of surface receptors leads to reversal of haemagglutination and release of virus from the cell surface. This is known as elution. After elution, the receptors are irreversibly damaged and cells are no longer agglutinable by that particular virus. The free virions are, however, unharmed.

Q. 3. Describe replication of viruses.

Ans. The genetic information necessary for viral multiplication is contained in the viral nucleic acid but the biosynthetic enzymes are lacking. They replicate by taking over the biochemical machinery of the host cell and redirecting it to the manufacture of virus components. The viral replication is divided into six stages.

1. Adsorption

The first event in the infection of a cell by a virus is the attachment of the virus particle to the cell surface. Virions come in contact with cells by random collision but adsorption or attachment is specific and is mediated by the binding of virion surface structures, known as ligands, to receptors on cell surface. In case of influenza virus, a surface glycoprotein (the haemagglutinin) binds specifically to sialic acid residue of glycoprotein receptor sites on the surface of respiratory epithelium. Destruction of receptor sites by neuraminidase (RDE) prevents viral adsorption.

In case of human immunodeficiency virus-1, surface glycoprotein gp120 acts as a ligand. It binds to the CD4 60kDa glycoprotein on the surface of mature T lymphocytes. Similarly, rabies virus binds to the acetylcholine receptor found on neural cells. Susceptibility to virus infection, therefore, depends upon the presence or absence of receptors on the cell surface. For example, the inability of poliovirus to infect non-primate cells is due to the lack of receptors on these cells.

2. Entry into the host cells

Viruses enter the cells by the following mechanism:

- After attachment nonenveloped viruses are engulfed by a mechanism resembling phagocytosis, a process known as viropexis. In case of enveloped viruses, the envelope fuses with the plasma membrane of the host cell and releases the nucleocapsid into the cytoplasm.
- Bacteria possess rigid cell walls. Bacteriophages, therefore, cannot penetrate into bacterial cells and only nucleic acid is introduced intracellularly by a complex mechanism.

3. Uncoating

This is the process of stripping the virus of its outer layers and capsid so that nucleic acid is released into the cell. With most viruses, uncoating is effected by the action of lysosomal enzymes of the host cells when the phagosome and lysosome fuse together.

4. Biosynthesis

This phase includes synthesis of:

- The viral nucleic acid.
- Capsid protein.
- Enzymes necessary in the various stages of viral synthesis, assembly and release.
- Certain regulatory proteins which serve to shut down the normal cellular metabolism and direct the sequential production of viral components.

Biosynthesis consists of following steps:

- Transcription of messenger RNA (mRNA) from viral nucleic acid.
- Translation of mRNA into '**early proteins**' or '**nonstructural proteins**'. These are enzymes and factors which initiate and maintain synthesis of virus components and induce shut-down of host protein and nucleic acid synthesis.
- Replication of viral nucleic acid.
- Synthesis of **late** or **structural proteins** which constitute daughter virion capsids.

5. Virion assembly

Assembly of the various viral components into virions occurs shortly after the replication of the viral nucleic acid and may take place in either the nucleus (herpes and adenoviruses) or cytoplasm (picorna and poxviruses). In case of enveloped viruses, the envelope is derived from the nuclear membrane if they assemble in the nucleus (herpesviruses), and from plasma membrane if they assemble in the cytoplasm of the host cell (orthomyxoviruses, paramyxoviruses and retroviruses). However, in this envelope virus encoded peplomers are also embedded.

6. Release

Release of completed viruses is the final step in virus multiplication. Viruses that exist as naked nucleocapsids may be released by:

- The lysis of the host cell (polioviruses) or they may be extruded by a process which may be called **reverse phagocytosis**.
- Enveloped viruses are released by a process of **budding** through special areas of host cell membrane (cytoplasmic or nuclear), where virus-specified transmembrane glycoproteins (peplomers) have been embedded.
- In case of bacterial viruses, the release of progeny virions takes place by **the lysis of the infected bacterium**.

Eclipse phase

From the stage of penetration till the appearance of mature daughter virions, the virus cannot be demonstrated inside the host cell. This period is known as eclipse phase. The time taken for a single cycle of replication in case of animal viruses is 15–30 hours and for bacteriophages it is 15–30 minutes.

Q. 4. Describe methods of isolation of viruses.

Ans. Viruses can replicate only in living cells, therefore, they cannot be grown on any of the inanimate culture media. Most of the viruses can be cultivated in laboratory animals, chick embryos or tissue cultures.

Laboratory animals

These animals have now almost disappeared from virus diagnostic laboratories, because simpler methods such as tissue cultures are available. However, suckling mice, less than 24 hours old, are still used for the isolation of arboviruses, rabies virus, and some of the group A coxsackieviruses. These are inoculated intracerebrally and/or intraperitoneally, then observed for up to 2 weeks for the development of pathognomic signs before sacrificing for histologic examination of affected organs.

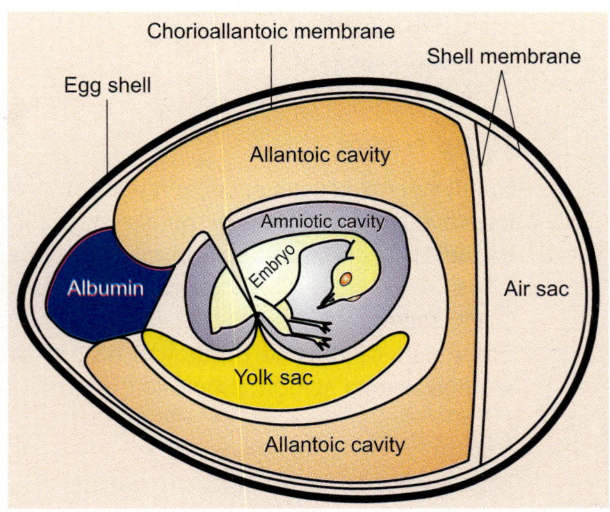

Fig. 37.2. Cross-section of an embryonated hen's egg.

Chick embryos

Embryonated eggs offer several sites for the cultivation of viruses. Chorioallantoic membrane (CAM), allantoic cavity, amniotic cavity and yolk sac (Fig. 37.2) of 8–11 day old eggs are inoculated and incubated for 2–9 days. The duration of incubation depends on the virus type and route of inoculation. Viruses may kill the embryo or may produce visible lesions like pocks on CAM, and haemagglutinating activity in the harvested amniotic and allantoic fluid. These effects help in the identification of the virus. Many viruses can be grown in eggs.

1. Chorioallantoic membrane (CAM)

Inoculation of CAM produces visible lesions (pocks). Pocks produced by different viruses have different morphology. Each infectious virus particle forms one pock. Pock counting, therefore, can be used for the assay of pock-forming viruses such as variola and vaccinia.

2. Amniotic cavity

Inoculation of amniotic cavity is used for primary isolation of the influenza virus.

3. Allantoic cavity

Inoculation of allantoic cavity provides a rich yield of influenza and some parainfluenza viruses. Allantoic inoculation is used for growing influenza virus for vaccine production. Other chick embryo vaccines are yellow fever (**17D strain**) and rabies (**Flury strain**) vaccines. Duck eggs are bigger than hen's eggs. Therefore, duck eggs provide a better yield of rabies virus and are used for the preparation of the inactivated nonneural rabies vaccines.

4. Yolk sac inoculation

Inoculation of yolk sac is used for the cultivation of some viruses, chlamydiae and rickettsiae.

Tissue culture

Three types of tissue culture are available:

1. Organ culture
2. Explant culture
3. Cell culture

Organ culture

Small bits of organs are maintained in tissue culture growth medium. Organ cultures are useful for the isolation of highly specialised viruses of certain organs. For example, the tracheal ring organ culture is employed for the isolation of coronavirus, a respiratory pathogen.

Explant culture

Fragments of minced tissue can be grown as 'explants' embedded in plasma clots. This method is now seldom employed in virology.

Cell culture

This is the type of culture routinely employed for diagnostic virology and for studying virus-cell interactions. Tissues are dissociated into component cells by the action of proteolytic enzymes such as trypsin or collagenase and mechanical shaking. The cells are washed, counted and suspended in a growth medium. The cell suspension is dispensed in glass or plastic bottles, tubes or petri dishes. The cells adhere to glass or plastic surface and on incubation, if culture conditions are suitable, they divide to form a confluent monolayer sheet of cells covering the surface within about a week. At this stage, cell division ceases due to contact inhibition. Cell culture is of three types (Table 37.1):

Table 37.1. Cell cultures in common use

1. Primary cell culture
   - Rhesus monkey kidney cell culture
   - Human amnion cell culture
   - Chick embryo fibroblast cell culture
2. Semi-continuous (diploid) cell strains
   - WI-38 Human embryonic lung cell strain
3. Continuous cell lines
   - HeLa Human carcinoma of cervix cell line
   - HEp-2 Human epithelioma of larynx cell line
   - KB Human carcinoma of nasopharynx cell line
   - McCoy Human synovial carcinoma cell line
   - Detroit 6 Sternal marrow cell line
   - Chang C/I/L/K Human conjunctiva, intestine, liver and kidney cell line
   - Vero African monkey kidney cell line
   - BHK-21 Baby hamster kidney cell line

1. Primary cell culture

These are normal cells freshly taken from the body and cultured. They are capable of very limited growth *in vitro* perhaps 5–10 divisions at the most. Because these cells have a normal diploid chromosome complement, therefore, they are preferred for cultivating viruses meant for vaccine production. Important examples of primary cell cultures are rhesus monkey kidney cell culture, human amnion cell culture and chick embryo fibroblast cell culture.

2. Semi-continuous (diploid) cell strains

These are cells of a single type, usually fibroblasts, that retain their original diploid chromosome number and karyotype. They can be subcultured for about 50 passages (serial subcultures) before the cells die off. Diploid cells developed from human fibroblasts are susceptible to a wide range of human viruses. They are useful for isolation of some fastidious pathogens and for the production of viral vaccines, e.g., rabies vaccine is produced by cultivation of the fixed rabies virus in WI-38 human embryonic lung cell strain.

3. Continuous cell lines

These are cells of a single type that are capable of indefinite propagation *in vitro*. Therefore, they are known as continuous cell lines. They have been derived from diploid cell lines or from malignant tissues. They invariably have altered and irregular numbers of chromosomes. Often they no longer bear any close resemblance to their cells of origin because of numerous sequential mutations during their long history in culture. Continuous cell lines such as HeLa, HEp-2 and KB derived from human carcinoma of cervix, human epithelioma of larynx, and human carcinoma of nasopharynx respectively, support the growth of a number of viruses. These cell lines have been used in the virus laboratories throughout the world for many years.

These cell lines may be maintained by serial subcultivation or stored at –70°C for use when necessary. Other cell lines (and their sources) in common use are McCoy (human synovial carcinoma cell line), Detroit 6 (sternal marrow cell line), Chang C/I/L/K (human conjunctiva, intestine, liver and kidney cell lines), Vero (African green monkey kidney cell line) and BHK-21 (baby hamster kidney cell line). The type of cell culture used for viral cultivation depends on the sensitivity of the cells to a particular virus.

Q. 5. Describe various methods for the detection of viral growth in cell culture.

Ans. Virus growth in cell culture can be detected by the following methods:

1. Cytopathic effect

Many viruses produce morphological changes in the cultured cells in which they grow. These changes are known as **cytopathic effects (CPE)** and viruses causing CPE are known as **cytopathogenic viruses**. Most CPE can be readily observed in unfixed and unstained monolayer of cells under low power of microscope. But fixation and staining of monolayer is essential in order to see details such as inclusion bodies and syncytia. Conventional haematoxylin and eosin is most suitable for this purpose. Fluorescent antibody staining is widely used to recognize viral antigens in such cultured cells. Following are the main types of CPE:

Rounding of cells: Viral replication may lead to nuclear pyknosis, rounding, refractility, degeneration and eventually complete or partial detachment of infected cells from the glass. This is seen in picornaviruses.

Rounding and aggregation: Some viruses may lead to cell rounding and aggregation into grape-like clusters which detach from the glass, leaving clear areas. It is seen in adenoviruses.

Syncytium formation: Some viruses (measles, respiratory syncytial virus and HIV) lead to syncytium formation in which infected cells fuse with neighbouring infected or uninfected cells to form giant cells containing several (up to 100) nuclei.

2. Haemadsorption

Orthomyxoviruses (influenza) and paramyxoviruses (parainfluenza, measles and mumps) code for red cell agglutinins which are incorporated into the cell membrane during infection, so that guinea-pig erythrocytes adhere to the infected cells. This adherence of erythrocytes to the infected cells is known as haemadsorption. It can be used to recognize infection with non-cytocidal viruses, as well as the early stage of cytocidal viruses. Sometimes virus can be detected by haemagglutination in the medium (culture fluid).

3. Interference

The multiplication of one virus in a cell usually inhibits the multiplication of a second virus, called **the challenge virus**, when it is added to the culture. This is because the first virus interferes with the replicative process of the challenge virus and is known as **interference challenge test**. This can be used for the detection of the growth of a non-cytopathogenic virus in cell culture.

A cell culture is inoculated with suspected clinical sample and incubated for several days. Then a standard dose of a known cytopathogenic challenge virus is introduced into the culture and after incubation, culture is observed for the CPE of challenge virus. If virus from original inoculum was replicating within the cells, replication of the challenge virus will be prevented and no CPE will be seen in the culture.

4. Transformation

Tumour-forming (oncogenic) viruses induce cell transformation and loss of normal contact inhibition, so that growth appears in a piled-up fashion producing **microtumours**. Some herpesviruses, adenoviruses, hepadnaviruses, papovaviruses and retroviruses (human T cell lymphotropic virus type 1) can transform cells.

5. Fluorescent antibody testing

Cells from virus infected cultures can be stained with fluorescein-conjugated antiserum and seen under fluorescence microscope for virus antigens. Both direct (DFA) and indirect (IFA) fluorescent antibody methods are useful in the identification of viral culture isolates. DFA testing is the most convenient method for identifying many viral isolates. It provides a complete identification in less than one hour.

6. Immunoperoxidase staining

Direct immunoperoxidase (DIP) staining method may also be used in identification of viruses isolated in cell culture.

7. Detection of viral enzymes

The virus isolate can be identified by detection of viral enzymes, such as reverse transcriptase in retroviruses, in the culture fluid.

8. Electron microscopy

Viruses have distinctive appearances and can be detected by electron microscopy of ultra thin sections of infected cells.

Q. 6. Describe morphology and life cycle of bacteriophage.

Ans. ***Morphology***

Bacteriophages that infect *Escherichia coli*, called the T-even phages (T2, T4, T6), have been studied in great detail. They serve as the prototypes in describing the properties of bacteriophages. They are tadpole shaped with a hexagonal head and a cylindrical tail (Fig. 37.3).

- **Head:** It consists of a tightly packed core of nucleic acid (double-stranded DNA) surrounded by a protein coat or capsid. The size of the head varies from 28–100 nm.
- **Tail:** It consists of a long hollow core surrounded by a contractile sheath and a terminal base plate. Attached to the base plate of the tail are six tail fibres and six tail pins. The virus uses the tail fibres to find a bacterium to infect and the tail pins on the base plate anchor the virus to the host cell during infection.

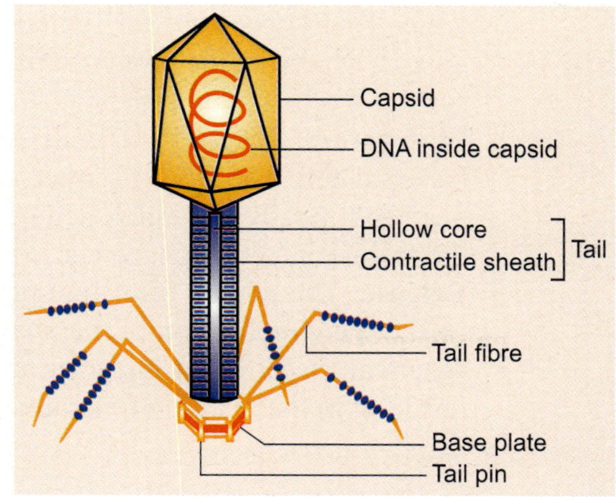

Fig. 37.3. Morphology of T4 phage particle.

Most of the phages possess double-stranded DNA, but single-stranded RNA or DNA and double-stranded RNA is present in some other phages.

Life cycle

Phages exhibit two different types of life cycle. In virulent or lytic cycle, there is intracellular multiplication of phages followed by lysis and release of progeny virions. In temperate or lysogenic cycle, the phage DNA becomes integrated with the bacterial genome replicating synchronously with it, causing no harm to the host cell.

1. Lytic cycle

The events between infection of a cell by a phage and its subsequent lysis to release daughter phage particles are similar for most phages. The lytic cycle of T-even phages is described below.

1. **Adsorption:** With the help of tail fibres and tail pins, phage particles attach to virus-specific receptors on the host cell. Adsorption is a specific process and depends on the presence of complementary chemical groups on the receptor sites on the bacterial surface and on the terminal base plate of the phage. Infection cannot occur in the absence of adsorption. Therefore, most phages are highly specific for a limited number of bacterial hosts and this constitutes the basis of bacteriophage typing of bacteria.
2. **Penetration:** Following adsorption, six tail pins make contact with the host cell surface and firmly attach the phage plate to it. The contractile tail sheath then contracts forcing the hollow interior tail tube about 12 nm into the bacterial cell wall. The phage DNA then passes through the hollow interior tail tube. Penetration may be facilitated by the presence on the phage tail of lysozyme which produces a hole on the bacterial cell wall for the entry of phage core. After penetration, phages leave their empty capsids and tails outside the bacteria.
3. **Synthesis:** Immediately after penetration of the phage nucleic acid , synthesis of phage components is initiated. The first products to be synthesized are **early proteins**. These

are enzymes necessary for synthesis of phage components. Subsequently, **late proteins** appear, which are the protein subunits of the phage head and tail. During this period, the synthesis of bacterial protein, DNA and RNA ceases.

4. **Maturation:** Phage DNA, head protein and tail protein are synthesized separately in the bacterial cell. The DNA is condensed into a compact polyhedron and packaged into the head and, finally, the tail structures are added. This assembly of phage components into the mature infective phage particles is known as maturation.
5. **Release:** The release of mature progeny phage particles occurs by lysis of the bacterial cell. During replication of the phage, the bacterial cell wall is weakened and assumes a spherical shape. Phage enzymes act on the weakened cell wall causing it to burst or lyse, resulting in the release of mature daughter phages.

2. Lysogenic cycle

Not all phage infections result in immediate progeny production and lysis of the host cell. There are many phages that, upon entering a sensitive cell, either undergo a lytic cycle like that described above or alternatively enter into a benign relationship with their hosts, called **lysogeny**. The phages that can develop both lytically and lysogenically are said to be **temperate phages**. In lysogenic state, the bacteriophage nucleic acid becomes integrated into the bacterial chromosome. The phage genome in this state is known as **prophage**. It replicates along with the bacterial chromosome. A bacterium that carries a prophage is known as a **lysogenic bacterium** or **lysogen**.

The prophage confers certain new properties on the lysogenic bacterium. This is known as **lysogenic** or **phage conversion**. Following are the examples of lysogenic conversion:

- **Toxin production** in *Corynebacterium diphtheriae* is determined by the presence in it of the prophage β. The elimination of this prophage abolishes the toxigenicity of the bacillus and nontoxigenic strains can be made toxigenic by lysogenization.
- *Clostridium botulinum* types C and D produce toxin only if these are infected with phage CE β and DE β respectively.
- A wide variety of temperate phages of *Salmonella* can **modify the antigenic properties** of somatic O antigen. The antigenic formula of *S.* Anatum is 3, 10:e, h:1, 6 but when it is lysogenised by a temperate phage its antigenic formula becomes 3, 15:e, h:1, 6 (*S.* Newington).

Occasionally, integrated prophage is excised from bacterial DNA, and phage multiplication and subsequent cell lysis ensues. This is known as **spontaneous induction of prophage**. It is a rare event but all lysogenic bacteria can be induced to shift to the lytic cycle by certain physical (UV rays) and chemical (nitrogen mustard) agents. A lysogenic bacterium is resistant to reinfection by the same or related phages. This is known as **superinfection immunity**.

Bacteriophages may act as **carriers of genes** from one bacterium to another. This is known as **transduction**. It has been discussed in the chapter on bacterial genetics.

Q. 7. Write short note on phage typing.

Ans. The limited host range of many phages enables them to be used as an epidemiological marker to discriminate between bacterial strains that are biochemically or serologically indistinguishable. This method has been used to trace outbreaks of infection caused by *Staphyolococcus* *aureus*, *S.* Typhi and *Vibrio cholerae*. The strain to be typed is inoculated on a plate of nutrient agar to produce a lawn culture. After drying, the phages are applied over marked squares in a fixed dose (**routine test dose**). Routine test dose is the highest dilution of the phage preparation that produces confluent lysis. After overnight incubation, the culture will be observed to be lysed by some phages but not by others. The phage type of the strain is expressed by the designation of the phage/phages that lyse it. For example, if a strain of *S. aureus* is lysed by phages 50, 52A and 80, then the phage type is expressed as 50/52A/80.

38

Virus-Host Interactions, Laboratory Diagnosis of Viral Infections, and Viral Vaccines

Q. 1. Describe virus-host interactions.

Ans. More than 2000 species of viruses have been described, with approximately 650 infecting humans and animals. Viral infection may cause a broad spectrum of effects ranging from no apparent cellular damage to rapid cell destruction. Some viruses like poliovirus cause **cell death** (**cytocidal effect**). Others may cause **cellular proliferation** (molluscum contagiosum) or **malignant transformation** (oncogenic viruses). In some instances, viruses remain as latent infections (herpes simplex virus). Some reactions of the host cells to viral infection are discussed below.

1. Inclusion bodies

A characteristic morphological change in cells infected by certain viruses is the formation of inclusion bodies (or inclusions) which can be seen by light microscope after fixation and staining. These may consist of aggregates of products of viral replication such as virus particles ready for release, overproduction of a particular viral protein or proteins or some aberrant cellular structure such as clumped chromatin. They may be present in the cytoplasm or in the nucleus or both of infected cells and may be acidophilic (stained by eosin) or basophilic (stained by hematoxylin), single or multiple, large or small and round or irregular. In general, those viruses that are assembled in the nucleus (usually DNA viruses) produce intranuclear inclusions, whereas cytoplasmic assembly (mainly RNA viruses) yields cytoplasmic inclusions.

Intracytoplasmic inclusion bodies

These are found in cells infected with rabies virus (**Negri bodies**), vaccinia (**Guarnieri bodies**), fowlpox (**Bollinger bodies**), molluscum contagiosum (**molluscum bodies**), paramyxoviruses and reoviruses.

Intranuclear inclusion bodies

These were classified into two types by Cowdry (1934):

- **Cowdry type A:** Inclusion bodies are of variable size and have a granular appearance (e.g., herpes virus, yellow fever virus).
- **Cowdry type B:** Inclusion bodies are more circumscribed and often multiple (e.g., adenovirus, poliovirus).

Both intranuclear and intracytoplasmic inclusion bodies

Some viruses, for example, measles virus and cytomegalovirus may produce both intranuclear and intracytoplasmic inclusion bodies (Fig. 38.1).

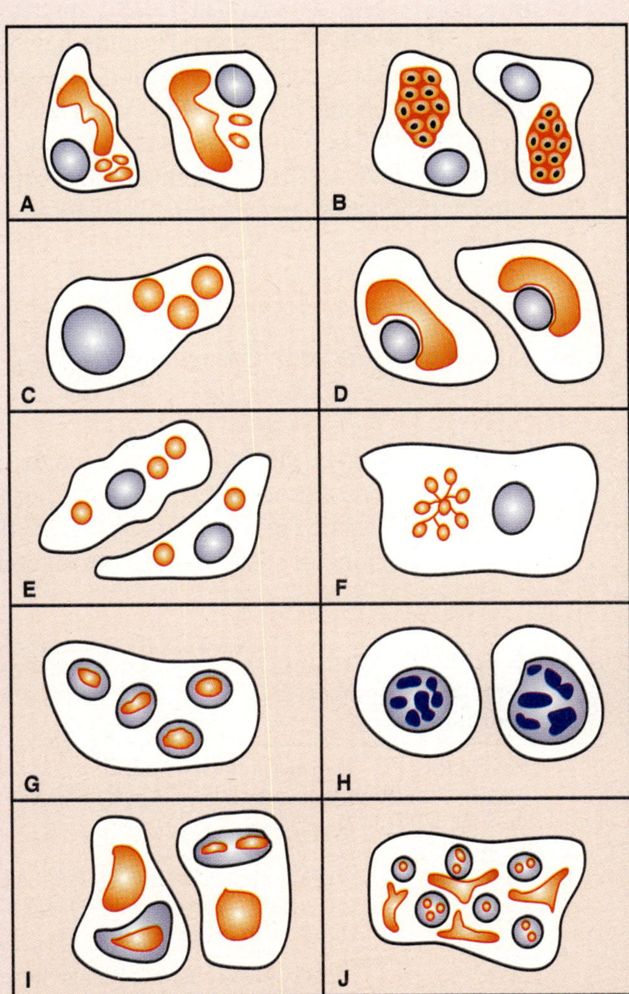

Fig. 38.1. Inclusion bodies in virus-infected cells. Intracytoplasmic (A–F): A, Vaccinia virus (Guarnieri bodies); B, Molluscipox virus (Molluscum body); C, Fowlpox virus (Bollinger bodies); D, Reovirus; E, Rabies virus (Negri bodies); F, Respiratory syncytial virus. Intranuclear (G–H): G, Herpes simplex virus; H, Adenovirus. Intracytoplasmic and intranuclear both (I–J) : I, Cytomegalovirus; J, Measles virus.

2. Cytocidal infection

Viruses like enteroviruses and reoviruses kill their host cells by inhibition of protein, RNA and DNA synthesis.

3. Latent and persistent infections

Viruses have evolved mechanisms to continue to survive in the face of a strong host immune response. For example, herpes simplex types 1 and 2 and varicella-zoster viruses, following primary infection, travel up the peripheral nerves to the sensory ganglia. The viruses remain latent in the ganglia, to be reactivated periodically in some individuals causing recurrent lesions. Similarly, cytomegalovirus (CMV) and Epstein-Barr virus (EBV) are also known to establish latent infection. Some viruses like hepatitis B virus (HBV) may cause chronic infections which may remain clinically inapparent for many years. However, it may lead to more serious consequences, such as **cirrhosis or hepatocellular carcinoma**.

Some viruses produce slow progressive infections. An important example of this type of persistent infection is **subacute sclerosing panencephalitis (SSPE)**. This disease develops between 1–10 years after recovery from measles virus infection. Other viruses that produce slowly progressive fatal diseases in man are human immunodeficiency virus (HIV) which causes acquired immunodeficiency syndrome, and kuru agent and Creutzfeldt-Jakob agent which cause slowly progressive encephalopathy.

4. Cell transformation

Infection of cells with human T cell lymphotropic virus type 1 (HTLV-1), HBV, hepatitis C virus (HCV), EBV and several papillomaviruses does not result in lytic infection and cell death, but leads to cell transformation. Transformed cells require the persistence of all or part of the viral genome to initiate the events leading to transformation and, in most cases, for the maintenance of the transformed state. Viral (or proviral) DNA in transformed cells is **integrated into the cell DNA**. The transformed cells acquire a capacity to divide unrestrictedly leading to tumour production and these cells express distinctive antigens called **tumour-associated antigens**.

Q. 2. Describe transmission of human virus infections.

Ans. Viruses enter the body through the following routes (Table 38.1):

1. Respiratory tract

Many viruses enter the body through inhaled droplets expelled from the nose or mouth of infected persons during talking, coughing or sneezing. This is the most important route of entry of viruses into the body. All viruses that infect the host via the respiratory tract probably do so by attaching to specific receptors on epithelial cells. Some viruses, such as *Influenza-*

Table 38.1. Transmission of human virus infections

Route of transmission	Viruses
Respiratory tract	**Respiratory viruses:** *Influenzavirus A*, *B* and *C*, parainfluenza types 1–4, RSV, *Rhinovirus*, *Coronavirus*, adenovirus and coxsackievirus A **Systemic viruses:** Measles, mumps, rubella, varicella-zoster, CMV and EBV
Alimentary tract	Many enteroviruses including poliovirus types 1–3, HAV, HEV, adenoviruses, rotaviruses, Norwalk and related viruses, *Coronavirus*, *Astrovirus*, coxsackievirus A and B and echovirus
Skin	**Minor abrasions:** Papillomaviruses, molluscum contagiosum, cowpox, orf, milker's nodes viruses, herpes simplex viruses and HBV **Insect bite:** Arboviruses **Animal bite:** Rabies virus, herpes B virus **Injection:** HBV, HCV, HIV-1, HIV-2, HTLV, CMV, EBV and Ebola virus
Genital tract	Papillomaviruses, herpes simplex viruses, HIV, HTLV, HBV, HCV
Conjunctiva	Some adenoviruses and a few enteroviruses

virus A, *B* and *C*, parainfluenza types 1–4, respiratory syncytial virus (RSV), *Rhinovirus*, *Coronavirus*, adenovirus and coxsackievirus A are restricted to respiratory tract where they multiply and produce local disease. These are known as **respiratory viruses**. Other viruses, such as measles, mumps, rubella, varicella-zoster, CMV and EBV multiply locally to initiate a silent local infection which is followed by lymphatic or haematogenous spread to other parts of the body where more extensive multiplication takes place before producing generalized disease.

2. Alimentary tract

Next to airborne infection, faecal-oral infection is the most important route of entry of viruses. They may either be swallowed or infect cells in the oropharynx and then be carried to the intestinal tract. The viruses that initiate infection of humans via the alimentary tract are many enteroviruses including poliovirus types 1–3, hepatitis A virus (HAV), hepatitis E virus (HEV), adenoviruses, rotaviruses, Norwalk and related viruses, *Coronavirus*, *Astrovirus*, coxsackie A and B and echovirus.

The protective mechanisms in the gastrointestinal tract include the acidity of the stomach, the alkalinity of the small intestine, the digestive enzymes found in saliva and pancreatic secretions, and the lipolytic action of bile. In addition, the intestinal tract is partially protected by mucus, which may contain specific secretory IgA antibodies. All these may inactivate viruses. However, viruses causing intestinal infections such as enteroviruses, rotaviruses, Norwalk and related viruses are acid- and bile-resistant. Polioviruses, HAV and HEV do not produce any intestinal symptoms, but cause generalized infection. HIV and HBV can be transmitted through rectum in homosexuals.

3. Skin

Viruses may enter the body through minor abrasions (papillomaviruses, molluscum contagiosum, cowpox, orf, milker's nodes viruses, herpes simplex and HBV), insect bite (arboviruses), animal bite (rabies virus) or injection (HBV, HCV, HIV, HTLV, CMV, EBV and Ebola virus). Some viruses like papillomaviruses, vaccinia, cowpox, molluscum contagiosum and orf replicate in the skin to produce local lesions.

4. Genital tract

Papillomaviruses and herpes simplex viruses are sexually transmitted and produce lesions on the genitalia and perineum. HIV, HTLV, HBV and HCV are also sexually transmitted but do not produce local lesions.

5. Conjunctiva

It may also act as a portal of entry of some adenoviruses and a few enteroviruses.

6. Congenital

Congenital infection may occur at any stage, from the development of the ovum up to birth. In acute systemic infections, congenital infection usually leads to foetal death and abortion. Congenital infection with rubella and cytomegalovirus may result in a large variety of congenital abnormalities or death of the foetus.

Q. 3. Describe host response to virus infection.

Ans. Host response to virus infection is influenced by the virulence of the infecting strain and resistance offered by the host. Many infections are subclinical or asymptomatic or inapparent but exposure gives rise to protection on re-exposure later in life, while others produce disease of varying degree of severity. The mechanism of host resistance may be immunological or nonspecific. Defence mechanisms which work to protect the individual from viruses and to eliminate them if an infection occurs are discussed below:

Nonimmunological responses

1. Age

Most virus infections tend to be most serious at the extremes of life, for example, coxsackieviruses are able to infect suckling but not adult mice. Similarly in man, rotaviruses and respiratory syncytial viruses cause severe disease only in infants in the first year or so of life. Transplacentally acquired maternal antibodies protect the infants against many viruses for first few months of life.

2. Hormones and pregnancy

Corticosteroid administration enhances most virus infections. Injudicious use of steroids in the treatment of herpetic keratoconjunctivitis may cause blindness. Coxsackievirus B1 does not normally cause disease in adult mice, but will induce a fatal infection in mice treated with cortisone. Normally mild infections such as varicella may be lethal in patients on cortisone. Pregnancy significantly increases the likelihood of severe disease following infection with certain viruses. It may be related to the hormonal changes associated with pregnancy. Latent herpesvirus infections are often reactivated during pregnancy contaminating the birth canal and leading to infection of newborn. The deleterious effect of cortisone may be due to its depression of the inflammatory and immune responses and inhibition of interferon synthesis.

3. Malnutrition

Nutritional deficiencies interfere with the generation of antibody- and cell-mediated immune responses, activity of phagocytes and the integrity of skin and mucous membranes. Therefore, malnutrition can exacerbate viral infections, for example, measles produces a much higher case fatality in malnourished than in well-fed children.

4. Fever

Most of the viral infections are accompanied by fever. It is mediated by interleukin-1 which is produced by macrophages. Fever may act as a natural defence mechanism against virus infections as most viruses are inhibited by temperature above 39°C. However, herpes simplex is usually reactivated by fever. *Herpes febrilis* is a frequent accompaniment of fevers caused by pneumococci, streptococci, influenza virus and malaria parasites.

5. Interferons (IFN)

Interferons (IFNs) are a family of regulatory proteins induced by many viruses, by some bacteria and protozoa and by double-stranded nucleic acids. They are classified into three types:

1. ***IFN-a:*** It is induced by virus infection and produced by leucocytes. It has antiviral activity by inhibiting protein synthesis.

2. ***IFN-β:*** It is induced by virus infection and produced by fibroblasts and epithelial cells. It has antiviral activity by inhibiting protein synthesis.
3. ***IFN-γ:*** It is produced by T lymphocytes and NK cells following antigen-specific and mitogenic stimulation. It is a lymphokine with immunoregulatory functions. It enhances MHC antigens and activates cytotoxic T cells, macrophages and NK cells.

Some IFNs especially β and γ display a certain degree of host species specificity, for instance, mouse interferons are ineffective in humans and vice versa. However, there is little or no viral specificity and IFN induced by one virus can confer protection against infection by the same or unrelated viruses.

Mechanism of antiviral effect

The synthesis of IFN (α and β) occurs when a cell becomes infected with a virus. It is released from the infected cell and binds to specific receptors on the plasma membrane of other cells. IFN-α and IFN-β share a common receptor while IFN-γ binds to its own specific receptor. On binding to the cell, IFNs α and β induce the production of three enzymes: RNase L (an endoribonuclease), 2-5A synthetase (2′,5′-oligoadenylate synthetase) and a protein kinase. These enzymes inhibit translation of viral mRNA into viral proteins, without affecting cellular mRNA.

Acquired immunity

Virions in general are good antigens and induce both antibody- and cell-mediated immunity (CMI), the primary mediators being B and T lymphocytes respectively. The activities of both these cells are regulated by T helper (Th) and T suppressor (Ts) lymphocytes, lymphokines and monokines. For some diseases such as poxviruses, measles, herpes simplex virus and CMV infections, CMI appears to be the main immunospecific defence, for others, such as enterovirus and arbovirus infections, antibody production appears to be the main immunospecific defence. However, some viruses have evolved strategies to evade detection and persist in their host.

Antibody-mediated immunity

IgG, IgM and IgA antibodies are produced in response to virus infection. IgG and IgM play a major role in blood and tissue spaces. IgA is a dimer, with four Fab fragments. Passing through epithelial cells, IgA acquires a 'secretory component' to become secretory IgA (sIgA), which is secreted through mucosae into the respiratory, intestinal and urogenital tracts. It is more resistant to proteases than other immunoglobulins and it is the principal immunoglobulin on mucosal surfaces, and in milk and colostrum. Therefore, it is important in resistance to infection of the respiratory, intestinal and urogenital tracts. There are several ways in which antibody against viral components can protect the host:

- Neutralization of infectious virus by preventing virus attachment, penetration or even subsequent events.
- Opsonization of virions for phagocytosis and killing by macrophages.
- Antibody may attach to viral antigens on the surface of the infected cells, rendering virus-infected cells prone to lysis by complement or destruction by phagocytes or killer (K) lymphocytes.

Cell-mediated immunity

Antibody can neutralize free virions but once these agents get into cells, cell-mediated immunity operates. It prevents infection of target organs and promotes recovery from disease by destroying virus and virus-infected cells by any of the following four different processes:

1. Cytolysis by Tc cells.
2. Cytolysis by NK cells.
3. Antibody-complement-mediated cytotoxicity.
4. Antibody-dependent cell-mediated cytotoxicity (ADCC).

Q. 4. Describe laboratory diagnosis of viral infections.

Ans. Laboratory diagnosis of viral infections can be carried out by the following methods:

I. Direct detection of virus, viral antigen or viral genome.
II. Virus isolation.
III. Detection of specific antiviral antibodies.
IV. Cytological or histological examination of cells from the site of infection.

I. Direct detection of virus, viral antigen or viral genome

1. Electron microscopy

Electron microscopy (EM) is one of the most useful tools for the direct demonstration of viruses in clinical specimens (Table 38.2). On the basis of their distinctive appearances, most of the viruses can be assigned to the correct family. Viruses that are difficult to culture (*Rotavirus*, astroviruses) can be recognized by electron microscopy. The clinical material can be negatively stained with potassium phosphotungstate or uranyl acetate and scanned by EM. Clinical applications of electron microscopy include detection of *Rotavirus* and hepatitis A virus in faecal specimens, poxviruses in vesicle fluid and herpesvirus in brain biopsy tissue. This method can also be used for the identification of virus isolates in cell culture.

2. Immunoelectron microscopy

EM as a diagnostic tool has low sensitivity. For satisfactory results, the specimen should contain 10^7 virions per ml. The sensitivity of electron microscopy can be increased by mixing specific antibody with the specimen to aggregate the virus particles. These aggregates can be sedimented by centrifugation, negatively stained and observed under EM.

Table 38.2. Detection of viruses in diagnostic electron microscopy

Disease	Specimen	Viruses detectable
Diarrhoea and vomiting	Faeces	*Rotavirus*, adenovirus, *Astrovirus*, *Calicivirus*, Norwalk virus, *Coronavirus*
Vesicular rash	Vesicular fluid	Herpes simplex, varicella-zoster
Warty lesions	Molluscum body	Molluscum contagiosum
Congenital anomalies	Urine	Cytomegalovirus
Meningitis	CSF	Enterovirus, mumps, varicella-zoster

3. Fluorescence microscopy

Virions or viral antigens can be detected in frozen tissue sections, acetone-fixed cell smears, cells from virus infected cultures or vesicle fluid by direct or indirect fluorescent antibody technique. Fluorescence microscopy of brain biopsy can be used for the diagnosis of herpes simplex encephalitis and subacute sclerosing panencephalitis (a late sequelae of measles) and for the verification of rabies in the brain of animals suspected to be rabid. This method is also useful for the rapid diagnosis of respiratory infections caused by paramyxoviruses, orthomyxoviruses, adenoviruses and herpesviruses.

4. Light microscopy

Viral antigens in infected cells can be detected by immunoperoxidase staining. Tissue section or smear of infected cells is stained with antibody coupled to horseradish peroxidase. Hydrogen peroxide together with a benzidine derivative is then added. It forms a coloured insoluble precipitate which can be seen under ordinary light microscope (LM).

5. Viral antigens

These may be detected by direct and indirect ELISA, radioimmunoassay and latex agglutination.

6. Nucleic acid probes

- Enzyme-labelled or radiolabelled nucleic acid (DNA or RNA) sequences complementary to unique regions in nucleic acid sequences of most viruses are now manufactured commercially. These labelled complementary sequences are known as nucleic acid probes. Two strands of the target DNA molecule in the clinical specimens are first separated by boiling, then, following cooling, allowed to hybridize with a labelled single-stranded DNA or RNA probe present in excess. Depending on the type of label attached to the probe, hybridized-labelled probe can be detected by radiography, gamma-counting or by a simple colourimetric evaluation (dot-blot hybridization).
- By use of nucleic acid probes cytomegalovirus, papillomavirus and Epstein-Barr virus have been identified.
- **In situ hybridization** may be used to detect integrated or nonintegrated copies of viral genome in persistent infections or viral cancers.
- **Southern blot hybridization and northern blot hybridization** can be used for detection of DNA and RNA respectively.

7. Polymerase chain reaction (PCR)

It is a DNA amplification system that allows molecular biologists to produce microgram quantities of DNA from picogram amounts of starting material. It is based on repeated cycles of high temperature template denaturation, oligonucleotide primer annealing and polymerase mediated extension. With the revolutionary PCR technique, a target DNA sequence can be amplified at least 100,000 folds in just a few hours, a sharp contrast to the days required for conventional amplification method (culture). Thus viral DNA extracted from a very small number of virions or infected cells can be amplified to the point where it can readily be identified using labelled probes in a hybridization assay. For the detection of viral RNA, it is first converted into DNA by reverse transcriptase.

PCR can be used for the diagnosis of infections caused by HIV-1, HIV-2, HTLV-1, cytomegalovirus, human *Papillomavirus*, herpes simplex viruses, HBV, HCV, HDV, HEV, rubella virus, Epstein-Barr virus, varicella-zoster virus, human herpesvirus 6 and 7, *Parvovirus* B19, enteroviruses, coxsackieviruses, echoviruses, rhinoviruses, measles virus and *Rotavirus* (Table 7.5).

II. Virus isolation

Most of the viruses can be cultivated in laboratory animals, chick embryos and cell cultures. The methods of cultivation and their identification are described in the previous chapter.

III. Detection of specific antiviral antibodies

Using panels of known antigens, a number of serological techniques may be used to detect specific viral antibodies. Paired sera should be collected from the patient, the 'acute-phase' serum sample collected as early as possible in the illness and the 'convalescent-phase' sample collected at least 2 weeks later. Antibodies in the serum samples can be detected by ELISA, RIA, western blot, latex agglutination, virus neutralization, haemagglutination inhibition, immunofluorescence, immunodiffusion and complement fixation tests.

IV. Cytological or histological examination of cells from the site of infection

Virus-induced histopathology (multinucleate giant cells and inclusion bodies) may be recognized by light microscopy. For example, demonstration of Negri bodies in the brain cells of animals is a useful method for presumptive diagnosis of rabies.

Q. 5. Write short note on viral vaccines.

Ans. Viral vaccines confer solid immunity and are, in general, more effective than bacterial vaccines. A number of viral vaccines have been outstandingly successful especially those directed against smallpox, yellow fever, poliomyelitis, measles and rubella. Smallpox vaccine has been used as a sole tool for global eradication of the disease. The World Health Organization is now determined on global eradication of poliomyelitis. No case of poliomyelitis has been reported from India after 11-02-2011. Viral vaccines are of three types (Table 38.3):

Table 38.3. Viral vaccines

I. Live-virus vaccines • Smallpox • Yellow fever (ITD) • Poliomyelitis (Sabin type) • Measles • Mumps • Rubella • Varicella
II. Inactivated virus and virus sub-unit vaccines or non-replicating vaccines • Poliomyelitis (Salk type) • Rabies • Influenza (Subunit vaccine) • Hepatitis A • Hepatitis B • Japanese encephalitis
III. Anti-idiotype and DNA vaccines

I. Live-virus vaccines

These are prepared from:

- Attenuated strains that are almost or completely devoid of pathogenicity.
- Temperature sensitive (ts) and cold-adapted (ca) mutants.
- Recombinant live viral or bacterial vectors.

Advantages of live-virus vaccines

1. A single dose is usually sufficient because they multiply in the human host and provide continuous antigenic stimulation over a period of time resulting in durable immunity.
2. They can be administered by the route of natural infection so that local immunity is induced.
3. They induce a wide spectrum of immunoglobulins including secretory IgA to whole range of viral antigens.
4. They also induce cell-mediated immunity.
5. They provide more effective long-lasting immunity than killed vaccines.
6. Some of them can be given as combined vaccines (measles-mumps-rubella vaccine).
7. Primary vaccine failures are uncommon and are usually the result of inadequate storage or administration.
8. They can, in general, be prepared more economically and more conveniently for mass immunization.

Disadvantages of live-virus vaccines

1. There is risk, however, remote, of reversion of virulence.
2. The vaccine may be contaminated with potentially dangerous viruses such as oncogenic viruses.
3. Interference by pre-existing viruses may sometimes prevent a good immune response following live vaccination.
4. Live-virus vaccines are heat-labile and have to be preserved under strict refrigeration.
5. Some live-virus vaccines may cause local remote complications.

Currently available live-virus vaccines are oral polio, measles, mumps, rubella, yellow fever and varicella vaccines. Polyvalent measles-mumps-rubella (MMR) vaccine is also available.

II. Inactivated virus and virus subunit vaccines or nonreplicating vaccines

Inactivated virus vaccines are prepared from virulent viruses by chemically destroying the infectivity while retaining the immunogenicity. Chemical agents used are β-propiolactone and formaldehyde. Subunit vaccines include purified viral proteins, purified proteins from cloned genes and synthetic peptides.

Advantages of nonreplicating vaccines

1. Safety.
2. Stability.

Disadvantages of nonreplicating vaccines

1. These vaccines need to be injected in large amounts. Primary course comprises of two or three injections. Thereafter, booster doses may be required at intervals over the succeeding years to revive waning immunity.
2. These vaccines have to be given by injections, therefore, local IgA immunoglobulins fail to develop.
3. Cell-mediated immunity is not induced.

Currently available nonreplicating viral vaccines include inactivated polio, rabies, influenza, hepatitis B, Japanese encephalitis and tick-borne encephalitis vaccines.

Q. 6. Write short note on antiviral therapy.

Ans. As viruses are obligate intracellular parasites, they are absolutely dependent on the biosynthetic mechanisms of the host cell for their replication. Hence, most agents that block the replication of viruses are lethal to the cell. However, it is now known that viral replication may be checked at the level of attachment, penetration, transcription of viral nucleic acid, translation of viral mRNA and inhibition of viral DNA polymerase and reverse transcriptase and replication of viral nucleic acid (Table 38.4).

Table 38.4. Major antiviral compounds used for treatment of viral infections

Drug	Viral spectrum
VIRAL POLYMERASE INHIBITORS	
Acyclovir	Herpes simplex, varicella-zoster
Cidofovir	Cytomegalovirus, herpes simplex
Foscarnet	Herperviruses, HIV-1, HBV
Ganciclovir	Cytomegalovirus
Valacyclovir	Herpesviruses
Vidarabine	Herpesviruses, vaccinia, HBV
BLOCKING OF VIRAL UNCOATING	
Amantadine	Influenzavirus A
HIV PROTEASE INHIBITORS	
Indinavir	HIV-1, HIV-2
Ritonavir	HIV-1, HIV-2
Saquinavir	HIV-1, HIV-2
REVERSE TRANSCRIPTASE INHIBITORS	
Lamivudine (deoxycytidine)	HIV-1, HIV-2, HBV
Nevirapine	HIV-1
Stavudine	HIV-1, HIV-2
Zidovudine (azidothymidine, AZT)	HIV-1, HIV-2, HBV
Zalcitabine (dideoxycytidine, ddC)	HIV-1, HIV-2, HBV
Didanosine (dideoxyinosine, ddI)	HIV-1, HIV-2
BLOCKING OF CAPPING OF mRNA	
Ribavirin	Respiratory syncytial virus, Influenzaviruses A and B, Lassa fever

Other question which may also be asked in the examination

Write short note on interferon.

For answer see pages 372–373.

39

HERPESVIRUSES

Q. 1. Classify herpesviruses, and describe morphology and cultivation of herpesviruses.

Ans. Herpesviruses have been divided into three subfamilies (Table 39.1).

Table 39.1. Human herpesviruses (HHV)

Subfamily	Common name	Scientific name
Alphaherpesvirinae	Herpes simplex virus type 1	Human herpesvirus 1
	Herpes simplex virus type 2	Human herpesvirus 2
	Varicella-zoster virus	Human herpesvirus 3
	Simian herpes B virus	Cercopithecine herpesvirus 1
Gammaherpesvirinae	Epstein-Barr virus	Human herpesvirus 4
	Kaposi's sarcoma-associated herpesvirus	Human herpesvirus 8
Bataherpesvirinae	Human cytomegalovirus	Human herpesvirus 5
	—	Human herpesvirus 6
	—	Human herpesvirus 7

Morphology

Herpesviruses are 120–200 nm in diameter. They comprise of four distinct structural elements – envelope, tegument, capsid and core (Fig. 39.1). Envelope is the outermost, it is composed of lipid with numerous small glycoprotein peplomers. Tegument is the electron-dense material present between envelope and capsid. It contains several proteins. Inner to the tegument is icosahedral capsid of 100 nm diameter. It has a total of 162 capsomers. Core, inside the capsid, consists of double-stranded, 124–235 kb DNA.

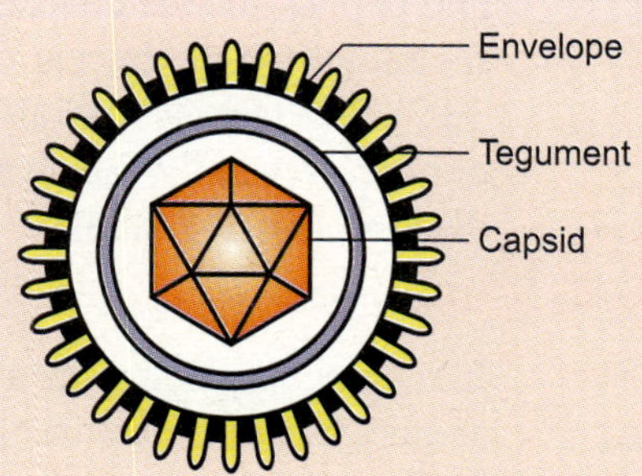

Fig. 39.1. Herpesvirus.

Cultivation

With the exception of Epstein-Barr virus, members of the family Herpesviridae can be cultivated in cell cultures and produce giant cells and Cowdry type A intranuclear inclusion bodies in infected cells.

Q. 2. Describe pathogenicity of herpes simplex viruses.

Ans. There are two types of herpes simplex virus – type 1 virus (HSV-1) and type 2 virus (HSV-2). Both these viruses share many characteristics, including DNA homology, antigen determinants, tissue tropism, and disease signs. HSV-1 infects primarily the mouth, the eye and the central nervous system (regions of the body above the waist), but it is also responsible for a proportion of cases of genital herpes. HSV-2 infects genital and anal regions. The infections caused by herpes simplex viruses can be divided into primary infection, latent infection, reactivation and recrudescence.

Primary infections

HSV is transmitted only by contact. The portal of entry in primary infection is the damaged skin or mucosa and the classic lesion is a vesicle beneath the keratinized squamous epithelial cells. The vesicle and surrounding tissue contain a dense infiltrate of inflammatory cells, mostly mononuclear. The vesicle drains and the lesion crusts before healing occurs, sometimes with residual scarring, and draining lymph nodes are commonly enlarged during this process.

Infections caused by HSV-1

1. Acute gingivostomatitis.
2. Herpetic whitlow.
3. Keratoconjunctivitis.
4. Eczema herpeticum.
5. Encephalitis.
6. Generalized infection.

1. Acute gingivostomatitis

It is the most common primary lesion. It leads to acute and painful ulcers, coated with a greyish slough, inside the mouth on the buccal mucosa and on the gums (Fig. 39.2). The lesions may also involve the tonsils, pharynx or nose. Normally, the disease is self-limiting and lesions disappear in 2–3 weeks.

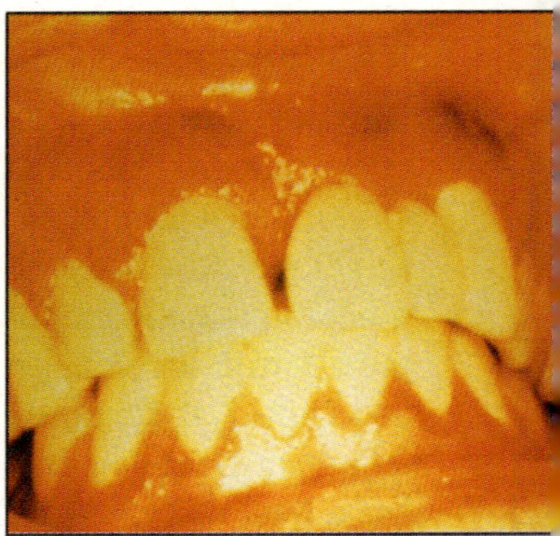

Fig. 39.2. Herpetic gingivostomatitis.

2. Herpetic whitlow

It is an occupational hazard of doctors and nurses, who acquire infection by implantation of virus from saliva and respiratory secretions of patients. The lesion is similar to staphylococcal whitlow, although the exudate is serous rather than purulent. Vesicles may also be produced on the skin of head and neck.

3. Keratoconjunctivitis

Infection of the eye by HSV-1 causes an extremely painful ulceration of cornea and vesiculation of the lids with associated conjunctivitis. In majority of the cases, the primary lesions heal in 2–3 weeks.

4. Eczema herpeticum

It is a superinfection of eczematous skin. It is mainly seen in young children. Crops of vesicles appear mainly on already eczematous areas with extensive ulceration.

5. Encephalitis

Both HSV-1 and HSV-2 can also infect central nervous system leading to herpes encephalitis. The main site of infection is temporal lobe where the disease causes necrosis.

6. Generalized infection

Rarely, primary infection with HSV-1 may lead to generalized disseminated infection. Patient develops acute gingivostomatitis, disseminated vesicular skin lesions, hepatitis and involvement of other organs.

Infections caused by HSV-2

1. Genital herpes.
2. Aseptic meningitis.
3. Neonatal infection.

It may rarely cause head and neck infections.

1. Genital herpes

HSV-2 causes one of the most prevalent forms of **sexually transmitted diseases**. It leads to the development of painful vesicles on the genitalia or anal regions with fever, malaise and tender, swollen lymph nodes. In the females, lesions may occur on the perineum, vagina, cervix or vulva. In the males, the lesions may occur on the glans, prepuce or shaft of the penis. HSV-2 proctitis has been reported in homosexual men. Majority (80%) of cases of genital herpes are due to HSV-2 and remaining cases are due to HSV-1. These cases are possibly due to orogenital sexual practices. HSV-2 may also be involved in oral infections. **It has also been blamed to cause cervical carcinoma.**

2. Aseptic meningitis

It may occur as a complication of HSV-2 genital infection.

3. Neonatal infection

It is acquired by the neonates usually from their mothers during passage through an infected birth canal, but in some cases it may be acquired in the immediate postnatal period from parents and nurses. Prenatally, a very few cases may acquire infection by viraemic transmission across the placenta or by ascending infection from the cervix. This may result in **abortions** or **congenital defects in the child**. If a woman has primary genital herpes at the time of delivery, the risk of neonatal herpes is 30–40%. Therefore, caesarean section is indicated in such mothers. Most of the cases of neonatal herpes are due to HSV-2, but those acquired postnatally may be due to HSV-1.

Neonatal herpes may present as:

- Disseminated disease, with a case fatality rate of 80%, most of the survivors being left with permanent neurologic or ocular sequelae.
- Encephalitis, with high mortality.
- Disease localized to mucocutaneous surfaces such as skin, eye and mouth.

Latent infection

During primary infection, the virus travels from the site of infection in the mouth to the trigeminal and probably other cranial and cervical ganglia. In genital herpes, HSV-2 travels to sacral ganglia. Within the sensory ganglia, viral DNA exists as a free circular episome perhaps about 20 copies per infected cells.

Reactivation and recrudescence

Reactivation of the virus is provoked by various stimuli such as common cold, fever, pneumonia, menstruation, exposure to sunlight, stress, etc. Infectious virions migrate along the nerve axon back to the nerve endings, where infection of epithelial cells may result in cluster of vesicles at the mucocutaneous junctions of the lips, in the nose, or eyes or on areas of skin that have experienced a primary infection. Reactivation recurs sporadically, sometimes often, throughout life.

Q. 3. Describe laboratory diagnosis and chemotherapy of herpes simplex infections.

Ans. Laboratory diagnosis

1. Specimens

Vesicle fluid, skin swab, saliva, conjunctival fluid, corneal scrapings, brain biopsy and CSF.

2. Microscopy

Diagnosis of HSV infection can be made by direct examination of clinical specimens by electron microscopy (EM), fluorescence microscopy (FM) and light microscopy (LM). Herpes virions may be demonstrated in the negatively stained smear of the specimen by EM. Viral antigens can be detected by FM in the cells scraped from the base of the lesions and tissue preparations stained by immunofluorescent staining. By LM, infected cell may be identified by characteristic changes, which include ballooning of cells, ground-glass nuclei, **eosinophilic intranuclear inclusions and multinucleated giant cells** (Figs. 38.1G and 39.3).

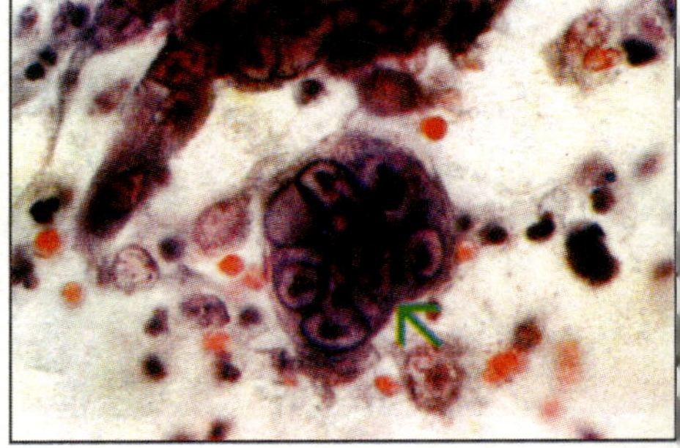

Fig. 39.3. Multinucleated giant cells with intranuclear inclusion bodies of herpes simplex virus.

3. Virus isolation

HSV can be isolated on human fibroblast or Vero cells although other mammalian cells also support its growth. Within 1–5 days distinctive foci of swollen, rounded cells appear. Some virus strains (particularly HSV-2 strains) may give rise to fusion of infected cells leading to

syncytium formation. Diagnosis can be confirmed within 24 hours by **immunofluorescent staining** of infected cell culture. Differentiation of HSV-1 and HSV-2 can be made by use of monoclonal antibodies in immunofluorescent staining or by **neutralization test** with specific antiserum.

4. Serology

Primary infections can be diagnosed serologically by detection of virus-specific IgM or of a rising IgG titre by complement fixation, neutralization, immunofluorescence, ELISA or RIA. However, serology is not widely used.

5. Polymerase chain reaction

Polymerase chain reaction may be used for detection of HSV DNA in CSF.

Chemotherapy

HSV infection can be successfully treated with acyclovir (acycloguanosine). It acts by interfering with viral DNA synthesis by inhibiting virus DNA-dependent DNA polymerase. For the treatment of ophthalmic herpes simplex infection, it may be used in the form of ointment. Oral acyclovir 200 mg 5 times daily for 10 days may be used for the treatment of primary herpes genitalis and orofacial herpes. For the treatment of herpes simplex encephalitis, neonatal herpes and disseminated infection in immunocompromised patients, intravenous acyclovir (10 mg/kg, 3 times daily for 2–3 weeks) may be given.

Q. 4. Describe pathogenicity and laboratory diagnosis of varicella-zoster virus. How will you treat varicella-zoster virus infection?

Ans. **Pathogenicity**

VZV causes varicella (chickenpox) in children and herpes zoster (shingles) in adults and immunocompromised patients. **Varicella follows primary infection in a nonimmune individual while herpes zoster is a reactivation of latent virus when immunity has fallen to ineffective levels.** A child can catch varicella from an elderly patient with herpes zoster, but the latter occurs only if the elderly or immunocompromised person had suffered from varicella in early part of his life.

Varicella

It is one of the common childhood exanthemata. Portal of entry of the virus is respiratory tract. Incubation period is about 2 weeks. The earliest manifestation is a **maculopapular rash** that progresses within a few hours to the vesicular stage. Vesicles characteristically are surrounded by a red rim. The lesions then rupture and crust or may become secondarily infected and pustular before healing.

Vesicles are centripetal in distribution, i.e., they are more profuse on the trunk followed by neck and proximal areas of limbs. Successive crops of vesicles appear over 2–5 days and as a result at any one time will have lesions at various stages of development on the same area of the skin. The accompanying fever is usually low grade. The incidence of complications in children is low, the most common problem being secondary infection of lesions and consequent scarring, a problem that can usually be solved by antibiotic treatment.

Infection of adults is generally more severe than in children; the vesicles heal more slowly, secondary bacterial infection and scarring are more common, and the accompanying fever is higher and more prolonged. Some patients of varicella may develop viral pneumonitis, encephalitis, Guillain-Barré syndrome and Reye's syndrome. **Varicella tends to be more serious in pregnancy**, if the patient has not been infected during childhood. **VZV can cross the placenta following viraemia** in the pregnant woman and infect the foetus. A syndrome of **congenital malformations** with hypoplasia of limbs, chorioretinitis and scarring of skin associated with maternal varicella in the first trimester may develop.

Herpes zoster

Herpes zoster or shingles is an **endogenous reactivation of virus** which has remained latent in one or more sensory ganglia following primary varicella many years earlier. Virus travels down the sensory nerves to produce painful vesicles in the area of skin (dermatome) enervated from the affected ganglion (Fig. 39.4). Thoracic nerves supplying the chest wall are most often affected. When the ophthalmic nerve of trigeminal ganglion is affected, the rash is distributed on the scalp and forehead. In about half of the patients, the eye is affected leading to corneal ulceration, stromal keratitis and anterior uveitis.

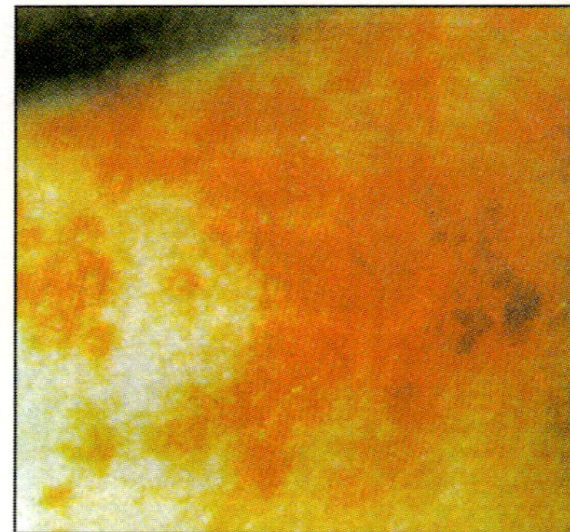

Fig. 39.4. Vesicles of varicella zoster infection on the left shoulder and neck.

The accompanying pain is often very severe for up to a few weeks, and in herpetic neuralgia, which occurs in half of all patients over 60 years of age, may persist for months which may require surgical ablation of the ganglion. Herpes zoster of the seventh cranial ganglion may lead to **Bell's palsy** and **Ramsay Hunt syndrome** which is characterized by facial nerve palsy with a rash on the tympanic membrane and the external auditory canal. Herpes zoster may also cause encephalitis. In immunocompromised and cancer patients, disseminated herpes zoster is sometimes seen.

Laboratory diagnosis

1. Direct examination of vesicle fluid by **electron microscopy** may reveal herpes virus particles.
2. Stained smears from the base of the lesion or sections from biopsy tissue show **multinucleated giant cells containing acidophilic intranuclear inclusion bodies**.
3. Rapid diagnosis is possible by using **monoclonal fluorescent antibody technique**.
4. VZV antigens can be detected in vesicle fluid by **ELISA**.
5. DNA can be extracted from virions in vesicle fluid, CSF and aqueous humour amplified by **PCR** and detected by nucleic acid hybridization.
6. The virus can be **isolated** from vesicle fluid in human embryonic lung fibroblasts, human amnion, HeLa or Vero cells. Cytopathic effect is focal with refractile ballooned cells. It develops slowly over a period of 2 or more weeks. However, VZV antigen can be demonstrated in nuclear inclusions by immunofluorescence with monoclonal antibody before the end of first week.

7. Recent infection can be diagnosed by **ELISA test** for varicella-zoster specific IgM antibody in patient serum.

Treatment

Acyclovir and vidarabine given intravenously are effective in the treatment of severe varicella and herpes zoster (e.g., in the immunocompromised patients).

Q. 5. Discuss pathogenicity of Epstein-Barr virus.

Ans. EBV has been named after the virologists (Epstein and Barr) who first observed it under electron microscope in cultures of lymphoblasts from Burkitt's lymphoma. EBV replicates in epithelial cells of nasopharynx and salivary glands, especially the parotid, lysing them and releasing infectious virions into saliva. B lymphocytes appear to become infected when they infiltrate infected nasopharyngeal mucosa. Inside B cells, EBV normally fails to replicate but establishes lifelong latency. In these cells, EBV genome persists as multiple full-length copies in the form of circular episomes. EBV has **oncogenic properties** and a proportion of infected B lymphocytes undergo transformations and transform cells *in vitro* too. Activated B lymphocytes secrete immunoglobulins especially IgM.

EBV possesses envelope glycoprotein gp350/220, which mediates attachment of the virus to CD21 receptors present on the susceptible cells. Most shedding of virus takes place in the oral cavity, therefore, transmission of virus requires salivary contact, either through kissing or contaminated eating utensils. Most infections are symptomless, especially when acquired during childhood. However, in adolescents it may cause infectious mononucleosis or glandular fever, infections in immunocompromised hosts and when EBV exerts its oncogenic potential, it may cause Burkitt's lymphoma, B cell lymphoma and nasopharyngeal carcinoma. In HIV-infected individuals, it may cause hairy leukoplakia and lymphocytic interstitial pneumonitis.

Infectious mononucleosis (Glandular fever)

It is a primary EBV infection seen mainly in the 15–25 years age group. EBV is commonly transmitted by infected saliva and initiates infection in the oropharynx. Viral replication occurs in epithelial cells of the pharynx and salivary glands.

After an incubation period of 4–7 weeks, patient presents with sore throat due to exudative tonsillitis, generalized lymphadenopathy, fever, malaise, headache, sweating, fatigue and gastrointestinal discomfort. In some cases spleen and liver are often enlarged. A faint transient morbilliform rash may be seen. A maculopapular rash may appear, especially following treatment with ampicillin due to immune complexes with antibody to ampicillin. The disease usually lasts for 2–3 weeks. However, some patients develop complications such as Guillain-Barré syndrome, Bell's palsy, meningoencephalitis, transverse myelitis, haemolytic anaemia, thrombocytopenia, carditis, nephritis, pneumonia and splenic rupture.

Infections in immunocompromised host

- EBV causes X-linked lymphoproliferative syndrome in male members of certain families with an X-linked recessive immunodeficiency with a reduced ability to synthesize interferon. About half of the boys die, within a month, from sepsis or haemorrhages and remainder develop and die from B cell lymphoproliferation with associated hypogammaglobulinaemia and later lymphoma.

- EBV may cause progressive lymphoproliferative disease in transplant recipients, immunodeficient children and AIDS patients.

EBV-associated malignancies

1. Burkitt's lymphoma

This lymphoma is a **malignant B cell lymphoma** (a tumour of the jaw) seen in regions of equatorial Africa and New Guinea where malaria is hyperendemic. EBV infection is acquired early in life. Malaria being immunosuppressive, may act as a co-factor by interfering with the immune responses that normally prevent reactivation of EBV from B cells thus enabling its full oncogenic potential to be expressed. The EBV genomic DNA is present in multiple copies, in the form of circular episomes, in each cell of most African Burkitt's lymphomas, but the cells do not produce virus unless induced to do so following cultivation *in vitro*. Tumour cells express viral antigens and sera from such patients contain elevated levels of antibody to virus-specific antigens.

2. B cell lymphoma

Immunodeficient patients, e.g., recipients of transplants and HIV-infected patients may develop EBV associated B cell lymphoma.

There has long been a suspicion that EBV may play some part in the induction of **Hodgkin's disease** and **T cell lymphoma**.

3. Nasopharyngeal carcinoma

It is also associated with EBV and viral DNA is regularly present in the malignant epithelial cells of the tumour. The patients have high levels of antibody to EBV. It shows a striking geographical and probably racial distribution, for example, the disease is common in people from Southern China, and in Eskimos and Greenlanders.

Oral hairy leukoplakia

This lesion is a wart-like growth that develops on the tongue in some HIV-infected patients and recipients of transplant (Fig. 39.5). It is an epithelial focus of EBV replication.

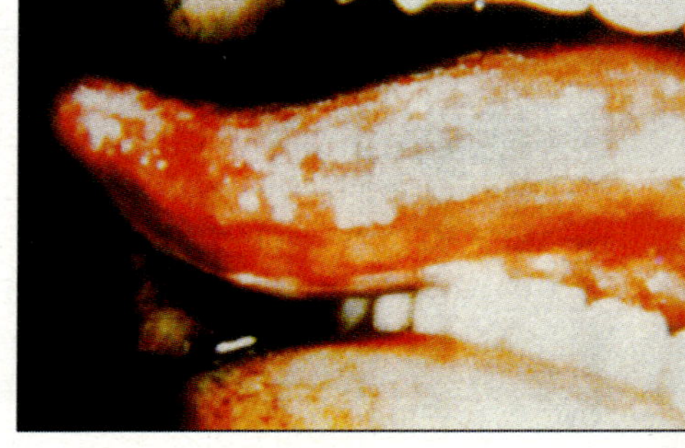

Fig. 39.5. Oral hairy leukoplakia in an AIDS patient.

Lymphocytic interstitial pneumonitis

EBV has also been associated with lymphocytic interstitial pneumonitis in HIV-infected children.

Q. 6. Describe laboratory diagnosis of infectious mononucleosis.

Ans. The clinical picture of infectious mononucleosis is so variable that laboratory confirmation is required. This can be carried out by:

1. Differential white blood cell count

By the second week of the illness patient develops leucocytosis (10,000–20,000/μl or more). Lymphocytes and monocytes account for 60–80%. Of these, 20% or more are **'atypical lymphocytes'**. The latter are large pleomorphic blasts with deeply basophilic vacuolated cytoplasm and lobulated nuclei. They persist for 2 weeks to several months.

2. Paul-Bunnell heterophile antibodies

Infectious mononucleosis is accompanied by production of **heterophile agglutinins**. These are heterophile IgM antibodies elicited by EBV infection. These antibodies appear in 85–90% of patients' sera during the acute phase of illness, reaching peak levels 2 weeks after the onset. Their titre decreases rapidly after fourth week and are not detectable after 3 months. Heterophile antibodies may be readily detected by a rapid slide agglutination test or Paul-Bunnell test. Agglutination of sheep or horse red cells by patient serum, adsorbed with guinea-pig kidney cells, to remove Forssman antibody, is the basis of this test.

3. EBV-specific antibodies

More reliable indicator of EBV infection is the demonstration of IgM antibody to the EBV viral capsid antigen by ELISA or indirect immunofluorescence. This antibody becomes detectable within 4 weeks and declines rapidly over the next 3 months or so.

4. Virus isolation

Saliva or throat washing and peripheral blood leucocytes can be inoculated onto umbilical cord lymphocytes. If the specimen contains EBV, it leads to immortalization of the cells to produce a lymphoblastoid cell line.

5. PCR and DNA hybridization

EBV can also be detected by PCR and DNA hybridization.

Q. 7. Describe pathogenicity and laboratory diagnosis of cytomegalovirus.

Ans. **Pathogenicity**

CMV is the largest virus in the family Herpesviridae, being 150–200 nm in size. The virus exhibits strict host-specificity. *In vivo*, CMV replicates in epithelial cells in salivary glands, kidneys and respiratory epithelium. The infected cells are enlarged and possess **inclusions in both the nuclei and cytoplasm**. *In vitro*, they can be isolated on human fibroblast cells. An individual infected with CMV carries the virus for life and may shed it intermittently in saliva, urine, semen, cervical secretions and breast milk. The virus is found in 0.3–2.4% of populations that have been sampled throughout the world. Infection is transmitted by close contact between individuals and blood transfusion. It may be acquired at any time, i.e. prenatal, perinatal and postnatal.

Prenatal (intrauterine) infection

CMV is the most common agent to cause intrauterine infection and prenatal damage to foetus leading to congenital abnormalities. Approximately 1% of all babies become infected in utero. Maternal viraemia following primary CMV infection or a reactivation during pregnancy may result in foetal infection. Majority (95%) of these are without obvious symptoms at the time of birth and 5% symptomatic infants have cytomegalic inclusion body disease. These infants show signs of growth retardation, hepatosplenomegaly, jaundice, thrombocytopenia, microcephaly, encephalitis and chorioretinitis. Of the remaining 95%, about 15% develop deafness and mental retardation.

Perinatal infection

This is acquired from infected maternal genital secretions or from breast feeding.

Postnatal infection

This may be acquired by kissing (from saliva), sexual intercourse or artificial insemination (from semen), blood transfusion and organ transplantation.

Infections acquired after birth are generally subclinical. However, it may cause hepatitis in young children. In adults and older children, it may cause a syndrome resembling EBV infectious mononucleosis, but with a negative Paul-Bunnell test and no pharyngitis or lymphadenopathy. CMV may cause widely disseminated infection in immunocompromised individuals such as graft recipients and AIDS patients leading to interstitial pneumonia, chorioretinitis, hepatitis, arthritis, chronic gastrointestinal infection, encephalitis, Guillain-Barré syndrome and transverse myelitis.

Laboratory diagnosis

1. Specimens

CMV can be isolated from urine, saliva, stool, breast milk, semen, cervical secretions and blood leucocytes.

2. Demonstration of cytomegalic cells

Cytomegalic cells can be demonstrated in centrifuged deposits of urine or saliva.

3. Isolation of virus

The specimens are inoculated on cultured human fibroblasts. The virus replicates very slowly, therefore, characteristic CPE of foci of swollen refractile cells with cytoplasmic granules may take 2–3 weeks to appear. When stained, these cells are **multinucleated giant cells containing acidophilic inclusions with perinuclear halo (owl's eye appearance) in the nuclei and cytoplasm** (Figs. 38.1I and 39.6). For precise identification, the cell line may be stained by immunofluorescence or immunoperoxidase technique using monoclonal antibody.

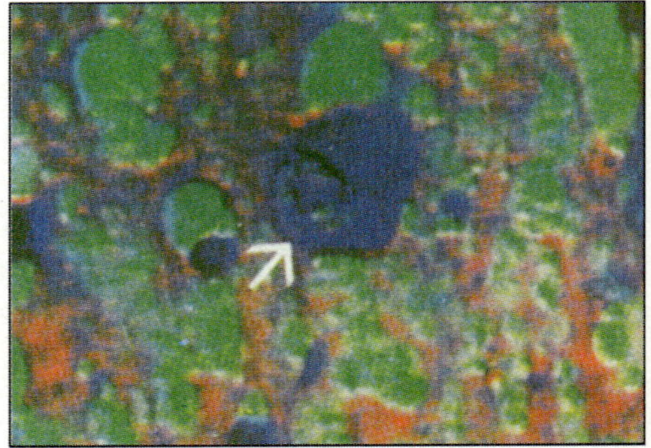

Fig. 39.6. Cytomegalovirus infection showing intranuclear inclusion bodies with perinuclear halo (owl's eye appearance).

4. Polymerase chain reaction (PCR)

CMV DNA, in the specimen, can be amplified by PCR.

5. Serology

CMV-specific IgM can be detected in the patient serum by ELISA.

40

Poxviruses, Adenoviruses, Parvoviruses, Papillomaviruses and Polyomaviruses

Q. 1. Name various genera of poxviruses and diseases produced by them in humans. Describe morphology, cultivation and pathogenicity of these viruses.

Ans. Four genera of poxviruses, *Orthopoxvirus*, *Parapoxvirus*, *Molluscipoxvirus* and *Yatapoxvirus*, cause diseases in humans (Table 40.1).

Table 40.1. Poxviruses producing disease in man

Genus	Disease
Orthopoxvirus	• Smallpox • Vaccinia • Buffalopox • Monkeypox • Cowpox
Parapoxvirus	• Milker's node • Orf
Molluscipoxvirus	• Molluscum contagiosum
Yatapoxvirus	• Yabapox • Tanapox

Morphology

Poxviruses are the largest animal viruses. They are large enough to be seen by light microscopy after special staining procedures. In most genera, the virions are **brick-shaped** with rounded corners, measuring 300 × 200 × 100 nm in size (Fig. 40.1). Nucleocapsids of these viruses do not conform to either of two types of symmetry found in most other viruses, hence, they are known as **complex viruses**. Poxviruses have a biconcave dumb-bell-shaped DNA core and two lateral bodies enclosed in a protein shell about 12 nm thick. It is known as outer membrane, surface of which consists of irregularly arranged tubules. Virions released from the cell are enclosed within an envelope which consists of host cell lipids and several virus-specified polypeptides, including the haemagglutinin.

Cultivation

Chick embryo

Variola and vaccinia viruses grow on chorioallantoic membrane of 11–13-day-old chick embryo, producing pocks in 48–72 hours. Variola pocks are small, shiny, white, convex, non-necrotic and non-haemorrhagic. In contrast, vaccinia pocks are larger, irregular, greyish, flat, necrotic and some of these are haemorrhagic.

Tissue culture

Variola and vaccinia viruses can be grown in monkey kidney, HeLa and chick embryo cells. Cytopathic effects are produced by vaccinia in 48–72 hours but variola takes longer to produce these changes. Intracytoplasmic, eosinophilic inclusion bodies – **Guarnieri bodies** – can be demonstrated in the stained preparation. Vaccinia, but not variola, produces plaques in chick embryo tissue culture.

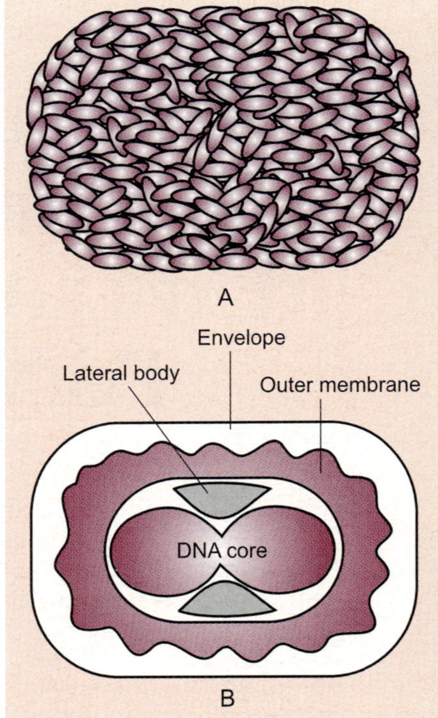

Fig. 40.1. The structure of vaccinia virion. (A) Surface structure of nonenveloped virus particle showing surface tubules; (B) Section of enveloped virion.

Human Orthopoxvirus infections

1. Smallpox (variola)

The virus causing classical smallpox was called variola major (fatal disease) and that causing alastrium (non-fatal disease) variola minor. Variola major and variola minor viruses are antigenically identical but differ in certain biological characteristics. In 1967 the World Health Organization (WHO) embarked on a Smallpox Eradication Campaign. The world's last naturally occurring case of smallpox was recorded in Merca, Southern Somalia, in October, 1977. On May 8, 1980, the WHO formally announced the **global eradication of smallpox**. Eradication of smallpox could be achieved because of:

- Its low communicability.
- No subclinical infection or carrier state.
- A single serotype virus which induced good immunity.
- An effective vaccine (originally discovered by Jenner in 1796).
- No animal reservoir.
- Aggressive surveillance-containment measures.

Although smallpox has been eradicated, two laboratories still hold stocks of smallpox virus (variola). These are the WHO collaboration centre in Atlanta, USA and Koltsovo, Russian Federation. Routine vaccination against smallpox has now been stopped.

2. Vaccinia

Origin of vaccinia virus is not known. It may have evolved from cowpox or smallpox virus. In the past, this virus was used for smallpox vaccination. Vaccinia virus is being used as a vector for incorporating genes for several different pathogens. Many genes have been inserted, including those coding for the antigens of HIV, hepatitis B virus and rabies virus. Because the large vaccinia genome can accommodate at least a dozen foreign genes, it is theoretically possible to construct a single recombinant virus as a vaccine capable of protecting against most of the common viral and nonviral infectious diseases of childhood.

3. Buffalopox

It occurs in buffaloes in India. It appears to be caused by vaccinia virus. It produces pustular lesions on the teats and udders of milking infected buffaloes. In man, lesions may develop on the hands and face of the milkers.

4. Monkeypox

Monkeypox virus was first isolated in 1958 from captive monkeys in Copenhagen. Human infections with this virus were discovered in the early 1970s. Human monkeypox occurs as a rare **zoonosis** in West and Central Africa, especially in Zaire. The outbreak in America occurred in 2003, in Wisconsin, affecting 11 local persons and many prairie dogs. Infection is probably acquired by handling infected animals (monkeys and squirrels). Person to person transmission is uncommon. Human monkeypox resembles mild smallpox. Patient develops a generalized pustular rash, fever and toxaemia. Diagnosis can be established by electron microscopy.

5. Cowpox

Rodents are the reservoir hosts of cowpox virus. From these animals the virus may occasionally spread to cats, cows, humans and various zoo animals. In cows, it produces ulcers on the teats and udders. It may spread to other cows and humans by the process of milking. Human infection presents as painful and haemorrhagic lesions on the hands and face. Pyrexia and constitutional disturbances are common. Cowpox virus resembles variola and vaccinia antigenically but can be differentiated by the haemorrhagic lesions it produces on CAM and rabbit skin.

Human Parapoxvirus infections

1. Milker's nodes

It primarily produces localized necrotic lesions on the teats of cows and ewes. In man, it produces localized, painless, nonulcerating, granulomatous lesions on the hand or face or both.

2. Orf

Orf is an infection of humans caused by virus of contagious pustular dermatitis of sheep and goats. In man, the disease occurs as a single chronic granulomatous lesion with a central ulcer, usually on hand or forearm or occasionally on the face. It heals without scarring.

Molluscipoxvirus infection

Molluscum contagiosum

Molluscum contagiosum is a common, self-limiting viral disease of skin caused by *Molluscipoxvirus*. Lesions are characterized by multiple discrete umbilicated nodules 2–5 mm in diameter, limited to the epidermis and occurring anywhere on the body except on soles and palms. Lesions are more commonly seen on the trunk and anogenital areas. Nodules are dome-shaped, waxy, pearly white or pink in colour and are painless (Fig. 40.2). A white caseous material can be squeezed from them. Lesions can persist for months and usually regress spontaneously.

The virus is transmitted by direct contact, perhaps through minor abrasions and sexually in adults. Extensive skin involvement is seen in AIDS patients. The cells in the nodules are greatly hypertrophied and contain large (up to 35 μm) hyaline acidophilic intracytoplasmic inclusion bodies which displace the nuclei to the margin. These are known as **molluscum bodies** (Figs. 38.1B and 40.3). These can be seen in cells of the stratum granulosum and the stratum corneum. Molluscum contagiosum virus has not so far been cultured.

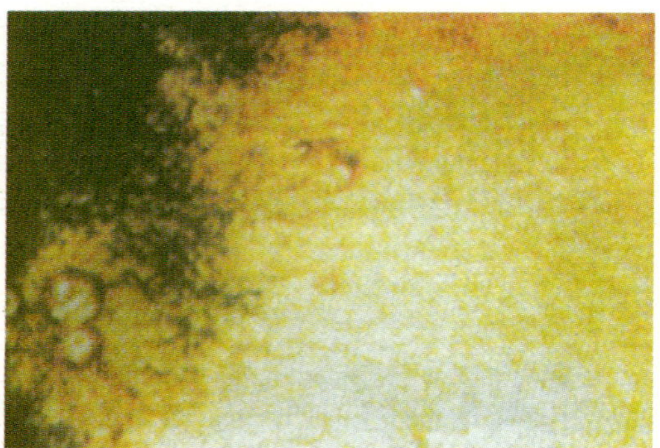

Fig. 40.2. Multiple lesions of molluscum contagiosum in the pubic area.

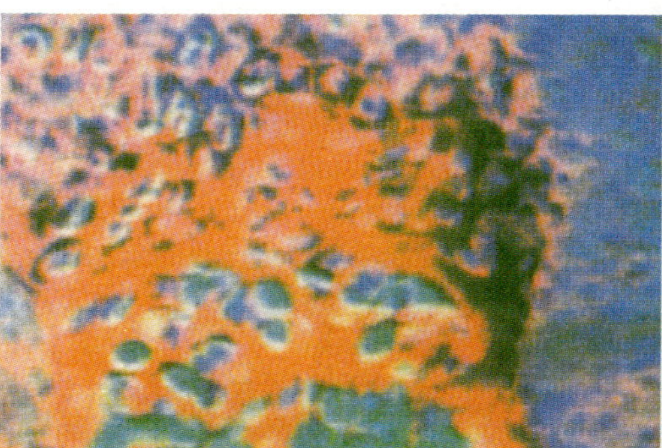

Fig. 40.3. Molluscum contagiosum. Horny layer shows numerous large, hyaline, acidophilic, intracytoplasmic inclusion bodies called molluscum bodies.

Human Yatapoxvirus infections

Yabapox

Yabapox virus produces large benign tumours in monkeys. Similar lesions have been reported, after accidental inoculation, in a laboratory attendant handling affected monkeys and in human volunteers.

Tanapox

Tanapox virus was first isolated from the cases of febrile illness that occurred along the Tana river in Kenya during 1950s. It is probably acquired by insect bite from a reservoir in wild animals of some unknown species. It produces single pock-like lesion on the skin which usually does not progress to pustules. The lesion is most commonly seen on the upper part of the body. The virus grows in human and monkey tissue culture but does not grow in embryonated egg culture. Epidemics of tanapox have been reported in East Africa.

Q. 2. Describe morphology, classification, cultivation, pathogenicity, clinical syndromes and laboratory diagnosis of adenoviruses.

Ans. ***Morphology***

Adenoviruses are icosahedral virions containing a single linear, double-stranded DNA. They

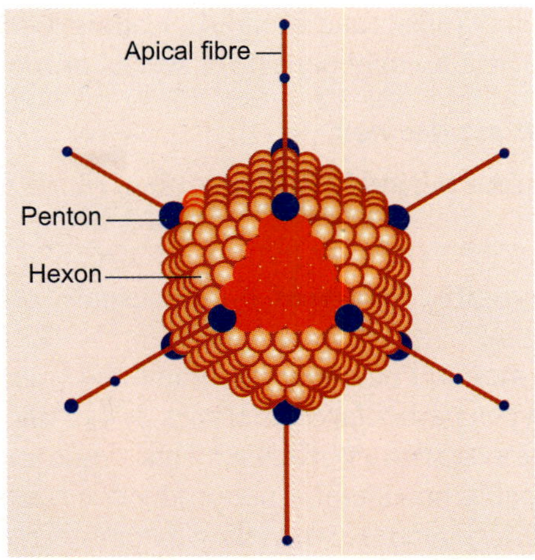

Fig. 40.4. Morphology of adenovirus.

measure 70–75 nm in diameter. Each capsid is composed of 252 capsomers – 240 hexons make up the 20 triangular faces of icosahedron and 12 pentons form the vertices. From each penton projects an apical fibre, 9–31 nm in length that serves to bind specifically to receptor sites on the host cell (Fig. 40.4).

Table 40.2. Classification of human adenoviruses

Species	Serotype	Total
A	12, 18, 31	3
B1	3, 7, 16, 21, 50	5
B2	11, 14, 34, 35	4
C	1, 2, 5, 6	4
D	8–10, 13, 15, 17, 19, 20, 22–30, 32, 33, 36–39, 42–49, 51	32
E	4	1
F	40, 41	2
G	52	1
	Total	52

Classification

The family comprises of two distinct genera – *Mastadenovirus* and *Aviadenovirus*. They possess mammalian and avian adenoviruses respectively. The genus *Mastadenovirus* comprises at least 52 serotypes which infect humans. On the basis of findings from deoxyribonucleic acid homology studies and the haemagglutination patterns, all of the 52 serotypes have been classified into seven (A–G) species (Table 40.2). Species B has been divided into two subspecies – B1 and B2.

Cultivation

Human adenoviruses can be grown in monolayers of HeLa, HEp-2, KB and human embryo kidney cells. Cytopathic effects may take several days to develop and consist of **cell rounding and aggregation in grape-like clusters**. Infected cells swell and become ballooned and show characteristic **basophilic intranuclear inclusions** in stained preparation.

Pathogenicity

Adenoviruses may infect via the conjunctiva or the nasal mucosa. Faecal-oral spread, particularly among children can also occur. They multiply initially in the conjunctiva, pharynx or small intestine and spread to preauricular, cervical and mesenteric lymph nodes. Most of the enteric and some of the respiratory infections are subclinical. In children, asymptomatic infection of tonsils and adenoids, leading to respiratory carriage, and Peyer's patches, leading to gut carriage, may persist for weeks or months.

Clinical syndromes

Incubation period is 5–8 days after which it may lead to:

I. Respiratory infections

- **Pharyngitis:** Serotypes 1–7 are usually responsible for pharyngitis particularly in young children.
- **Pneumonia:** Pneumonia in infants and young children may be caused by any of the common serotypes particularly serotypes 3, 4, 7 and 21.
- **Acute respiratory disease:** This syndrome is characterized by fever, chills, pharyngitis, cervical lymphadenitis, nonproductive cough and malaise. This occurs usually in outbreaks in military recruits when they assemble in camps. It is generally caused by serotypes 4, 7, 14 and 21.

II. Ocular infections

- **Pharyngoconjunctival fever:** This syndrome of febrile pharyngitis and conjunctivitis occurs in outbreaks in children. It is usually caused by serotypes 1, 2, 3, 4, 5 and 7.
- **Epidemic keratoconjunctivitis:** It is a severe and highly contagious infection involving all age groups. It often occurs in epidemic form and is characterized by follicular conjunctivitis and progresses to involve the cornea. It is generally caused by serotypes 8, 9, 11, 19, 35 and 37.

III. Genitourinary infections

- **Cervicitis and urethritis:** These venereal infections are caused by serotype 37.
- **Acute haemorrhagic cystitis:** It is mainly seen in infants and young children and is caused by serotypes 11 and 21.

IV. Enteric infections

- **Infantile gastroenteritis:** Serotypes 40 and 41 may cause infantile gastroenteritis in up to 10% of the cases.

Some human adenoviruses produce **carcinomas** if injected into newborn hamsters, mice or rats. Infection of cultured hamster or rat cells, *in vitro*, also results in **transformation**. However, there is no evidence that this can occur in man too.

Laboratory diagnosis

1. Specimens

Throat swab, nasopharyngeal aspirate, transtracheal aspirate, bronchial lavage, conjunctival swab, corneal scraping, urine, anal swab, faecal swab, genital secretions, and biopsy and autopsy materials.

2. Light microscopy

Adenovirus-infected cells can be visualized by light microscopy as 'smudge cells' in hematoxylin and eosin or Wright-Giemsa-stained tissues, fluid sediments, or cultures. Smudge cells are large, late-stage-infected cells containing solitary, central, intranuclear, basophilic inclusions composed of adenoviral particles.

3. Electron microscopy

Virus particles may be seen directly in stool extracts by **electron microscopy** and **immuno-electron microscopy**.

4. Immunofluorescence

Viral antigens in the cells from respiratory tract, eye, urine, biopsy or autopsy material and infected cell cultures may be demonstrated by **immunofluorescence** using polyclonal or monoclonal antibodies.

5. Detection of enteric adenoviruses

Enteric adenoviruses may be detected by **latex agglutination** method using latex particles coated with specific antibody to each virus.

6. Detection of antigen

Viral antigens in faeces and nasopharyngeal secretions may be detected by **ELISA** using monoclonal or polyclonal antibodies.

7. Detection of viral DNA

Viral DNA in the faeces may be detected by **polyacrylamide gel electrophoresis**.

8. Virus isolation

Virus from the clinical specimens, may be isolated on HeLa, HEp-2, KB and human embryo kidney cells.

9. DNA probes and polymerase chain reaction

DNA probe and polymerase chain reaction are used to identify enteric adenovirus serotypes 40, 41 and 42 directly in stool specimens, which do not grow in cell cultures.

10. Serology

For serological diagnosis, rise in titre of antibodies should be demonstrated in paired sera. Examination of a single sample of serum is inconclusive as adenovirus antibodies are so common in the population.

Q. 3. Describe briefly general properties of parvoviruses.

Ans. Family *Parvoviridae* comprises very small (20–25 nm) nonenveloped, icosahedral viruses containing a linear single-stranded DNA, 4–6 kb in size. There are five genera in this family – *Parvovirus*, *Erythrovirus*, *Dependovirus*, *Amdovirus* and *Bocavirus*. Members of the genus *Dependovirus* are defective and require co-infection with a helper virus for their own replication. They are usually found in association with an adenovirus and are known as **'adeno-associated viruses' (AAV)**. They have not yet been associated with any human disease. Genus *Parvovirus* is capable of replication without the aid of a helper virus. They cause disease in animals but some may cause diarrhoea in humans. Parvovirus B19 has now been allocated to a separate genus, *Erythrovirus*.

Q. 4. Describe pathogenesis and laboratory diagnosis of Parvovirus B19.

Ans. ***Pathogenesis***

Parvovirus B19 is highly contagious. It is transmitted by respiratory secretions and close contact. Other routes of transmission are transplacental and via blood transfusion. It can cause:

Erythema infectiosum

It is a common childhood febrile illness with rash. It is characterized by an **erythematous skin eruption of the cheeks** ('slapped cheek') and a reticulated lace-like eruption on the trunk and extremities. The rash usually resolves in 1–2 weeks. The rash may be preceded by fever, headache, malaise and myalgia.

Chronic anaemia in immunodeficient patient

If parvovirus B19 infects patients with acute leukaemia on chemotherapy, AIDS patients, children with congenital immunodeficiency syndrome and bone marrow transplant recipients, it may lead to chronic anaemia.

Arthropathy

Most of the adults are immune, but susceptible persons may develop arthritis or arthralgia.

Transient aplastic crisis

Parvovirus B19 has an affinity for immature red blood cell precursors. It can lead to transient aplastic crisis in patients with a variety of conditions that require increased red cell production, including sickle cell anaemia, thalassemia, hereditary spherocytosis and acute blood loss.

Erythroblastosis foetalis

If a pregnant woman develops primary parvovirus B19 infection, fatal erythroblastosis foetalis with hydrops may result.

Laboratory diagnosis

1. Virus isolation and detection

Parvovirus B19 may be cultured in cells from human bone marrow or foetal liver in the presence of erythropoietin and interleukin-3. By electron microscopy, it can be detected in the patient serum.

2. Nucleic acid detection

Viral nucleic acid can be detected by nucleic acid hybridization or by polymerase chain reaction.

3. Antigen detection

Antigen can be detected in serum and other specimens by ELISA, RIA or indirect immunofluorescence.

4. Antibody detection

Most successful diagnostic assay is the detection of IgM antibodies or a significant rise in IgG antibodies by ELISA or RIA.

Q. 5. Describe general properties, pathogenicity and laboratory diagnosis of papillomaviruses.

Ans. ***General properties***

Papillomaviruses are small (55 nm in diameter), nonenveloped and have an icosahedral capsid composed of 72 capsomers. The genome is a supercoiled dsDNA molecule of 7.2–8 kilobase pairs. They are host species-specific and infect the squamous epithelia and mucous membranes of higher vertebrates, including man. There are over 100 types of human papillomaviruses (HPV). These are distinguished on the basis of the homology between their genomes. **Papillomaviruses cannot be grown in cell cultures.**

Pathogenicity

HPV are not only host species-specific but also display a predilection for the skin and certain mucous membranes. They cause cutaneous warts, genital warts, recurrent respiratory papillomatosis, oral papillomatosis and cancer. The infection is transmitted by indirect or direct contact including sexual contact.

Papillomaviruses infect both cutaneous and mucosal epithelium of the skin, oral cavity, conjunctiva, anus, and lower genital tract of men and women, with no systemic, or blood-borne phase. Consequently, transmission occurs via direct epithelium-to-epithelium contact and not by exposure to bodily fluids as in the case of hepatitis and human immunodeficiency virus infections. Infection is thought to occur only in basal epithelial cells, which are presumably accessed through microtrauma incurred during sexual activity, which can occur both through penetrative and nonpenetrative epithelial abrasive contact.

1. Cutaneous warts

These are generally caused by HPV types 1, 2, 4, 7, 26 and 29. Virus penetrates the skin through an abrasion and infects the basal cell layer leading to hypertrophy of all the layers of the dermis and hyperkeratosis of the horny layer. Incubation period is 2 years. Cutaneous warts are raised papillomas with a rough surface and are commonly found in children. They disappear within 2 years of the onset. Recurrence is believed to be due to persistence of the virus in the skin surrounding the original wart.

2. Genital warts

These lesions are also known as **condyloma acuminata** and are common in sexually active adults. In women they are found on the vulva, within vagina and on the cervix. In men, the lesions generally appear on the shaft of the penis, perianal skin and anal canal. Genital warts are generally caused by HPV types 1, 2, 6, 10, 11, 16, 30, 44 and 45.

3. Recurrent respiratory papillomatosis

HPV types 6 and 11 may lead to benign squamous papillomas on the mucosa of respiratory tract, particularly on the larynx. Children below 5 years of age acquire the disease by passage through an infected birth canal. Adults after the age of 15 may acquire the disease by orogenital contact with an infected sexual partner. **Malignant conversion** of laryngeal papillomas has been reported.

4. Oral papillomatosis

Infection is usually acquired by orogenital contact with infected sexual partner. It is caused by HPV types 6, 7, 13, 16 and 32. Multiple papillomatous lesions may develop on the buccal mucosa, a condition known as oral florid papillomatosis. **Oral papillomas sometimes progress to malignancy.** HPV-16 DNA has been reported in a minority of oral carcinomas. HPV (and also Epstein-Barr virus) has also been blamed to cause **hairy leukoplakia** on the tongue in patients infected with human immunodeficiency virus.

5. Cancer

HPV types 11, 16, 18, 31, 33, 35 and 42–45 have been blamed to cause invasive cancers of the skin, larynx and genital tract, mainly of cervix and also of penis, vulva, vagina, perineum and anus. HPV 16 is found in over 50% of cases of cervical carcinoma followed by type 18 (24%), type 45 (8%), and type 31 (5%).

Laboratory diagnosis

It can be carried out by:

1. Histopathology and cytopathology

These reveal hypertrophy of all layers of the dermis and hyperkeratosis of the horny layer.

2. Electron microscopy

Papillomavirus particles can be readily seen by electron microscopy in most warts but are less in number in genital warts.

3. Immunocytochemistry

The HPV capsid antigen in paraffin sections of tissues or in cell smears can be detected by an immunoperoxidase test using a commercially available antiserum prepared by immunization of rabbits with bovine *Papillomavirus* particles disrupted with sodium dodecyl sulphate. It detects all the genital HPV types. However, monoclonal antibodies that can differentiate the genital types have now been produced and may be used as diagnostic tools.

4. Detection of viral nucleic acid

Viral DNA in fresh tissues, fixed tissues and exfoliated cells can be detected by DNA hybridization and polymerase chain reaction.

Q. 6. Describe morphology, pathogenicity and laboratory diagnosis of polyomaviruses.

Ans.

Morphology

Polyomavirus (*poly:* many, *oma:* tumour) virions are nonenveloped, 40–45 nm in diameter with a 72 capsomer icosahedral capsid. Viral genome, like that of papillomaviruses, is a double-stranded supercoiled loop of DNA molecule with a molecular weight of 3.4 million daltons.

Pathogenicity

1. Mouse polyomavirus

It causes only harmless inapparent infections in mice when spread by natural routes. However, when injected into infant rodents such as hamsters it induces many different types of malignant tumours.

2. Simian virus 40 (SV40)

It causes subclinical infection in monkeys, but when inoculated into baby rodents it leads to tumour formation.

3. JC polyomavirus

It causes infection in man. It was first isolated from the brain of a male patient with Hodgkin's disease who developed progressive multifocal leukoencephalopathy (PML). It was designated by the initials of the person from whom it was isolated. The virus persists for life in the kidneys and is shed in urine sporadically and more frequently during pregnancy and immunosuppression.

PML is a rare, fatal, subacute demyelinating disease of nervous system that results from JC polyomavirus infection of oligodendrocytes in the brain. It is seen mainly as a complication of advanced disseminated malignant conditions such as Hodgkin's disease or chronic lymphocytic leukaemia and primary or secondary immunodeficiency syndromes, especially AIDS or following immunosuppression for organ transplantation.

4. BK polyomavirus

It was isolated from the urine of a renal transplant recipient and was named after his initials. It causes subclinical infection of children before the age of 10. It may, however, cause upper respiratory symptoms. The virus persists for life in kidneys. Reactivation may occur during last trimester of pregnancy and following immunosuppression for organ transplantation leading to asymptomatic shedding of virus in urine.

Laboratory diagnosis

1. Electron microscopy

Human polyomaviruses can be detected by electron microscopy of diseased brain tissue from cases of PML (JC polyomavirus) and in the urine of a renal allograft recipient (BK polyomavirus).

2. Cytopathology

Cytological examination of exfoliated urinary epithelial cells shows the presence of the enlarged deeply staining basophilic nuclei, with a single inclusion.

3. Virus isolation

BK polyomavirus can be isolated from urine in human diploid fibroblasts, and JC polyomavirus from urine or brain in human foetal glial cell culture. These two viruses can be differentiated by haemagglutination inhibition.

4. Detection of viral antigen

Viral antigen in urine can be detected by **ELISA**. Following brain biopsy or autopsy, JC polyomavirus antigen can be detected by **immunofluorescence**.

5. Detection of viral nucleic acid

It can be carried out by nucleic acid hybridization and **PCR**. Following brain biopsy or autopsy, JC polyomavirus DNA can be demonstrated by **in situ hybridization**.

41

PICORNAVIRUSES

Q. 1. Describe general characters and classification of family Picornaviridae.

Ans. Family Picornaviridae (*pico:* small, *rna:* RNA genome, *viridae:* viruses) comprises of a large number of very small RNA viruses with a diameter of 27–30 nm. The capsid is a naked icosahedron made up of 60 protein subunits (protomers). The genome consists of a single linear molecule of single-stranded RNA of positive polarity with 7–8 kilobase pairs. The Picornaviridae is divided into six genera, four of which, *Enterovirus*, *Rhinovirus*, *Hepatovirus* and *Parechovirus* possess human pathogens (Table 41.1).

Q. 2. Describe general characters of enteroviruses.

Ans. Enteroviruses are among the most stable viruses. They can remain viable for years at –20°C or –70°C and for months at 4°C. In faeces, at room temperature, the virus can remain infective for several weeks. Being nonenveloped they are insensitive to ether and chloroform. The virus is readily killed by moist heat at 50–55°C, but in food stuffs the virus may survive exposure to 60°C and holder method of pasteurization. Enteroviruses are rapidly inactivated by ultraviolet light, drying, formaldehyde (0.3%), hydrochloric acid (0.1 M) or free residual chlorine (0.3–0.5 ppm). However, higher concentrations of chlorine are necessary to inactivate virus in the presence of organic matter because the latter diminishes the activity of chlorine.

Q. 3. Describe morphology, antigenic properties, pathogenicity, clinical features, laboratory diagnosis and prophylaxis of polioviruses.

Ans. ***Morphology***

The virion is 27–30 nm in diameter. Capsid is composed of 60 capsomers arranged in icosahedral symmetry. Each capsomer is composed of four viral proteins (VP1–VP4). The genome is a single strand of positive sense RNA.

Table 41.1. Human picornaviruses

Genus	Species	Major disease
Enterovirus	Polioviruses 1–3	Paralytic poliomyelitis, aseptic meningitis
	Coxsackieviruses A1–24 except 23	Aseptic meningitis, herpangina, conjunctivitis (A24)
	Coxsackieviruses B1–6	Aseptic meningitis, fatal neonatal disease, pleurodynia, myocarditis or pericarditis
	Echoviruses 1–34 except 8, 10, 22, 23 and 28	Aseptic meningitis, rashes, febrile illness
	Enteroviruses 68–72	Conjunctivitis (enterovirus 70), polio-like illness illness (enterovirus 71), pneumonia and bronchitis
Rhinovirus	Rhinoviruses 1–100	Common cold
Hepatovirus	Hepatitis A virus	Hepatitis
Parechovirus	Echoviruses 22 and 23	

Antigenic properties

On the basis of neutralization tests, polioviruses can be divided into three serotypes. Type 1 is the common epidemic type, type 2 is usually associated with endemic infections and type 3 occasionally causes epidemics. Each type contains two type-specific antigens C and D (C: coreless or capsid; and D: dense). C antigens of all types are cross reactive but D antigen is type-specific.

Pathogenicity

Polioviruses have affinity for nervous tissue and narrow host range. Only man and some primates like cynomolgous and rhesus monkeys are susceptible. These monkeys can be infected by the oral route and develop paralysis.

Natural infection occurs only in man. The virus is spread from man to man by faecal-oral route and because early multiplication occurs in both the oropharynx and the intestinal mucosa, therefore, the virus is also spread by pharyngeal secretions (droplet infection) during first week of illness. No intermediate host is known.

On entering the body of a new host the virus multiplies in the tonsils and Peyer's patches of the ileum. Spread to regional lymph nodes (cervical and mesenteric) leads to a viraemia, enabling the virus to become disseminated throughout the body including spinal cord and brain.

In the central nervous system, the virus multiplies selectively in the neurons and destroys them. The lesions are mostly in the anterior horns of the spinal cord, causing flaccid paralysis, but posterior horns and intermediate columns may also be involved to some extent. In some cases encephalitis occurs, primarily involving the brain stem but extending upto the motor and premotor areas of the cerebral cortex.

Predisposing factors

1. Neural spread may occur in children with inapparent infection at the time of tonsillectomy. Poliovirus present in the oropharynx may enter nerve fibres exposed during surgery and spread to brain resulting in bulbar paralysis.

2. A similar mechanism of viral spread via neural pathways may be responsible for paralysis of a limb recently injected with inflammatory injections such as diphtheria-pertussis-tetanus (DPT) vaccine. This is probably associated with the irritant properties of the adjuvant.
3. Pregnancy increases the incidence of paralysis.
4. Muscular activity during the paralytic phase of the illness may lead to paralysis of the limbs used.

Clinical features

There are four types of poliovirus infection:

1. **Asymptomatic illness:** Patient does not have any symptom but the virus may be isolated from stool or throat or both. This is seen in 90–95% individuals.
2. **Minor illness:** Patient develops mild, transient 'influenza-like' illness. This is seen in 4–8% cases.
3. **Non-paralytic poliomyelitis or aseptic meningitis:** In addition to 'influenza-like' illness patient also develops headache, neck stiffness and back pain that may indicate some degree of aseptic meningitis. The illness lasts 2–10 days with rapid and complete recovery. This is seen in 1–2% individuals.
4. **Paralytic poliomyelitis or the major illness:** Patient develops paralysis during the course of the illness. It is uncommon, occurring in 0.1–2% poliovirus infections. On the basis of the site of involvement the paralysis may be spinal, bulbar or bulbospinal.

Laboratory diagnosis

Specimens

Virus can be isolated from blood, faeces and throat swab taken early in the disease. It can seldom be isolated from CSF but can be obtained from the spinal cord and brain, postmortem.

Virus isolation

It can be cultivated on monkey kidney, human amnion, HeLa, HEp-2 and other cell cultures. A cytopathic effect is usually seen in the cells within 48 hours. It consists of cell retraction, increased refractivity, cytoplasmic granularity and nuclear pyknosis. The identification of the serotype is carried out by neutralization tests. A wild virulent virus can be differentiated from an attenuated vaccine strain in the following ways:

1. Virulence tests in the monkeys.
2. Because the nucleotide sequences of all vaccine strains and prevalent wild strains are now known, the two can be readily distinguished by nucleic acid hybridization.

Prophylaxis

Two effective vaccines are available:

- Inactivated polio vaccine (Salk vaccine), and
- Live attenuated oral polio vaccine (Sabin vaccine).

Inactivated polio vaccine (IPV)

IPV (Salk vaccine) for parenteral injection was developed by Jonas Salk in 1953. The vaccine contains formalin inactivated strains of the three serotypes of virus grown in monkey kidney cell culture. The vaccine is given by deep subcutaneous or intramuscular injection. Three injections are given with intervals of 6–8 weeks between the first and second doses and 4–6 months between the second and third doses. IPV produces long-lasting immunity to all three poliovirus types. It is not associated with local or general reactions. The injection of this vaccine stimulates the production of IgG antibodies in the serum. It does not induce detectable levels of secretory IgA in the gut and therefore would not be expected to prevent alimentary tract infections. Following infection, a virulent virus is neutralized as it enters the blood stream, thus preventing involvement of the central nervous system. The absence of live virus makes it safe to administer to immunocompromised individuals.

Live attenuated oral polio vaccine (OPV)

OPV (Sabin vaccine) was developed by Albert Sabin in 1962. It contains live attenuated strains of the three serotypes of poliovirus grown either in cultures of monkey kidney cells or human diploid cells. The vaccine is administered orally and parallels natural infection. It stimulates both local secretory IgA antibodies in the pharynx and alimentary tract and humoral IgG antibodies. Virus is excreted in the faeces for several weeks, during which time the vaccine may spread to close contacts, inducing or boostering immunity in them.

Theoretically, a single dose should be sufficient to establish infection and immunity but in practice three doses are given to ensure that all three types of vaccine virus multiply in the intestine, overcoming interference among themselves and other enteric viruses. It has been recommended that in the tropics the number of doses of vaccine be increased to five, in order to enhance seroconversion in the vaccinees.

At the age of 1½ months first dose of OPV is given along with DPT. Second, third and fourth doses of these vaccines are given at the ages of 2½, 3½ and 16–24 months, respectively. With multiple rounds of replication in the vaccine and after transmission to the contact, there is a theoretical possibility that the vaccine virus may revert to neurovirulence. The risk of vaccine-associated poliomyelitis has been estimated at between 0.5 and 3.4 cases per million.

Ideally, it is desirable to vaccinate all children aged 0–5 years in the whole community at one time so that natural dissemination is prevented. The strategy of administering the vaccine to all children in a region on the same day (**pulse immunization**) has been found to be useful in the developing countries. By global immunization with OPV it was considered possible to eradicate the disease by the year 2000. However, progress in immunization in many countries has been a setback to this objective. Following are the causes of poor response to OPV:

- Interference by other enteroviruses so common in the tropics.
- Frequent diarrhoeal diseases preventing colonization by the vaccine virus.
- Breast-feeding immediately before or after the vaccine is given (vaccine virus may be neutralized by antibodies in the breast milk).
- Vaccine virus may also be neutralized by some other inhibitory agent in the saliva and intestinal secretions.

With the programme of pulse polio, it has now been eradicated from India. It was declared on 11-02-2014. Since 11-02-2011, no case of poliomyelitis has ben reported from India. Thanks to Sabin.

Q. 4. Classify coxsackieviruses. Describe pathogenicity and laboratory diagnosis of coxsackieviruses.

Ans. These viruses are typical enteroviruses and were named so because the first isolation was made from Coxsackie village in New York by Dalldrof and Sickles (1948). Based on the pathological changes produced in suckling mice, coxsackieviruses are classified into two groups, A and B (Table 41.2). Group A viruses are associated with diseases involving vesicular lesions (e.g., herpangina), whereas group B viruses (B for body) are most frequently associated with myocarditis and epidemic myalgia.

Table 41.2. Coxsackieviruses

	Group A	Group B
Pathological changes induced by inoculation of suckling mice	Generalized myositis Flaccid paralysis Death within a week	Patchy focal myositis Spastic paralysis Localized lesions in the liver, pancreas, myocardium, brain and brown fat pads
Number of types by neutralization test	23 (1–24 except 23*)	6 (1–6)

* Coxsackievirus 23 is now classified as echovirus 9.

Pathogenicity

Like other enteroviruses, coxsackieviruses inhabit the alimentary canal primarily and are spread by faecal-oral route. They may cause following lesions:

Group A viruses

These viruses give rise to:

1. **Aseptic meningitis:** It may be caused by most group A and all group B viruses. A maculopapular rash may be present. Occasionally, clinical picture may resemble paralytic poliomyelitis.
2. **Herpangina (vesicular pharyngitis):** It is caused by several types of group A viruses and is not related to a herpesvirus infection. It is usually seen in young children. Outbreaks may be seen in nurseries and schools. There is an abrupt onset of fever and sore throat. The illness is self-limited and requires only symptomatic management.
3. **Hand-foot-and-mouth disease:** It is usually caused by types 5 and 16 and is predominantly a childhood illness. The disease presents as a painful stomatitis with a vesicular rash on the hands and feet. The patient is mildly febrile, and illness subsides in a few days.

Group B viruses

1. **Epidemic myalgia (Bornholm disease):** It is so called because it was first described on the Danish island of Bornholm. It is a febrile disease with stitch-like pains in the muscles of the chest (intercostals), epigastrium or hypochondrium. Involvement of diaphragm leads to abdominal pain.

2. **Myocarditis and pericarditis:** Group B viruses may lead to severe and often fatal myocarditis in newborn infants. Myocarditis and pericarditis may also occur in children and adults.
3. **Aseptic meningitis:** Group B viruses may cause aseptic meningitis sometimes with paralysis.
4. **Juvenile diabetes:** Coxsackievirus B4 may cause juvenile diabetes.
5. **Orchitis:** Coxsackievirus may also cause orchitis.
6. **Neonatal infection:** Transplacental transmission of type B viruses has been demonstrated. It results in hepatitis, meningoencephalitis and adrenocortical involvement.
7. **Post-viral fatigue syndrome:** Type B viruses have been associated with post-viral fatigue syndrome, but neither the condition nor the association have been clearly defined.

Laboratory diagnosis

Animal inoculation

Specimens from the lesions or faeces may be inoculated by intracerebral and/or intraperitoneal routes into newborn mice (under 24 hours of age). The animals are then observed for illness, sacrificed and subjected to histologic examination.

Tissue culture

Human diploid embryonic lung fibroblasts and monkey kidney cell line support the growth of some coxsackieviruses. Cytopathic effects resemble those of poliovirus, but develop more slowly, commencing with foci of rounded refractile cells which then lyse and fall off the glass.

The isolate in the animal or cell culture can be identified by neutralization test with reference antisera.

Q. 5. Describe briefly echoviruses.

Ans. These were originally isolated from the faeces of persons who had no clinical illness and caused a cytopathic effect in cell culture. Therefore, these viruses were given the name of **enteric cytopathogenic human orphan viruses (echoviruses)**.

Properties

They resemble other enteroviruses in their properties. On the basis of the presence of a type-specific neutralizing antigen in their capsid, echoviruses have been subdivided into 32 (1–34 except 10 and 28, the former becoming a reovirus and the latter a rhinovirus) types. Like other enteroviruses, they inhabit the alimentary tract and spread by faecal-oral route.

Clinical features

Most of the echoviruses produce asymptomatic infections but some have been associated with clinical syndromes such as aseptic meningitis, paralysis, fever with rash, respiratory disease (pneumonia, bronchiolitis and upper respiratory tract illness), infantile diarrhoea, pericarditis and myocarditis.

Laboratory diagnosis

Isolation of virus

Echoviruses can be readily isolated from nose and throat swabs, stools or CSF on human diploid embryonic lung fibroblasts and monkey kidney cell line. The cytopathic effect is similar to that of coxsackieviruses. Identification of virus type is done by neutralisation tests.

Serology

Serological diagnosis is not practicable due to the existence of large number of serotypes, except in case of epidemics where the causative serotype has been identified.

Q. 6. Write short note on enteroviruses 68–71.

Ans. Of the four enteroviruses 68–71, three are associated with disease in human beings (Table 41.3).

Table 41.3. Diseases produced by enteroviruses 68–71

Enterovirus type	Disease
68	Pneumonia and bronchitis
69	—
70	Acute haemorrhagic conjunctivitis, meningoencephalitis and paralysis
71	Meningoencephalitis and paralysis

Enterovirus 70

In 1969, a pandemic of acute haemorrhagic conjunctivitis (AHC) spread widely involving several parts of Africa, the Middle East, India, Southeast Asia, Japan and Europe. AHC is highly infectious, has an incubation period of about 24 hours and the symptoms are sudden swelling, congestion, watering and pain in the eyes. Although subconjunctival haemorrhage is a characteristic feature, most cases recover in 3–7 days. Sometimes enterovirus 70 may cause meningoencephalitis and paralysis. It can be isolated on human embryonic kidney and HeLa cells.

Q. 7. Describe properties, cultivation, pathogenicity and laboratory diagnosis of rhinoviruses.

Ans. Rhinoviruses are causative agents of common cold. They can be isolated from nose and throat.

Properties

Rhinoviruses are small RNA viruses, morphologically and biochemically similar to other members of the family Picornaviridae. They can be differentiated from the enteroviruses on the basis of their acid lability (thus their inability to infect the intestinal tract) and their optimal temperature for replication (33°C). They are inactivated below pH 5. They are relatively stable in temperature range of 20–37°C and can survive on environmental surfaces such as door knobs for several days. Some rhinoviruses may survive heating at 50°C for 1 hour. They are resistant to 20% ether and 5% chloroform but are sensitive to aldehydes and hypochlorites. They can be preserved at –70°C.

On the basis of a type-specific antigen in their capsid, rhinoviruses have been subdivided into more than 100 serotypes.

Cultivation

They are fastidious, growing only at 33°C (temperature of the nose), instead of the usual 37°C in human embryonic kidney cells, human embryonic nasal or tracheal epithelium, human diploid cell lines and HeLa cells with cytopathic changes, if good oxygenation (achieved by rolling), low pH (around 7) and low temperature (33°C) are provided. Some strains grow in both monkey and human cell lines, these are designated as M strains, those which grow only in human cells are known as H strains and those which grow only in nasal or tracheal ciliated epithelium are known as O strains.

Pathogenicity

Rhinoviruses are the major cause of common cold accounting for about half of all colds. Other viruses which may also cause common cold include coronaviruses, some enteroviruses particularly coxsackieviruses A21 and A24 and echoviruses 11 and 20, respiratory syncytial virus, parainfluenza viruses and the low numbered adenoviruses. Rhinoviruses are transmitted by inhalation of droplets expelled from the nose of a patient during sneezing and coughing.

The virus attaches to receptors on nasal ciliated epithelial cells, enters and replicates within them, spreading to other cells. The cilia and cells are damaged and the epithelium is subjected to bacterial infection. During the acute phase of the illness high concentrations of virus are present in nasal secretions which may contaminate hands, fingers, handkerchiefs or paper tissues, door knobs, etc. and the normal individuals who touch these, contaminate their fingers which may touch the eye or nasal mucosa leading to "cold". For rhinoviruses, hand contact seems to be the prime mode of transmission. *Rhinovirus* infections are observed throughout the year, but the incidence of "cold" in temperate climates increases in the autumn and spring and in the tropics the peak incidence occurs in the rainy season.

After an incubation period of 2–4 days, patient develops profuse watery discharge (rhinorrhoea) with nasal obstruction, sneezing, sore throat, cough, headache, malaise and little or no fever. On an average, symptoms subside in about a week but in a proportion of the cases the symptoms may be prolonged for 2 weeks or longer. Sinusitis or otitis media may supervene, particularly if secondary bacterial infection occurs. The illness is generally worse in smokers. Recovery is mediated by endogenous interferons, locally synthesized IgA antibodies and serum IgG antibodies.

Immunity to rhinoviruses is transient and unlikely to prevent subsequent infection because of the numerous serotypes of the virus. Both nasal secretory IgA and serum IgG antibody are induced by a primary rhinovirus infection and can be detected within a week of infection. The secretory IgA response dissipates quickly, and immunity begins to wane approximately 18 months after infection. Cell-mediated immunity is not likely to play an important role in controlling rhinovirus infection.

Laboratory diagnosis

Isolation of virus

Rhinoviruses may be isolated from nose and throat swabs or nasopharyngeal aspirate on human and monkey cell lines incubated at 33°C.

Demonstration of antigen

Virus antigen, in nasal washings, may be demonstrated by ELISA.

Demonstration of virus RNA

Virus RNA, in nasal washings, may be demonstrated by PCR.

42

RHABDOVIRUSES

Q. 1. Describe morphology, host range and growth characteristics, pathogenicity, clinical features and immune response of rabies virus.

Ans. Morphology

Rabies virus is **bullet-shaped** 180 × 75 nm, with one end rounded or conical and the other plane or concave (Fig. 42.1). **The core of the virion consists of a negative sense 11–12 kilobase, single-stranded RNA enclosed in a helically wound nucleocapsid.** RNA-dependent RNA polymerase enzyme which is essential for the initiation of replication of the virus, is enclosed within the virion in association with the ribonucleoprotein core. The latter is surrounded by **matrix protein** (viral membrane) which may be invaginated at the plane end. The matrix protein in turn is surrounded by a **lipoprotein envelope** which carries glycoprotein peplomers (spikes). The spikes do not cover the plane end of the virion.

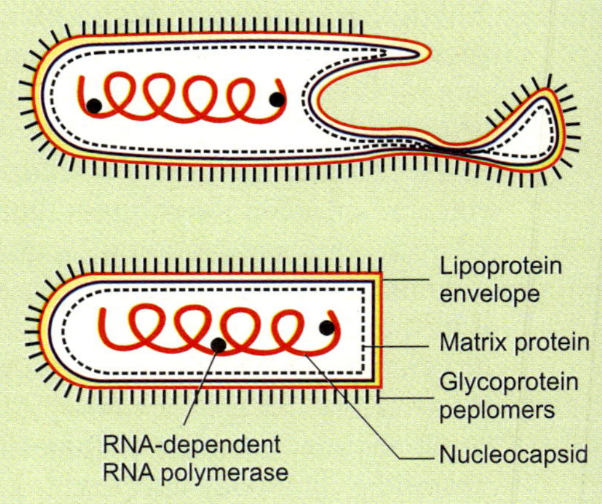

Fig. 42.1. Rabies virus.

Host range and growth characteristics

1. Animals

All warm-blooded animals of which rabbits, guinea-pigs, rats and mice are useful for primary isolation are susceptible to rabies infection. Some species such as cattle, cats and foxes are highly susceptible, whereas skunks, opossums and fowl are relatively resistant. Man and dog occupy intermediate position. Pups are more susceptible than adult dogs.

Street virus

Freshly isolated virus from natural human or animal infection is termed street virus. It produces fatal encephalitis in laboratory animals, inoculated by any route, after a **long and variable incubation period** of 1–12 weeks. Intracytoplasmic inclusion bodies (**Negri bodies**) can be demonstrated in the brains of animals dying of street virus infection.

Fixed virus

After several serial intracerebral passages in rabbits, the virus undergoes certain changes and becomes what is called fixed virus. It is more neurotropic and much less infective by other routes. After intracerebral inoculation, it produces fatal encephalitis after a **short and fixed incubation period** of 5–8 days and Negri bodies are usually not demonstrable in the brains of animals dying of fixed virus infection. It produces paralytic rather than furious symptoms. It is used for **vaccine production**.

2. Chick embryo

Rabies virus can be grown in the yolk sac of chick embryo. Serial propagation in chick embryos has led to the development of attenuated vaccine strains like Flury and Kelev. Strains adapted to duck eggs which give high yields of virus have been used for preparation of inactivated vaccines.

3. Tissue culture

Rabies virus can be grown in several cell cultures including baby hamster kidney, human diploid lung fibroblasts, chick embryo fibroblasts and Vero monkey kidney cells with minimal cytopathic effects. The last three are used in vaccine production.

Pathogenicity

Rabies is probably the most feared of all human diseases. It is the classic zoonotic infection. It is a natural infection of dogs, foxes, wolves, skunks, cats and bats. Rabies virus is excreted in the saliva of affected animals. Man acquires infection by the bite of rabid dog or other animals. Rarely, infection can occur following licks on abraded skin and intact mucosa. Infection has occurred through the inhalation of massive virus aerosols generated in bat caves and in laboratory accidents. Oral infection has been induced experimentally in some animals, but no evidence so far suggests that these are common routes of natural infection.

Infection by bite of rabid animal results in deposition of rabies-infected saliva in the wound (Fig. 42.2). The virus replicates in the muscles, connective tissue or nerves at the site of deposition. After it reaches a sufficient concentration, it infects peripheral nerves in the muscle or skin. Once within the nerve fibres, it is out of reach of any circulating antibody and it travels along the axon towards the central nervous system **at a speed of 3 mm per hour**. In the central nervous system, it multiplies and produces encephalitis. The virus then spreads outwards along the nerve trunks to various parts of the body including the salivary glands. **It multiplies in the salivary glands and is shed in the saliva.** There is little evidence that haematogenous or other modes of spread are involved.

The presence of virus in the saliva, and the irritability and aggression brought on by the encephalitis ensure the transmission and survival of the virus in nature. The virus ultimately reaches virtually every tissue in the body and is almost invariably present in the cornea and the skin of face and nape of the neck of the patient because of their proximity to the brain. This provides a method for the antemortem diagnosis of rabies. The virus may also be shed in the milk and urine.

Exposure of humans to rabies virus does not necessarily result in infection. *Contrary to popular belief, man is not highly susceptible to the virus*. The incidence of human rabies after bites by known rabid dogs is about 15%. However, the incidence ranges from 1% after contamination of minor wounds to more than 60% after severe bites on the face.

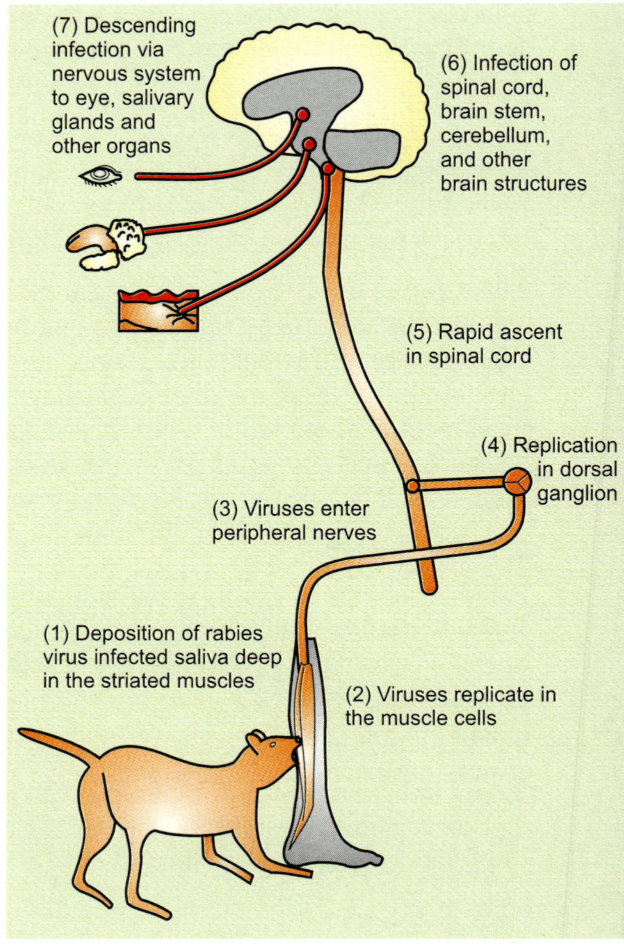

Fig. 42.2. Pathogenesis of rabies virus.

Clinical features

Following the bite of a rabid animal, the **incubation period** is usually between 1–2 months. However, it may be as short as 9 days and rarely as long as a year or more. It is shorter in children than in adults and shorter in persons bitten on the face or head and longer in those bitten on the legs. This is related to the distance the virus has to travel to reach the brain.

After a prodromal phase of malaise, headache, fever and paraesthesia at and around the site of bite, muscles become hypertonic and the patient becomes anxious, with episodes of hyperactivity, aggression and convulsions. **Patient develops difficulty in drinking, together with intense thirst. Patient may be able to swallow dry solids but not liquids.** Attempts to drink bring on painful spasm of pharynx and larynx producing choking and gagging. Thereafter, mere sight or sound of water precipitates distressing muscular spasm leading to **hydrophobia** (fear of water). **The rabies in animals does not have this peculiar feature.**

The furious form of rabies, gradually subsides into delirium, convulsions, coma and death. Sometimes only the **dumb form** is seen, with symmetrical ascending paralysis followed by coma and death. The disease, once developed, is almost always fatal in 4–14 days. However, there are rare reports of survival after prolonged intensive treatment.

Rabies virus may be secreted in the saliva, urine and other secretions of human rabies victims as in that of animals. Man to man transmission of rabies is rarely recorded. Some cases of inter-human transmission have been reported following cornea transplant from donors with undiagnosed rabies.

Immune response

Rabies virus ascends to the brain along the nerves and does not come in contact with immune system of the body. It is only after the virus spreads from CNS along the nerve trunks to different parts of the body that antibodies are produced. But by this time it is too late, irreversible damage of the neurons has already been caused and patient dies of respiratory paralysis. However, antibody is certainly protective when present before exposure and prompt vaccination after exposure induces resistance which is associated with antibody production.

Q. 2. Describe laboratory diagnosis, postexposure treatment and prophylaxis of rabies.

Ans. **Laboratory diagnosis**

1. Demonstration of Negri bodies

Sections or impression smears of brain stained by Seller's technique may reveal inclusion bodies, known as **Negri bodies**. These are intracytoplasmic, round or oval, eosinophilic with basophilic inner granules (Fig. 42.3). Negri bodies vary in size, from 3–27 μm in diameter and are seen mainly in the pyramidal cells of Ammon's horn, in Purkinje cells of hippocampus, brain stem and cerebellum. Negri bodies may be absent in about 20% of the cases.

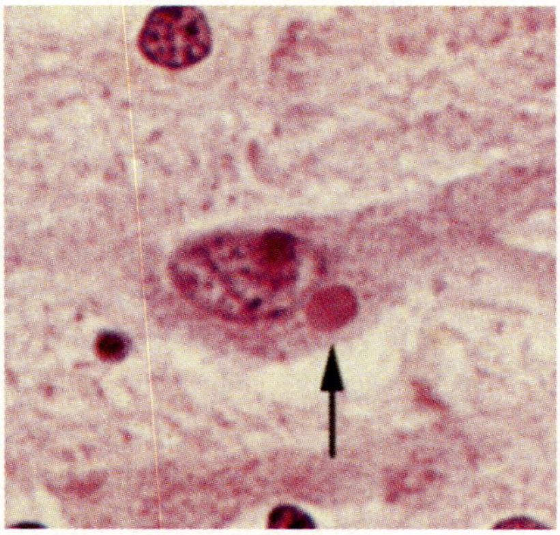

Fig. 42.3. Intracytoplasmic eosinophilic inclusion body in cells infected with rabies virus (Negri body).

2. Demonstration of rabies antigen by direct immunofluorescence

(a) Ante mortem

In salivary, corneal or conjunctival smears or skin biopsy from the nape of the neck by direct immunofluorescence using antirabies serum tagged with fluorescein isothiocyanate.

(b) Post mortem

In impression smears of the cut surface of the salivary gland, hippocampus, brain stem or cerebellum by direct immunofluorescence using antirabies serum tagged with fluorescein isothiocyanate.

3. Detection of genomic RNA and viral mRNA

It is carried out by PCR and dot-blot hybridization assay with ^{32}P-labelled cDNA probes on skin biopsy, corneal impression or saliva.

4. Virus isolation

(a) Mouse inoculation

Rabies virus can be isolated by intracerebral inoculation of saliva or cerebral fluid (ante mortem) and salivary gland or brain tissue extract (post mortem) in suckling mice. The animals die in 7–21 days. However, they may be killed after five days and brain smears stained with fluorescent antibody.

(b) Isolation in cell culture

Rabies virus can be grown in baby hamster kidney, human diploid lung fibroblasts, chick embryo fibroblasts and Vero monkey kidney cells. No cytopathic changes are observed but rabies antigen can be detected by fluorescent antibody staining 18–24 hours after inoculation.

5. Detection of rabies antibodies

Rabies antibodies can be detected in the serum and CSF of the patient by ELISA. **High titre antibodies are present in the CSF in rabies but not after immunization.** Their demonstration can, therefore, be used for diagnosis.

Postexposure treatment and prophylaxis

Postexposure treatment in a previously unvaccinated person consists of:

1. **First-aid treatment** to eliminate virus from the site of infection by prompt cleansing of wound with plenty of soap and water or solutions of quaternary ammonium compounds (such as cetavalon) and running water for 5 minutes followed by application of 40–70% alcohol or tincture or aqueous solution of iodine. **Soap and water, and quaternary ammonium compounds destroy the virus effectively**. Scrubbing should be avoided and suturing delayed if possible.
2. **Human rabies immunoglobulin** 20 IU/kg body weight or heterologous (equine) anti-rabies serum 40 IU/kg body weight – up to half the dose should be administered intramuscularly in the gluteal region and the remaining half should be infiltrated around the bite. Passive immunization is essential in cases of severe bites notably on face, neck, thorax and arms and in cases of licking of the mucous membranes because the period of incubation in such cases may be limited to one week and vaccination even when given on the same day of bite, offers solid immunity only after 2 weeks. In such cases if antibody is not given then the virus may reach the target organ (CNS) and get fixed to neurons before antibody is produced and patient may develop rabies and die.
3. **Cell culture vaccine** (see below): One ml of the vaccine should be given intramuscularly on days 0, 3, 7, 14, 30 and 90 in the **deltoid region**. The dose of cell culture vaccines is not age or body weight dependent. Rabies antibody test may be done on day 30 to ensure that the patient has developed a satisfactory response. In abbreviated multisite schedule, the 2–1–1 regimen, one dose is given in the right arm and one dose in the left arm at day 0, and one dose given in the deltoid muscle on days 7 and 21. The 2–1–1 schedule induces an early antibody response and may be particularly effective when post-exposure treatment does not include administration of rabies immunoglobulin.
4. Adequate **tetanus prophylaxis** should be given.

5. Treatment may be discontinued if the animal involved (dog or cat) remains healthy throughout an observation period of 10 days, or if the animal is killed humanely and found to be negative for rabies by laboratory examination. Any biting animal suspected of being rabid should be immediately killed humanely and tissues examined using appropriate laboratory techniques.

Q. 3. Describe briefly rabies vaccines.

Ans. **Rabies is the only human disease that can be prevented by active immunization after infection**, because a long incubation period of the disease allows time for immunity to develop before the onset of symptoms. *An estimated 1.4 million people in India receive postexposure treatment from animal bites both in public and private sector.*

I. Neural vaccines

Vaccination after exposure to rabies was introduced by Pasteur in 1885. He injected a young boy, bitten by a rabid dog, with ground-up spinal cords of rabies infected rabbits. The infected spinal cords had been dried for various lengths of time to partially inactivate the virus. After this came the vaccines (Table 42.1) which consisted of rabies-infected sheep brain in which virus was inactivated with phenol (Semple vaccine) or beta-propiolactone (BPL vaccine).

Table 42.1. Rabies vaccines

I. Neural vaccines
1. Semple vaccine
2. Beta-propiolactone (BPL) vaccine
3. Suckling mouse brain vaccine

II. Non-neural vaccines
- A. Duck egg vaccine
- B. Cell culture vaccines
  - Human diploid cell (HDC) vaccine
  - Purified chick embryo cell (PCEC) vaccine
  - Purified Vero cell (PVC) vaccine

1. Semple vaccine

It was developed by Semple (1911) at Central Research Institute, Kasauli (India). It is 5% suspension of sheep brain infected with fixed virus and inactivated with phenol at 37°C, leaving residual live virus.

2. Beta-propiolactone vaccine

This is a modification of Semple vaccine in which BPL is used as the inactivating agent instead of phenol. It is believed to be more antigenic.

The dose schedule of neural vaccines require repeated and painful injections and their potency is low. Moreover myelin component of the neural vaccines sensitizes 1 in 500 vaccinees leading to neuroparalytic accidents.

3. Suckling mouse brain vaccine

Since the brain tissues of newborn animals contain little myelin, therefore, a vaccine prepared from suckling mouse brain and inactivated with BPL was used, but was discontinued because of its poor immunogenicity.

II. Non-neural vaccines

A. Duck egg vaccine

Vaccine prepared from virus grown in duck embryos and inactivated with BPL was used for many years. It has been discontinued because of its poor immunogenicity.

Live attenuated chick embryo vaccine

Two types of vaccine were developed – low egg passage (LEP) and high egg passage (HEP) at 40–50 egg passage level and at 180 egg passage level respectively. LEP was used for dogs and HEP for cattle and cats. Since this vaccine contains live virus, therefore, it is not recommended for humans.

B. Cell culture vaccines

(a) **Human diploid cell (HDC) vaccine:** This vaccine consists of fixed rabies virus grown on human diploid lung fibroblasts and inactivated with BPL or tris-*n*-butyl phosphate. It is highly antigenic and free from serious side effects but there may be local reaction in around 15% vaccinees. Because of the greater potency of HDC vaccine, quantity administered is much less than that of neural vaccines. Only five or six doses given intramuscularly in the **deltoid region** in 1.0 ml volumes on days 0, 3, 7, 14, 30 and 90 after exposure are recommended. The last dose is optional. *HDC vaccine should not be injected in gluteal region because high fat content in this region retards the absorption of vaccine.*

(b) **Purified chick embryo cell (PCEC) vaccine and purified Vero cell (PVC) vaccine:** Because of its high cost, HDC vaccine is not available to majority of the patients in developing countries where rabies is a major public health problem. Therefore, to reduce the cost, a number of other cell culture vaccines have been developed using cells more easily grown in bulk than human diploid cells. This has allowed the cost of vaccine to be reduced. Rabies vaccines with a similar potency to HDC vaccine have been produced in chick embryo fibroblasts and Vero cells. The vaccines produced in these cell cultures are known as purified chick embryo cell (PCEC) vaccine and purified Vero cell (PVC) vaccine respectively. *No problems have arisen from a change of vaccine mid course and rabies antibody titres have been satisfactory in those people who were given more than one type of cell culture vaccine.*

Q. 4. Write short note on pre-exposure immunization against rabies.

Ans. Preexposure immunization should be offered to persons at high risk of exposure, such as laboratory staff working with rabies virus and handling infected material, veterinarians, animal handlers, wildlife officers, and other individuals who are living in or travelling to areas where rabies is endemic.

Three injections of tissue culture vaccine, 1.0 ml intramuscularly, should be given on days 0, 7 and 28 or on days 0, 28 and 56. Further boosters are recommended at intervals of 1–3 years as long as the person remains at risk. The presence of virus-neutralizing antibodies in vaccinated individuals should be ascertained, where feasible, using serum samples collected 1–3 weeks after the last dose. If the titre is less than 0.5 IU per ml, booster doses should be administered till the antibody level reaches more than 0.5 IU per ml. Such individuals on getting exposed to rabies virus after successful preexposure immunization shall require only two booster doses of the vaccine, given on days 0 and 3 without any antirabic serum.

43

Orthomyxoviruses

Q. 1. Describe morphology, haemagglutination reaction, elution and haemadsorption of influenza viruses.

Ans. ***Morphology***

Influenzavirus A and *Influenzavirus B* are morphologically similar, but *Influenzavirus C* differs from them in certain respects, particularly in having **only a single type of glycoprotein spike**. The virions are spherical, 80–120 nm in diameter, but larger pleomorphic and filamentous forms 1,000 nm or more in length may be abundant. The nucleocapsid (Fig. 43.1) has helical symmetry. Influenza A and B viruses have eight RNA segments, and influenza C virus has seven segments. Gene segments range from 800–2500 nucleotides in length, and the entire genome ranges from 10–14.6 kb. The segmented genome of influenza viruses allows the exchange of one or more gene segments between two viruses when both infect a single cell. This exchange is known as **genetic reassortment** and results in the generation of new strains containing a mix of genes from both parental viruses. Genetic reassortment between human and avian influenza virus strains led to generation of H2N2 (1957), H3N2 pandemic strains (1968), H5N1 (1997) and H1N1 virus (2009).

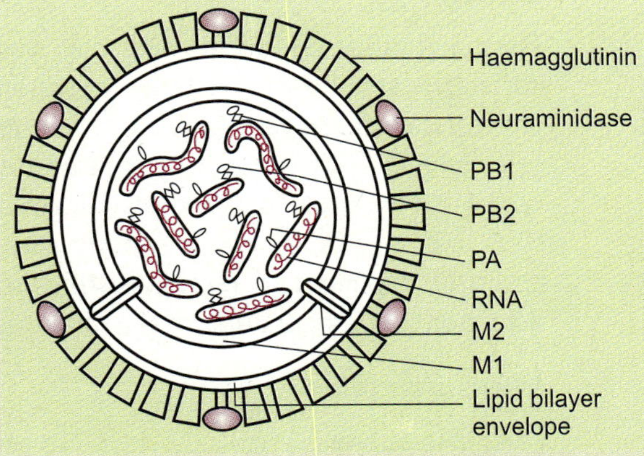

Fig. 43.1. Influenza virus.

RNA segments are associated with nucleoprotein and 3 large **polymerase proteins**, an acidic (PA) and 2 basic (PB1 and PB2). RNA with associated nucleoprotein is known as ribonucleoprotein (RNP). Three polymerase proteins are associated with RNP at its end. They are responsible for RNA replication and transcription. The nucleocapsid is surrounded by a protein layer or **matrix protein (M1)**, which in turn, is enclosed in host plasma membrane derived **lipid bilayer envelope**. The **M2 protein** projects through the envelope to form ion channels which allow pH changes in the endosome.

Attached to the lipid envelope of *Influenzavirus A* and *B* are two types of glycoprotein peplomers or spikes, the haemagglutinin (HA) and the neuraminidase (NA). HA peplomers exist as 500 tapered projections, 10 nm in length, with their broadest (5 nm) ends outermost and their narrow ends inserted in the lipid membrane. NA peplomers are 100 mushroom-shaped projections per virion measuring 9 nm in length.

Haemagglutination reaction

The virus particles bind to the host cell receptors (sialic acid) by haemagglutinin peplomers. The haemagglutinin activity of influenza virus results from the ability of the haemagglutinin peplomers present on the surface of the virus to attach to the sialic acid present on glycoproteins on the surface of erythrocytes causing them to agglutinate. The haemagglutination reaction is important in laboratory work because it provides a simple and rapid method for detection of viruses in egg or tissue culture fluid. Influenza viruses can agglutinate erythrocytes of fowl, guinea-pig, man and others.

Elution

Haemagglutination is followed after a time by the detachment of the virus from the cell surface, reversing the haemagglutination. This is known as elution and is caused by the enzyme neuraminidase present in the neuraminidase peplomers. The enzyme acts on the cell receptor, destroying it by splitting off N-acetylneuraminic acid from it. Virus particles which have eluted from red cells are still capable of agglutinating fresh red cells but red cells that have been acted on by the virus are not susceptible to agglutination by the same strain of the virus. **Haemagglutination inhibition** offers a convenient method for the detection and quantitation of the antibody to the virus in patient sera.

Haemadsorption

Plasma membrane of cells in which virus is multiplying contains haemagglutinins. Therefore, RBCs get adsorbed to the surface of such cells. This is known as haemadsorption, a technique by which the growth of influenza virus can be identified in cell culture.

Q. 2. Describe system of nomenclature of influenza viruses.

Ans. *Influenzavirus A* is divided into subtypes, all of which share nucleoprotein and matrix proteins but differ in their haemagglutinins and/or neuraminidase. Sixteen subtypes of haemagglutinins (H1–H16) and nine of neuraminidase (N1–N9) are known in birds, some of which have also been found in various combinations in humans. Human viruses show 3 HA (H1, H2, H3) and 2 NA (N1, N2) types. All non-human influenza viruses belong to type A while types B and C viruses are exclusively human viruses. System of nomenclature includes *Influenzavirus* genus *A* or *B*, host of origin, place of isolation, strain number, year of first isolation, followed in parentheses by HA and NA subtypes, e.g., A/swine/Iowa/3/70 (H1N1). If isolated from a human host, the origin is omitted, e.g., A/Shangai/24/90 (H3N2).

Genome of *Influenzavirus C* contains only seven RNA segments and no neuraminidase activity. The receptor-binding and receptor-destroying enzyme functions of *Influenzavirus C* are distinct from those of *Influenzavirus A* and *B* and both activities seem to reside on the same surface glycoprotein. *Influenzavirus C* shares no antigens with *Influenzavirus A* or *B*.

Q. 3. Describe briefly antigenic structure and antigenic variation of influenza viruses.

Ans. ***Antigenic structure***

The influenza viruses have following antigens:

1. **Ribonucleoprotein (RNP):** It is genus-specific, and all strains of a genus possess the same antigen. It is stable and does not exhibit any significant antigenic variation.
2. **Matrix (M1) protein:** Like RNP antigen, it is also genus-specific.
3. **Haemagglutinin (HA):** It is a glycoprotein composed of two polypeptides – HA1 and HA2. It is strain-specific and is capable of great variation. Antihaemagglutinin antibodies are produced following infection and immunization.
4. **Neuraminidase (NA):** It is a glycoprotein enzyme which destroys cell receptors by hydrolytic cleavage. Like haemagglutinin it is strain-specific, exhibits variation and anti-neuraminidase antibody is formed following infection and immunization.

Antigenic variation

Influenza virus is capable of undergoing antigenic variation due to frequent changes in the antigenicity of HA and NA. This is of great importance in the epidemiology of the disease. Incidence of antigenic variation is highest in *Influenzavirus A*, less in *B* and it has not been demonstrated in *Influenzavirus C*. Depending on the degree of antigenic change of HA and NA, two distinct forms of antigenic variation are known.

1. Antigenic drift

The gradual sequential change in the antigenic structure occurring regularly at frequent intervals is known as antigenic drift. It results from mutations in *H* or *N* genes. This process occurs every 2–3 years, causing local outbreaks of influenza A and B infection. The new antigens acquired though different from the previous are yet related to them so that they can still react with antisera to the predecessor virus strain to some extent.

2. Antigenic shift

It is an abrupt, drastic, discontinuous variation in the antigenic structure resulting in a new virus strain unrelated antigenically to predecessor strain. It may involve HA or NA or both. Antibodies to predecessor virus strains do not neutralize the new variants, therefore, they can spread widely in the population leading to major epidemics and pandemics. Drastic changes in the sequence of surface glycoproteins are unlikely to be due to mutation. They result from gene reassortment (recombination) of genomes of different strains, including animal strains in doubly infected cells. This process occurs only with influenza A virus. In contrast to influenza A, influenza B is predominantly a human virus and does not undergo antigenic shift.

Q. 4. Describe methods of cultivation of influenza viruses.

Ans. *Animal inoculation*

The virus can produce experimental infection in ferrets and mice by intranasal inoculation.

Chick embryo inoculation

Influenzavirus A, *B* and *C* can be isolated in the **amniotic cavity** of 13-day-old chick embryos incubated at 33–35°C for 2–3 days. After a few egg passages, *Influenzavirus A* and *B* grow well in allantoic cavity also, whereas *Influenzavirus C* can be grown only in amniotic cavity. Virus growth is detected by the appearance of haemagglutinin in the amniotic and allantoic fluids.

Tissue culture

Influenza virus can also be isolated on primary monkey kidney or human embryo kidney cells. Madin-Darby canine kidney (MDCK) cells, a continuous line, may also be used to isolate influenza viruses, provided trypsin (2 μg/ml) is present in the medium to cleave the haemagglutinin of progeny virions and enable spread to other cells. Cytopathic effects are not prominent and virus growth is detected by haemadsorption or demonstration of haemagglutinin in culture fluid.

Q. 5. Describe pathogenicity and laboratory diagnosis of and immunity against influenza viruses.

Ans. ***Pathogenicity***

Influenza viruses are transmitted from person to person primarily via droplets generated by sneezing, coughing and speaking. Direct or indirect (fomites) contact with contaminated secretions and small-particle aerosols are other potential routes of transmission. In case of human infections caused by avian strains of influenza virus, direct contact with infected birds is the most common factor of transmission. There has been concern about the pandemic potential of avian strains of influenza A/H5N1 virus since 1997, when several human cases occurred in Hong Kong in association with a large poultry outbreak. The outbreak was controlled by slaughtering all poultry in Hong Kong.

Influenza A/H5N1 virus again caused outbreaks in poultry in China in 2003 and in several Southeast Asian countries in 2004 and 2005. By late 2005 and early 2006, the virus had spread to other parts of Asia, as well as to parts of Europe, Africa, and the Middle East. Human cases of A/H5N1 have been directly associated with outbreaks in poultry. Up to 2010, more than 500 human infections have been documented. In 2009, a swine-origin influenza A/H1N1 virus was identified.

Very small doses, three viable particles or more can initiate infection. The viral neuraminidase facilitates infection by hydrolyzing the mucus film lining the respiratory tract and exposing the cell surface receptors for virus adsorption. Ciliated epithelial cells of respiratory tract are the main sites of virus infection. The death and sloughing of these cells renders the respiratory tract vulnerable to secondary bacterial infection. Viraemic phase is extremely rare.

Incubation period is short varying from 1–4 days. The illness is characterized by a sudden onset of systemic symptoms such as chills, fever, sore throat, rhinorrhoea, nasal congestion, nonproductive cough, myalgia, headache and malaise. The uncomplicated illness usually lasts for 3–7 days. Worldwide, severe influenza infections occur in 3–5 million people annually, and 250,000–500,000 deaths occur.

Complications

1. Young children may develop croup, pneumonia or middle ear infection.
2. Elderly people may develop secondary bacterial pneumonia usually due to *Staphylococcus aureus*, *Streptococcus pneumoniae* and *Haemophilus influenzae*.
3. Influenza may produce various cardiac complications ranging from temporary changes in electrocardiogram patterns to inflammatory changes in the heart muscles.
4. **Reye's syndrome:** It is characterized by a severe encephalomyelitis accompanied by liver degeneration. It is thought to be associated with influenza B and less certainly with influenza A virus infection in children.
5. Worsening of metabolic state in diabetics who suffer from influenza. Influenza deaths among them are not uncommon.

Laboratory diagnosis

Electron microscopy

Influenza viruses may be detected in clinical specimens by visualization of their typical morphological appearance by electron microscopy (EM). Immune EM is the most sensitive EM method and allows differentiation of virus type and subtype when specific hyperimmune sera are used in the assay. However, large number of viruses (> 10^5–10^6 per ml) must be present in the clinical sample for successful detection using this diagnostic approach.

Fluorescence microscopy

Smears of nasopharyngeal secretions and nasal swab or centrifuged deposit of throat garglings are stained with fluorescein-tagged influenza antiserum and seen under fluorescence microscope. Fluorescent antibody test using monoclonal antibodies, can detect 70–100% of cases diagnosed by culture.

Nucleic acid analyses

Molecular methods are increasingly being used for both the detection and the characterization of influenza viruses. The most commonly used molecular method is reverse transcription PCR (RT-PCR).

Virus isolation

Influenza viruses can be isolated during first 2–3 days of illness. Throat garglings are collected using suitable buffered salt solution. The specimen should be processed immediately. If short delay is expected then store it at 4°C and if long delay is expected then store it at –70°C. The specimen is treated with antibiotics to destroy bacteria and inoculated into amniotic cavity of chick embryos, primary monkey kidney, human embryo kidney cells or MDCK cells.

Procedure: Influenza virus isolation procedures should be performed under biosafety level 2 (BSL-2). The material is inoculated into the **amniotic cavity** of 11–13-day-old eggs, using at least six eggs per specimen. After incubation at 35°C for three days, the eggs are chilled and the amniotic and allantoic fluids harvested separately. The fluids are tested for haemagglutination using guinea pig and fowl RBCs in parallel at room temperature and at 4°C. Some strains of influenza virus type A agglutinate only guinea pig cells on initial isolation. The type B virus agglutinates both cells, while type C strains agglutinate only fowl cells.

Inoculated cell cultures are incubated at 33°C in roller drums and the virus growth can be identified by testing the culture fluid for haemagglutination or by haemadsorption.

Serological tests

Serological diagnosis of influenza is based upon demonstrating a four-fold or higher increase in antibody titre between acute-phase and convalescent-phase sera. Complement fixation, haemagglutination inhibition and neutralization tests are done for this purpose. Since serological diagnosis is retrospective, therefore, it is of limited use.

Haemagglutination inhibition (HAI) is a convenient and sensitive test for the serological diagnosis of influenza. The major drawback is the frequent presence in the sera of non-specific inhibitors of haemagglutination. The sera suitably treated for the removal of nonspecific inhibitors are diluted serially in haemagglutination plates and the influenza virus suspension containing 4 HA units added to each cup. Fowl red cells are then added. The highest dilution of serum that inhibits haemagglutination is its H1 titre.

Complement fixation test with the RNP antigen of influenza virus is very useful as the antibodies are formed during infection, but not following immunisation with inactivated vaccines.

Immunity

An attack of influenza confers protection effective for one to two years. Following infection and immunisation, circulating antibodies are formed against the various antigens of the virus. However, local concentration of antihaemagglutinin (IgA) is more relevant in protection. The apparent short duration of immunity is due to the antigenic variation that the virus undergoes frequently.

When an individual suffers from repeated infections with different antigenic variants of influenza virus type A, he forms antibodies not only against each infecting strain, but also against the strain he first came into contact with. The dominant antibody response will be against the strain that caused the earliest infection. This phenomenon is known as the doctrine of **'original antigenic sin'**.

Q. 6. Describe influenza vaccines.

Ans. Vaccination is the main method of preventing influenza, but major difficulty in immunoprophylaxis is the frequent change in the antigenic structure of influenza virus. Vaccines are of two types:

1. Inactivated vaccines

Influenza virus is grown in allantoic cavity of chick embryos. These are inactivated with formalin or β-propiolactone, then purified by zonal ultracentrifugation and disrupted with detergents. The resulting polyvalent inactivated vaccine is used every autumn. This vaccine can be further purified to contain only haemagglutinins and neuraminidases. This is known as **subunit vaccine**. The vaccine is administered parenterally in a single dose. Inactivated vaccines induce the formation of circulating antibodies. The level of antibodies in the respiratory mucosa is only a fraction of the serum level.

2. Live attenuated vaccines

Temperature-sensitive (ts) mutants of influenza virus may be used as live vaccine. They can grow at lower temperature of the nasopharyngeal mucosa (32–34°C) but not in lungs (37°C). Live vaccine is administered by **aerosol spray or intranasally**. It stimulates the production of local IgA antibodies. Circulating antibodies of IgM and IgG classes are not raised to the same extent as when killed vaccine is injected.

Q. 7. Describe pathogenesis, epidemiology and laboratory diagnosis of avian influenza (bird flu).

Ans. ***Pathogenesis and epidemiology***

Avian influenza is a contagious disease caused by virus that normally infects only birds and less commonly pigs. First evidence of direct transmission from birds to humans was observed in 1997, when an unusual case of human respiratory illness caused by influenza A (H5N1) was identified in Hong Kong, China. Later that year, more cases began to be seen. Eventually, a total of 18 human illnesses, one third fatal, were found in children and young adults. Immediate containment measures and the slaughter of all (over 1.6 million) chickens and other poultry species in Hong Kong stopped the danger before the strain developed person-to-person transmissibility, which could have initiated a pandemic.

A number of other episodes of human illness due to avian influenza subtypes – H7N7 (Great Britain, 1995; Netherlands, 2003; Hong Kong, 2003), H9N2 (Hong Kong, 1999), and H7N3 (Canada, 2004) were identified producing both respiratory disease and conjunctivitis. Investigations of these events suggested they resulted from direct contact with infected avian hosts without evidence of human-to-human transmission. Such transmission is considered an essential feature for a virus to have pandemic potential.

In late 2003, cases of human avian influenza due to influenza A (H5N1) once again were recognized, this time in Vietnam and then in Thailand. In contrast to previous limited episodes, these illnesses were more geographically scattered and were accompanied by evidence of widespread circulation of the implicated virus in poultry, where it was highly pathogenic, and in migratory birds. Similar to the 1997 Hong Kong episode, the human disease associated with this strain occurred mostly in children and young adults and produced unusually severe illness with high case fatality rates. These findings have sharply increased concerns that influenza A (H5N1) represents the next global pandemic strain.

Since its emergence in 2003, influenza A (H5N1) has remained in continuous circulation in migratory birds, producing devastating epizootics in domesticated poultry, in some wildlife avian species, in animals, and in humans. It has been detected throughout Asia, Europe, and Africa, carried on avian migratory routes.

Between 2003 and 2008, WHO received reports of 395 human illnesses caused by influenza A (H5N1). These illnesses have been reported from 15 countries in Asia, Africa, and Europe, with largest number in Indonesia (141 cases), Vietnam (107 cases), and Egypt

(51 cases). Among the human cases, the resulting illness has been extremely severe: 250 (63%) have been fatal.

Certain water birds such as waterfowls and migratory birds act as reservoir of avian influenza viruses, and usually only get asymptomatic infection. They carry the virus in their intestines and shed it in their faeces. Avian influenza viruses are spread to susceptible birds through inhalation of influenza particles in nasal and respiratory secretions and from contact with the faeces of infected birds. The disease can spread from country to country through international trade in live poultry. Migratory birds, including waterfowl, sea birds, and shore birds can also carry the virus for long distances and have, in the past, been implicated in the international spread of highly pathogenic avian influenza.

The symptoms can vary from a mild disease with little or no mortality to a highly fatal, rapidly spreading epidemic depending on the infecting virus strain and host factors. Domestic poultry including chickens and turkeys are particularly susceptible to epidemics of rapidly fatal influenza. Decreased food consumption and drops in egg production are some of the earliest and most predictable signs of the disease. Other signs may include coughing, sneezing, ruffled feathers, swollen heads and diarrhoea. In some cases, birds die rapidly without clinical signs of disease.

The reported symptoms of avian influenza in humans have ranged from typical influenza-like symptoms (fever, cough, sore throat and muscle aches) to eye infections, pneumonia and acute respiratory distress.

Laboratory diagnosis

It is not always possible to clinically distinguish human influenza caused by a seasonal influenza virus from those due to avian influenza infections, especially in the early phase of the infection. Therefore, laboratory confirmation is required to establish the aetiology of clinical influenza. Furthermore, laboratory diagnosis will also contribute to the early detection and characterization of viruses that have undergone genetic changes favourable to the emergence of a pandemic strain. Hence, if the laboratory diagnosis is not performed, there is a risk of failure to detect and warn the global community of potential pandemic strains of avian influenza and to initiate timely public health interventions to avert such an epidemic.

Specimens

A variety of specimens are suitable for the diagnosis of avian influenza. These include nasal swab, nasopharyngeal swab, nasopharyngeal aspirate, nasal wash and throat swab. In addition to swabs from upper respiratory tract, invasive procedures can be performed for the diagnosis of virus infections of lower respiratory tract where indicated. These include transtracheal aspirate, bronchoalveolar lavage and lung biopsy.

Laboratory diagnosis of avian influenza in humans can be carried out by:

1. *Detection of antigen by:*
   - Immunofluorescence test.
   - Antigen capture ELISA with monoclonal antibody to the nucleoprotein.
   - Polymerase chain reaction.
2. *Virus isolation in:*
   - Cell line Madin-Darby canine kidney cells.
   - Egg inoculation.

Q. 8. Write short note on H1N1 (swine flu) virus.

Ans. H1N1 (Swine flu) virus is a swine origin influenza A virus. This new virus was first detected in the United States in April 2009. Other countries, including Mexico and Canada, have also reported people sick with this new virus. It spreads from person-to-person probably in much the same way that regular seasonal influenza viruses spread.

Existing vaccines against seasonal flu provide no protection. It is more contagious than seasonal flu and is believed to spread from human to human in much the same way as seasonal flu. The most common mechanism by which it spreads is by droplets from coughs and sneezes of infected people and also by touching a surface or the hands of a person contaminated with the virus and then touching one's eyes, nose or mouth. Unlike seasonal flu, H1N1 can infect cells deep in the lungs. Most people infected with this virus suffer a mild illness, but only a small minority are often severely ill. H1N1 destroys the lung alveoli, often causing acute respiratory distress. People at high risk for developing flu-related complications include:

- Children younger than 5, but especially younger than 2-years-old.
- Adults 65 years of age and older.
- Pregnant women.

Patient develops fever, cough, sore throat, running or stuffy nose, body aches, chills and fatigue. Some people may have vomiting and diarrhoea. From April 2009 to November 2009, in the US, 3,900 people died of the H1N1 pandemic virus. Existing vaccines against seasonal flu provide no protection.

Laboratory diagnosis

Specimens

Samples should be taken from deep nostrils (nasal swab), nasopharynx (nasopharyngeal swab), nasopharyngeal aspirate, and throat or bronchial aspirates. Acute and convalescent serum specimens should be used for the detection of rising antibody titres.

Molecular diagnostics

Molecular diagnostics are currently the method of choice for pandemic (H1N1) virus. Important gene targets are – type A influenza matrix gene; haemagglutinin gene specific for pandemic (H1N1) 2009 virus; and haemagglutinin gene specific for seasonal influenza A H1/H3. Protocols currently available are – influenza A type-specific conventional and real time PCR; pandemic (H1N1) 2009 virus-specific conventional and real time PCR; CDC realtime RT-PCR (rRT-PCR) protocol for the detection and characterization of pandemic H1N1 2009; and seasonal influenza A (H1N1 and H3N2); and avian influenza A (H5, H7 and H9) realtime RT-PCR.

Virus isolation

Current protocols for virus isolation of seasonal influenza viruses using MDCK cells and egg inoculation can be used. Turkey, chicken, guinea pig and human red blood cells agglutinate with pandemic (H1N1) 2009 virus.

Immunofluorescence

Immunofluorescence tests designed for direct detection of influenza A viruses do not differentiate seasonal influenza from pandemic (H1N1) 2009 virus.

Serology

Haemagglutination inhibition and microneutralization tests using pandemic (H1N1) 2009 virus are expected to be able to detect antibody responses following infection.

Prophylaxis

- Wash your hands with soap and water. If soap and water are not available, use an alcohol-based hand rub.
- Avoid touching your eyes, nose or mouth.
- Try to avoid contact with sick people.
- If you are sick with flu-like illness, you stay home for at least 24 hours after your fever has disappeared except to get medical care.

44

PARAMYXOVIRUSES, CALICIVIRUSES, ASTROVIRUSES AND CORONAVIRUSES

Q. 1. Tabulate differences between various paramyxoviruses.

Ans. Differentiation of various paramyxoviruses is given in Table 44.1.

Table 44.1. Differentiation of various paramyxoviruses

Property	Parainfluenza virus	Mumps virus	Measles virus	Respiratory syncytial virus
Fusion (F) protein	+	+	+	+
Haemagglutinin	+	+	+	–
Neuraminidase	+	+	–	–

Q. 2. Describe morphology, pathogenesis and laboratory diagnosis of parainfluenza, mumps and measles viruses.

Ans. ***Morphology***

Parainfluenza, mumps and measles viruses are indistinguishable under the electron microscope. They range from 150–300 nm or more in diameter, occasionally there are filamentous forms and giant forms up to 800 nm in diameter. They are enclosed by a lipid envelope derived from plasma membrane of the host cell. The envelope of parainfluenza and mumps viruses contains HN and F glycoprotein peplomers 12–14 nm long and 2–4 nm wide. The former carries both haemagglutinating and neuraminidase functions and latter causes fusion of cell membranes leading to the formation of syncytia. The spikes on the measles virus envelope carry a haemagglutinin but not a neuraminidase. The inner surface of the envelope is lined by matrix (M) protein. Within the virion, there is a nucleocapsid of helical symmetry. It contains a single-stranded, negative sense RNA genome as a single piece, 16–20 kb in size, and an RNA-dependent RNA polymerase (Fig. 44.1).

Parainfluenza viruses

There are four types of parainfluenza viruses – types 1, 2, 3 and 4.

Pathogenesis

Parainfluenza viruses are highly transmissible and are acquired by droplets and by contact with respiratory secretions. **Incubation period varies from 2–6 days.** All parainfluenza viruses produce upper respiratory tract infections. In infants and children, these viruses may invade the lower respiratory tract, causing **pneumonia**. In older children (6 months to 5 years), parainfluenza virus type 1 and to some extent, type 2 may cause **laryngotracheobronchitis or croup**. The patient presents with fever, cough and respiratory distress that may need emergency tracheostomy. Type 3 infects infants within first year or two of life. Type 4 produces only mild illness.

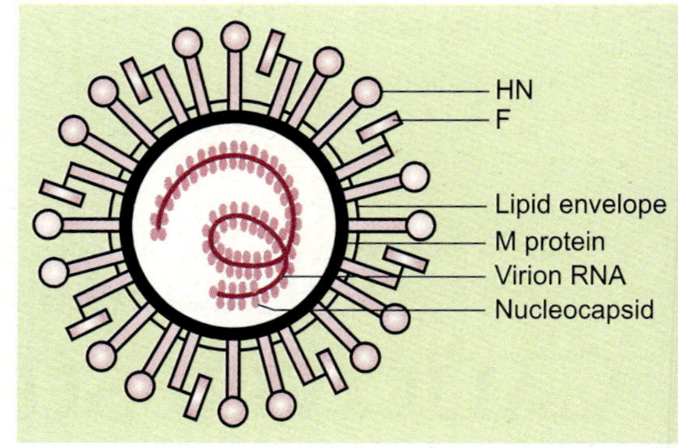

Fig. 44.1. Schematic diagram of parainfluenza and mumps viruses.

Laboratory diagnosis

Microscopy

Electron microscopy can easily demonstrate the presence of parainfluenza viruses, but these and other paramyxoviruses appear the same.

Immunofluorescent staining

Viral antigens can be demonstrated in exfoliated cells aspirated from respiratory tract by immunofluorescent straining using monoclonal antibodies. It is used for rapid diagnosis.

Detection of free antigen

Detection of free antigen in mucus by ELISA and RIA.

Virus isolation

Parainfluenza viruses may be isolated in primary human or monkey kidney cells or in continuous cell lines such as H292 derived from human lung mucoepidermoid carcinoma. They produce little cytopathic effect, except type 2 which induces syncytia. Viral growth can be detected by haemadsorption of guinea-pig red cells or by use of specific immunofluorescent antibody.

Serology

Type-specific antibody may be detected by neutralization, ELISA and complement fixation test. A four-fold rise in titre is indicative of infection with a parainfluenza virus.

Mumps virus

Morphology

Morphology of mumps virus is the same as described under morphology of parainfluenza and measles viruses.

Pathogenesis

Mumps is predominantly a disease of childhood. The mumps virus is transmitted by way of respiratory and oral secretions, and **respiratory tract is the portal of entry**. It multiplies in the upper respiratory tract and in local lymph nodes. The virus then enters the blood stream and the infection spreads to many organs of the body. The major manifestation is **painful swelling of one or both parotid glands** occurring 14–18 days after exposure. It may also cause meningo-encephalitis, orchitis, oophoritis, pancreatitis, arthritis, myocarditis and renal dysfunction.

Immunity

There is **only one serotype of mumps virus**. Infection with this virus leads to **lifelong immunity**.

Laboratory diagnosis

Microscopy

Microscopic examination of affected salivary glands reveals an oedematous interstitium diffusely infiltrated by macrophages, lymphocytes, and plasma cells, which compress acini and ducts. Neutrophils and necrotic debris may fill the ductal lumen, causing focal damage to ductal epithelium.

Antigen detection

Mumps virus antigen may be detected by immunofluorescence staining of throat swab specimens.

Nucleic acid detection

Mumps virus RNA may be detected by RT-PCR in oral fluid, CSF, saliva, and urine.

Virus isolation

Virus can be isolated from saliva from affected gland, throat swab, CSF and urine on primary monkey kidney cells, H292 and HEp-2 cells. It produces little cytopathic effect but virus can be detected by immunofluorescence and haemadsorption (of guinea-pig or chicken red cells) which can be inhibited by specific antiserum.

Serology

For rapid diagnosis, ELISA is useful for detecting mumps-specific IgM antibodies in the serum.

Prophylaxis

A live attenuated vaccine, derived by passage in chick fibroblasts, offers 95% protection which lasts for 12 years. It can be given by subcutaneous injection in combination with attenuated measles and rubella strains (MMR vaccine). This vaccine is administered to children of both sexes, aged 15 months.

Measles virus

Morphology

Measles virus resembles parainfluenza viruses and mump virus in morphology.

Pathogenesis

Measles is the **commonest highly contagious childhood disease** spread by respiratory secretions. Virus gains access to the human body via the respiratory tract, where it multiplies locally. The infection then spreads to the regional lymphoid tissue, where further multiplication occurs. This leads to **primary viraemia**. It disseminates the virus, which then replicates in the reticuloendothelial system, followed by **secondary viraemia**. It seeds the epithelial surfaces of the body, including skin, respiratory tract, and conjunctiva where focal replication occurs.

After an **incubation period of 10–12 days**, patient develops upper respiratory tract infection with high fever, rhinitis, cough and conjunctivitis. **Koplik's spots**, which are small, 1–3 mm in diameter, bluish white spots surrounded by erythema can be seen on the buccal mucosa during this stage and are pathognomonic of measles. After 1–2 days, the acute symptoms decline with the appearance of characteristic **maculopapular rash** which appears first on the neck and then spreads to the rest of the body. **The rash is due to type IV hypersensitivity to viral antigens.** In next 10–14 days, rash fades with considerable desquamation and sometimes by discolouration of the skin. There is **only one antigenic type of measles virus. Infection confers lifelong immunity**.

Since measles decreases the resistance of the respiratory epithelium, therefore, patient may develop secondary bacterial infections like sinusitis, otitis media, bronchitis, bronchiolitis, croup and bronchopneumonia. Giant cell pneumonia may occur most frequently in those with impaired cell-mediated immunity. In addition, acute postinfectious encephalitis and subacute sclerosing panencephalitis (SSPE) may occur in 1 in 1000 and 1 in 300,000 cases of measles respectively.

Subacute sclerosing panencephalitis is a rare and late complication of measles infection. The disease begins insidiously **5–15 years after a case of measles**. It is characterized by progressive mental deterioration, involuntary movements, muscular rigidity, and coma. It is invariably fatal. Patients with SSPE exhibit high titres of measles antibody in cerebrospinal fluid and serum, and defective measles virus in brain cells. With the widespread use of measles vaccine, SSPE has become less common.

Laboratory diagnosis

Specimen collection and transport

For successful virus isolation specimens should be collected early in the acute phase of infection, when the virus is present in high concentrations, and transported to a laboratory under conditions that maintain the infectivity of labile viruses. Suitable samples for isolation of measles virus or for detection of viral antigens are whole blood, serum, throat and nasopharyngeal secretions, urine, and in special circumstances, brain and skin biopsy samples. Specimens should be processed as soon as possible after collection and are best kept at 4°C rather than frozen; since freezing causes significant loss of recoverable virus.

Direct microscopy

Giemsa-stained smears of nasal secretions show multinucleated giant cells.

Immunofluorescence

The measles virus antigen can be detected in the infected cells of nasal secretions by immunofluorescence.

Virus isolation

The measles virus can be isolated, though with some difficulty, from throat washings, blood, urinary sediment, etc. on monkey kidney, primary human embryo kidney and human amnion cells. Cytopathic changes may take 7–10 days to develop. The appearance of multinucleated giant cells containing numerous acidophilic inclusions in cytoplasm and nuclei, in the cultured cells, suggests the presence of measles virus (Fig. 38.1J), but earlier diagnosis is possible by immunofluorescent staining with monoclonal antibody.

Serology

Measles antibody in the patient serum can be detected by IgM capture ELISA. Complement fixation test can be carried out on acute and convalescent sera. A rise in antibody titre is diagnostic. Demonstration of high titres of measles antibody in the CSF is diagnostic of SSPE.

Polymerase chain reaction (PCR)

Reverse transcriptase PCR is a sensitive and specific method of diagnosis.

Prophylaxis

Children of the age of 15 months are given MMR vaccine, followed by a booster at the age of 4–6 years.

Q. 3. Write short note on respiratory syncytial virus.

Ans. Respiratory syncytial virus (RSV) is pleomorphic and ranges in size from 150–300 nm. The viral envelope has two glycoproteins – the G protein by which the virus attaches to cell surfaces and the F (fusion) protein that induces fusion of infected cells that leads to formation of large multinucleated syncytia from which the virus gets its name. RSV differs from other paramyxoviruses in not possessing haemagglutinating and neuroaminidase activities. The diameter of nucleocapsid of RSV is less (13 nm) than that of other paramyxoviruses.

RSV is **highly contagious**. It is the most important respiratory pathogen of childhood. It is responsible for nearly half the cases of **bronchiolitis** and a quarter of all cases of **pneumonia** occurring during the first few months of life. Virus is shed in respiratory secretions for several days or weeks. Infection is transmitted by contact with contaminated hands and surfaces. **Nosocomial infections** are frequent in nurseries and paediatrics wards. Incubation period of the disease is 4–5 days. The virus multiplies in the mucous membranes of the nose and throat. RSV infecting infants younger than 6 months of age frequently results in lower respiratory tract infections, causing pneumonia or bronchiolitis. Older children and adults may be reinfected, however, unlike primary infections, reinfections do not usually involve the lower respiratory tract. Disease in them may cause no more than a cold. In elderly and immunosuppressed transplant recipients, it may lead to severe pneumonia.

Laboratory diagnosis

Detection of viral antigens

Viral antigens can be detected in nasopharyngeal aspirates by:

- Immunofluorescence using monoclonal antibody.
- ELISA technique.

Isolation of virus in cell culture

Virus can be isolated from nasopharyngeal secretions by inoculation of HeLa cells and HEp-2 cells. Characteristic syncytia are produced in 2–10 days. However, definitive identification can be carried out by immunofluorescence.

Q. 4. Write short note on caliciviruses.

Ans. Family Caliciviridae contains nonenveloped spherical virions. They possess single-stranded positive sense RNA genome of 7.5–7.7 kb. It is surrounded by icosahedral capsid. The latter is made up of 90 capsomers and 32 cup-shaped (*calix*, cup) surface depressions which give the family its name. This family has a single genus *Calicivirus* which includes human caliciviruses and hepatitis E virus.

Human caliciviruses

Human caliciviruses are of two types:

1. **Typical caliciviruses:** They are 30–35 nm icosahedral virions with cup-shaped depressions.
2. **Norwalk virus:** It is an amorphous round virion measuring 27–40 nm in diameter. It has an indistinct ragged or feathery outline.

Pathogenesis

Caliciviruses cause **gastroenteritis** primarily in infants and young children. Outbreaks have been reported in schools, orphanages and hospital paediatric wards. Calicivirus infection leads to a self-limited vomiting and diarrhoea. Recovery takes place in 4–10 days.

After an **incubation period of 24–48 hours**, Norwalk virus leads to nausea, vomiting, diarrhoea, abdominal cramps, headache, myalgia and low grade fever. Norwalk agent and caliciviruses are excreted in the faeces and/or vomit of the infected person. Infection is acquired via faecal contamination of water and food.

Laboratory diagnosis

Human caliciviruses have not been grown on cultured cells. Virus can be detected in the faeces by immunoelectron microscopy. Radioimmunoassay (RIA) and ELISA are also used to detect the virus and viral antigens in stool.

Q. 5. Write short note on astroviruses.

Ans. Astroviruses are small (28–30 nm in diameter) spherical virions with a characteristic five- or six-pointed **star-shaped** outline by negative staining. The genome consists of a single linear 7 kb single-stranded RNA molecule of positive polarity. This family has only one genus, *Astrovirus* which has five serotypes. Astroviruses can be isolated, in the presence of trypsin, in cultures of primary human embryonic kidney cells.

Astroviruses have been found in the faeces of humans, calves and lambs suffering from enteritis. They are transmitted by the faecal-oral route from person to person and via contaminated food or water. After an **incubation period of 1–4 days** patient develops **watery**

diarrhoea lasting 1–4 days or more, vomiting and abdominal discomfort. It occurs principally in young children.

The virus in the faeces can be detected by immunoelectron microscopy and ELISA test.

Q. 6. Write short note on coronaviruses.

Ans. Coronaviruses are enveloped, 120–160 nm in diameter. They contain an unsegmented genome of single-stranded positive sense RNA (27–30 kb), the largest genome among RNA viruses. The nucleocapsid is helical measuring 9–11 nm in diameter. This is enclosed within a lipoprotein envelope which carries large (20 nm long) club- or petal-shaped projections that are widely spaced on the outer surface of the envelope (Fig. 44.2), resembling a solar corona (hence the name, coronaviruses). Coronaviruses are sensitive to heat, lipid solvents, non-ionic detergents, formaldehyde and oxidizing agents.

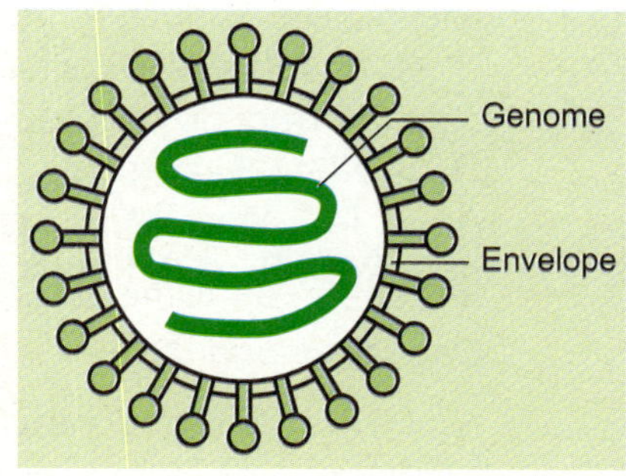

Fig. 44.2. *Coronavirus.*

Human coronavirus infects the respiratory tract by the inhalation of droplets or aerosols generated by cough and sneezes of infected individuals. Up to 30% of common colds are caused by coronaviruses. The typical coronavirus cold is marked by nasal discharge and malaise. Cough and sore throat are generally not as prominent as in rhinovirus infection, and there is little or no fever. The incubation period of the disease varies from 2–5 days and symptoms persist for about a week. The coronaviruses have also been reported to cause gastroenteritis in children and adults.

Laboratory diagnosis

Virus isolation

Nasopharyngeal aspirate/washings are used for the isolation of virus. Human coronaviruses can be cultured in human foetal tracheal organ culture. Some strains may be isolated more readily in human diploid cells derived from human embryonic lung or intestine.

Detection of virus antigen and antibody

Coronavirus antigens, in nasopharyngeal aspirates and nasal swabs, and antibodies in serum may be detected by ELISA test. Serologic diagnosis of infections with human coronavirus 229E is possible using a passive haemagglutination test in which red cells coated with coronavirus antigen are agglutinated by antibody-containing sera.

Q. 7. Describe pathogenesis, causative agent, laboratory diagnosis and treatment of severe acute respiratory syndrome.

Ans. ***Pathogenesis***

Severe acute respiratory syndrome (SARS) is an **emerging viral infectious disease**. It is an atypical pneumonia characterized by high rate of transmission to healthcare workers. It originated in November 2002 in the Guangdong Province of China and, by February 2003, had spread to Hong Kong and subsequently to 32 other countries or regions.

According to World Health Organization (WHO) a **suspected case** of SARS is defined as documented fever (temperature 38°C), lower respiratory tract symptoms, and contact with a person believed to have had SARS or history of travel to an area of documented transmission during the 10 days prior to onset of symptoms. A **probable case** is a suspected case with chest radiographic findings of pneumonia, acute respiratory distress syndrome (ARDS), or an unexplained respiratory illness resulting in death with autopsy findings of ARDS.

As on July 4, 2003, a total of 8439 probable cases and 812 deaths due to SARS have been reported from 30 countries. The affected areas are Toronto (Canada), Singapore, Beijing, Hong Kong, Guangdong, inner Mongolia, Shanxi, Tianjin, Taiwan Province, and Manila. As on 14th May, 2003, 3 probable cases of SARS have been reported from India, one each from West Bengal, Karnataka and Gujarat.

Causative agent

A newly discovered variant of *Coronavirus* (SARS-CoV) is the causative agent of this syndrome. SARS virus has fulfilled the Koch's postulates. It has been successfully cultivated *in vitro* (in Vero cell line) as well as *in vivo* (experimental infection has been established in monkeys). The genome of SARS virus is 29,727 nucleotides in length and the genome organization is somewhat similar to that of other coronaviruses. SARS virus can survive after drying on plastic surfaces for up to 48 hours. It can survive in faeces for at least 2 days and in urine for up to 24 hours.

The incubation period is usually 2–7 days but may extend up to 10 days. SARS virus appears to spread most commonly by close person-to-person contact involving exposure to infectious droplets, and possibly by direct contact with infected body fluids. Persons having close contact with the cases, especially the healthcare workers and family members, are at higher risk. WHO estimates that case fatality rate ranges from 0–50% depending on the age group affected, with an overall estimate of about 15%.

Laboratory diagnosis

Specimens

The following specimens should be collected from suspected/probable cases of SARS:

1. Acute and convalescent serum for serology.
2. Throat swab in viral transport medium.
3. Nasopharyngeal swab or aspirate in viral transport medium.
4. Stool, fresh or in viral transport medium.

Detection of viral RNA genome

The method of choice is detection of the viral RNA genome in respiratory and stool samples by RT-PCR.

Virus isolation

Virus isolation of SARS-CoV requires stringent biosafety level 3 (BSL-3) conditions. Virus in clinical specimens from SARS patients can be cultured on Vero cells.

Electron microscopy (EM)

EM can be used to detect coronavirus-like particles in stool specimens.

Antibody detection

Serology using enzyme-linked immunosorbent assay can be used to evaluate acute and convalescent sera.

Treatment

As of now, there is no vaccine or specific treatment available for SARS. However, good supportive treatment has been found effective in many cases. Ribavarin and steroids have been shown to be useful in treating critically ill patients. Ribavarin may be given 8 mg/kg every 8 hours intravenously or 1.2 g every 12 hours orally, with an oral loading dose of 4 g for those with normal renal functions. Administer for 7–14 days depending upon the response. Give hydrocortisone 2 mg/kg every six hours or 4 mg/kg every 8 hours intravenously. Tail of over one week when there is clinical improvement. For severe and rapidly deteriorating cases give methyl prednisolone 10 mg/kg every 24 hours intravenously for two days, and then continue with hydrocortisone as above. Antibiotics treatment (coverage for typical and atypical agents for 7–14 days using drugs such as levofloxacin and macrolides) is advocated to prevent superadded infection. Investigation to exclude other causes of pneumonia should be carried out. All suspect or probable cases of SARS must be treated in isolation with barrier nursing, and universal precautions should be taken by the healthcare workers to prevent the further spread of disease.

45

ARBOVIRUSES: TOGAVIRIDAE, FLAVIVIRIDAE AND BUNYAVIRIDAE

Q. 1. Write short note on morphology and classification of family Togaviridae.

Ans. ***Morphology***

Virions of the family Togaviridae are spherical, 50–70 nm in diameter and have an icosahedral capsid surrounded by a lipid envelope containing glycoprotein peplomers. The genome consists of a molecule of single-stranded positive sense RNA 11–12 kb in length.

Classification

The family Togaviridae has two genera – *Alphavirus* (previously group A arboviruses) and *Rubivirus*. The former has 32 species, of which 13 have been shown to cause disease in humans. **They are arthropod-borne (arboviruses), principally by mosquitoes.** Genus *Rubivirus*, which contains rubella virus, **is not arthropod-borne**. It is transmitted both horizontally and vertically between vertebrate hosts, frequently causing congenital malformation after transplacental infection.

Q. 2. Describe pathogenesis and laboratory diagnosis of alphaviruses.

Ans. ***Pathogenesis***

Alphaviruses are transmitted to humans, horses and birds by the bite of bloodsucking mosquitoes. The infected female mosquito introduces its proboscis directly into a capillary beneath the skin and injects saliva containing viruses. Viral multiplication takes place in the vascular endothelium, blood monocytes and macrophages in lymph nodes, bone marrow, spleen and liver followed by viraemia. The disease process may halt here or may progress to involve more organs causing rash, arthritis, hepatitis, nephritis and encephalitis.

Fever is associated with haemorrhagic phase. Skin rash is due to swelling of capillaries, and perivascular oedema and haemorrhages are due to thrombocytopenia. In encephalitis, pathologic features include neuronal necrosis with neuronophagia and intense perivascular and interstitial mononuclear inflammatory infiltration. Vertebrate reservoir, vector mosquitoes, disease produced and geographical distribution of important alphaviruses is given in Table 45.1.

Table 45.1. Human diseases caused by alphaviruses

Virus	Vertebrate reservoir	Vector mosquitoes	Disease	Geographic distribution
Encephalitis group				
Eastern equine encephalitis (EEE)	Wild birds	*Culiseta, Aedes, Culex Coquillettidea*	Encephalitis	North, Central and South America, Caribbean
Western equine encephalitis (WEE)	Wild birds	*Culex*	-do-	North and South America
Venezuelan equine encephalitis (VEE)	Horses	*Aedes, Culex*	-do-	South and Central America
Febrile illness group				
Chikungunya	Monkeys, humans	*Aedes*	Fever, arthralgia myalgia, rash	Africa, India, Southeast Asia
O'nyong-nyong	Humans	*Anopheles*	-do-	Africa
Mayaro	Monkeys	*Haemagogus*	-do-	South and Central America
Ross river	Marsupials, rodents	*Culex, Aedes*	-do-	Australia, Fiji
Sindbis	Wild birds	*Culex, Culiseta, Aedes*	-do-	Africa, Europe, India, Malaysia

Encephalitis viruses

Three members of this group – Eastern, Western and Venezuelan equine encephalitis viruses – cause encephalitis in horses and humans. Vertebrate reservoirs, vector mosquitoes and geographical distribution of these viruses is given in Table 45.1. Formalinised vaccines have been developed for Eastern equine encephalitis and Western equine encephalitis and a live attenuated vaccine for Venezuelan equine encephalitis.

Viruses causing febrile illness

Chikungunya

Chikungunya virus was first isolated from patients and mosquitoes during an epidemic in the Newala district of Tanzania in 1952/53. It first appeared in India in 1963, when along with dengue, it caused very extensive epidemic in Kolkata, Chennai and other areas. The name 'Chikungunya' is derived from the native word for the disease in which the patient lies 'doubled up' due to severe joint pains. In Africa, a sylvatic transmission cycle occurs between wild primates and *Aedes* mosquitoes, while urban chikungunya epidemics in India and Southeast Asia causing hundreds-of-thousands of cases involve *Aedes aegypti* transmission in a human-mosquito-human cycle. It has frequently been isolated from humans and mosquitoes during epidemics in India, Southeast Asia, Southeast Africa and sub-Saharan

Africa. Unlike dengue, which is endemic in many of the Asian cities, chikungunya disappears and reappears at regular intervals. The mechanism of virus maintenance during inter-epidemic periods or re-introduction is unknown.

After an **incubation period of 2–4 days**, patient develops fever, crippling joint pains, chills, flushed face, headache, myalgia, backache, photophobia, rash, anorexia and constipation with recovery in 5–7 days. Clinical picture resembles that of dengue fever, with which it is often confused.

In India and Southeast Asia, this virus has been implicated in outbreaks of haemorrhagic fever, often in association with dengue viruses. However, chikungunya is not a cause of severe haemorrhagic disease. It is transmitted by *Aedes aegypti* and *A. africanus*.

Sindbis

Sindbis virus was isolated from *Culex* mosquitoes in the Sindbis district of Egypt in 1952. It occurs in Africa, India, tropical Asia, Australia and Europe. It causes febrile illnesses. It is maintained in enzootic cycles involving a variety of birds and mosquito species of the genera *Culex*, *Aedes* and *Culiseta*.

O'nyong-nyong virus

This virus was first isolated from Uganda. It is confined to Africa. It is closely related to the chikungunia virus antigenically and causes a similar disease. This is transmitted by *Anopheles* species.

Laboratory diagnosis

Specimens

Blood collected during the acute phase of the disease. CSF is collected in encephalitis cases, but the best specimen for such cases is the brain. For serological diagnosis serum is collected.

Virus isolation

- **Suckling mice:** Specimens are inoculated intracerebrally into suckling mice. The animal develops fatal encephalitis.
- **Tissue culture:** Some viruses may also be isolated in tissue cultures. Vero cells, BHK21 and mosquito cell lines are inoculated with the specimens. Isolates are identified by haemagglutination inhibition, complement fixation, immunofluorescence, ELISA or neutralisation with appropriate antisera.

Serology

- Using an IgM capture ELISA, serotype specific IgM antibody may be detected in the patient serum within 1–3 days after the onset of illness.
- The detection of a four-fold or greater rise of antibody titre by ELISA test on paired sera collected during the initial week and several days later also provides a good evidence of infection.

Q. 3. Describe morphology, pathogenicity, laboratory diagnosis and prohylaxis of rubella virus.

Ans. ***Morphology***

Rubella virus is a pleomorphic, roughly spherical, 50–70 nm in diameter, with a single-stranded RNA genome. It is surrounded by an envelope carrying haemagglutinin peplomers. The virus agglutinates goose, pigeon, one-day-old chick and human erythrocytes at 4°C.

Pathogenicity

Rubella or German measles is primarily a mild childhood fever. It may be acquired congenitally or postnatally. It is not transmitted by arthropods.

A. Postnatal rubella

Rubella virus is excreted in oropharyngeal secretions and infection is acquired by inhalation. Virus multiplies locally in the upper respiratory tract and in the cervical lymph nodes, followed by dissemination throughout the body by the way of the blood stream. After an **incubation period of 2–3 weeks**, patient develops fine, pink, discrete macules of the erythematous rash which first appear on the face, then spread to the trunk and limbs. Fever is usually inconspicuous, but a characteristic feature is that postauricular, suboccipital and posterior cervical lymph nodes are enlarged and tender from very early in the illness.

The illness is of short duration and recovery is usually complete within 3–4 days after appearance of rash. Nearly half of infections in children are asymptomatic but asymptomatic rubella is less common in adults. Mild polyarthritis usually involving hands occurs in about 60% adult women. Complications like thrombocytopenic purpura, postinfectious encephalopathy and rubella panencephalitis though rare are sometimes observed.

B. Congenital rubella

Rubella virus can cross the placental barrier, particularly in early pregnancy, and infect the foetus, where it disseminates and grows in every foetal organ. It may result in a large variety of **congenital abnormalities or death of the foetus**. Congenital abnormalities may include total or partial neurosensory deafness, cataract, glaucoma, microphthalmia or retinopathy leading to blindness, congenital heart disease especially patent ductus arteriosus, sometimes accompanied by septal defects and pulmonary artery stenosis, microcephaly with mental retardation, thrombocytopenic purpura and hepatosplenomegaly. This is known as **congenital rubella syndrome** (CRS).

About 20% of all infants infected in utero during the first trimester of pregnancy are born with severe and usually multiple congenital abnormalities and many of the remainder have milder defects. Severe congenital abnormalities may lead to intrauterine death with abortion or stillbirth. If rubella occurs in the fourth month of pregnancy, the risk reduces to approximately 5% and the only abnormality likely to be seen is neurosensory deafness. If infection occurs after fourth month of pregnancy, congenital abnormalities are very infrequent.

Laboratory diagnosis

Virus isolation

Rubella virus can be isolated from adult throat swab, and from the throat, urine, CSF or leucocytes of a newborn infant with CRS on RK13 (rabbit kidney), SIRC (rabbit cornea) and Vero cells. CPE is inconspicuous, therefore, rubella virus, in cell culture, is detected by **interference** with the CPE of a challenge virus (coxsackievirus A9) and by **immunofluorescence** or **immunoperoxidase staining** for detection of antigen in such cells.

Serology

- Recent infection with rubella virus can be diagnosed by the demonstration of rubella IgM antibody in a single sample of blood by ELISA, radioimmunoassay and haemadsorption inhibition test.
- In case of rubella IgG antibody, four-fold or more rise in titre in paired sera has a diagnostic value. Antibodies of IgM class generally do not persist beyond 4–5 weeks after onset of illness, but IgG antibodies usually persist throughout life.

In a newborn baby, demonstration of rubella IgM antibody is diagnostic of congenital rubella as IgM antibodies do not cross the placenta. However, many babies have rubella IgG antibodies, acquired transplacentally.

Prophylaxis

A live attenuated MMR vaccine is recommended for all infants in the second year of life, followed by a booster at the age of 4–6 years.

Q. 4. Classify viruses belonging to the family Flaviviridae. Name syndromes produced, the vectors transmitting viruses, and geographical distribution, and describe morphology of virions of family Flaviviridae.

Ans. The original group B arboviruses have been assigned the generic name of *Flavivirus* of the family Flaviviridae. Non-arthropod-borne viruses of this family belong to two genera – *Pestivirus* (which contains viruses of veterinary importance but no human pathogen) and *Hepacivirus* (hepatitis C virus). Genus *Flavivirus* possesses more than 70 member viruses of which 13 are capable of causing human disease (Table 45.2). Some are mosquito-borne while others are tick-borne.

Morphology

Virions of the family Flaviviridae are spherical, 40–50 nm in diameter. They possess a molecule of single-stranded, positive sense RNA of 10.5–11 and 9.5 kb in case of *Flavivirus* and hepatitis C virus respectively. Inner viral core is surrounded by a lipid bilayer envelope covered with glycoprotein peplomers and a matrix or membrane protein.

Q. 5. Write short note on yellow fever.

Ans. Yellow fever occurs in tropical Africa and tropical Central and South America and despite the presence of the mosquito *Aedes aegypti* it has not been reported from Asia including India. It is transmitted by mosquito from monkey to man and man to man. Virus infection occurs in two forms. Urban cycle where man is the reservoir and *Aedes aegypti* is the vector. The second form, forest or sylvatic cycle, involves monkeys and forest-dwelling mosquitoes, e.g., *Haemagogus* and *Sabethes* in South America and *Aedes africanus* in East Africa.

Liver is the major target organ with virus replicating in Kupffer cells and massive necrosis of hepatocytes leading to jaundice and decreased formation of prothrombin. After an **incubation period of 3–6 days**, patient develops fever of acute onset with chills, headache, backache, myalgia and vomiting. Some patients develop severe jaundice, haematemesis and melaena. The pulse rate is slow despite the high fever and the blood pressure falls, resulting in albuminuria, oliguria and anuria. Death occurs in 20–50% cases of severe form of the disease within 6–7 days of onset.

Table 45.2. Clinical syndromes caused by flaviviruses

Syndrome	Vector	Virus	Geographical distribution
Encephalitis	Mosquito	Japanese encephalitis Murray Valley encephalitis St. Louis encephalitis Rocio encephalitis	Asia Australia, New Guinea Americas Brazil
	Tick	Louping-ill Powassan Tick-borne encephalitis	British Isles Canada, United States, Russia Russia, Eastern Europe, Scandinavia
Yellow fever	Mosquito	Yellow fever	Tropical Africa and tropical Central and South America
Dengue	Mosquito	Dengue 1, 2, 3, 4	Entire tropical zone
Haemorrhagic fever	Mosquito	Dengue 1, 2, 3, 4	India, the Philippines
	Tick	Kyasanur Forest disease Omsk haemorrhagic fever	Southwest India Siberia
Miscellaneous tropical fevers	Mosquito	Ilheus West Nile	Caribbean, South America Africa, Central Asia, India, Mediterranean area

Q. 6. Write short note on dengue.

Ans. Dengue virus has four serotypes – dengue-1, dengue-2, dengue-3 and dengue-4, all of which are endemic throughout the tropics, particularly in Asia, the Caribbean, the Pacific and some areas of West Africa. During 1996, there was a large outbreak of dengue and dengue haemorrhagic fever reported from Delhi when 10,252 cases and 453 deaths were reported to the state directorate.

Considerable cross-reactivity is observed among the different serotypes and recovery from an infection by one type does not provide complete immunity against infection by other types. Thus, individuals can have as many as 4 dengue infections in their life, one with each serotype. The virus is transmitted from person to person by several species of mosquitoes of the genus *Aedes* principally *A. aegypti*. Humans and the *Aedes* mosquito are recognized reservoir and vector respectively, however, as in yellow fever, monkey may also serve as a major reservoir.

Clinical features

Dengue may occur in two forms – classic dengue and dengue in more serious forms, with haemorrhagic manifestations.

Classic dengue

Classic dengue usually affects older children and adults. After an **incubation period of 5–8 days**, patient develops fever of sudden onset and often biphasic (saddle back) with severe headache, chills, retrobulbar pain, conjunctivitis and severe pain in the back, muscles and joints ('*breakbone fever*'). A **maculopapular rash** generally appears on the trunk in 3–5 days of illness and spreads later to the face and extremities. Petechiae may sometimes be seen on the dorsum of the feet, legs, hands, axillae and palate. **The disease lasts for about 10 days** after which recovery is generally complete.

More serious forms of dengue

Dengue may also occur in more serious forms, with haemorrhagic manifestations. These are known as **dengue haemorrhagic fever** (DHF) and **dengue shock syndrome** (DSS). DHF/DSS appears to result from *antibody-dependent enhancement of dengue virus infection*. When a patient having antibodies against a particular serotype of dengue virus (provided by an earlier encounter with that serotype or by transmission of maternal antibodies) develops infection with another serotype, these antibodies are not sufficient to neutralize newly acquired virus but bind to the same and opsonize it. It is more avidly taken up, via Fc receptors, by monocyte/macrophage in which it replicates best. Thus antibody promotes the efficient binding and entry of virus into the cell, thus accelerating the process.

DHF/DSS occurs primarily in two age ranges namely 6–9 months, who are born to dengue immune mothers, and 5–10 years, who are immune to one of the dengue virus serotypes and are undergoing an infection by a second serotype.

Q. 7. Write short note on Japanese encephalitis.

Ans. Japanese encephalitis (JE) virus was first isolated from the brain of a fatal case of encephalitis in Tokyo, Japan. It has emerged as a disease of major public health importance in India since 1970.

Pathogenesis

The mosquito, *Culex tritaeniorhynchus*, breeding in irrigated rice fields is the main vector. It transmits the virus to man from water birds and pigs, which act as amplifying hosts. Infection in man is the dead end of the transmission. Man to man transmission has not been documented.

Clinical features

Incubation period varies from 5–15 days. The disease has an abrupt onset with fever, headache and vomiting. After 1–6 days, signs of encephalitis set in with neck rigidity, convulsions, altered sensorium and coma. Residual neurological damage may persist in up to 50% of survivors.

Prophylaxis

Preventive measures include mosquito control and locating piggeries away from human dwellings. Inactivated vaccines prepared in mice and hamster kidney cell cultures, and a live attenuated vaccine are available.

Q. 8. Write short note on Kyasanur Forest disease.

Ans. Kyasanur Forest disease (KFD) is an Indian haemorrhagic disease. It appeared in Kyasanur Forest in Shimoga district in Karnataka, India in 1957 as a fatal epizootic affecting wild monkeys, along with a severe prostrating illness in some of the villagers in the area. The causative virus was isolated, from the patients and dead monkeys, in National Institute of Virology, Pune. It is antigenically related to TBE virus.

Pathogenesis

Forest birds and small mammals are believed to be the reservoirs of the virus. It is transmitted by the bite of tick (*Haemaphysalis spinigera*). As infection in monkeys leads to fatal disease, therefore, they are unlikely to be the reservoirs, but only amplifier hosts. However, ticks may act as the reservoir to some extent as transovarial transmission of the virus has been demonstrated in them.

Clinical features

After an incubation period of 3–7 days, patient develops fever of sudden onset with headache, vomiting, myalgia, conjunctivitis and severe prostration. Massive haemorrhage in alimentary canal, chest cavity and epistaxis may occur in some cases. Case fatality is about 10%. An inactivated vaccine is available.

Q. 9. Describe laboratory diagnosis of infections caused by flaviviruses.

Ans. *Virus isolation*

Virus can be isolated by intracerebral inoculation of newborn mice and by inoculation of cultured mosquito or vertebrate cells, from blood collected as early as possible during the course of dengue and yellow fever, from the brain in case of encephalitis, the liver in yellow fever, and from the vectors. The viral isolates can be identified by immunofluorescence of the cultured cells, haemagglutination inhibition and neutralization tests.

Serology

In primary dengue infection, circulating IgM antibody to the viral coat proteins is detected 5–6 days after the onset of illness, and gradually decreases within 1–2 months of onset. IgG antibody to dengue virus is detected approximately 14 days after onset in primary infection. In secondary infection, IgM antibody may reappear but gradually diminishes, while IgG antibody persists, often at high titre. These patterns of dengue antibody development permit serological differentiation of primary and secondary infections. Patients with secondary infection generally have higher IgG levels. Acute or recent infections are identified by a rise in antibody titre as well as high IgM levels. ELISA is used for detection of both IgG and IgM antibodies. There is substantial cross-reactivity among flaviviruses, due to the presence of common antigenic determinants. The four dengue serotypes cross-react among themselves, but there are also unique determinants for each serotype.

Q. 10. Describe general characters, morphology, pathogenicity, clinical syndromes and laboratory diagnosis of family Bunyaviridae.

Ans. ***General characters***

Family Bunyaviridae has more than 300 members. Most of them are arthropod-borne. Many of the virus species are transmitted transovarially by an arthropod vector. Bunyaviruses infecting vertebrates belong to four genera – *Bunyavirus*, *Phlebovirus*, *Nairovirus* and *Hantavirus*. They have at least 160, 50, 30 and 6 viruses respectively. Bunyaviruses are transmitted predominantly by mosquitoes, nairoviruses by ticks and phleboviruses by sandflies, gnats or ticks. The genus *Hantavirus* has non-arthropod-borne viruses. They are maintained in nature by chronically infected rodents, especially of the family Muridae, and are thought to be transmitted most commonly among rodents by bite and aerosol, and to humans by aerosol.

Morphology

The virions of the family Bunyaviridae are 90–120 nm in diameter. They possess a lipid envelope with glycoprotein peplomers enclosing three circular nucleocapsids of helical symmetry. The genome consists of three linear segments of ssRNA, designated large (L), medium (M) and small (S), of approximately 7, 4 and 1–2 kb respectively. They replicate in the cytoplasm.

Pathogenicity

The geographical distribution, vectors, reservoir hosts and human diseases caused by various members of the family Bunyaviridae is given in Table 45.3. Hantaviruses are not arboviruses. They are transmitted to humans from rodent hosts by inhalation of aerosolized rodent urine or by direct contact with rodent excreta or contaminated fomites.

Most of the Bunyaviridae are arboviruses and possess many of the same pathogenic mechanisms as the togaviruses and flaviviruses. The viruses are spread by an arthropod vector and are injected into the blood to initiate a viraemia. Dissemination of the virus can deliver the virus to target sites typically involved in that particular viral disease, such as central nervous system, liver, kidney, and vascular endothelium. As mentioned above, genus *Hantavirus* has non-arthropod-borne viruses.

Many Bunyaviridae cause encephalitis. Some of these may cause hepatic necrosis (Rift Valley fever), leakage of plasma and erythrocytes through the vascular endothelium (Crimean-Congo haemorrhagic fever, and Hantaan haemorrhagic disease). In the latter infection, these changes are most prominent in the kidney and are accomplished by haemorrhagic necrosis of the kidney.

Clinical syndromes

Mosquito-borne bunyaviruses usually cause a nonspecific febrile flu-like illness. The incubation period of these illnesses is approximately 48 hours, and the fever typically lasts 3 days. Most patients have mild illness.

- **Encephalitic illnesses** (e.g., La Cross virus) are sudden in onset after an incubation period of approximately 1 week. Patient develops fever, headache, lethargy, and vomiting. Seizures occur in 50% of patients with encephalitis. Signs of meningitis may also be present. The illness lasts for 10–14 days.
- **Haemorrhagic fevers**, such as Rift Valley fever, are characterized by petechial haemorrhages, ecchymosis, epitaxis, haemtemesis, malena, and bleeding of the gums. Death occurs in as many as half of the patients with haemorrhagic disease.

Table 45.3. Virions of family Bunyaviridae causing disease in humans

Genus	Virus	Geographical distribution	Vector	Reservoir host	Human disease
Bunyavirus	La Crosse	USA	Mosquito	Chipmunk, squirrel	Encephalitis
	Oropouche	Caribbean, South America	Mosquito	Sloths, monkeys	Fever, arthralgia, myalgia
Phlebovirus	Rift Valley fever	Northern, Eastern and Southern Africa	Mosquito	Sheep, cattle, buffalo, goats	Fever, myalgia, retinitis, haemorrhagic fever
	Sandfly fever	European and North African countries surrounding the Mediterranean Sea, extending eastward through Israel and Iran to West Pakistan, Central India	Sandfly	Man	Dengue-like fever, myalgia, conjunctivitis
Nairovirus	Crimean-Congo haemorrhagic fever	Asia, Eastern Europe, Central and Southern Africa	Tick	Sheep, cattle, goats	Haemorrhagic fever
Hantavirus	Hantaan	Japan, Korea, China, Russia	Nil	Rodents	Haemorrhagic fever, nephro-pathy
	Belgrade	Balkans	Nil	Rodents	Haemorrhagic fever, nephro-pathy
	Seoul	Worldwide	Nil	Rats	Nephropathy, sometimes haemorrhagic fever
	Puumala	Scandinavia	Nil	Rodents and humans	Nephropathy
	Muerto Canyon	USA	Nil	Rodents	Fever, myalgia, respiratory failure

Laboratory diagnosis

1. Virus isolation

- By intracerebral inoculation of suckling mice.
- By inoculation of cultured cells like Vero-E6 or BHK-21 or *Aedes* mosquito cell line. Growth of virus in cell culture can be detected by immunofluorescence.

2. Polymerase chain reaction (PCR)

Detection of viral RNA by reverse transcriptase polymerase chain reaction (RT-PCR) has become the accepted method for detecting and identifying bunyaviruses.

3. Serology

- **Detection of antibody:** IgM antibody and rising titre of antibody can be detected by ELISA, neutralization, complement fixation and immunofluorescence tests.
- **Detection of antigen:** ELISA may detect antigen in clinical specimens from patients with an intense viraemia (e.g., Rift Valley fever, haemorrhagic fever with renal syndrome, Crimean-Congo haemorrhagic fever) or from mosquitoes.

46

FILOVIRUSES, ARENAVIRUSES AND REOVIRIDAE

Q. 1. Describe morphology, cultivation, pathogenicity, clinical features and laboratory diagnosis of filoviruses.

Ans. ***Morphology***

The members of the family Filoviridae (filoviruses) are long filamentous (*filo:* filament or thread), enveloped, single-stranded, negative sense RNA virions. They are 80 nm in diameter and 800–1000 nm in length. Particles as long as 14,000 nm in length have also been reported. The envelope is composed of lipid bilayer covered with peplomers. It surrounds a helically wound tubular nucleocapsid. The RNA of the virion is 19 kb in size.

Cultivation

Virus can be cultured in Vero cells and in many other cell types. Virus multiplies in the cytoplasm forming large inclusion bodies. Progeny virions are released from the plasma membrane by budding.

Pathogenicity

Filoviruses (Marburg and Ebola viruses) are highly virulent with infections usually ending in death. They are transmitted to man from primates by aerosol route and by direct contact with blood, organs or tissue cultures. However, secondary spread between humans occurs by:

- Contact with body fluids from an acute case.
- The use of contaminated injection equipment.
- Aerosols.
- Sexual intercourse.

The liver is the major site of infection, although the virus can infect most tissues in the body.

Clinical features

After an **incubation period of 3–15 days**, patient develops headache, high fever, conjunctivitis, bradycardia, myalgia, abdominal pain, vomiting, diarrhoea, proteinuria, severe haemorrhages (haematemesis, melaena or passage of fresh blood in stools, bleeding from nose, gums and vagina, and subconjunctival haemorrhages) and profound hypotension. The mortality rates of the outbreaks of Marburg, Ebola-S and Ebola-Z viruses were found to be 25%, 60% and 90% respectively. The cases arising out of man to man transfer do not have such a high mortality. The cause of death is shock due to fluid or blood loss into the tissues. Bleeding is due to abnormal platelet function.

Laboratory diagnosis

Electron microscopy

Filamentous viruses can be seen in the blood and in the cytoplasm of the affected cells particularly of liver, lungs and kidneys by electron microscopy. A large number of virions can be seen in the damaged hepatocytes and in the bile canaliculi.

Virus isolation

Virus can be isolated from the blood during the febrile phase, by inoculation of Vero cells. The viral isolate is identified by electron microscopy and direct immunofluorescence. However, *filoviruses are classified as Biosafety Level 4 pathogens*, therefore, virus culture must only be attempted in maximum security laboratories.

Polymerase chain reaction

A recently described reverse transcriptase polymerase chain reaction (RT-PCR) test amplifying a conserved region of the *L* gene has proved to be the most sensitive and specific method for rapid diagnosis.

Immunofluorescence

Antibodies in the patient serum can be detected by indirect immunofluorescence, 7–10 days after the onset of the disease.

Serology

ELISA techniques are available for detection of either viral antigen or specific IgM.

Q. 2. Describe morphology, pathogenicity and laboratory diagnosis of arenaviruses.

Ans. ***Morphology***

The family Arenaviridae derives its name from the sand-sprinkled appearance when viewed in the electron microscope (*arena:* sand). This is due to the incorporation within virions of the ribosomes of the host cell during assembly. The virions are pleomorphic, 110–130 nm in diameter. They possess host plasma membrane-derived envelope into which are embedded glycoprotein peplomers. The envelope encloses two circular nucleocapsid segments. The genome consists of ssRNA of negative sense. It exists as two molecules, large (L) and small (S) of 7.2 kb and 3.4 kb respectively.

Pathogenicity

Family Arenaviridae has only one genus *Arenavirus*. Arenaviruses causing human disease are given in Table 46.1.

Arenaviruses have rodents as their natural hosts, in which they cause persistent infection with chronic viraemia and virus shedding in urine which contaminates their environment and then spread to humans by contact through abraded skin and by aerosol.

Table 46.1. Vertebrate hosts and geographic distribution of arenaviruses pathogenic to man

Virus	Geographic distribution	Vertebrate host	Human disease
Lymphocytic choriomeningitis	Worldwide	*Mus musculus*	Influenza-like illness, aseptic meningitis and rarely severe encephalomyelitis
Lassa	West Africa	*Mastomys natalensis*	Haemorrhagic fever
Junin	Argentina	*Calomys laucha*, *Calomys musculinus* and *Akadon azarae*	Argentine haemorrhagic fever
Machupo	Bolivia	*Calomys callosus*	Bolivian haemorrhagic fever
Guanarito	Venezuela	*Sigmodon* spp.	Venezuelan haemorrhagic fever

Lymphocytic choriomeningitis (LCM)

Human infection with LCM virus is often inapparent but may present as:

- An influenza-like illness characterized by fever, malaise, coryza, myalgia and bronchitis.
- Less often as aseptic meningitis.
- Rarely as severe encephalomyelitis.

Incubation period varies from 1–2 weeks. Man acquires infection probably from the excreta of rodents.

Lassa fever

Lassa fever was first noticed in 1969 in an American Mission station in Lassa, Nigeria. Rodent excreta probably act as the source of infection. Man to man transmission may also occur by droplet infection. After an **incubation period of 3–16 days**, patient develops high fever of insidious onset, headache, muscle and joint pain, abdominal and retrosternal pain, pharyngitis, conjunctivitis, dysphagia, diarrhoea, vomiting, oedema of the face and neck, lymphadenopathy, and bleeding from nose, gums, intestines and vagina. It is due to platelet dysfunction. Lymphocyte and platelet counts fall. Mortality rate varies from 27–44%. Death is due to hypotension, peripheral vasoconstriction, anuria and cardiac arrest.

South American Arenavirus haemorrhagic fevers

Three South American *Arenavirus* haemorrhagic fevers viz. Argentine, Bolivian and Venezuelan haemorrhagic fevers are caused by Junin, Machupo and Guanarito viruses respectively. After an **incubation period of 1–2 weeks**, patient develops 'flulike' prodromal illness. Serious cases develop petechiae, haemorrhages from gastrointestinal tract, thrombocytopenia, leucopenia, hypotension and oliguria. Mortality rate varies from 5–30%. Death is due to hypovolemic shock.

Laboratory diagnosis

Virus isolation

For the laboratory diagnosis of infections caused by arenaviruses, Biosafety Level 4 containment is required. However, in case of LCM virus level 3 suffices. Arenaviruses can be isolated from blood, CSF, throat washings, pleural fluid, urine and autopsy specimen by inoculation of suckling mice, hamsters and guinea-pigs. They can also be isolated by inoculation of Vero E6 and BHK-21 cells. The growth is obtained in 2–3 days and the virus isolate can be identified by indirect immunofluorescence.

Genome detection

Genome detection is by RT-PCR amplification, with or without confirmation by DNA hybridization. RT-PCR is highly sensitive and specific, and is particularly valuable for early diagnosis.

Antigen detection

Antigen detection from blood by immunofluorescence assay (IFA) or ELISA is useful for early diagnosis and prognosis. Early IFA positivity is correlated with risk of death.

Antibody detection

For antibody detection, ELISA is the most useful test and can be adapted to detect a specific IgM response.

Q. 3. Write short note on classification and morphology of Reoviridae.

Ans. Family Reoviridae contains nine genera of which *Coltivirus*, *Orbivirus*, *Orthoreovirus* and *Rotavirus* contain human pathogens. They are nonenveloped spherical virions possessing an inner core surrounded by two concentric icosahedral capsids. *Rotavirus* is 70 nm in diameter, and *Orthoreovirus* and *Coltivirus* are 80 nm in diameter. The genome of these viruses possess 11, 10 and 12 segments of dsRNA respectively.

Q. 4. Write short note on coltiviruses.

Ans. These viruses possess a genome of 12 segments of dsRNA. They can be isolated from ticks, mosquitoes, rodents and humans. Coltiviruses cause Colorado tick fever. It is endemic in the Rocky Mountain region of the USA and Canada. In insect vector (ticks of many species) Colorado tick fever virus (CTFV) infects the midgut from which it spreads to other organs including salivary glands. Infection is transmitted to the rodents and occasionally man by the bite of the infected ticks. As rodents have prolonged CTF viraemia they seem to be the main reservoir for tick infection in nature.

After an incubation period of 3–6 days, humans develop fever, headache, retrobulbar pain, myalgia, leucopenia and rash. More serious forms of the disease, notably meningo-encephalitis and haemorrhagic fever, occur in 5% cases mainly in children. Rarely, it may cause haemorrhagic form of the disease (purpura, epistaxis and gastrointestinal bleeding).

Virus can be isolated from red blood cells in continuous cell lines (Vero, BHK-21), or detected inside red blood cells by immunofluorescence. It seems that the virus multiplies in erythrocyte precursors in bone marrow, then persists in the mature red cells throughout its life-span, protected from antibody.

Q. 5. Write short note on orbiviruses.

Ans. The genus *Orbivirus* consists of 19 species and at least 130 subspecies. These viruses possess a genome of 10 segments of dsRNA. They commonly infect insects, and many are transmitted by insects to vertebrates. None of these viruses causes serious clinical disease in humans, but they may cause mild fevers. Serious animal pathogens include bluetongue virus (BTV) of sheep and African horse sickness virus (AHSV). Antibodies to orbiviruses are found in many vertebrates, including humans.

Q. 6. Write short note on orthoreoviruses.

Ans. The *Orthoreovirus* (reovirus) genome consists of 10 segments of dsRNA. These viruses are found worldwide in a wide range of vertebrates (mammals, including humans and birds). There are three distinct but related types of reovirus. It has been suggested that there is an association of reovirus infections with enteritis in infants and children, upper respiratory tract infections and possibly neonatal biliary atresia. By 3 years of age, more than 70% of children have antibodies against all 3 types of reoviruses. These viruses replicate well in many types of cell culture. CPE is slow to develop and not particularly striking, however, on staining, characteristic crescentic perinuclear acidophilic inclusions are seen in the cytoplasm.

Q. 7. Describe morphology, pathogenicity and laboratory diagnosis of rotaviruses.

Ans. ***Morphology***

Rotavirus (*rota*, meaning wheel) has two concentric icosahedral shells, resembling a wheel with short spokes radiating from a wide hub to a clearly defined outer rim. The genome consists of double-stranded segmented RNA. The complete or double-shelled virus measures 70 nm in diameter and has a smooth surface. The incomplete or single-shelled virus is smaller, about 60 nm, with a rough surface. It is a rotavirus that has lost the outer shell. Empty particles without RNA core are also seen.

Pathogenicity

Rotaviruses are classified as members of family Reoviridae genus *Rotavirus*. These were discovered as the cause of infantile human gastroenteritis in 1973, although they were then already well-known as the cause of acute gastroenteritis in young animals. Since their discovery, human rotaviruses have been found to be the main aetiological agents of gastroenteritis in infants and young children worldwide. Mature rotavirus particles are about 70 nm in diameter and are nonenveloped. They are classified into seven serogroups, (A–G). Groups A to C rotaviruses infect both humans and animals, with the group A rotaviruses infecting humans most frequently and causing disease mainly in children. Group D to G rotaviruses are mainly animal pathogens. Other viruses that produce diarrhoea in children and adults include enteric adenoviruses, Norwalk virus, caliciviruses and astroviruses.

Rotaviruses are excreted in large numbers in the faeces and infection occurs by ingestion. Since the virus is resistant to chlorination, water-borne epidemics involving adults also occur.

Rotaviruses infect epithelial cells at the tips of the villi of small intestine. As a result of infection, the cells are destroyed and virus is released in large numbers in the intestinal lumen which may involve the entire length of small intestine and sometimes colon. Cellular damage leads to malabsorption resulting in fluid accumulation in the lumen of the gut, vomiting and diarrhoea which may lead to severe dehydration. **Incubation period is 1–2 days and illness lasts for 4–5 days.**

Laboratory diagnosis

Rotavirus particles in the faeces can be detected by:

- Latex agglutination test, using latex particles coated with rotavirus-specific antibody.
- Reverse passive haemagglutination.
- ELISA.
- Electron microscopy.
- Immunoelectron microscopy.

A concentration of 10^7 or more particles per ml is necessary for the virus to be seen in faeces by electron microscopy. The sensitivity of electron microscopy can be increased by mixing specific antibody with the faeces to aggregate the virus particles. These aggregates can be sedimented by centrifugation, negatively stained and observed under electron microscope.

Human Immunodeficiency Virus: AIDS

Q. 1. Describe morphology, viral genes and antigens, antigenic variation, resistance and modes of transmission of human immunodeficiency viruses.

Ans. Morphology

Human immunodeficiency viruses are enveloped positive-stranded RNA viruses. Mature viral particles measure 80–120 nm in diameter and have a conical core. The core contains two identical copies of single-stranded RNA, 9.2 kb each associated with reverse transcriptase, which are surrounded by structural proteins that form nucleo-capsid, matrix protein shell and host cell membrane derived lipid bilayer envelope from which project 72 glycoprotein peplomers (Fig. 47.1).

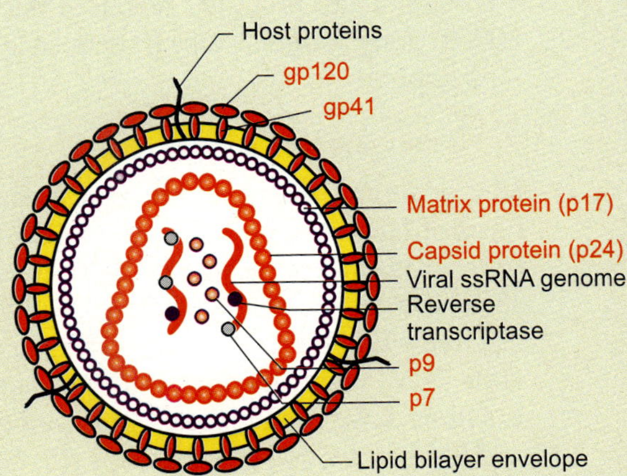

Fig. 47.1. Schematic representation of a mature HIV virion showing the localization of viral proteins.

Viral genes and antigens

The genome of HIV contains three structural genes (*gag*, *env* and *pol*) characteristic of all retroviruses, as well as other non-structural and regulatory genes specific to the virus. The products of these genes, both structural and non-structural, act as antigens. The sera of infected persons contain antibodies to them. Detection of these antigens and antibodies is useful in the diagnosis and prognosis of HIV infection.

Gene coding for structural proteins

1. The *gag* (group-specific antigen) gene encodes a precursor protein p55. It is cleaved into three proteins – p24 (core and capid protein), p15 and p17 (matrix protein).

2. The *env* gene determines the synthesis of envelop glycoprotein (gp160) which is cleaved into the two envelope components – gp120 which forms the suface spike and gp41 which is the transmembrane anchoring protein.
3. The *pol* gene encodes polymerase reverse transcriptase and other viral enzymes, such as protease and endonuclease. It is expressed as precursor protein which is cleaved into proteins p31, p51 and p66.

The proteins (p) and glycoproteins (gp) are indicated by their molecular weight expressed in kilodaltons.

Non-structural and regulatory genes

Structural genes are present in all retroviruses while non-structural and regulatory genes are specific to HIV only.

- *tat* (transactivating gene) enhances the expression of all viral genes.
- *nef* (negative factor gene) down-regulates viral replication.
- *rev* (regulator of virus gene) enhances the expression of structural proteins.
- *vif* (viral infectivity factor gene) influences the infectivity of viral particles.
- *vpu* (only in HIV-1) and *vpx* (only in HIV-2) enhance maturation and release of progeny virus from cells.
- *vpr* stimulates promoter region of the virus.
- LTR (long terminal repeat) sequences, one at either end, give promoter, enhancer and integration signals.

Antigenic variation

HIV undergoes frequent antigenic variation of core and envelop antigens. Two antigenic types of HIV have been identified. HIV-1 represents the original LAV/HTLV-3. HIV-2 was isolated from West Africa in 1986. It causes similar spectrum of disease. It displays only about 40% nucleotide sequence similarity (homology) with HIV-1, therefore, it is only weakly reactive with HIV-1 antiserum. HIV-2 is more closely related to simian immunodeficiency virus (SIV) with which it has 75% homology. It is largely confined to West Africa, though isolations have been reported from some other areas, including western and southern India.

HIV-1 is divided into 3 groups (M, N and O). Group M (major) is responsible for global epidemic. Group O (outlier) is less common. It is mostly confined to West Africa. Group N (non-M, non-O) represents a few strains of HIV-1 isolated from Cameroon. Group M has been further divided into nine subtypes, or clades, designated A, B, C, D, F, G, H, J and K. Subtype A is most prevalent, being worldwide, while B is the most common in the Americas and Europe. **Subtype C is most prevalent in India and China.** The common subtypes in Africa are A, C and D. In Asia, the common subtypes are B, C and E. HIV-2 is divided into six subtypes (A–F)

Resistance

HIV is a delicate virus. It is thermolabile, being inactivated at 56°C in 30 minutes and in seconds at 100°C. At room temperature in dried blood, it may survive for up to seven days. It withstands lyophilisation. It is susceptible to common disinfectants. It can be inactivated in 10 minutes at room temperature by treatment with 35% isopropyl alcohol,

70% ethyl alcohol, 1% lysol, 5% formaldehyde, 2% glutaraldehyde, 3% hydrogen peroxide, 0.5% household bleach, 0.5% sodium hypochlorite and 2.5% Tween-20. Because of its lipid membrane envelope, it is highly susceptible to detergents, therefore, standard washing with detergents and hot water are adequate for decontaminating clothes and household utensils. For treatment of contaminated medical instruments, 2% solution of glutaraldehyde is useful.

Modes of transmission of the virus

There are three modes of transmission of HIV –**sexual**, **parenteral** and **perinatal**. Of these, unprotected, penetrative sexual mode of transmission is the most important. AIDS in 80% of the patients is due to sexual mode of transmission and in 10% each, it is due to parenteral and perinatal mode of transmission. During sexual intercourse virus gets transmitted from man to man, man to woman and woman to man. The risk of transmission is higher to the passive (receptive) partner and higher following anal intercourse (1% per episode) than vaginal intercourse (0.1% per episode) because mucosal tears are very frequent during anal intercourse and virus-laden lymphocytes in the semen can directly enter through these tears. It has been observed that 75% of HIV infections in India are occurring through heterosexual contact.

Presence of other sexually transmitted diseases (STD) facilitates the acquisition and transmission of HIV infection. There is 10-fold increased risk for HIV transmission in patients with genital ulcers caused by syphilis, chancroid and herpes. The risk of transmission of HIV in patients with genital discharge caused by gonorrhoea, chlamydial infection, trichomoniasis and vaginosis is 4-fold. Thus early diagnosis and effective treatment of STD can contribute significantly to the control of HIV infection. There is mounting evidence that some STD pathogens are more virulent in the presence of HIV related immunodeficiency. Risk of acquisition of HIV infection is also greatly enhanced if the sexual partners are more than one.

Parenteral transmission may occur through blood transfusion. Therefore, each unit of blood should be tested for AIDS and if found positive, it should be incinerated. Transmission of HIV has been recorded in a few recipients of blood transfusion even when the blood transfused was found negative for HIV antibodies. This occurs when blood is collected in the '**window period**', i.e., the interval between the time of exposure to the virus and development of detectable levels of antibodies. This period varies from 1–3 months. Therefore, screening of blood is not 100% safe (How safe is safe?).

Infection can also be transmitted by blood products like plasma, serum and cells from HIV-positive individuals and AIDS cases. It can also be transmitted from the donors of bone marrow, semen and organs like cornea, kidney, heart, etc. Therefore, donors of various fluids and organs should be screened for AIDS before they donate them. AIDS can also be transmitted by sharing blood contaminated syringes. Therefore, HIV is more common in intravenous drug users who share syringes and needles. HIV can also be transmitted by the use of unsterile syringes and needles, needle-stick injury and through the barber's razor.

The third mode of transmission of infection is **perinatal, i.e., vertical transmission** from mother to the baby. Infection may be transmitted across the placenta before birth. Some of those who do not develop this infection before birth may develop it from the genital secretions during birth and from mother's milk after birth. In the absence of therapeutic intervention, the risk of mother-to-child transmission ranges from 15–30% and is further increased in the setting of breast-feeding. However, the risk can be significantly reduced to below 2% if antiretroviral therapy is administered to women during pregnancy and labour. Antiretroviral treatment of the mother and infant after birth can also significantly decrease the risk of HIV-1 infection in newborn. Table 47.1 shows the efficiency of different routes of transmission of HIV.

Table 47.1. Efficiency of different routes of transmission of HIV

Route	Efficiency
Blood transfusion	> 90%
Perinatal	13–40%
Sexual intercourse	
• Anal intercourse	1% per episode
• Vaginal intercourse	0.1% per episode
Intravenous drug use	0.5–1%

Q. 2. Describe replication, pathogenicity and clinical features of human immunodeficiency viruses.

Ans. **Replication of HIV**

HIV attaches via its gp120 envelope glycoprotein (surface spike) to the CD4 antigen complex which is the primary HIV receptor on CD4+ (helper/inducer) T lymphocytes and cells of the macrophage lineage. The CD4 molecule has binding avidity for gp120 of HIV. Then by pinocytosis, the nucleocapsid of the virion enters into host cell. The envelope of the same does not enter into the cell. After entry into the cell, the nucleocapsid releases its RNA into the cytoplasm. The viral reverse transcriptase, acting as an RNA-dependent DNA-polymerase, makes a DNA copy of the genomic RNA. The ssDNA is made double-stranded by the same enzyme, now acting as a DNA-dependent DNA-polymerase.

This dsDNA moves to the nucleus, and several such molecules become integrated as provirus at random sites in the host cell chromosome causing a latent infection. The integrated provirus is transcribed by cellular RNA polymerase II either for the production of mRNAs which are translated into proteins or for the production of genomic RNA for insertion into progeny virions (Fig. 50.5).

HIV establishes a latent infection with or without an initial productive phase. In this state, the integrated proviral DNA remains silent without transcription or expression of most viral proteins. Certain factors, however, can activate the virus and convert the latent state into productive HIV infection. During viral replication, naked virus buds from the surface of the infected cell and acquires a lipoprotein envelope which contains lipid derived from the host cell membrane and glycoproteins which are virus-coded.

Pathogenicity

AIDS is a unique sexually transmitted disease without local genital manifestations at any time during infection but with grave systemic manifestations. The first cells to become infected may be resident tissue macrophages or submucosal lymphocytes in the genital tract or rectum. The virus is then transported to the draining lymph nodes, where it replicates extensively.

Two or three weeks after infection, most patients develop viraemia, fall in CD4+ T lymphocytes and **glandular fever-like illness**. Since HIV infects cells expressing CD4 antigen, therefore, in the circulation the virus is found in CD4+ T lymphocytes and also in monocyte-macrophage cells, which may act as a reservoir for virus. Macrophages are also important in carrying the virus into the central nervous system across the blood-brain barrier.

Virus is also present in the plasma. It is probably derived from the lysis of activated lymphocytes. Within one month or so, viraemia declines to a near undetectable level and illness subsides. This is brought about by CD8+ cytotoxic T lymphocytes, natural killer (NK) cells and antibody-dependent cell-mediated cytotoxicity (ADCC).

This is followed by a **long asymptomatic period** of 1–15 years (average 10 years). During this period, only a small number of circulating CD4+ cells are producing virus and only low titres of virus are present in the blood. However, many infected cells can be detected in the lymph nodes. Follicular hyperplasia develops in these and other lymphoid organs. When CD4+ T cell count falls below 400/μl, a large number of virions spill over from the degenerating lymph nodes into the blood and opportunistic infections with various microorganisms may develop. Cause of death is the opportunistic infections, malignancy and cachexia-like state. Fall in CD4+ T cell count is due to:

1. Viral cytolysis of CD4+ T cells.
2. Infected CD4+ T cells can fuse, via gp120, with up to 100 uninfected CD4+ T cells forming a unit called syncytium. This will lead to the death of the entire unit.
3. Immune cytolysis of infected T cells by cytotoxic T cells, NK cells, ADCC and antibody/complement-mediated lysis.
4. HIV may also infect stem cells, so that there is no replacement.
5. AIDS may be an autoimmune disease, causing autoimmune destruction of infected CD4+ T cells.

Table 47.2. Classification of HIV infection and AIDS (Centers for Disease Control, USA)

Group I	Acute HIV infection or HIV seroconversion illness
Group II	Asymptomatic infection
Group III	Persistent generalized lymphadenopathy
Group IV	Symptomatic HIV infection
A	Constitutional disease
B	Neurological disease
C	Secondary infectious disease
C1	Specified infectious diseases listed in the CDC surveillance definition for AIDS, such as *Pneumocystis jirovecii* pneumonia, cryptosporidiosis, toxoplasmosis, generalized strongyloidiasis, cryptococcosis, CMV or herpes diseases
C2	Other specified secondary diseases, such as oral hairy leukoplakia, *Salmonella* bacteremia, nocardiosis, tuberculosis, thrush
D	Secondary cancers, such as Kaposi's sarcoma, lymphomas
E	Other conditions

Clinical features

The Centers for Disease Control in Atlanta, USA have classified the clinical course of HIV infection under various groups (Table 47.2).

I. Acute HIV infection

Two to six weeks after infection, most patients develop acute-onset fever with or without night-sweats, malaise, headache, myalgia, arthralgia, lethargy, diarrhoea, depression, sore throat, lymphadenopathy, skin rash, mucocutaneous ulcerations and sometimes meningoencephalopathy. Spontaneous resolution occurs within one month. There is a temporary fall in CD4+ and CD8+ T cells, followed by CD8+ lymphocytosis. Virus, viral nucleic acid or viral p24 antigen may be detected during this illness. Tests for HIV antibodies are usually negative at the onset of the illness but become positive during its course. Therefore, acute HIV infection is also known as **seroconversion illness**.

II. Asymptomatic infection

The asymptomatic period, which usually lasts several years, is the period between primary infection and the development of clinical immunodeficiency. During this period, the number of CD4+ lymphocytes declines slowly and virus continues to replicate, albeit at a relatively stable level. During this clinical latency period, high titres of virus can be found in lymphoid and other tissue compartments. The length of the clinical latency period varies considerably but is 10 years on average. In rapid progressors, AIDS develops within 1–2 years. In contrast, 5–10% of HIV-infected individuals are long-term nonprogressors and remain symptom-free for longer than 20 years. They show positive HIV antibody tests during this phase and are infectious. However, autoimmune conditions like Guillain-Barré syndrome, chronic demyelinating neuropathy, idiopathic thrombocytopenia, Reiter's syndrome, polymyositis, cranial nerve palsy and Sjogren's syndrome may occur during this period.

III. Persistent generalized lymphadenopathy (PGL)

Twenty five to thirty per cent of patients who are otherwise asymptomatic develop enlarged lymph nodes, at least 1 cm in diameter, in two or more noncontiguous extrainguinal sites, that persist for at least three months. PGL must be distinguished from other causes of lymphadenopathy such as the lymphomas.

IV. Symptomatic HIV infection

Following features indicate disease progression:

1. Downward trend of CD4+ T cells in successive samples.
2. The ease of virus culture.
3. The presence of p24 antigen in the plasma.
4. The loss of antibody to p24 antigen.

When CD4+ T cell count falls below 400/µl, the patient may develop constitutional symptoms like fever, night sweats, diarrhoea, weight loss and opportunistic infections which generally are not life-threatening. The latter include infections of skin and mucous membranes such as oral hairy leukoplakia, oral and oesophageal candidiasis, gingivitis, seborrhoeic dermatitis, bacterial folliculitis, chronic sinusitis, warts and molluscum contagiosum. Gastrointestinal infections caused by *Candida albicans* and *Cryptosporidium* and reactivation of herpes simplex and varicella-zoster infections also occur. In these patients, mycobacterial infections are also common.

When CD4+ T cells drop below 200/µl, their number generally begin to decline at an accelerated rate, the titre of virus in blood increases markedly and there is irreversible breakdown of immune defence mechanisms, leaving the patient a prey to progressive opportunistic infections and malignancies (Table 47.3). Most of the patients with HIV disease die of infections other than HIV. Tuberculosis is the commonest opportunistic infection.

Table 47.3. Opportunistic infections and malignancies commonly associated with HIV infection

I. BACTERIAL
1. *Mycobacterium avium* complex
2. *M. tuberculosis* – disseminated or extrapulmonary
3. *Salmonella* – recurrent septicaemia

II. VIRAL
1. Cytomegalovirus
2. Herpes simplex virus 1, 2
3. Varicella-zoster virus
4. Epstein-Barr virus
5. Human herpesvirus 6
6. Human herpesvirus 8

III. FUNGAL
1. Candidiasis
2. Cryptococcosis
3. Aspergillosis
4. *Pneumocystis jirovecii* pneumonia
5. Histoplasmosis
6. Coccidioidomycosis

IV. PARASITIC
1. Toxoplasmosis
2. Cryptosporidiosis
3. Isosporiasis
4. Microsporidiosis
5. Generalized strongyloidiasis

V. MALIGNANCIES
1. Kaposi's sarcoma
2. B cell lymphoma and non-Hodgkin's lymphoma

VI. SLIM DISEASE

Q. 3. Describe laboratory diagnosis of AIDS.

Ans. Serum samples are used routinely for standard HIV antibody and antigen detection, although plasma samples are also acceptable. The serum/plasma should be promptly separated from the clot/cellular elements and refrigerated at 2–8°C. If testing will not be performed within 7 days, the serum specimen should be frozen at –20°C or lower. Serum/plasma specimens can be transported either refrigerated (if transport takes place within 7 days of collection) or frozen in screw-cap plastic vials. Laboratory tests employed for the diagnosis of HIV infection may be classified into three groups (Table 47.4).

Table 47.4. Laboratory tests for the diagnosis of HIV infection

1. Screening (E/R) tests
- (a) ELISA
- (b) Rapid tests
  - Dot blot assays
  - Particle agglutination (gelatin, RBC, latex, microbeads)
  - Dip stick and comb tests (ELISA technology based)
  - Immunochromatography based tests

2. Supplemental tests
- (a) Western blot assay
- (b) Immunofluorescence test

3. Confirmatory tests
- (a) Virus isolation
- (b) Detection of p24 antigen
- (c) Detection of viral nucleic acid
  - In situ hybridization
  - Polymerase chain reaction

1. Screening (E/R) tests

These are serological tests which are used to screen antibodies against HIV. These tests are of two types.

(a) ***ELISA:*** It is a highly sensitive and specific test and a standard procedure for diagnosing HIV infection. The sensitivity and specificity of ELISA is 99.7% and 95% or more respectively. If two ELISAs are used then accuracy is 99.93%. If one ELISA and western blot is used then accuracy is 99.99%. ELISA test usually takes 2–3 hours to yield result.

(b) ***Rapid tests:*** These tests have a total reaction time of less than 30 minutes and do not require expensive equipment.

2. Supplemental tests

These tests also detect antibodies against HIV. These tests are recommended for validation of the positive results of the screening tests. Supplemental tests are often referred to as confirmatory tests which is not a correct nomenclature as these tests do not confirm the results of screening tests but provide additional information only. These include:

(a) ***Western blot assay:*** Western blot is highly specific and sensitive assay. In this assay, HIV proteins from detergent disrupted purified virions are separated according to their electrophoretic mobility and molecular weight by polyacrylamide gel electrophoresis, then blotted onto nitrocellulose membrane by standard blotting procedure. The membrane is then cut into strips having a full complement of viral proteins.

A serum sample found positive by screening test is reacted with the strip followed by washing. Antibodies which attach to separated viral antigens on the strip are detected by anti-human gammaglobulin antibody to which enzyme has been tagged. Enzyme substrate is subsequently added which indicates positive test. The substrate changes colour in the presence of enzyme and permanently stains the strip. The position of the band on the strip indicates the antigen with which the antibody has reacted.

(b) ***Immunofluorescence test:*** In this test, HIV infected cells are acetone fixed onto glass slides and then reacted with test serum followed by fluorescein conjugated anti-human gammaglobulin. A positive reaction appears as apple-green fluorescence of cell membrane under fluorescence microscope.

3. Confirmatory tests

These are the tests which confirm HIV infection in an individual who is either seropositive or has equivocal results from various serological tests. These include:

(a) ***Virus isolation:*** HIV can be isolated from patient's peripheral blood lymphocytes by co-cultivation with normal healthy donor's lymphocytes in the presence of mitogens and T cell growth factor (interleukin-2). Isolation of the virus is a slow process taking 3–6 weeks and must be conducted under conditions of strict biocontainment. Therefore, virus isolation is carried out only in certain research and reference laboratories. The presence of the virus is detected by **assays for reverse transcriptase and p24 antigen in the culture fluid**. Less readily HIV can also be isolated from plasma, CSF, genital secretions and various organs such as brain and bone marrow.

(b) ***Detection of p24 antigen:*** p24 antigen can be detected in the serum by ELISA in 30% patients during 'window period', 10% of asymptomatic patients and 50–60% of AIDS patients. As the antibody response builds up, antigen tests become negative. Late in infection p24 antigen may reappear.

(c) ***Detection of viral nucleic acid:*** Viral nucleic acid can be detected by **in situ hybridization and polymerase chain reaction**. The latter is the most sensitive assay. It can detect a single copy of RNA or proviral DNA from infected cells. Viral load assays, which measure the quantity of HIV-1 RNA present in plasma, are used as prognostic markers, to monitor response to therapy, and to determine infectiousness. HIV-1 plasma viral load is a strong predictor of the rate of disease progression. But HIV-1 RNA load assays are most commonly used to guide HIV treatment decisions.

Q. 4. Write short note on antiretroviral therapy.

Ans. The care of the human immunodeficiency virus-infected patient has changed dramatically in the last few years. Potent new antiretroviral drugs combined with updated treatment strategies have now achieved efficient inhibition of HIV replication in most patients. Classes of drugs include both nucleoside and nonnucleoside inhibitors of the viral enzyme reverse transcriptase, and inhibitors of the viral protease (Table 47.5). With the use of combinations of drugs that target different proteins involved in HIV pathogenesis, a treatment strategy known as **highly active antiretroviral therapy (HAART)**, rates of death and illness have been dramatically reduced. Although the death rate due to AIDS in Europe and North America has fallen by 80% since HAART was introduced, relatively few people in poor countries have reaped these benefits.

Table 47.5. Currently available antiretroviral agents

Nucleoside Reverse Transcriptase Inhibitors (NRTIs)	Nonnucleoside Reverse Transcriptase Inhibitors (NNRTIs)	Protease Inhibitors (PIs)
Abacavir – ABC licensed	Delavirdine – DLV licensed; rarely used	Amprenavir – APV licensed, largely replaced by fosamprenavir
Didanosine – ddI licensed	Efavirenz – EFV licensed	Atazanavir – ATV licensed
Emtricitabine – FTC licensed	Etravirine – TMC125 Phase III trials	Darunavir – TMC114 licensed
Lamivudine – 3TC licensed	Nevirapine – NVP licensed	Fosamprenavir – FPV licensed
Stavudine – d4T licensed	**CCR5 Inhibitors**	Indinavir – IDV licensed
Tenofovir – TDF licensed	Maraviroc – Licensed in US	Lopinavir/ritonavir – LPV/RTV licensed
Zidovudine – AZT, ZDV licensed	Selzentry	Nelfinavir – NFV licensed
Fusion Inhibitors	Vicriviroc – Phase III trials	Ritonavir – RTV licensed; mostly used in low doses to boost other PIs
Enfuvirtide – T-20 licensed	**Maturation Inhibitors**	Saquinavir – SQV licensed
Integrase Inhibitors	Bevirimat – PA-457 Phase II trials	Tipranavir – TPV licensed
Elvitegravir – GS-9137 Phase II trials		
Raltegravir – 0518 Phase III		
Isentress MK – Licensed		

48

HEPATITIS VIRUSES

Q. 1. Describe morphology, resistance, cultivation, pathogenesis, clinical features, laboratory diagnosis and prophylaxis of hepatitis A virus.

Ans. Hepatitis A virus (HAV) was previously classified as enterovirus type 72, but it has now been accorded the status of a separate genus, *Hepatovirus* of the family Picornaviridae.

Morphology

HAV is a nonenveloped 27 nm icosahedral virus containing linear, single-stranded RNA, 7.5 kb in length and of positive polarity (Table 48.1). It has only one serotype.

Resistance

HAV is one of the most stable viruses infecting humans. It can withstand heating at 60°C for one hour and treatment with 20% ether, acid (pH 1.0 for 2 hours) and many disinfectants. Inactivation of viral activity can be achieved by boiling for 1 minute, by contact with formaldehyde and chlorine, or by ultraviolet irradiation.

Cultivation

It can be transmitted to chimpanzees and several species of marmoset monkeys and can be grown in cell cultures of primate and human cells. **HAV is the only one of the human hepatitis viruses that can be cultivated in cell culture.** It has also been cloned.

Pathogenesis

HAV is shed early in the stools of infected individuals, 1–2 weeks prior to the onset of symptoms, and persists for the first several days after the transaminase levels peak. There is very little virus in the serum and hardly any at all in other body fluids which explains the epidemiology of the disease as **faecal-oral enteric infection**. Transfusion-associated hepatitis A is exceedingly rare. It probably multiplies first in the intestinal epithelial cells and then spreads to the liver via the blood. **Viral antigens can be seen in the cytoplasm of hepatocytes.**

HAV occurs throughout the world and is endemic in countries with substandard hygiene and sanitation, so the vast majority of native population have detectable anti-HAV by the age of 10 years. In developed countries, acute hepatitis A tends to be a sporadic overt febrile illness. Overall, hepatitis A accounts for about 25% of clinically evident acute hepatitis worldwide.

Clinical features

Hepatitis A is an acute self-limiting disease with an incubation period of 2–6 weeks. The onset is abrupt with fever, malaise, anorexia, nausea and lethargy which comprise the prodromal (preicteric) stage. Hepatomegaly, due to cell necrosis, causes blockage of the biliary excretions resulting in jaundice. It may also produce pain in the right upper abdominal quadrant. The fulminant form of hepatitis A and liver failure can occur in less than 0.5% cases. Complete recovery occurs in 8–12 weeks. Hepatitis A has no apparent adverse effect on the outcome of pregnancy. Transmission during birth by exposure to maternal faeces or by breast-feeding has been reported.

The severity of the disease varies with age. Only 5% of the children under 3 years of age develop jaundice, while more than 50% of adults develop it. Fatality rate is also more in adults. **In contrast to hepatitis B, hepatitis A infection does not produce extrahepatic manifestations, no carrier state and is not associated with cirrhosis or hepatocellular carcinoma.**

Laboratory diagnosis

Biochemical tests

Serum levels of both alanine and aspartate aminotransferase are markedly raised.

Immunoelectron microscopy

Virus particles can be demonstrated in faecal extracts by immunoelectron microscopy.

Serology

- Faecal HAV may be detected by **ELISA**.
- Detection of IgM anti-HAV by **ELISA or RIA** is the method of choice for the diagnosis of HAV infection. It is detectable in the serum for 2–6 months after the onset of symptoms. It is followed by the appearance of IgG anti-HAV which persists for many years and is a useful indicator of immunity.

Virus isolation

Virus, from the faeces, may be cultured on continuous cell lines of monkey kidney cells or human fibroblasts or hepatoma.

Polymerase chain reaction (PCR)

Trace amounts of HAV in food or water can be detected by PCR.

Prophylaxis

1. Proper collection, treatment and disposal of sewage.

2. Bathing and cultivation of shellfish for human consumption should not be allowed near sewerage outlets.
3. **Passive immunization** with normal human immunoglobulin (NIG) gives protection to seronegative individuals for a period of 4–6 months. It is recommended for the personnel travelling to highly endemic areas of the tropics and for the control of outbreaks in institutions such as homes for the mentally handicapped.
4. **Hepatitis A vaccine** consisting of formalin inactivated preparation of virions grown in human fibroblasts or monkey kidney cell lines, adsorbed to alum as an adjuvant, can be used for active immunization. Two doses injected one month apart with or without a booster after 6 months elicit a good immune response in 99% of vaccinees lasting for some years. Because of the low yield of virus from cultured cells the vaccine is costly. It may be given to high risk individuals like long-term visitors to countries in which HAV is endemic, sewage workers, sexually active homosexual men and intravenous drug users.

Q. 2. Tabulate differentiating features of various hepatitis viruses.

Ans. See Table 48.1 on page 463.

Q. 3. Describe morphology, cultivation and stability, and pathogenesis of hepatitis B virus.

Ans. Morphology

HBV or **Dane particle** is a complex 42 nm double shelled particle (Fig. 48.1 and Table 48.1). The outer surface or envelope contains **hepatitis B surface antigen (HBsAg)**. It is

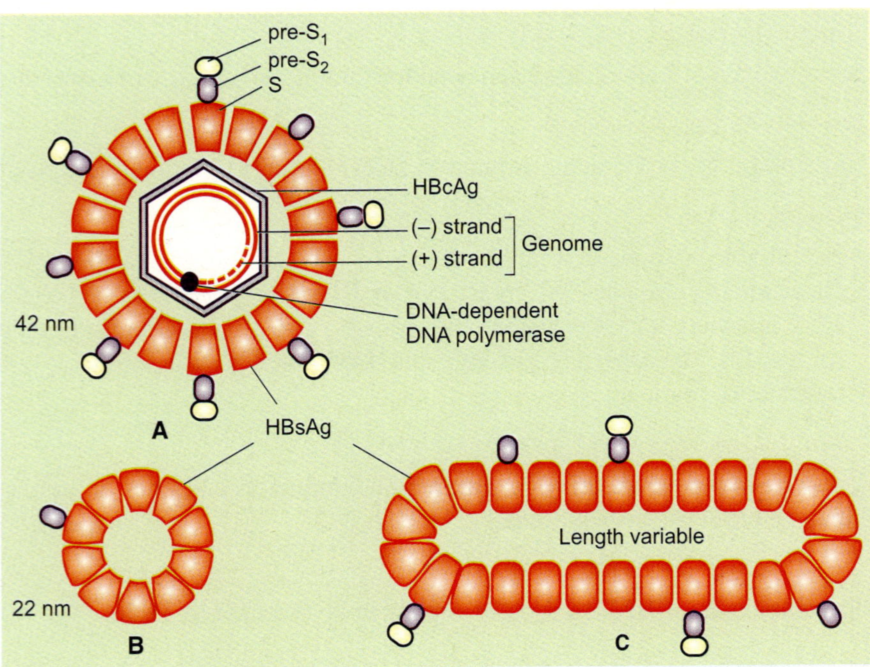

Fig. 48.1. Schematic diagram of hepatitis B virus particles: A, Dane particle; B, spherical particle; and C, tubular particle.

Table 48.1. Hepatitis viruses

Feature	Hepatitis A virus	Hepatitis B virus	Hepatitis C virus	Hepatitis D virus	Hepatitis E virus	Hepatitis G virus
Previous designation	Infectious hepatitis	Serum hepatitis	Non-A, non-B hepatitis (NANBH)	Delta hepatitis	Enterically transmitted epidemic NANBH	GBV non-A, non-E hepatitis (NANEH)
Year of identification	1973	1965	1989	1977	1980	1995
Family	Picornaviridae	Hepadnaviridae	Flaviviridae	Unclassfied	Caliciviridae	Flaviviridae
Genus	*Hepatovirus*	*Orthohepadnavirus*	*Hepacivirus*	*Deltavirus*	Unnamed	*Hepacivirus*
Genome	ssRNA	dsDNA	ssRNA	ssRNA	ssRNA	ssRNA
Genome size	7.5 kb	3.2 kb	9.5 kb	1.7 kb	7.6 kb	9.4 kb
Virion	27 nm, icosahedral	42 nm, spherical	50–60 nm, spherical	36–38 nm, spherical	27–38 nm, icosahedral	?
Envelope	No	Yes (HBsAg)	Yes	Yes (HBsAg)	No	?
Stability	Heat- and acid-stable	Acid-stable	Ether- and acid-sensitive	Acid-sensitive	Heat-stable	?
Transmission	Faecal-oral	Parenteral, sexual	Parenteral, sexual	Parenteral, sexual	Faecal-oral	Parenteral, sexual
Vertical transmission						
• Intrauterine	No	Yes	Possible but rare	Possible but rare	Yes	?
• Perinatal	No	Yes	Yes	Yes	Yes	Yes
• Early postnatal infection	Possible but rare	Possible but rare	Possible	?	?	?
Incubation period	2–6 weeks	6 weeks–6 months	6–8 weeks	6 weeks–6 months	2–8 weeks	?
Onset	Acute	Insidious or acute	Insidious	Insidious or acute	Acute	?
Age preference	Children, young adults	Young adults, babies, toddlers	Any age but more common in adults	Any age	Young to middle-age adults	?
Antigens	HAV	HBsAg, HBcAg	HCV	HBsAg, HDAg	HEVAg	?
Antibodies	Anti-HAV	Anti-HBs, Anti-HBc, Anti-HBe	Anti-HCV	Anti-HBs, Anti-HD	Anti-HEV	?
Chronic carrier state	No	5–10%	50%	>50%	No	?
Chronic hepatitis, cirrhosis	No	1–5%	20%	>50%	No	?
Hepatocellular carcinoma	No	Yes	Yes	No	No	?

?, data not yet available.

made up of lipid, protein and carbohydrate. It encloses an inner icosahedral 27 nm nucleocapsid (core), which contains **hepatitis B core antigen (HBcAg)**. Inside the core is the genome of HBV and a DNA-dependent DNA polymerase. The HBV genome (Fig. 48.2) consists of a 3.2 kilobase pair molecule of circular partially dsDNA of most unusual structure. The plus strand is incomplete leaving 15–50% of the molecule single-stranded. The minus strand is complete and contains four overlapping open reading frames (genes) coding for multiple proteins (Fig. 48.2):

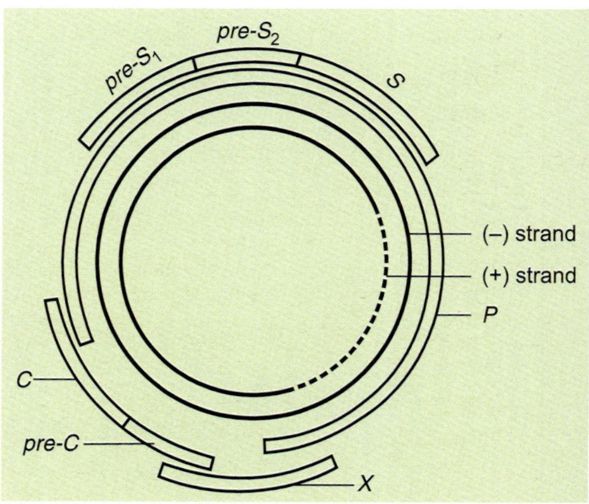

Fig. 48.2. Gene organization of HBV DNA.

1. The ***P* gene** (or *POL*), which comprises 80% of the genome and overlaps all the other genes, encodes DNA polymerase enzyme.
2. The ***S* gene** encodes the envelope protein, which occurs in three forms (Fig. 48.1): a large protein, translated from *pre-*S_1, *pre-*S_2, plus *S* regions of the genome and occurs in the envelope of infectious virions; a middle-sized protein comprises the product of *pre-*S_2 plus *S*; and finally the most abundant product is the S protein, the basic constituent of non-infectious HBsAg particles, the product of *S* gene only.
3. The ***C* gene** has two initiation sites that divide it into a *pre-C* and a *C* region, producing two distinct proteins, HBeAg and HBcAg respectively.
4. The ***X* gene**, spanning the cohesive ends of the genome encodes for HBxAg, which can transactivate the transcription of cellular and viral genes, its clinical relevance is not known.

Along with the mature virions (Fig. 48.1A), two subvirion morphological forms are formed in large excess:

1. Spherical particles with a diameter of 22 nm (Fig. 48.1B), and
2. Elongated tubules of similar diameter (Fig. 48.1C).

Both these pleomorphic structures are composed of HBsAg, are devoid of HBcAg and nucleic acid. They are not infectious and consist solely of surplus virion envelope. They normally occur in large (100- to 1,000-fold) excess over the mature 42 nm virions.

HBsAg carries a group-specific antigen '**a**' and two type-specific antigens, '**d**' or '**y**' and '**w**' or '**r**'. Thus there are four antigenic types of HBsAg – **adw**, **adr**, **ayw** and **ayr**. Type **ayw** is predominant in Africa, Russia and India, particularly in parenteral drug users. Type **adw** is predominant in Europe and USA particularly in homosexual men and type **adr** is predominant in Asia. The *w* antigen has additional four variants and additional antigens such as '**q**', '**x**' and '**g**' have been identified, but they have not been characterized. HBV is present in the blood mainly in the form of HBsAg and to smaller extent as Dane particles.

Cultivation and stability

HBV has not been cultivated in the laboratory. The chimpanzee is susceptible to experimental infection and can be used as a laboratory model. Experiments on chimpanzee inoculation reveal that the virus gets inactivated by heating at 60°C for 10 minutes and by treatment with hypochlorite (10,000 ppm available chlorine) and 2% glutaraldehyde in 10 minutes.

Pathogenesis

HBV infection is prevalent worldwide, representing a global public health problem. The WHO estimates that >2 billion people are infected with HBV, and approximately 600,000 people die each year due to acute or chronic HBV infection. The majority of these individuals live in Asia and Africa. Approximately one-fourth of infected children will die as adults from liver cirrhosis or hepatocellular carcinoma linked to HBV.

There are three important modes of transmission of HBV infection – parenteral, perinatal and sexual.

1. Parenteral transmission

HBV is present in the blood and in body fluids such as semen, vaginal secretions, menstrual discharge, saliva, colostrum and breast milk. The concentration of HBV in blood and body fluids is much greater than HIV. Less than 1 ml of blood contaminating a syringe or needle, can readily transmit hepatitis B from one individual to another. Transmission of infection may result from accidental inoculation of minute amounts of blood or fluid containing HBV during medical, surgical or dental procedures.

Needle-stick injuries, use of contaminated needles and syringes, intravenous and percutaneous drug abuse, ear and nose piercing, tattooing, acupuncture, sharing of shaving razor and kissing can transmit HBV infection. HBsAg has been demonstrated in several species of mosquitoes and bedbugs, but transmission of infection by arthropods has not been authenticated. Professionals occupationally at risk include dentists, surgeons, pathologists, mortuary attendants and technicians working in serology, haematology, blood bank, biochemistry, microbiology and haemodialysis units.

2. Perinatal transmission

HBV can be transmitted from carrier mothers to their babies during the perinatal period. Transmission probably occurs when maternal blood contaminates the mucous membranes of the newborn during birth. Infection may also result from haematogenous **transplacental transmission**, **breast-feeding** and **close postnatal contact** between infant and the infected parent. Perinatal infection and infection during the first year of life have important consequences because 90% of these infants become chronic carriers, as compared to 10% of those infected after the age of 6 years. **Such chronicity increases the risk of cirrhosis and hepatocellular carcinoma.**

3. Sexual transmission

Since HBV is present in semen and vaginal secretions, therefore, it can be transmitted by sexual contact. Sexually promiscuous individuals particularly male homosexuals are at very high risk. Most of the HBV infections are subclinical, particularly in childhood.

The course of acute HBV infection can be divided into three phases – preicteric, icteric and convalescent.

1. Preicteric (prodromal) phase

After an **incubation period** of 6 weeks to 6 months patient develops malaise, anorexia, weakness, myalgia, nausea, vomiting and pain in the right upper abdominal quadrant. A minority of patients develop arthralgia, urticarial or maculopapular rash, polyarteritis nodosa and glomerulonephritis. These features may be related to circulating immune complexes.

2. Icteric phase

Two days to two weeks following the initial symptoms patient develops jaundice, pale stools and dark urine (bilirubinuria). Hepatocellular damage is detectable biochemically before the onset of jaundice and persists after it has resolved.

3. Convalescent phase

This phase is long and drawn out with malaise and fatigue lasting for several weeks. The duration of uncomplicated hepatitis is rarely more than 8–10 weeks, but mild symptoms may persist for more than one year.

HBV infection occurs virtually in every country of the world. **The carrier rate in India is estimated to be 5%.** Mild cases that do not result in jaundice are termed anicteric. Less than 1% of the icteric cases die of fulminant hepatitis, 90–95% recover with complete regeneration of the damaged liver within 2–3 months. The remaining patients progress to **chronic active hepatitis, cirrhosis** and **hepatocellular carcinoma** (HCC). **HCC is one of the 10 most frequent tumours in the world, and there is considerable evidence that 80% are caused by chronic infection with HBV.** Thus, the highest rates of HCC are found in areas where HBV is highly endemic and where infection occurs at a very early age. This is necessary as there may be interval of 30–40 years between infection and tumour development, although shorter intervals are seen. Hepatoma cells often contain HBV DNA, but the patient is usually negative for HBcAg and other indications of ongoing viral replication. Integration of HBV DNA fragments into the hepatocyte genome is a frequent event during HBV infection.

Q. 4. Write short note on hepatitis B carriers

Ans. About 5–10% of HBV infections result in chronic carrier state. The latter may be defined as **persistence of HBsAg in the circulation for more than six months**. Carriers are of two types:

1. Super carriers

They have HBeAg, high titres of HBsAg and DNA polymerase in their blood. HBV may also be demonstrable in their blood. Very minute amount of serum or blood from such carriers can transmit the infection.

2. Simple carriers

These are more common types of carriers who have low level of HBsAg, and no HBeAg, HBV and DNA polymerase in the blood. They transmit the infection only when large volumes of blood are transferred as in blood transfusion.

Q. 5. Describe laboratory diagnosis and prophylaxis of hepatitis B virus infection.

Ans. Laboratory diagnosis

1. Biochemical tests

Levels of serum transaminases (aminotransferases) are increased 5- to 100-fold. Both alanine aminotransferase and aspartate aminotransferase rise together late in the incubation period. Peak level is obtained about the time jaundice appears and reverts to normal in next 2 months. Serum bilirubin levels may rise up to 25-fold.

2. Detection of viral markers

Specific diagnosis of hepatitis B can be carried out by serological demonstration of the viral markers (Table 48.2).

Table 48.2. Serological markers of hepatitis B infection

Clinical condition	Serological marker						
	HBsAg	HBeAg	Anti-HBs	Anti-HBe	Anti-HBc		HBV DNA
					IgM	IgG	
Incubation period	+	+	–	–	–	–	+
Acute hepatitis	+	+	–	–	+	+	+
Chronic active hepatitis	+	+	–	–	+	+	+
Asymptomatic carrier state	+	–	–	+	–	+	–
Past infection	–	–	+	–	–	+	–
Immunization without infection	–	–	+	–	–	–	–

- **HBsAg** is the first marker to appear in blood after infection. It is detectable in blood even before elevation of transaminases and onset of clinical illness. Peak levels of HBsAg are seen in the preicteric phase of disease. It remains in circulation throughout the icteric or symptomatic course of the disease. It disappears with recovery from clinical disease in most patients, but may sometimes last for six months and even beyond. Antibody to HBsAg (anti-HBs) appears after disappearance of HBsAg and persists for very long periods. Anti-HBs is the protective antibody.
- **HBcAg** is not demonstrable in serum because it is enclosed within the HBsAg coat. Anti-HBc antibody appears in serum a week or two after the appearance of HBsAg. It is the earliest antibody to appear in the blood. It persists lifelong, therefore, it serves as a useful indicator of prior infection with HBV, even after all viral markers become undetectable. Initially anti-HBc is predominantly IgM, but after about six months, it is mainly IgG. Therefore, selective tests for IgM or IgG anti-HBc enable distinction between recent or remote infection respectively.
- **HBeAg** appears in blood along with HBsAg or soon afterwards. Circulating HBeAg is an indicator of active intrahepatic viral replication. **The presence in blood of DNA polymerase,**

HBV DNA and virions indicates high infectivity. The disappearance of HBeAg coincides with the fall of transaminase levels in blood. It is followed by the appearance of anti-HBe.

3. Viral DNA polymerase

Viral DNA polymerase appears transiently during preicteric phase.

4. Polymerase chain reaction (PCR)

HBV DNA can be detected in serum by PCR. It is highly sensitive test.

Prophylaxis

Measures for the control of HBV infection are similar to those for HIV infection, i.e., screening of blood donors, use of sterile disposable syringes and needles by the medical personnel and parenteral drug users, reduction of the number of sexual partners, the use of condoms, etc. Medical personnel should wear gloves, gowns, masks and eyeglasses to prevent exposure to blood and body fluids, avoidance of mouth-pipetting, eating or smoking in the place of work and proper hand washing after work. Blood spills should be cleaned up with 2% glutaraldehyde or 1% sodium hypochlorite. Disposable equipment should be incinerated and other equipment should be properly sterilized.

Passive immunization

Hepatitis B immune globulin (HBIG) is prepared from donors with high titres of anti-HBs. It can be given in the doses of 300–500 IU in 3 ml intramuscularly after accidental exposure, as may occur by needle-stick injury or by splashing of blood from an HBsAg positive patient. HBIG should be administered as early as possible after exposure and preferably within 48 hours. A second dose is usually given 4 weeks after the first. Passive immunization is also effective in reducing the risk of the carrier state in babies born to infectious mothers. **HBIG must be given as early as possible but not later than 12 hours after birth.** When this is repeated at monthly intervals for up to six months, the proportion of babies who become carriers can be reduced by about 70%.

Active immunization

Immunization against HBV is required for high risk individuals like:

- Health care personnel, especially those in direct contact with blood and sharp instruments.
- Patients and health care personnel of institutions for the mentally retarded.
- Patients requiring repeated transfusion of blood and blood products.
- Patients on maintenance dialysis.
- Patients receiving prolonged inpatient treatment.
- Patients who require frequent tissue penetration.
- Parenteral drug users.
- Sexually promiscuous individuals and prostitutes.
- Spouses of those known to be infected with HBV.

Following vaccines are available:

1. Plasma-derived hepatitis B vaccine

It consists of purified 22 nm particles of HBsAg, prepared from the plasma of symptomless carriers. The particles are separated by ultracentrifugation and treated with proteinase, 8M urea and formaldehyde. The product is immunogenic but becomes unacceptable because its source is human plasma, limited in availability, and not totally free from possible risk of unknown pathogens.

2. Recombinant yeast hepatitis B vaccine

It is currently preferred vaccine. It is produced by cloning the *S* gene of HBV in yeasts *Saccharomyces cerevisae* and the HBsAg particles produced are extracted and purified for use as vaccine. This vaccine is safe, antigenic, free from side effects and as immunogenic as plasma-derived vaccine. It is adsorbed with aluminium hydroxide as adjuvant, **stored in cold but not frozen** and are injected intramuscularly into the **deltoid region** in a course of three doses given at 0, 1 and 6 months. Care should be taken to avoid injection into fat as this may produce poorer seroconversion rates.

3. Recombinant chinese hamster ovary (CHO) cell hepatitis vaccine

Expression system of CHO cells has been successfully used and the product is commercially available. This is the first vaccine using mammalian cell expression system.

4. Synthetic peptide vaccines

As the name indicates these are chemically synthesized polypeptide vaccines. These are safe and cheap. These are still under experimental stage.

Combined immunization

Greater protection is provided by combined passive and active immunization in postexposure prophylaxis. It is advisable to give the injections into different sites. Babies also respond to vaccine. The protective efficacy of the combined treatment is 90%.

Q. 6. Describe morphology, cultivation, pathogenesis and clinical features of hepatitis C virus.

Ans. ### Morphology

A virus of growing importance, hepatitis C virus (HCV), belongs to the genus *Hepacivirus* in the family Flaviviridae. The HCV viral particle is 50–60 nm in diameter and consists of an envelope derived from host cell membrane into which are inserted the virally encoded glycoproteins (E1 and E2) surrounding a nucleocapsid and a positive-sense, single-stranded RNA genome of about 9,500 nucleotides.

The virus shows extensive genome heterogeneity and has been classified into six genotypes or clades (1–6) and more than 80 subtypes. Genotype 1 is the main HCV genotype prevalent worldwide and accounts for 40–80% of all isolates. Genotypes 2 and 3 are also found globally but to a lesser extent. HCV can be inactivated by exposure to chloroform, ether and other organic solvents and by detergents.

Cultivation

HCV has not been grown in culture, but has been cloned in *Escherichia coli*.

Pathogenesis

HCV transmission occurs by needle-stick injuries or cuts with sharps, use of contaminated blood, and sexual intercourse. HCV can be transmitted in utero, during parturition and by breast milk. Transmission by saliva and tears cannot be excluded. HCV transmission from a conjunctival blood splash has also been reported.

Liver is the major site of virus replication *in vivo*. The levels of viral proteins and RNA in liver are very low and thus cannot be easily detected. Apart from liver cells there is enough evidence to show that HCV also replicates in peripheral blood mononuclear cells.

The virus attaches to the host cell by binding to host cell receptors. CD81 has been identified as the putative HCV receptor and E2 glycoprotein carries the ligand which binds to HCV receptor, as E2 specific antisera can block binding to cells. The role of E1 glycoprotein in binding is not clear, it may act as fusion protein.

Exposure to HCV infection can cause acute hepatitis in majority (about 80%) of the patients, of whom 10–20% progress to **liver cirrhosis** with an increased risk of **hepatocellular carcinoma (HCC)**. HCC is the most serious outcome of HCV infection. HCV has reached epidemic proportions with 200 million people infected worldwide. According to an estimate by CDC, HCV contributes to about 12,000 deaths every year in the US alone. It is gradually being realized that **HCV is also an important health problem in India as well**. HCV antibody prevalence varies from 0.4% to 2% in different parts of the world. In India, prevalence rate is between 1.5–2%.

The virus causes liver cell damage either by immune-mediated mechanism against the virus infected hepatocytes or by direct cytopathic effect. T4 and cytotoxic T cells play a dominant role in the immune-mediated injury. This results in necroinflammatory changes in the liver, which may resolve after the acute infection. However, in some of the patients, low-grade necroinflammation continues leading to chronic HCV infection. The dominant morphological changes in the liver in chronic HCV infection are necroinflammatory changes, regeneration and fibrosis, which causes distortion of architecture and can lead to cirrhosis.

Extrahepatic manifestations of chronic HCV infection

Autoimmune thyroiditis is the most common disorder in patients with chronic HCV infection. It also causes lymphocytic sialadenitis with xerostomia, thrombocytopenic purpura, non-Hodgkin lymphoma, diabetes mellitus and polyarteritis nodosa in 8–36%, 88%, 20–40%, 14% and 5–50% of patients with chronic HCV infection respectively.

HCV and hepatocellular carcinoma

The most serious late outcome of chronic HCV infection is HCC. HCV is frequently detected in patients with HCC with high rates being found in Southern Europe and Japan, intermediate in Australia, Taiwan and Saudi Arabia, and low in the United States and South Africa. In India, HCV is the cause in only 4% of HCC, while a dual infection with HBV and HCV is the cause in 8% cases. HBV alone is the cause in 71% patients.

Clinical features

Incubation period of hepatitis C averages 6–8 weeks though it may range up to several months. As compared to hepatitis B, clinical infection with hepatitis C is generally less severe, has shorter preicteric period, milder symptoms, absent or less marked jaundice, and the case fatality rate from fulminant hepatitis is 1% or less.

However, about 80% of the acute HCV infections become chronic. The affected individuals have persistence of the virus in their blood, elevated ALT levels for at least a year or two or more and they are at risk, just as in hepatitis B, of developing cirrhosis and hepatocellular carcinoma.

The mechanisms through which HCV evades the immune response and persists in the host are not completely understood. It has been proposed that:

1. The HCV-specific immune response is too weak to clear HCV from all infected hepatocytes. This may be due to either inefficient induction of the primary immune response during acute HCV infection or the inability to maintain T cell response at high enough levels.
2. The display of HCV antigens on cell surface is relatively low and HCV primarily infects hepatocytes which, unlike antigen-presenting cells such as dendritic cells (DCs), do not express high enough levels of co-stimulatory molecules.
3. Many recent reports indicate an active and direct role of HCV proteins in suppressing the immune response.
4. Another possible explanation of HCV persistence is the high genetic variability of the virus.

Q. 7. Describe laboratory diagnosis and prophylaxis of hepatitis C virus.

Ans. Laboratory diagnosis

Diagnosis of HCV infection can be established by:

- detection of anti-HCV by ELISA,
- viral genome by PCR and by immunofluorescence, and
- in situ hybridization on biopsy and autopsy specimens.

In acute hepatitis C, there is peak increase in serum ALT and presence of antibody to HCV. In 30–40% of the patients, anti-HCV is not detectable until 2–8 weeks after onset of symptoms. However, HCV RNA is detectable during early acute phase. Chronic hepatitis C is characterized when anti-HCV is present and serum ALT levels remain elevated for more than 6 months. Antibodies to various HCV antigens are nearly universally present in patients who are chronically infected with HCV. Testing for HCV RNA by PCR confirms the diagnosis and documents that viraemia is present.

Prophylaxis

HCV infection can be prevented by screening of blood donors, avoidance of use of unsterile needles for injections, and tattooing. Many of the public health measures adopted to prevent transmission of human immunodeficiency virus and HBV by parenteral routes will assist efforts at controlling HCV.

No effective vaccine has been developed to prevent HCV infection. Therefore, vaccine against hepatitis C designed to either prevent new infections or treat existing chronic infections remains the highest priority for future research. However, there are many challenges in the path to a successful HCV vaccine:

1. The lack of a suitable *in vitro* culture system makes production of vaccine quantities of whole virus impractical.
2. The genetic diversity of the virus and the high level of mutability also complicate vaccine development. Some regions of viral genome are specially prone to mutation and this allows the virus to escape immune surveillance.

3. Even within the same infected person, closely related but divergent HCV genomes are found and this evolution of new quasispecies is a continuous process.
4. HCV manages to persist in chronically infected persons in spite of broadly reactive antibody and T cell response.

Q. 8. Write short note on hepatitis D virus.

Ans. The HDV is a defective satellite virus requiring HBV as helper virus. It is spherical, 36–38 nm in diameter with HBsAg coat and HDAg nucleoprotein (Fig. 48.3). The genome consists of a single small circular molecule of minus sense RNA of 1.7 kilobase pairs (Table 48.1). It encodes its own nucleoprotein, the **delta antigen** or HDAg, but the outer capsid (HBsAg) of HDV virion is encoded by the genome HBV coinfecting the same cell. Replication of HDV requires the concomitant expression of HBV gene products, therefore, HBV is necessary for the production of HDV virions. It belongs to the genus *Deltavirus*.

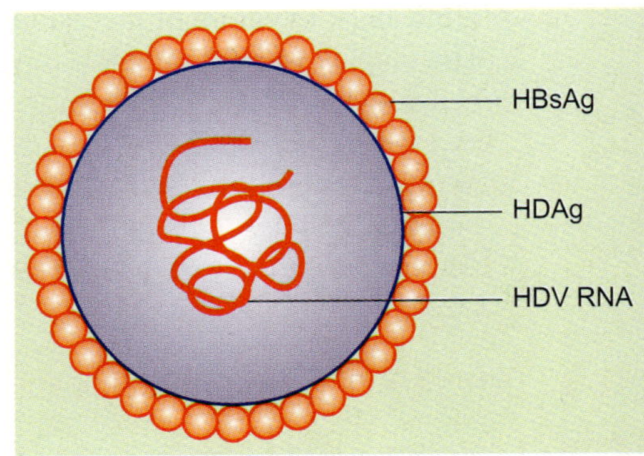

Fig. 48.3. Hepatitis D virus.

Pathogenesis

HDV is transmitted principally by blood and blood products, but also by sexual contact. Vertical transmission is also possible (Table 48.1).

Two types of HDV infections are possible:

1. **Simultaneous coinfection with HBV and HDV in the same inoculum.** It most commonly results from parenteral transmission, for example, in intravenous drug users. The clinical and biochemical features of such infection resemble those of acute hepatitis B alone. However, coinfection with HBV and HDV may be more severe than the disease caused by HBV alone.
2. **Superinfection of an HBsAg carrier by HDV.** It is commoner and more serious because a large number of hepatocytes are already producing HBsAg, and HDV can replicate without delay with a relatively short incubation period. It leads to severe liver damage, fulminant HBsAg positive hepatitis and elevated mortality (up to 20%).

In simultaneous acute HBV and HDV infections, IgM anti-HBc will be detectable, while in acute HDV infection superimposed on chronic HBV infections, anti-HBc will be of IgG class.

Laboratory diagnosis

The delta antigen is primarily expressed in liver cell nuclei, where it can be demonstrated by **immunofluorescence**. It is only occasionally present in serum. In patients with HBV-HDV coinfection, shortly before the end of incubation period, HBsAg appears in the serum and towards the end of incubation period HDAg appears which can be detected by **ELISA** or **immunoblotting**, and HDV RNA can be detected by **hybridization to a radiolabelled**

RNA probe. Two to three weeks after infection, anti-HD IgM appears followed by anti-HD IgG. However, in chronic infection, the IgM antibody persists for years. It can be detected by **ELISA**.

Prophylaxis

HDV infection can be prevented by prevention of coinfection with HBV or of superinfection of HBV carriers and hence requires all the measures that apply to the prevention of HBV infection, including vaccination against HBV. HBV vaccine is effective as HDV cannot infect persons immune to HBV.

Q. 9. Write short note on hepatitis E virus.

Ans. Hepatitis E virus belongs to the family Caliciviridae.

Morphology

Virions of HEV are spherical, nonenveloped and 27–38 nm in diameter. They possess single-stranded positive sense RNA genome of 7.6 kb which is surrounded by icosahedral capsid with characteristic surface depressions.

Pathogenesis

A substantial proportion of cases of acute viral hepatitis occurring in young to middle-aged adults in Asia and the Indian subcontinent appear to be caused by HEV. Hepatitis E has been shown to occur in epidemics, endemics and sporadic forms almost exclusively in the less developed parts of the world. It is primarily associated with **ingestion of faecally contaminated drinking water**. It was first documented in New Delhi, India, in 1955, when 29,000 cases of icteric hepatitis were identified following widespread faecal contamination of the city's drinking water. A similar epidemic of hepatitis E occurred between December 1975 and January 1976 in Ahmedabad city, India, again due to contaminated water supplies. Many similar water-borne outbreaks have been recorded subsequently from Indian sub-continent (Nepal and Pakistan), Southeast Asia (Myanmar and Indonesia), Central Asia (Kirgiz Republic and China), Africa (Algeria, Ivory Coast, Chad, Sudan and Somalia) and North America (Mexico).

Incubation period of hepatitis E ranges from 2–8 weeks, with an average of 5–6 weeks. It occurs predominantly in the 15–40 years age group. Clinically, the disease closely resembles that of hepatitis A. However, bilirubin levels tend to be higher and jaundice deeper and more prolonged. The case-fatality rate is 0.5–3% but in infected pregnant women it varies from 10–20%. In contrast to HAV, HEV has considerable implications in pregnancy. It may cause intrauterine and perinatal infections. HEV infection during pregnancy may cause a high rate of abortion and intrauterine death and increased perinatal mortality in babies born to women with fulminant hepatitis. **Like hepatitis A, hepatitis E does not progress to chronic hepatitis, cirrhosis, cancer or carrier state.**

Laboratory diagnosis

1. **Exclusion of hepatitis A** by IgM serology and hepatitis B by absence of HBsAg and IgM anti-HBc.

2. **Immunoelectron microscopic examination** of patient faeces for aggregated calicivirus-like particles using monoclonal antibodies.
3. **ELISA** tests for IgM and IgG anti-HEV.
4. A **Western blot assay** for IgM and/or IgG anti-HEV.
5. **Polymerase chain reaction (PCR) assay** for the detection of HEV RNA (as cDNA) in patient faeces or in acute-phase sera.

Prophylaxis

Hepatitis E can be prevented by improved standards of sanitation and provision of chlorinated water throughout the developing world. During the epidemic, take boiled water and only cooked food. No vaccine or effective antiviral drugs exist.

Q. 10. Write short note on hepatitis G virus.

Ans. Hepatitis G virus (HGV) was first isolated from a patient with chronic hepatitis in 1996. Along with HCV it has been placed in family Flaviviridae genus *Hepacivirus*. The genome of HGV consists of 9.4 kb molecule of ssRNA of positive polarity. Its structure resembles that of HCV, but it has <25% homology with HCV. HGV replicates in peripheral blood cells, however, its replication in the liver is not known. The virus is transmitted parenterally (exposure to blood through transfusions, haemodialysis, or sharing equipment in injecting drug use), sexually, and from mother to child (Table 48.1). More than 30% of transfusion recipients and up to 80% of injecting drug users are HGV marker positive. HGV and human immunodeficiency virus (HIV) share same infection routes, and a significant proportion of HIV-infected subjects are HGV-coinfected.

The virus is present worldwide. Majority of the individuals with HGV infection have no detectable evidence of liver disease. There have been, however, cases of acute, fulminant and chronic hepatitis where HGV is presently the only explanation for their liver disease. There is no evidence of a causal relationship between HGV infection and hepatocellular carcinoma. HGV infection results frequently in chronic viraemia. It often subsides after several years and anti-HGenv antibody develops.

Laboratory diagnosis

HGV infection is mainly detected by reverse transcriptase polymerase chain reaction (RT-PCR). Recently, an immunoassay has been developed to detect anti-HGenv. Serum HGV RNA indicates viraemia, whereas anti-HGenv is associated with recovery. These can be found respectively in <2% and 9% of healthy blood donors. Prevalence increases in association with HCV or HBV infection.

Prophylaxis

HGV infection can be prevented by employing the same measures as for HBV, HCV and HIV.

49

Oncogenic (Tumour) Viruses, Slow Virus Infections and Prions

Q. 1. Define oncogenic viruses. Describe changes associated with transformed cells and types of oncogenic viruses.

Ans. Viruses that produce tumours in their natural hosts or in experimental animals, or induce malignant transformation of cells on culture are known as oncogenic viruses. Changes associated with transformed cells include:

1. Alterations in cell growth patterns

Increased rate of growth, decreased requirement for serum growth factors, decreased cell adhesion to a substrate, enhanced ability to grow in semisolid medium, and loss of 'contact inhibition'. Because of loss of contact inhibition, the transformed cells are no longer inhibited by contact with other cells, as normal cells are, but tend to pile up to form a 'focus'. Induction of foci provides the basis for a quantitative assay for certain tumour viruses.

2. Alterations in cell surface

Increased rate of transport of cell nutrients, increased secretion of proteases and protease activators, increased agglutinability by plant lactins, and changes in composition of glycoproteins and glycolipids, sometimes including the presence of virus-encoded proteins.

3. Alterations in intracellular components and biochemical processes

Increased metabolic rate, increased glycolysis, altered levels of cyclic nucleotides, activation or repression of certain cellular genes, presence of viral DNA, mRNA and viral coded proteins; and changes in cell cytoskeleton, often resulting in a more rounded cell shape.

4. Tumourogenicity

Production of tumours when transformed cells are injected into appropriate test animals, especially immunologically deficient animals.

The development of a tumour is usually a rare outcome of virus infection but it has nevertheless been estimated that up to 20% of human tumours have a viral risk factor.

Types of oncogenic viruses

All known oncogenic viruses either have a DNA genome (DNA viruses) or generate a DNA provirus (RNA viruses) after infection of cells. DNA tumour viruses belong to the families Papovaviridae, Herpesviridae, Hepadnaviridae and Poxviridae. With the exception of hepatitis C virus which belongs to the family Flaviviridae all other RNA oncogenic viruses belong to the family Retroviridae. Oncogenic viruses associated with human and animal neoplasia are given in Tables 49.1 and 49.2, respectively.

Q. 2. Write a short note on permissive and nonpermissive host cells for a given virus replication.

Ans. Host cells are either permissive or nonpermissive for replication of a given virus. Permissive cells support viral growth and production of progeny virus; nonpermissive cells do not. Especially with the DNA viruses, permissive cells are not transformed unless the viral replicative cycle that normally results in death of the host cell is blocked in some way. DNA viruses replicate in certain cells of their natural host but rarely, if ever, produce tumours in those hosts. On the other hand, they are usually unable to replicate in heterologous host cells but can, on occasion, transform them. For example, simian virus 40 (SV40) naturally infects rhesus monkeys. This virus replicates in monkey kidney cells but does not transform these cells. This virus cannot replicate in cells of rodent origin but is able to transform them at low efficiency. However, RNA tumour viruses can both replicate in and transform homologous cells. Thus, RNA tumour viruses differ from DNA tumour viruses in that the former can transform both permissive and nonpermissive cells.

Q. 3. Write short note on mechanism of oncogenesis.

Ans. *1. Viral oncogenes*

Retroviruses carry RNA-directed polymerase (reverse transcriptase) that forms a DNA copy of the RNA genome of the virus. The DNA copy (provirus) becomes integrated into the DNA of the infected host cell and replicates. During this process the viral genome incorporates sequences which in the host cell under normal condition is concerned with normal cell growth. This process is termed transduction. Coming now under the control of viral genes, this proto-oncogene becomes abnormal, i.e., viral oncogene (*V-onc*), which upon entering a new cell brings about transformation of the cell. Generally, very few copies (perhaps one) of the viral genome are integrated in a transformed cell.

2. Cellular oncogenes

Proto-oncogenes are genetic sequences in the cell nuclei controlling normal cell growth. When a viral DNA is juxtaposed to a proto-oncogene, the latter can be activated, and becomes a cellular oncogene (*C-onc*), a process termed insertional mutagenesis. Transduction and insertional mutagenesis require oncogenic viruses.

3. Oncogenes of DNA tumour viruses

The transforming genes of the oncogenic DNA viruses bear no close relationship to cellular

Table 49.1. Oncogenic viruses associated with human neoplasia

Virus family	Virus	Associated tumours
DNA VIRUSES		
Papovaviridae	Human papillomaviruses	Genital tumours (cervical, vulvar and penile cancers), squamous cell carcinoma
Herpesviridae	Epstein-Barr virus	Nasopharyngeal carcinoma, Burkitt's lymphoma, B cell lymphoma, Hodgkin's disease, immunoblastic lymphoma
	Herpes simplex virus (types 2 and 1)	Cervical neoplasia
	Cytomegalovirus	Cervical neoplasia
	Human herpesvirus 8	Kaposi's sarcoma
Hepadnaviridae	Hepatitis B virus	Hepatocellular carcinoma
Poxviridae	*Molluscipoxvirus*	Molluscum contagiosum
RNA VIRUSES		
Retroviridae	Human T cell leukaemia (lymphotropic) virus-I	Adult T cell leukaemia
Flaviviridae	Hepatitis C virus	Hepatocellular carcinoma

Table 49.2. Oncogenic viruses associated with animal neoplasia

Virus family	Virus	Associated tumours
DNA VIRUSES		
Papovaviridae	Bovine papillomavirus	Dermal and oesophageal papillomas, and squamous cell carcinoma
	Polyomavirus of rodents	Mouse adenocarcinomas, fibrosarcomas
	Simian virus 40	Sarcoma (rodents)
Herpesviridae	Frog herpesvirus	Renal adenocarcinoma
	Marek's disease virus	Neurolymphomatosis (fowl)
Hepadnaviridae	Woodchuck hepatitis virus	Hepatocellular carcinoma (woodchuck)
Poxviridae	Shope fibroma virus	Fibroma (rabbit)
	Yaba virus	Nodular fibromatous hyperplasia (monkey)
Adenoviridae	Adenovirus types 2, 5, 12	Fibrosarcomas (hamster)
RNA VIRUSES		
Retroviridae	Mouse mammary tumour virus	Mammary adenocarcinomas, T cell lymphoma
	Avian leucosis viruses Rous sarcoma virus	Various sarcomas, some carcinomas, lymphomas and leukaemias
	Avian reticuloendotheliosis virus	Lymphomas and leukaemias
	Murine leukaemia and sarcoma viruses	Lymphomas, leukaemias and sarcomas
	Feline leukaemia and sarcoma viruses	Lymphosarcomas (mainly T cell), myeloid leukaemias, fibrosarcomas
	Bovine leukaemia virus	B cell leukaemias

gene products. They are integral components of the viral genome and provide important functions early in replicative cycle.

4. Antioncogenes

In addition to oncogenes there are certain genes which have been found to reduce the frequency of genetic mutations. These are the suppressor genes or antioncogenes. Deletion of their suppression effect can lead to oncogenesis.

Q. 4. Describe briefly slow virus infections.

Ans. The term 'slow virus infections' is applied to several viral infections of animals and human beings that have a very long incubation period leading to a slowly progressive, invariably fatal disease. They have predilection for involvement of the central nervous system. These include visna and maedi in sheep, and subacute sclerosing panencephalitis (SSPE) and progressive multifocal leukoencephalopathy in humans (Table 49.3).

Table 49.3. Slow virus diseases

Disease	Virus	Host	Incubation period	Disease
Visna	Retrovirus	Sheep	About 2 years	Demyelinating disease of sheep
Maedi	Retrovirus	Sheep	2–3 years	Slowly progressive fatal haemorrhagic pneumonia of sheep
Subacute sclerosing panencephalitis	Measles virus	Humans	2–20 years	Chronic sclerosing panencephalitis
Progressive multifocal leukoencephalopathy	Papovavirus	Humans	Years	Central nervous system demyelination

Characteristics of slow virus infections

1. Long incubation period ranging from months to years.
2. Course of illness lasting for years. Predilection for involvement of central nervous system.
3. Absence of immune response.
4. Genetic predisposition.
5. Fatal termination.

Visna

Visna is a demyelinating disease of sheep with an incubation period of about 2 years. It is caused by a retrovirus. This virus infects all the organs of the body of the infected sheep, however, pathologic changes are confined primarily to the brain, lungs, and reticuloendothelial system. The disease has an insidious onset with paresis, progressing to total paralysis and death.

During the long-term persistent infection, the virus undergoes antigenic variations. Many mutations occur in the structural gene that codes for viral envelope glycoproteins. Infected animals develop antibodies to the virus. These can be detected in the cerebrospinal fluid as well as in the serum of sick animals.

Maedi

It is a slowly progressive fatal haemorrhagic pneumonia of sheep. The incubation period is 2–3 years. It is also caused by a retrovirus.

Subacute sclerosing panencephalitis

Subacute sclerosing panencephalitis (SSPE) is a rare, fatal, slowly progressive degenerative disease of the CNS. It is generally seen in children or early adolescents aged 6–8 years who have had measles early in life, usually under 2 years of age. It occurs in only 1 in 300,000 cases and has become very rare, following the reduction in measles itself by widespread immunization of children. Boys are more likely to develop SSPE than the girls. Under electron microscope, large numbers of viral nucleocapsid structures are visible in neurons and glial cells. There is restricted expression of the viral genes (*M*, *F*, *H*) that encode envelope proteins. Therefore, the virus in persistently infected neural cells lacks components essential for assembly and budding of mature infectious particles. Defective measles virus has been recovered from brains of patients with SSPE by co-cultivation of brain cells with susceptible cells. Such isolates are mutated in one or more viral proteins. Patients with SSPE have high titres of measles antibody in both serum and cerebrospinal fluid. However, antibody to the M protein is frequently lacking.

The course of SSPE is variable and usually starts with a generalized intellectual deterioration, which may last for weeks or months, until definite neurological signs or motor dysfunctions such as generalized convulsions, aphasia, visual disturbances and mild repetitive simultaneous myoclonic jerks appear. Viral invasion of retina may lead to chorioretinitis, often affecting macular area, followed by blindness. Finally, the disease proceeds to progressive cerebral degeneration, leading to coma and death. Disease generally lasts for 1–3 years.

Progressive multifocal leukoencephalopathy

(See JC polyomavirus).

Q. 5. Describe briefly general characters of prions.

Ans. ***General characters***

Prions may be defined as **small proteinaceous infectious particles**. They do not contain nucleic acid genome. However, viruses, viroids, bacteria, fungi and parasites all have nucleic acid genomes that code for their progeny. The prion protein (PrP) is encoded by the host's chromosomal DNA. An abnormal isoform of this protein is the only known component of the prion and is associated with transmissibility. This abnormal isoform differs physically from the normal cellular isoform by its high beta-sheet content, its insolubility in detergents, its propensity to aggregate, and its relative resistance to proteolysis.

The causative agents of the subacute spongiform encephalopathies are composed largely of a protein designated as the scrapie isoform of the prion protein (PrP^{sc}) which is a pathogenic conformer of the cellular isoform (PrP^{c}). PrP^{sc} has the same amino acid sequence as PrP^{c} found in the membrane of normal neurons of the host, but differs in conformation. The genes for the prion proteins of human reside on the short arm of chromosome 20. The genes for the infectious prion proteins of all the subacute spongiform encephalopathies have been sequenced.

The mechanism of reproduction of prions is not known. One hypothesis is that PrP^{sc} forms a heterodimer with PrP^{c}, serving as a template which alters the folding of the latter to that of PrP^{sc}. In contrast to PrP^{c}, PrP^{sc} is highly resistant to proteolysis. Because of their resistance to digestion, these abnormal isoforms accumulate. Prions lack nucleic acid. Their infectivity is very resistant to inactivation by a variety of physical and chemical treatments that inactivate viruses, including nucleases, UV-irradiation, formalin, mild proteolysis, and even boiling. They do not elicit an immune response in the host. Prions are resistant to conventional inactivation methods:

1. Dry heat

They are extremely resistant to dry heat. A treatment of 360°C for one hour has been reported not to be completely effective.

2. Wet heat

They are more resistant to steam than conventional transmissible agents (bacteria and their spores, fungi and viruses). Steam has been found to be effective if a temperature of 134–138°C is maintained for 18 minutes.

3. Chemicals

Sodium hypochlorite (25% available chlorine) treatment at room temperature for one hour inactivates the agent. They are also sensitive to phenol (90%), household bleach, ether, acetone, urea (6 mol/l), 10% sodium dodecyl sulphate and iodine disinfectants. A number of other chemicals like aldehyde, potassium permanganate, hydrogen peroxide, ethylene oxide, β-propiolactone, ethanol, proteases, deoxycholate and ionizing irradiation have been found to be ineffective. **Formalin fixed tissue should be considered infective and treated with special care.**

Q. 6. Describe spongiform encephalopathies of humans and animals.

Ans. Prions produce slow infections with long incubation periods (months to years), followed by progressive disease, which leads to death from a degenerative condition of the brain characterized by a spongiform appearance. Prion diseases of humans are kuru, Creutzfeldt-Jakob disease (CJD), Gerstmann-Sträussler-Scheinker (GSS) syndrome, and fatal familial insomnia (FFI) in humans. Prion diseases of animals are scrapie of sheep and goats, bovine spongiform encephalopathy (BSE) of cattle, mink and feline encephalopathy and wasting disease of deer and elk (Table 49.4).

Table 49.4. Prion diseases (spongiform encephalopathy) of humans and animals

Diseases of humans	Diseases of animals
Kuru	Scrapie of sheep and goats
Creutzfeldt-Jakob disease	Bovine spongiform encephalopathy of cattle
Gerstmann-Sträussler-Scheinker syndrome	Mink and feline encephalopathy
Fatal familial insomnia	Wasting disease of deer and elk

Characteristics of prion diseases

Following are the characteristics of diseases caused by prions:

1. The prion diseases are infectious, inherited and sporadic disorders.
2. They are confined to the nervous system.
3. The basic lesion is a progressive vacuolation in neurones, an extensive astroglial hypertrophy and proliferation, and spongiform change in the grey matter.
4. Prion protein accumulates within the central nervous system both as diffuse deposits and in the form of amyloid plaques.
5. Long incubation periods (months to decades) precede the onset of clinical illness and are followed by chronic progressive pathology (weeks to years).
6. Diseases are always fatal.
7. Host shows no inflammatory response.
8. Prions do not appear to be antigenic, therefore, host shows no immune response.
9. Interferon is not produced.
10. There is no effect on host B or T cell function.
11. Between 10% and 15% cases of prion diseases are inherited whilst the remaining cases are sporadic.

Scrapie

Scrapie is an infection of sheep, usually transmitted from ewe to lamb vertically, less often by contact. The incubation period is very long (up to 3 years). The affected animals are irritable and develop intense pruritis, scraping themselves against trees and rocks, hence the name scrapie. The disease progresses slowly but invariably to paralysis and death.

Bovine spongiform encephalopathy

A disease similar to scrapie, designated bovine spongiform encephalopathy or 'mad cow disease' emerged in cattle in Great Britain in 1986 and by 1995 there had been 150,000 cases. This outbreak was traced to infection of cattle with scrapie agent via feed that contained bone meal from sheep carcasses that had been treated in a fashion that failed to destroy the infectivity or scrapie agent.

Kuru

Kuru (meaning tremor) was first described in 1957. It occurs only in a particular tribe in the remote New Guinea highlands, the women and children of which practised ritualistic cannibalism of their own deceased relatives. It occurs more frequently in women than in men, because the remains of dead relatives were handled and eaten primarily by women and children. **The incubation period is 5–10 years.** Patient develops progressive cerebellar ataxia and tremors, ending fatally in 3–6 months. Following the abandonment of this macabre custom the incidence of the disease has decreased. Brain material from patients who died from kuru can produce similar disease when injected into chimpanzees, and the serial passage of diseased chimpanzee brain into healthy chimpanzees or rodents transfers the illness.

Creutzfeldt-Jakob disease

Creutzfeldt-Jakob disease (subacute presenile dementia) is the most common prion disease in humans. It develops gradually, with progressive dementia, ataxia and somnolence, and leads to death in 8–12 months. The histologic lesions resemble those of kuru and scrapie, including the presence of amyloid plaques. CJD has a worldwide incidence of about one case per million population annually. These sporadic cases do not appear to have been due to infection, although a number of cases of iatrogenic transmission of CJD have been traced to dura mater grafts, implantation of cerebral electrodes, corneal transplants and administration of human growth hormone derived from pituitary glands, presumably from the donors who had the infection.

CJD can be thought of as the equivalent of a rare somatic mutation, due not to change in the nucleotide sequence of the prion protein, but to the spontaneous generation of the PrP^{sc} isoform from the host PrP^{c} by a rare stochastic event, with an incidence of one per million. A protein similar to the scrapie PrP^{sc} is present in brain tissue infected with CJD. It has been speculated that the agent of CJD was derived originally from scrapie-infected sheep and transmitted to humans by ingestion of poorly cooked sheep brains. As in case of kuru, brain material from patients who died from CJD can produce similar disease when injected into chimpanzees, and the serial passage of diseased chimpanzee brain into healthy chimpanzees or rodents transfers the illness.

Gerstmann-Sträussler-Scheinker syndrome (GSS) and fatal familial insomnia (FFI)

GSS and FFI are two familial forms of CJD, due to autosomal dominant genes. Patients suffering from GSS have a single amino acid substitution in the normal cellular prion protein, PrP^{c}, due to a mutation in codon 102, which increases the likelihood of the production of PrP^{sc}.

Diagnosis of human prion diseases

Human prion disease should be considered in any patient who develops a progressive subacute or chronic decline in cognitive or motor function. They typically involve adults between 40 and 70 years of age. A definitive diagnosis of human prion disease, which is invariably fatal, can often be made by the examination of brain tissue.

Medical Mycology

Q. 1. Describe morphological classification of fungi.

Ans. On the basis of morphology, there are four groups of fungi:

1. **Yeasts:** Yeasts are round, oval or elongated unicellular fungi. These organisms remain in the yeast form at both room temperature and body temperature (37°C). Most of them reproduce by an asexual process called **budding** in which the cell develops a protuberance which enlarges and eventually separates from the parent cell (Fig. 50.1A and B). Some reproduce by fission. They form moist or mucoid colonies. *Saccharomyces cerevisae* and *Cryptococcus neoformans* are the examples of nonpathogenic and pathogenic yeasts respectively.
2. **Yeast-like:** In some yeasts, like *Candida*, the bud remains attached to the mother cell and elongates, followed by repeated budding forming chains of elongated cells known as **pseudohyphae**. These can be differentiated from true hyphae because they have constriction at the septa and the septa are also present at the branching point (Fig. 50.1C). Some species like *C. albicans* also produce true hyphae.

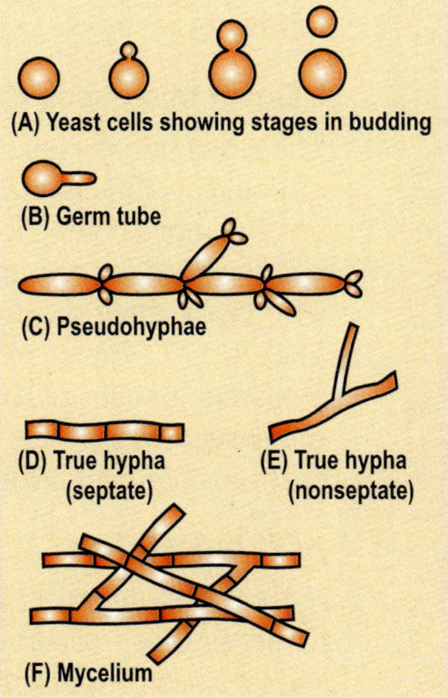

Fig. 50.1. Basic fungal morphology.

3. **Molds:** In molds, spores germinate to produce branching filaments called **hyphae** (singular hypha). They are 2–10 μm in diameter (Fig. 50.1D and E). They may be septate or nonseptate (coenocytic). The hyphae continue to grow (Fig. 50.1F) and branch to form tangled mass of growth called **mycelium** (pl., mycelia). In the culture medium, the part

of the mycelium which projects above the surface is called **aerial mycelium** and the part growing in the medium is called **vegetative mycelium**. They reproduce by the formation of different types of sexual and asexual spores. Dermatophytes, *Aspergillus*, *Penicillium*, *Mucor* and *Rhizopus* are the examples of molds.

4. **Dimorphic fungi:** Many fungi pathogenic to man like *Histoplasma capsulatum*, *Sporothrix schenckii*, *Blastomyces dermatitidis*, *Coccidioides immitis*, *Paracoccidioides brasiliensis*, and *Penicillium marneffei* have a yeast form in the host tissue and *in vitro* at 37°C on enriched media, and hyphal (mycelial) form *in vitro* at 25°C.

Q. 2. Describe laboratory diagnosis of mycoses.

Ans. Specimens for the diagnosis of mycoses include skin scrapings, oral scrapings, vaginal scrapings, corneal scrapings, hair and nails, bone marrow, blood, cerebrospinal fluid, urine, sputum, bronchial lavage specimens, mycetoma grains, pus and tissues. Specimen should be collected under aseptic conditions, i.e., after appropriate cleaning and decontamination of collection site and rapidly transported to the laboratory. If delay in processing is unavoidable, the specimen for fungal culture may be stored at 4°C for a short time. **Specimens not likely to contain contaminating microorganisms, e.g., cerebrospinal fluid, should not be refrigerated.** Causative agents of mycoses can be identified by following methods:

I. Direct microscopic examination of specimens

The direct microscopic examination of clinical specimen may be as simple as placing a drop of liquid specimen on a clean glass slide and examining it with light microscope, or it may involve more complex procedures, including staining of tissues. Although the Gram stain performed in the routine microbiology laboratory often gives the first evidence of infection with yeast, other direct stains give more specific information concerning a mold infection. The types of direct examination used in identification of fungal infections include wet preparation such as KOH preparation, KOH with calcofluor white, India ink, and tissue stains such as periodic acid-Schiff (PAS) stain, Gomori methenamine silver (GMS) stain, Giemsa stain, and haematoxylin and eosin (H&E) stain.

KOH preparation

A 10–20% solution of KOH is useful for detecting fungal elements in skin, hair, nails, and tissue. In this procedure, KOH is mixed in equal proportions with the specimen on a slide and the specimen material is teased with two inoculating needles. A coverslip is placed over it and heated gently. Preparation with KOH clears the tissue and cellular debris from all types of clinical specimens without damaging the fungal cells. This clearing process requires only 5–10 minutes, after which one can observe the fungal morphology as well as the pigment of the fungal cell wall under a phase-contrast or bright-field microscope, using low-power followed by high-power objectives.

KOH with calcofluor white

A drop of 0.1% calcofluor white solution (fluorescent reagent) can be added to the KOH preparation prior to placing coverslip over it. Calcofluor white binds to polysaccharide present in the chitin of the fungus or to cellulose. Fungal elements fluoresce apple green or blue-white, depending on the combination of filters used. The actual fungal structure must be seen before a positive preparation is reported.

India ink

India ink preparations may be used for detecting encapsulated yeast *Cryptococcus neoformans* in cerebrospinal fluid (CSF). A drop of India ink is mixed with a drop of centrifuged deposit of CSF, and the preparation is examined under high power. With this negative stain, budding yeast surrounded by a large clear area against a dark background is presumptive evidence of *C. neoformans*.

Tissue stains

The diagnosis of fungal diseases should preferably be established on the basis of histopathologic evidence combined with cultural evidence, because detection of fungi in tissue and confirmation of tissue invasion are required in diagnosing many opportunistic fungal infections. For example, isolation of common fungi such as *Aspergillus*, *Penicillium*, and *Rhizopus* species from sputum does not establish pulmonary infection by these fungi unless there is also histopathological evidence. Moreover, certain mycoses, e.g., rhinosporidiosis, lobomycosis and *Pneumocystis jirovecii* infection can only be diagnosed by histologic studies since growth conditions of the fungi causing these infections have not been defined.

Histopathologic procedures are rapid and relatively inexpensive. Because of the size, characteristic morphology, and staining properties of many fungi, histopathologic studies often yield a presumptive diagnosis. There are several mycoses in which etiologic agents can be identified to the generic level because the morphologic characteristics are distinctive to the genus involving several species – aspergillosis and candidiasis.

Haematoxylin and eosin (H&E) stain used routinely in the pathology laboratory is often not adequate for detecting fungal elements. Many fungi stain poorly and some fungi do not stain at all with H&E. However, with this stain the tissue response can be demonstrated better than with any special stain and the innate colour of the fungal elements, whether dematiaceous or hyaline, can be determined.

- **The Gomori methanamine silver (GMS) staining procedure** provides better contrast between the fungi and background tissue. This procedure results in the brownish black colouration of all forms of viable and non-viable fungal cells. The GMS stain is the best special fungal stain for screening and H&E is the best stain for studying the tissue response to etiologic agents.
- **The Gridley fungus (GF) stain** colours fungal cells purplish red with a yellow background.
- **The PAS stain** is one of the most widely used stains for fungal histopathology. Aldehydes produced by the oxidation of fungal polysaccharide react with periodic acid and colour the fungi pinkish red.
- **Giemsa stain** is used primarily to detect *Histoplasma capsulatum* in blood or bone marrow.
- **Mayer's mucicarmine and alcian blue procedures** stain the mucopolysaccharide capsule of *Cryptococcus* species red and blue respectively.

II. Culture

Most pathogenic fungi are easy to grow in culture. **Sabouraud's dextrose agar** (SDA) and **4% malt extract agar** are most commonly used. These may be supplemented with chloramphenicol (50 mg/l) to minimize bacterial contamination and cycloheximide (500 mg/l) to reduce contamination with saprophytic fungi. Cycloheximide should not be added to all media because the growth of *Cryptococcus* spp., *Candida* spp., *Trichosporon* spp., *Aspergillus* spp., Mucorales, hyalohyphomycetes, yeast phase of *Histoplasma capsulatum*, *Blastomyces dermatitidis* and *Paracoccidioides brasiliensis* are completely or partially inhibited by it. Special (differential) media may be used for isolation and to help rapid identification when the identity of a particular fungus is strongly suspected. For example, *C. neoformans* develops black colonies on **bird seed agar**. Specimens for the isolation of fungi are inoculated on slants or agar plates. When slants are used, the culture tube should be large enough (2 × 15 cm) to provide a wide surface area for growth. The screw caps should be left loosened during incubation to permit an adequate supply of oxygen.

Many fungal pathogens have an optimum growth temperature below 37°C. With some dimorphic pathogens, enriched media such as **brain-heart infusion** or **blood agar** are used to promote growth of yeast phase. Many fungi grow relatively slowly and cultures should be retained for at least 2–3 weeks (in some cases up to 6 weeks) before being discarded. Growth of *Candida*, *Aspergillus*, *Mucor* and *Rhizopus* species appears within 24–72 hours. Therefore, culture should be examined for growth daily for the first week.

Once an organism has grown, it is examined for characteristic gross and microscopic structures, so that identification can be made. Pigment on the reverse side of the colony or in aerial mycelium is noted. For microscopic examination **slide mounts** should be made in **lactophenol cotton blue** (LCB). On occasion, a slide culture may be prepared, when the initial isolate fails to show conidial morphology. Characteristics that should be observed are septate versus nonseptate hyphae, hyaline or dematiaceous hyphae and the types, size, shape, and arrangement of conidia.

III. Serological tests

Positive fungal cultures can be difficult to obtain – the yield being low, growth often slow, and taking biopsy from a deep infected site may be difficult or impossible. Therefore, serological tests have been developed for the diagnosis of fungal infections. Tests for antibody have an established diagnostic use in coccidioidomycosis, paracoccidioidomycosis, aspergillosis, blastomycosis, and in some patients with histoplasmosis.

The most widely used is the assay for the detection of *Histoplasma* antigen. The test has proven useful for the detection of antigenemia in patients having disseminated disease, particularly those with acquired immunodeficiency syndrome. Serological tests have been developed commercially for detecting cryptococcal and *Candida* antigens. Detection of polysaccharide cryptococcal antigen in serum and cerebrospinal fluid by latex agglutination is a method of choice for the rapid diagnosis of meningitis and disseminated infection caused by *C. neoformans*. Latex agglutination test kits for detecting *Candida* antigens in serum are also commercially available.

IV. Molecular testing

In situ hybridization

One of the simplest approaches used has been in situ hybridization using specific nucleic acid probes for identification of organisms in patient specimens.

Polymerase chain reaction

Amplification assays using the polymerase chain reaction allow for the detection of small amounts of target DNA in clinical specimens. Specific primers with or without specific probes have been used with some success. Assays have been developed to detect DNA of *Candida*, *Aspergillus*, *Fusarium*, *Cryptococcus*, *Histoplasma*, *Blastomyces*, *Paracoccidiodes*, *Pneumocystis jirovecii*, and *Penicillium marneffei*.

Q. 3. Describe classification of mycoses.

Ans. Infection caused by fungus is known as mycosis (pl., mycoses). It can be divided into four categories:

I. Superficial mycoses

These are strictly surface infections involving skin, hair, nail and mucous membrane. These include:

- Infection of skin, hair and nail caused by dermatophytes.
- Infection of skin, nail and mucous membrane caused by *C. albicans*.
- Infection of skin caused by *Malassezia furfur* complex (pityriasis versicolor) and *Hortaea werneckii* (tinea nigra).
- Infection of hair caused by *Piedraia hortae* (black piedra) and *Trichosporon* spp. (white piedra).

II. Subcutaneous mycoses

Mycoses of the skin, subcutaneous tissues and bones result from the inoculation of saprophytic fungi of the soil or decaying vegetation leading to progressive local disease with tissue destruction and sinus formation. The lesion may spread via lymphatics. These occur mainly in the tropics and subtropics. The principal subcutaneous mycoses are mycetoma, chromoblastomycosis, sporotrichosis and rhinosporidiosis.

III. Systemic mycoses

Systemic mycoses are caused by inhalation of airborne spores/conidia produced by the fungi which are present as saprophytes in soil and on plant material. From the lungs the fungus may disseminate to CNS, bone and other internal organs. Systemic mycoses include blastomycosis, histoplasmosis, coccidioidomycosis and paracoccidioidomycosis.

IV. Opportunistic mycoses

The opportunistic mycoses are infections attributable to fungi that are normally found as human commensals or in the environment. Virtually any fungus can serve as an opportunistic pathogen, and the list of those identified as such becomes longer each year. The most common opportunistic mycoses include aspergillosis, penicilliosis, mucormycosis, candidiasis, cryptococcosis and pneumocyctosis.

I. SUPERFICIAL MYCOSES

Q. 4. Describe pathogenicity, causative agent and laboratory diagnosis of pityriasis versicolor.

Ans. Pityriasis versicolor is a mild, chronic superficial fungal infection of the stratum corneum characterized by white-brown or fawn-coloured discrete to confluent lesions covered with thin scales localized in upper trunk. It has a worldwide distribution, though it is more frequent in tropical climates. The incidence in temperate climates is much lower. It affects mainly young adults of both sexes. In tropical zones, it is also very common in infancy and even in babies.

It is caused by *Malassezia furfur* complex which are lipophilic yeast-like fungi. On the basis of their morphological features these are classified in the phylum Basidiomycota. These are common members of the normal skin flora and most infections are thought to be endogenous. The lesions may appear hypo- or hyperpigmented, depending on the degree of pigmentation of the surrounding skin. The commonest sites involved include chest, back, abdomen, neck and upper arms.

Laboratory diagnosis

KOH preparation

Scales are scraped with a scalpel and placed in a drop of 10% KOH. It is heated gently, covered with coverslip and seen under microscope. Clusters of round or oval yeast cells 2–7 μm in diameter along with short, curved and occasionally branched hyphae 2.5–4 μm in diameter can be seen (Fig. 50.2).

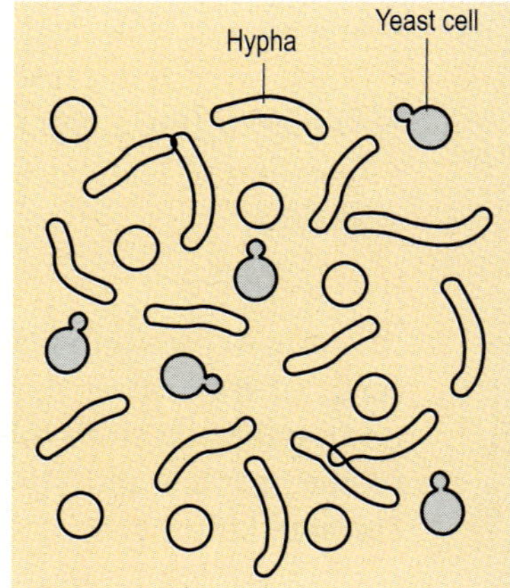

Fig. 50.2. *Malassezia furfur* complex.

Histopathology

In biopsy specimens, they can be seen with H&E stain but are best demonstrated by special stains for fungus, preferably PAS.

Culture

The fungus can be isolated from skin scrapings by inoculating it on SDA containing chloramphenicol and cycloheximide. The etiologic agent, *M. furfur* complex, will grow only on a medium that has been overlaid or supplemented with olive oil or another long chain fatty acid. Creamy colonies develop in 5–7 days at 30°C. Lactophenol cotton blue (LCB) wet mount of the colonies shows yeast-like cells measuring 1.5–4.5 × 2–6.5 μm in diameter. These cells are unique in being round at one end and bluntly cut off at the other, where budlike structures form singly on a broad base. There is no constriction at the point of conidiation. Hyphal elements are usually absent but sparse rudimentary forms may occasionally develop. Since *M. furfur* complex are part of the normal flora of the skin, therefore, positive culture does not always indicate infection.

Q. 5. Describe pathogenicity, causative agent and laboratory diagnosis of tinea nigra.

Ans. Tinea nigra is a superficial mycosis of the stratum corneum caused by traumatic inoculation from soil, wood or compost. No invasion of living tissue occurs. It is common in tropical regions of Central and South America, Africa and Asia. In Southeast Asia, this has been reported from Sri Lanka, India, southern China, Java, Sumatra and other adjoining countries. It is more common in females and the infection is more evident in young people and children.

It is characterized by single, discrete, painless, brown to black (due to an accumulation of melanin-like substance), non-scaly macules or patches affecting thickly keratinized sites such as palms and soles, and rarely other skin surfaces. Tinea nigra is so superficial that it can be scraped off with vigorous effort.

It is caused by melanized ascomycete, *Hortaea* (*Phaeoannellomyces*) *werneckii*. This organism has also been described as *Exophiala werneckii*.

Laboratory diagnosis

KOH preparation

The diagnosis is made by scraping the stratum corneum and examination of 10% KOH wet mount. It shows darkly pigmented, branched, septate, narrow hyphae (1.5–3.0 µm wide) usually accompanied by elongated budding cells (1.5–5.0 µm in diameter) (Fig. 50.3).

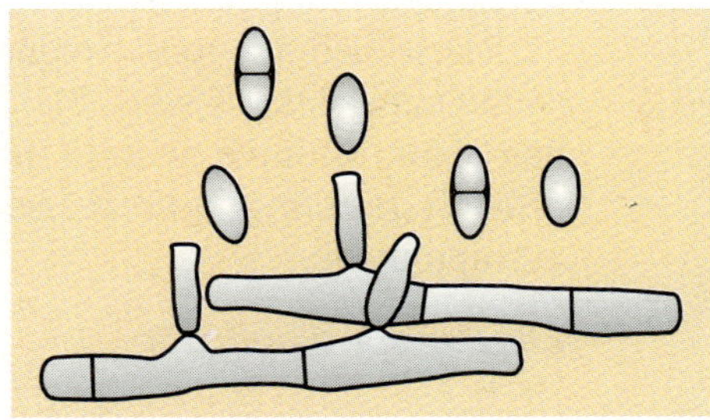

Fig. 50.3. Darkly pigmented, septate hyphae and budding cells of *Hortaea werneckii* in 10% KOH preparation.

Histopathology

A biopsy specimen can be obtained painlessly from a patient infected with tinea nigra by carefully scraping off the stratum corneum with a scalpel blade.

The organism stains well with special fungal stains, but the natural pigmentation can be best seen with H&E stain. Tissue reaction reveals mild to moderate hyperplasia and/or hyperkeratosis in the epidermis. A minimal mononuclear cell infiltrate may occur in dermis.

Fungal culture

H. werneckii can be cultured on SDA with cycloheximide. It is incubated at 25–30°C. Growth usually appears in 2–3 weeks. The colony is at first yeast-like and white to grey but quickly changes to olive or greenish-black. Microscopic examination reveals budding yeasts with 0–1 septa and hyphae. Hyphae are up to 6 µm wide, becoming thick walled, olivaceous-black, and densely septate at maturation. Conidia are produced laterally from hyphae or from the poles of budding cells by annellidic conidiogenesis. Annellated zones are conspicuous and 1–2 µm wide, with clearly visible annellations. Conidia are initially hyaline and one-celled but soon become olivaceous. After liberation they inflate and develop transverse and occasionally oblique septa. Liberated cells are converted into budding cells or chlamydoconidia-like cells.

Q. 6. Describe briefly causative agents, pathogenicity and laboratory diagnosis of black piedra and white piedra.

Ans. Piedra, meaning stone in Spanish, is an asymptomatic fungal infection of the hair shaft, resulting in the formation of **nodules** of different hardness on the infected hair. The infection is also known as **trichomycosis nodularis**. The nodules are concretions of hyphae and fruiting bodies of the fungus from which fungal spores are released. Both sexes and people of all ages are equally affected. Two varieties of piedra are seen – black piedra and white piedra.

1. Black piedra

It is caused by *Piedraia hortae*, an **ascomycetous fungus**. It occurs in the tropical and subtropical areas of Africa, Asia and South America. The fungus is believed to exist in the soil and affects monkeys as well as man. It is characterized by the presence of discrete, black, gritty, hard nodules which are composed of a mass of fungus cells on the hair shaft. The nodules vary in size from microscopic to a millimetre or more and are adherent to the hair shaft. Infection is normally restricted to scalp hair but may involve hairs of the beard, moustache and pubic hair with fungal activity limited to the cuticle.

Black piedra is more frequent than white piedra. As nodules are gritty to feel, metallic sound may be heard when hair are combed or brushed. The nodules cannot be pulled off the hair shaft. Multiple nodules may be present on a single hair, weakening the hair shaft and possibly resulting in breakage. Patients do not experience pruritis and they are otherwise asymptomatic.

Laboratory diagnosis

KOH preparation

Crushing the nodule in 10% KOH reveals dark septate hyphae around the surface of the hair with round or oval asci containing 2–8 hyaline, nonseptate banana-shaped ascospores. *P. hortae* produces sexual spores in its parasitic phase.

Fungus culture

It grows on SDA at 25°C. Growth is slow. It matures in 21 days. Colonies are small, adherent, compact, somewhat raised, and dark greenish-brown to black and may be glabrous or covered with very short aerial hyphae. Reverse is black. Microscopic examination shows closely septate, dark, and thick-walled hyphae with many intercalary chlamydoconidium-like cells. Asci may be produced in culture. The walls of the asci readily dissolve, releasing single-celled, curved ascospores (5–10 × 30–35 μm) that taper at the ends to form whiplike extensions (Fig. 50.4). Ascospores are more likely to be seen on direct microscopic examination of the specimen than on culture.

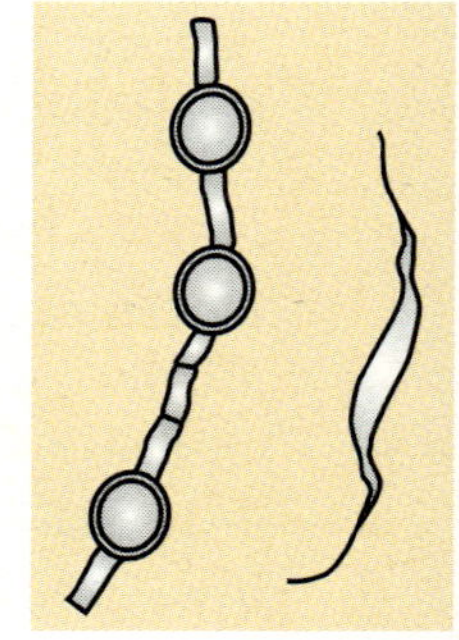

Fig. 50.4. *Piedraia hortae.*

2. White piedra

White piedra is a superficial infection of the hair shaft of the scalp, face, axillary or pubic regions. It is characterized by white, yellow or green nodules composed of hyaline septate hyphae and arthroconidia. Nodules are adhered less firmly and are softer as compared to black piedra. These vary in size from microscopic to 1 mm in diameter, and can be easily detached from the hair. The fungus grows both within and outside the hair shaft, and the hair shaft may be weakened and break off.

White piedra is caused by several *Trichosporon* species. It is considered as a basidiomycetous yeast. Genus *Trichosporon* is characterized by the production of true hyphae, pseudohyphae, arthroconidia and blastoconidia (budding yeast cells). This genus has undergone extensive taxonomic revision in 1992. Partial sequencing of the small and large subunits of the rRNA have clearly delineated numerous species. Some are soil borne and others are associated with animals and humans. Six species are of clinical significance – *T. ovoides*, *T. inkin*, *T. cutaneum*, *T. asteroides*, *T. asahii* and *T. mucoides*.

Infection of the scalp hair is caused by *T. ovoides* whereas *T. inkin* infects the pubic hair. *T. asteroides* and *T. cutaneum* have been associated with superficial skin lesions. *T. asahii* causes systemic infection with predilection for haematogenous dissemination. *T. mucoides* causes systemic infection with preference for central nervous system. The infection occurs in South America, Africa, Central and Eastern Europe, and Japan. The horse and certain species of monkey may be affected.

Laboratory diagnosis

KOH preparation

Hair mounted in 10% KOH mount reveal intertwined hyphae around the shaft which fragment into arthroconidia or produce blastoconidia 2–8 μm in diameter. The mycelial elements are held together in a cement-like substance.

Fungus culture

On SDA, *Trichosporon* spp. form cream-coloured, dry wrinkled colonies within 48–72 hours upon incubation at room temperature. The fungus is composed of septate hyphae that fragment into oval or rectangular arthroconidia. Blastoconidia are also produced (Fig. 50.5). Most *Trichosporon* species are inhibited by cycloheximide, therefore, this antibiotic should be excluded from the culture medium.

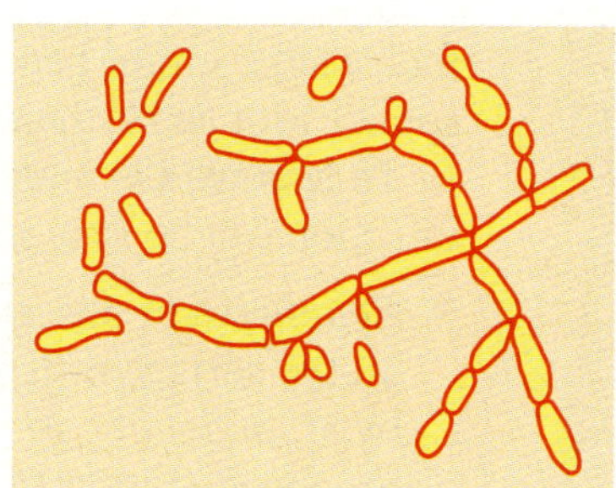

Fig. 50.5. Septate hyphae, oval or rectangular arthroconidia and blastoconidia of *Trichosporon* spp. in culture.

Q. 7. What do you understand by the term dermatophytosis? Enumerate various genera and species of dermatophytes, classify these and describe briefly their pathogenicity.

Ans. Dermatophytosis, tinea or ringworm is the most common type of superficial mycosis seen in human beings. It infects keratinized tissues of the skin, hair and nails. Dermatophytosis is caused by 41 species of dermatophytes which belong to three genera (*Trichophyton*-24, *Microsporum*-16 and *Epidermophyton*-1). Dermatophytes are filamentous fungi that are able to digest and obtain nutrients from keratin (the primary component of skin, hair and nails) by a unique enzymatic activity (keratinase).

On the basis of their natural habitats and host preferences, the dermatophytes can be classified into three groups:

1. Geophilic species

They occur as saprophytes of keratinous material (e.g., hair, feathers, horns, hooves, nails, etc.) in soil, and occasionally cause infection in man and animals. Examples are *Microsporum gypseum* and *Trichophyton ajelloi.*

2. Zoophilic species

Zoophilic dermatophytes are those whose natural hosts are animals but which may also infect man. Man acquires infection by direct and indirect contact with domestic animals (cats and dogs) and occasionally with wild animals. Examples are *T. verrucosum* and *M. canis*.

3. Anthropophilic species

A few dermatophytes have become adapted to human hosts and are termed anthropophilic. These are believed to have evolved from zoophilic fungi and are confined to man as a host. They are unable to colonise other animals and have no other environmental sources. Examples are *T. rubrum*, *M. mentegrophytes* and *Epidermophyton floccosum*.

Dermatophytes grow only on the keratinized layers of skin and its appendages and do not ordinarily penetrate the living tissues. Hypersensitivity to fungus antigens may lead to secondary eruptions occurring in sensitized patients because of circulation of allergenic products from the primary site of infection. It is known as **dermatophytid** or **id reaction**.

The *Trichophyton* spp. usually infect skin, hair and nails, *Microsporum* spp. infect skin and hair, and *Epidermophyton* spp. infect skin and nails. Clinically, ringworm can be classified depending on the site involved. Tinea corporis, tinea capitis, tinea barbae, tinea cruris, tinea manuum, tinea unguium and tinea pedis involve body, shaft of hair of scalp, beard and moustache, groin, hands, nail plates and feet respectively. The lesions are circular which spread with an erythematous border with variable degree of scaling and inflammation.

In lesions, dermatophytes appear as hyphae and arthroconidia. Three types of hair infection can be seen in 10% KOH wet mounts:

1. ***Ectothrix:*** In this, the fungus is present on the surface of hair shaft. It is caused by *M. audouinii*, *M. canis* and *T. mentagrophytes* (Fig. 50.6A).
2. ***Endothrix:*** In this, the arthroconidia are present within the hair completely filling the hair shaft without a conspicuous external sheath of arthroconidia. This is caused by *T. tonsurans* and *T. violaceum* (Fig. 50.6B).
3. ***Favus:*** In this, there is sparse hyphal growth and formation of air bubbles or tunnels and fat droplets within the hair shaft. This is caused by *T. schoenleinii* (Fig. 50.6C).

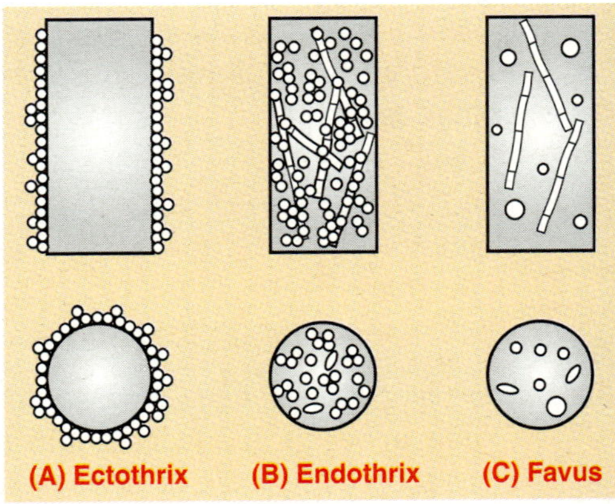

Fig. 50.6. Hair invasion of dermatophytes in longitudinal and transverse sections. (A) Ectothrix; (B) Endothrix; (C) Favus.

Q. 8. Describe laboratory diagnosis of dermatophytosis.

Ans. *KOH preparation*

The direct microscopic examination of a properly collected specimen is one of the most rapid and effective methods of detecting dermatophytes. Skin scrapings, hair stubs, and nail clipping or scrapings are collected. A drop of 10% KOH is placed on a slide, a small amount of specimen is added to the drop, a coverslip is placed over it and the preparation is gently heated. KOH softens and clears the specimen for easier detection of hyphae by digesting any proteinaceous debris and disrupting the keratin cellular sheets, thereby rendering the more biochemically resistant fungus more visible as highly refractile, septate branched or unbranched hyphae (2–4 μm in diameter) and arthroconidia.

In hairs, fungal elements may appear as arthroconidia on the outside (ectothrix invasion) of the hair shaft, or within the hair completely filling the hair shaft (endothrix), or they may appear as hyphae co-occurring, with bubbles and channels (favic invasion). Fungal hyphae must be differentiated from a variety of hypha-like artifacts such as cotton wool and synthetic fibres and from so-called mosaic fungus. The last artifact consists of cholesterol crystals deposited around the periphery of epidermal cells. It can be recognized by its regularity of outline and abrupt changes in width.

Calcofluor white stain

Calcofluor white stain, a fluorescent dye, binds to chitin and cellulose in fungus cell wall and fluoresces on excitation by long-wave ultraviolet rays or short-wave visible light. This increases the sensitivity of the direct examination; however, this requires a fluorescence microscope. Calcofluor white can be combined with KOH for rapid clearance of the specimens. Although background elements may also fluoresce, the fungal components are generally brighter and readily recognizable.

Culture method

Culture is available adjunct to direct microscopy. The clinical specimen should be inoculated on Sabouraud dextrose agar (SDA) with cycloheximide and chloramphenicol, and dermatophyte test medium (DTM). Both these media contain cycloheximide to inhibit saprophytes contaminating molds, e.g., *Penicillium* and *Aspergillus*. DTM incorporates gentamicin, and chlortetracycline to inhibit bacteria and a phenol red indicator that changes colour from yellow to red within 14 days when the medium becomes alkaline as a result of growth of dermatophytes. However, many non-dermatophytes also turn this medium red giving false-positive results, and isolates often exhibit atypical colonial and microscopic characteristics when grown on DTM. It cannot be used to study pigment production because of the intense red colour of the indicator.

In cultures on SDA, dermatophytes form characteristic colonies consisting of septate hyphae and two types of asexual spores, microconidia and macroconidia. Sexual spores of some species have also been identified. The differentiation of the three genera is based mainly on the nature of macroconidia (Table 50.1 and Fig. 50.7).

Trichophyton

Colonies may be powdery, velvety or waxy with pigmentation characteristic of different species. Macroconidia are usually rare but microconidia are abundant. The latter are arranged

Table 50.1. Generic characteristics of dermatophyte macroconidia

Genus	Frequency	Size	Number of septations	Thickness of wall	Surface of wall	Manner of attachment
Microsporum	Very numerous (except *M. audouinii*)	5–100 × 3–8 µm	3–15	Thick (except *M. gypseum* and *M. nanum*)	Rough	Singly
Trichophyton	Usually rare	20–50 × 4–6 µm	2–8	Thin	Smooth	Singly
Epidermophyton	Numerous	20–40 × 6–8 µm	2–4	Both thin and slightly thick	Smooth	Singly or in clusters

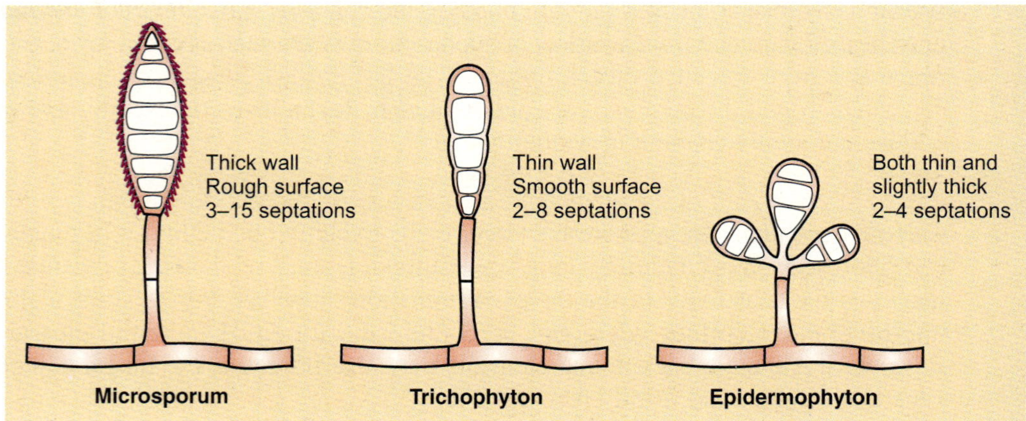

Fig. 50.7. Macroconidia in the three genera of dermatophytes.

in clusters along the hyphae or borne on conidiophores. Some species possess special types of hyphae, i.e., spiral hyphae, racket hyphae and favic chandeliers (Fig. 50.8). Fungi of this genus can infect skin, hair and nails. ***T. rubrum* is the most common species infecting man.**

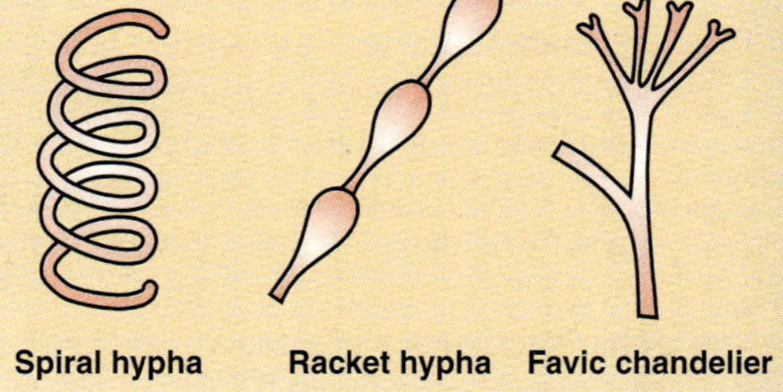

Fig. 50.8. Special types of hyphae in dermatophytes.

Microsporum

Colonies of the fungi of this genus are cottony, velvety or powdery with white to brown pigmentation. Macroconidia are very numerous and microconidia are relatively scanty. They infect skin and hair but not the nails.

Epidermophyton

Colonies are powdery and greenish-yellow. Microconidia are absent and macroconidia are club-shaped and are arranged in groups of two or three. It infects skin and nails but not the hairs.

Hair perforation test

Hair perforation test is useful in differentiating *T. rubrum* from *T. mentagrophytes*. To observe hair perforation, short (5–10 mm) strands of human hair (ideally hair from an under 18-month-old child) are placed in a petri dish with 20 ml of distilled water and autoclaved. Two to three drops of 10% sterilized yeast extract are added to the petri dish and hair strands are inoculated with small fragments of test fungus grown on SDA. It is incubated at 25–30°C and the hair strands are removed and microscopically examined in lactophenol cotton blue at weekly intervals for up to 1 month. ***T. rubrum* which may be morphologically similar to *T. mentagrophytes*, usually causes only surface erosion of hair shafts in this test, whereas *T. mentagrophytes* causes wedge-shaped perforation perpendicular to the hair shaft** (Fig. 50.9).

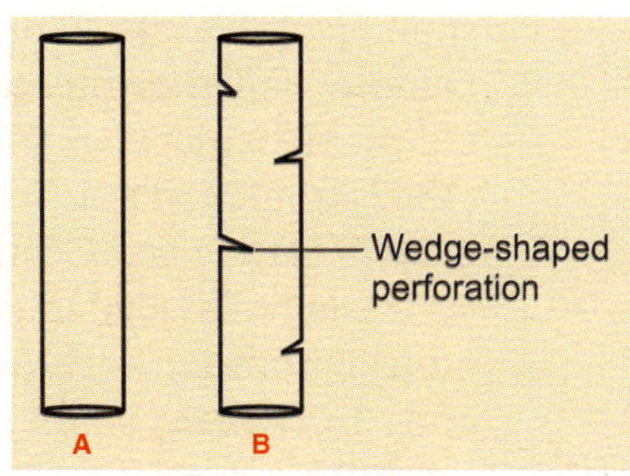

Fig. 50.9. Hair perforation test: (A) Normal hair; (B) Hair showing wedge-shaped perforations.

Urease test

Urease test is useful for distinguishing isolate of *T. mentagrophytes* from that of *T. rubrum*. Urease splits urea in Christensen's medium, producing ammonia which raises the pH and causes a colour shift of the phenol red indicator from amber to bright pink. For example, *T. mentagrophytes* produces a bright pink colour (positive), while *T. rubrum* produces no colour change (negative). A tube of Christensen's urea agar is very lightly inoculated with the dermatophyte and incubated at 25–30°C for 7 days. A positive reaction is indicated by a change of the original colour to bright pink.

II. SUBCUTANEOUS MYCOSES

Q. 9. What do you understand by the term mycetoma? Describe briefly its pathogenicity, types, causative agents and laboratory diagnosis.

Ans. Mycetoma is a chronic granulomatous infection usually of exposed parts of the body especially feet and hands (Figs. 50.10 and 50.11). Infection follows traumatic inoculation of

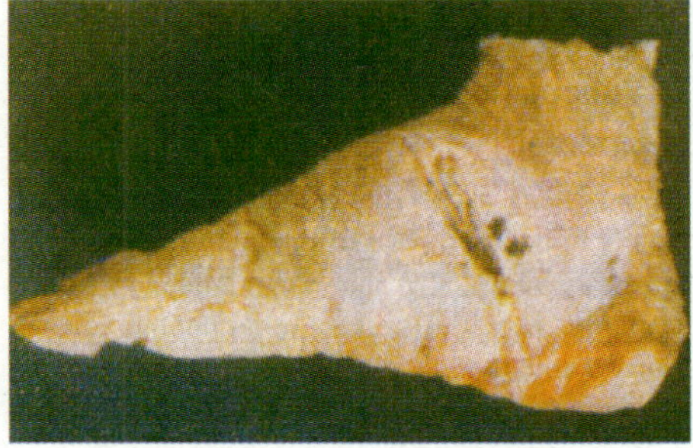

Fig. 50.10. Mycetoma foot showing black granules.

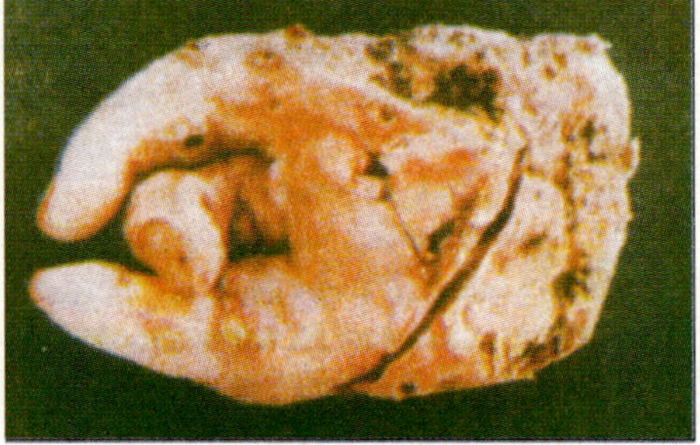

Fig. 50.11. Mycetoma hand showing black granules.

the organism into the subcutaneous tissue from soil or vegetable sources, e.g., thorns or splinters and results in **tumefactions, deformities and draining sinuses discharging fungal colonies called grains or granules (triad of symptoms)**. Granules are white, yellow, pink, red or black depending upon the species of etiologic agent. It was first reported by Gill (1842) from Madurai, South India. The disease is prevalent in tropical and subtropical regions of Asia, Africa and Central America.

It can be divided into three types, **eumycetomas**, **actinomycetomas** and **botryomycosis**. Important causative agents of these are given in Table 50.2. Grains can be mounted in a drop of 10% KOH on a slide and crushed under a coverglass. Observation of the colour of the grains, and the size and septations of the hyphae allow differentiation between actinomycetoma and eumycetoma. In actinomycetoma, the grains are composed of very thin filaments (0.5–1 µm in diameter) with coccoid and bacillary elements while in eumycetoma they are broad (2–6 µm in diameter), septate and often have large, globose swollen cells (up to 15 µm or more) at the margin. Grains are crushed between two slides and then heat fixed. Filaments of the actinomycotic grain are Gram-positive and the cement substance and peripheral fringe are Gram-negative. However, Gram stain, in general is of limited value in demonstrating the presence of eumycetes, though some eumycetes are Gram-positive. *Madurella mycetomatis* and *Actinomadura madurae* are the most common causes of eumycetoma and actinomycetoma respectively.

Table 50.2. Important causative agents and colour of the grains of various types of mycetoma

Causative agent	Colour of the grains
A. ***Eumycetoma***	
• *Madurella mycetomatis*	Brown to black
• *M. grisea*	Brown to black
• *Exophiala jeanselmei*	Brown to black
• *Curvularia geniculata*	Brown to black
• *Leptosphaeria senegalensis*	Brown to black
• *Pseudallescheria boydii*	White to yellow
• *Acremonium falciforme*	White to yellow
• *Aspergillus nidulans*	White
• *Fusarium* species	White
B. ***Actinomycetoma***	
• *Actinomadura madurae*	White to yellow
• *A. pellitieri*	Red to pink
• *Nocardia asteroides*	White to yellow
• *N. brasiliensis*	White
• *Nocardiopsis dassonvillei*	Cream
• *Streptomyces somaliensis*	Yellow
C. ***Botryomycosis***	
• *Staphylococcus aureus*	White
• *Escherichia coli*	White
• *Proteus* species	White
• *Pseudomonas aeruginosa*	White

Q. 10. What do you understand by the term chromoblastomycosis? Enumerate its causative agents, pathogenicity and laboratory diagnosis.

Ans. Chromoblastomycosis is a chronic, localized fungal infection of skin and subcutaneous tissue, characterized by crusted, warty lesions usually involving lower legs. It is caused by several darkly pigmented, soil inhabiting phaeoid (dematiaceous) fungi. These include *Phialophora verrucosa*, *Fonsecaea pedrosoi*, *F. compacta*, *Cladosporium carrionii* and *Rhinocladiella aquaspersa*. Infection occurs following a wound or slight abrasion of the skin which is contaminated with soil or vegetable matter containing any of these fungi. The disease has been reported from most parts of the world, but it is more common in tropical and subtropical regions of the Americas and Africa. The causative organisms have been isolated from soil and decaying vegetation in high-prevalence areas. It more often involves males and those who work outdoor without footwear. Lesions develop most commonly on the distal lower extremities, a location compatible with exposure of damaged skin to soil.

- **The primary skin lesion** is a small papule that gradually enlarges over weeks to months to form a superficial nodule with an irregular, friable surface. Lesions continue to evolve over many years.
- **The verrucous lesions** are warty and hyperkeratotic.
- **Tumorous lesions** are larger than nodular lesions, with raised surface projections that may be covered by crusting and epidermal debris. These lesions can become very large, and their surface texture has been compared with that of cauliflower.
- **Plaque lesions**, the least common type, are flat, reddish and scaly.
- **Cicatricial (scarring) lesions** have irregular borders and expand at their periphery with central healing and scarring. "Black dots" may be observed on the surface of lesions. Samples of material from these areas are particularly useful for microscopic examination.

Tissue reaction in skin shows a characteristic pseudoepitheliomatous hyperplasia with hyperkeratosis and parakeratosis. Inflammation is generally granulomatous. It is often accompanied by a suppurative reaction, possibly from a secondary reaction, causing satellite microabscesses.

Laboratory diagnosis

1. Superficial crusts scraped from the lesions, preferably from an area containing "black dots", contain long, brown, branching hyphae (3–5 μm in diameter) which are easily seen upon microscopic examination after digestion in potassium hydroxide.
2. In pus, granulation tissue obtained by curettage, or in biopsy specimens of epidermis and subcutaneous tissue, the fungus is present in the form of rounded, thick walled, brown cells with a diameter of 5–12 μm. They have horizontal and/or vertical septations. They reproduce by equatorial splitting and not by budding. They are known as **sclerotic bodies** (Fig. 50.12). These structures were at one time thought to be budding yeast cells, resulting in the name chromoblastomycosis (*chromo*: coloured, *blasto*: budding, *mycosis*: fungal infection). Sclerotic bodies are seen within giant cells, rarely in macrophages or extra-cellularly in microabscesses. **The fungi typically migrate to the surface of the skin and are seen as "black dots" in the keratin scales.**

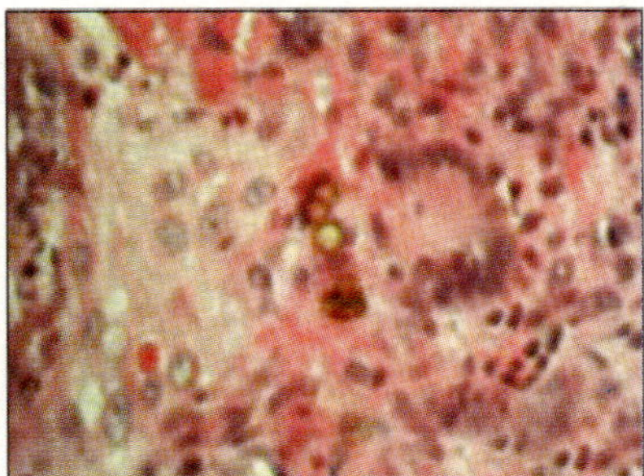

Fig. 50.12. Chromoblastomycosis showing sclerotic bodies.

3. Because the causative agents cannot be distinguished on the basis of histologic features, culture of lesion material is necessary. Crusts, pus, and biopsy material are inoculated on culture media both with and without antibiotics because of the possibility of bacterial contamination, and inoculated plates should be incubated at both 25°C and 30°C. In most cases colonies are formed within 2 weeks; but cultures should be held for 4 weeks before being reported as negative.

Q. 11. Write short note on phaeohyphomycosis.

Ans. It is a mycotic infection caused by phaeoid (dematiaceous, brown-pigmented) fungi where the tissue morphology of the causative organism is mycelial. This separates it from other clinical types of disease involving brown-pigmented fungi where the tissue morphology of the organism is a grain (eumycotic mycetoma) or sclerotic body (chromoblastomycosis). Phaeohyphomycosis may be divided into four disease categories – superficial (tinea nigra and black piedra), cutaneous and corneal, subcutaneous, and systemic.

Common causative agents of subcutaneous phaeohyphomycosis are *Cladosporium bantiana*, *Ochroconis gallopavum*, *Wangiella dermatitidis*, *Curvularia* spp., *Bipolaris* spp., *Exophilia jeanselmei*, *Nattrasia mangiferae*, *Alternaria* spp. and *Exserohilum* spp.

Laboratory diagnosis

The diagnosis of phaeohyphomycosis is established in the laboratory by KOH mount, histopathology and culture. There are no available serologic tests to diagnose infection with these fungi.

KOH mount

The aspirates from cysts, curettings from the cutaneous and corneal lesions, and biopsy material are examined in KOH wet mount. In case of phaeohyphomycosis, the fungus is present in the form of darkly pigmented septate hyphae 2–6 µm in diameter.

Histopathology

The pathological features are similar regardless of the etiologic agent. In systemic phaeohyphomycosis lesions of a given organ may occur as single or multiple abscesses. The abscesses are usually circumscribed and encapsulated granulomas, the walls of which comprise epithelial histiocytes and giant cells surrounded by connective tissue. The centre of the granulomas contain necrotic debris, fibrin, and degenerated polymorphonuclear cells.

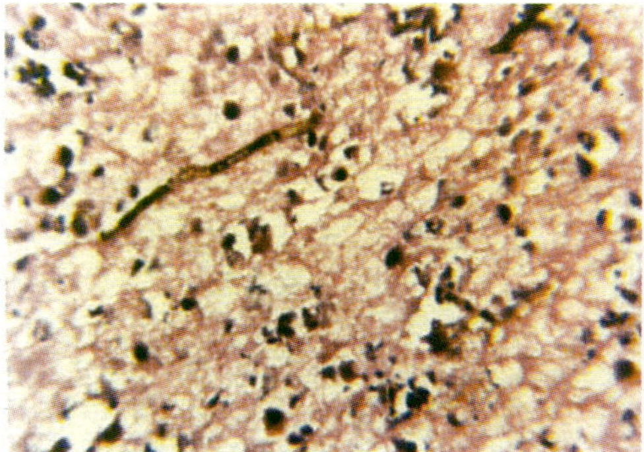

Fig. 50.13. Phaeohyphomycosis showing brown septate fungal hypha.

Within the necrotic debris and inflammatory infiltrates, as well as in the giant cells, fungal elements can be observed. The fungus in the tissue is present in the form of darkly pigmented, septate hyphae (2–6 µm in diameter) (Fig. 50.13) and pseudohyphae. Large, bizarre, thick-walled vesicular swellings (up to 25 µm in diameter), resembling chlamydoconidia may be seen along, or at the end of the hyphae. Yeast-like cells producing buds singly or in chains are also commonly present. **Special fungal stains such as Gomori methenamine silver and periodic acid-Schiff mask the natural colour of the hyphae, but in haematoxylin and eosin sections the brown colour may be obvious.** In some cases, however, the hyphae appear unpigmented and a specific stain for melanin, Masson Fontana stain, must be used to reveal the presence of the fungal pigment.

Q. 12. Describe pathogenicity, causative agent and laboratory diagnosis of rhinosporidiosis.

Ans. Rhinosporidiosis is a chronic granulomatous disease characterized by the development of pedunculated or sessile, red, spongy, friable, polypoid, granulomatous growths in the nose, conjunctiva and occasionally in ears, larynx, bronchus, penile urethra, vagina, rectum and skin. It was thought to be caused by a fungus, *Rhinosporidium seeberi*, but all attempts at isolation from clinical material failed. On the basis of modern molecular based studies, it is now considered to be a **hydrophilic protistan** hence called pseudofungal organism.

Taxonomically, it is now included, along with some fish and amphibian pathogens, in a new clade – **Mesomycetozoa**. It is known to infect not only humans but a large variety of domestic and wild animals in all the continents except Australia. More than 90% of cases have been reported from India, Sri Lanka and South America. In India, sporadic cases occur all over but endemic foci exist in parts of Orissa, Andhra Pradesh, Kerala, Chennai and Raipur (Chhatisgarh). Very rarely, there is haematogenous spread with metastatic lesions in the lungs, brain and bones.

***Rhinosporidium seeberi* has not been cultured and animal inoculation is also not successful.** Nothing definite is known about the mode of transmission of infection. However, it has been suggested that the organism is transmitted in dust or water. It is believed that fish may be the natural hosts of *R. seeberi*. Infection is more common in:

- Persons bathing in muddy stagnant pools of water.
- Those who dive into streams to collect sand from riverbeds.
- Paddy cultivators.
- In dry areas, after dust storm and eye injuries.

Laboratory diagnosis

The definitive diagnosis of rhinosporidiosis depends on the histopathological examination of biopsied or resected tissues. The infected tissue shows hyperplasia with a chronic granulomatous inflammatory response. Lymphocytes, plasma cells, macrophages, giant cells and, rarely eosinophils are usually found around the spherical phenotypes of *R. seeberi*. **Large numbers of sporangia at different stages of development are a main feature of the histopathologic tissue sections.** Active macrophages are also seen with engulfed endoconidia. However, sufficient numbers of endoconidia evade elimination to become immature and mature sporangia.

R. seeberi can be identified in haematoxylin and eosin stained sections, but sometimes one may need special stains such as Gomori methenamine silver (GMS) and periodic acid-Schiff (PAS) stains to demonstrate the causative agent. Sporangia can be seen with the naked eye as small white dots. The mature sporangium measures 100–500 μm in diameter and contains hundreds of endoconidia 5–20 μm in diameter (Fig. 50.14).

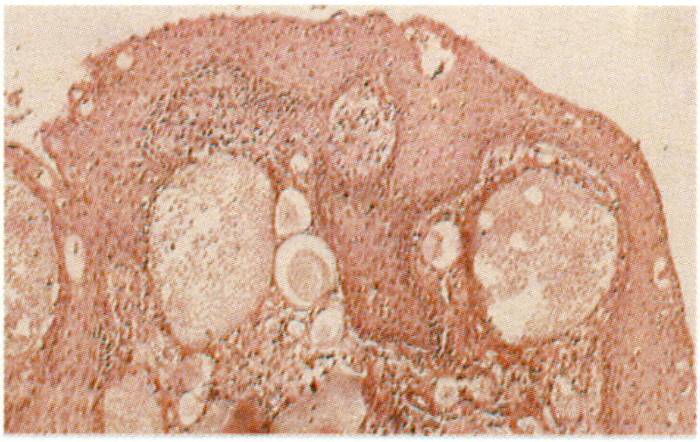

Fig. 50.14. Rhinosporidiosis showing sporangia and endoconidia.

Q. 13. Describe pathogenicity, causative agent and laboratory diagnosis of sporotrichosis.

Ans. Sporotrichosis is a chronic pyogranulomatous infection of the skin and subcutaneous tissues, although it may become disseminated by lymphatic spread. It is caused by *Sporothrix schenckii*, a dimorphic fungus. It occurs all over the world.

The fungus is found in soil, decaying wood, thorns and on infected animals, including horses, cats, rats and dogs. Infection with *S. schenckii* typically occurs by direct skin inoculation from contaminated soil or thorny plants. **Sporotrichosis is a recognized occupational hazard of farmers and gardeners.**

The initial lesion is a small ulcerated nodule commonly on the hand or the forearm. Nodules and abscesses occur along the draining lymphatics and the regional lymph nodes enlarge, suppurate and ulcerate. The primary lesion may remain localized or disseminate to involve the bones, joints, lungs and rarely CNS particularly in debilitated or immunosuppressed individuals.

In infected tissues, *S. schenckii* appears in the form of round, oval (4–6 μm), elongated or cigar-shaped yeast-like cells with irregular budding (Fig. 50.15A). With ordinary stains, they are difficult to find. The use of PAS or GMS stains and fluorescent antibody technique facilitates detection of these organisms. The abscesses may show the **asteroid body**. This consists of central budding yeast cell with eosinophilic Splendore-Hoeppli material (antibody complex) radiating from it (Fig. 50.16). In most human lesions very few yeast-like organisms can be seen. However, their number can be increased by inoculating pus from human sporotrichosis into an experimental animal such as mouse or rat.

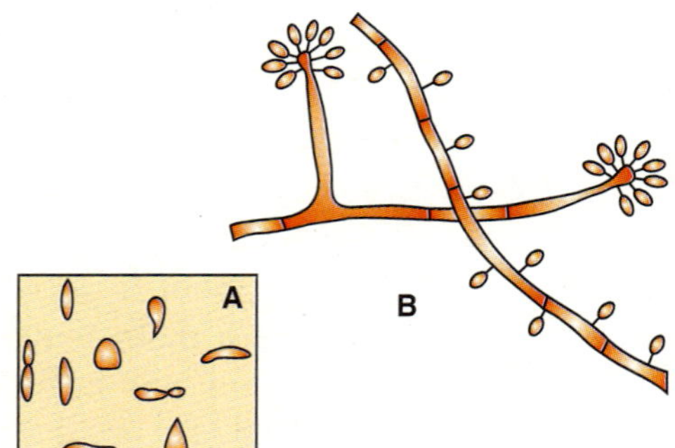

Fig. 50.15. *Sporothrix schenckii*: (A) yeast phase; and (B) mycelial phase.

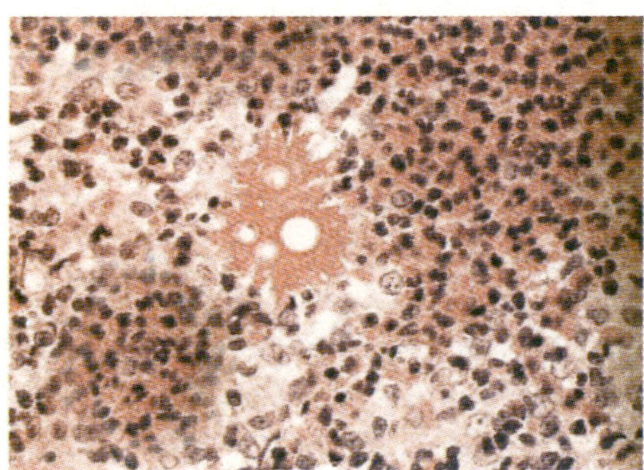

Fig. 50.16. Asteroid body in sporotrichosis. The yeast-like cells are surrounded by eosinophilic Splendore-Hoeppli material (haematoxylin and eosin stain).

The diagnosis is confirmed by isolation of the causative organism by culture of swabs from the ulcerated lesions or pus aspirated from subcutaneous nodules or biopsy material. *S. schenckii* grows well on routine agar media, and at room temperature (25–30°C). The young colonies are blackish and shiny, becoming wrinkled and fuzzy with age. Strains vary in pigmentation from shades of black and grey to whitish.

Microscopic examination reveals thin, delicate hyphae bearing conidia developing in a 'rosette' pattern at the ends of delicate conidiophores. Conidia are also produced along the sides of the hyphae (Fig. 50.15B). To induce mycelial to yeast conversion, the fungus is inoculated on blood agar tubes and incubated at 37°C. The formation of yeast colonies may require several subcultures. Complete conversion seldom occurs, but a portion of the colony will develop cigar-shaped yeast-like cells.

A **latex agglutination test**, for detection of antibodies against *S. schenckii*, is available for the diagnosis of the extracutaneous forms of sporotrichosis.

A **skin test** with sporotrichin antigen is positive in all patients with cutaneous sporotrichosis.

III. SYSTEMIC MYCOSES

Q. 14. Describe pathogenicity, epidemiology, causative agent and laboratory diagnosis of histoplasmosis.

Ans. Histoplasmosis is an intracellular mycosis of reticuloendothelial system involving lymphatic tissues, lungs, spleen, liver, adrenals, kidneys, skin, central nervous system and other organs of the body. It is caused by a dimorphic fungus, *Histoplasma capsulatum*. Taxonomically, *H. capsulatum* has been divided into three varieties – *H. capsulatum* var. *capsulatum*, *H. capsulatum* var. *duboisii*, and *H. capsulatum* var. *farciminosum*. Histoplasmosis caused by these fungi is known as histoplasmosis capsulati, histoplasmosis duboisii and histoplasmosis farciminosi respectively.

The most important clinical entity is caused by *H. capsulatum* var. *capsulatum*. It is cosmopolitan, being endemic in all the continents of the world. The *duboisii* variety is restricted to the central part of the African continent between the tropics of Cancer and Capricorn, and to the offshore island of Madagascar in the Indian Ocean. The *farciminosum* variety is endemic in Africa, eastern Europe, the Middle East, Asia and the Far East. All the three varieties occur as saprophytes in the soil.

Pathogenicity

H. capsulatum var. *capsulatum* grows in soil with high nitrogen content. The growth of the fungus appears to be most frequently associated with soil enriched by excreta of bats, chickens and other birds. This provides high nitrogen content. The organism has been isolated from bat caves, bird roosts, chicken houses and similar environments. Bat and bird excreta provide an excellent medium for enrichment of *H. capsulatum* var. *capsulatum*.

Disturbances of such sites create aerosols laden with infectious propagules of *H. capsulatum* var. *capsulatum*. When inhaled, these aerosols result in infections. Histoplasmosis is ordinarily an asymptomatic or relatively mild, self-limiting pulmonary infection, although chronic or acute disseminated disease with poor prognosis may occur. In addition, it may also involve lymph nodes, spleen, liver, adrenals, kidneys, skin, CNS and other organs of the body. Granulomatous and ulcerative lesions may develop on the skin and mucosa.

In tissues, *H. capsulatum* var. *capsulatum* is present inside phagocytic cells in yeast phase. They are round or oval, yeast-like cells, 2–5 μm in diameter with budding on a narrow base at the smaller end. They reproduce within monocytes or macrophages. They fill the cytoplasm of macrophages, monocytes and occasionally polymorphonuclear leucocytes.

Some organisms may be found free in the tissues also. With Giemsa or Wright stains, the cell wall and the cell protoplasm stain light blue and dark blue respectively.

With H&E staining, only a central protoplasmic mass surrounded by a halo is seen (Fig. 50.17). Only a dark staining can outline the cell wall. In the PAS stain, the wall is stained pink to purplish red with pallor coloured protoplasm filling the cell. In the GMS stain the cell wall stains intense black (Fig. 50.18). The so called 'capsule' of *H. capsulatum* var. *capsulatum* is considered to be an artifact resulting from the shrinkage of the protoplasm within the cell wall. The yeast phase of *H. capsulatum* var. *capsulatum* should be carefully differentiated from other intracellular parasites such as *Toxoplasma gondii*, *Leishmania* spp., and *Trypanosoma cruzi*.

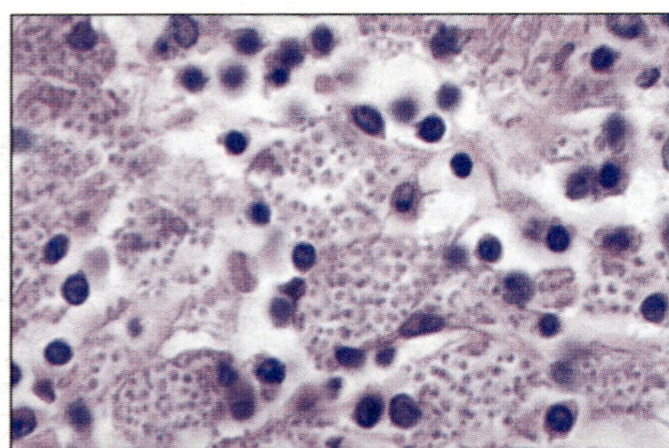

Fig. 50.17. Section of skin stained with haematoxylin and eosin showing *Histoplasma capsulatum* surrounded by clear halo filling the cytoplasm of phagocytes.

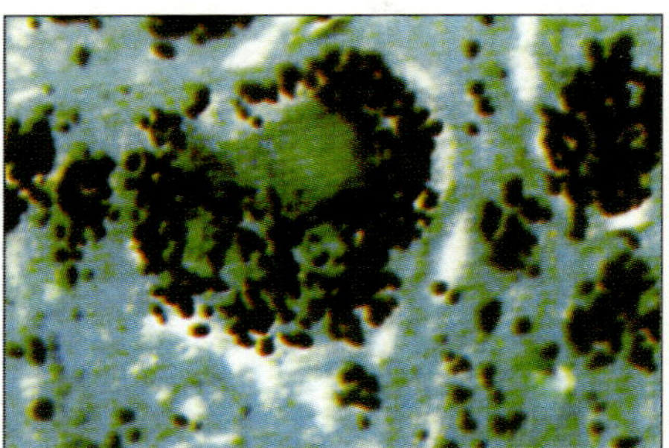

Fig. 50.18. Section similar to that demonstrated in Fig. 50.21 but stained with Gomori methanamine silver staining. It shows black budding yeast cells.

Culture

On SDA, at 25–30°C, it forms white to tan fluffy colony with septate branching hyphae with two types of unicellular, asexual spores:

1. Large round, tuberculate macroconidia (8–14 μm) are most prominent and are diagnostic.
2. Small spores or microconidia usually appear first. They are sessile or stalked, smooth-walled, round to pyriform, 2–5 μm in diameter (Fig. 50.19A). The yeast phase cells (2–5 μm) can also be produced *in vitro* by culture at 35–37°C on brain-heart-infusion agar (Fig. 50.19B).

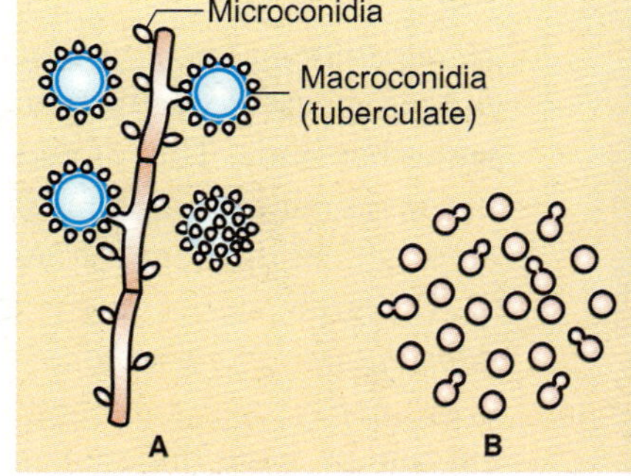

Fig. 50.19. *Histoplasma capsulatum*: (A) mycelial phase; and (B) yeast phase.

Laboratory diagnosis

Diagnosis may be made by microscopic examination of sputum or pus smear stained by Wright or Giemsa procedures. Blood smears may be positive for *H. capsulatum* var. *capsulatum*, especially in patients with AIDS. Liver or lung biopsies stained with PAS or GMS may provide a rapid diagnosis of disseminated histoplasmosis in some patients. *H. capsulatum* var. *capsulatum* is seen as small, oval yeast cells, typically packed within macrophages or monocytes. Specimen should be cultured on SDA at 25–30°C to obtain the mycelial phase. Mold cultures of *H. capsulatum* var. *capsulatum* are a hazard to laboratory staff and consequently test-tube slopes rather than petri dishes should be used for isolation.

Serological tests like latex agglutination, precipitation and complement fixation become positive two weeks after infection. Tests for antigen detection by radioimmunoassay or ELISA are useful but are not widely available. Delayed hypersensitivity to the fungus can be demonstrated by histoplasmin skin test.

Q. 15. Write short note on *Histoplasma capsulatum* var. *duboisii* or African histoplasmosis.

Ans. African histoplasmosis is caused by *H. capsulatum* var. *duboisii*. It is mainly restricted to the continent of Africa. It primarily involves skin, subcutaneous tissue and bones with little evidence of involvement of lungs. *H. capsulatum* var. *duboisii* is morphologically identical to *H. capsulatum* var. *capsulatum* in its mycelial phase but differs in the yeast phase both *in vivo* and *in vitro*. In parasitized tissues and in cultures on brain-heart-infusion agar incubated at 35–37°C it forms thick-walled (upto 1.5 µm) yeasts measuring 12–15 µm in diameter that are distinct from those of *H. capsulatum* var. *capsulatum* (2–5 µm in diameter).

Q. 16. Write short note on *Histoplasma capsulatum* var. *farciminosum* or histoplasmosis farciminosi.

Ans. *Histoplasma capsulatum* var. *farciminosum* causes histoplasmosis farciminosi. It causes subcutaneous and ulcerated lesions of the skin, particularly of the front legs and neck, and at the site of the injury. The mycosis involves the lymphatics and may be disseminated to many organs. Diagnosis can be made by detection of the tissue-form cells of the dimorphic *H. capsulatum* var. *farciminosum*. The fungus in tissue is similar to *H. capsulatum* var. *capsulatum*. They measure 2.5–3.5 × 2.0–3.0 µm and are found intracellular within phagocytes. It can be cultured on a variety of fungal media including enriched SDA with 2.5% glycerol, and brain-heart-infusion agar with or without 5% sheep blood. This organism grows as a mycelium at cooler temperatures. The colonies grow slowly and develop in 2–8 weeks at 25°C. They are dry, granular, wrinkled and grayish-white, becoming brown as they age.

On microscopic examination the hyphae are hyaline, septate, branched and pleomorphic. A variety of conidia including arthroconidia, blastoconidia and chlamydoconidia may be found, but *H. capsulatum* var. *farciminosum* does not produce the large, round, thick-walled macroconidia often seen in *H. capsulatum* var. *capsulatum* culture.

Mycelial phase can be converted to yeast phase by growing the isolates at 37°C on brain-heart-infusion agar with or without 5% sheep blood. The yeast phase forms colonies that are flat, raised, wrinkled, white to grayish brown and pasty. Complete conversion occurs only after repeated serial transfers to fresh media.

Q. 17. Describe pathogenicity, causative agent and laboratory diagnosis of blastomycosis.

Ans. Blastomycosis, formerly known as North American blastomycosis, is a chronic infection of the lungs which may spread to other tissues, particularly skin, bone and genitourinary tract.

Chest radiograph may resemble that of tuberculosis or carcinoma. Disseminated blastomycosis may develop in immunosuppressed patients including those with AIDS. It is caused by *Blastomyces dermatitidis*, a dimorphic fungus.

The infectious particles of *B. dermatitidis* are its mycelial fragments and conidia. The respiratory tract is the portal of entry for all forms of blastomycosis except direct transcutaneous inoculation. In the alveoli, the organism transforms into the yeast and induces an acute inflammatory response that includes neutrophils and macrophages, resulting in granuloma formation.

The most common clinical presentation is a pulmonary infiltrate in association with a variety of symptoms indistinguishable from other acute lower respiratory infections. Patients can also present with chronic pneumonia.

Culture

In tissue or culture on brain-heart-infusion agar at 37°C, *B. dermatitidis* grows as a thick-walled multinucleated spherical yeast (8–15 μm) that usually produces single buds. The bud and the parent yeast are attached with a broad base (Fig. 50.20A), and the bud often enlarges to the same size as the parent yeast before it becomes detached. The yeast colonies are wrinkled, waxy, and soft. When grown on Sabouraud dextrose agar at 25°C, a white or brownish colony develops, with branching hyphae bearing spherical, ovoid, or pyriform conidia (2–10 μm in diameter) on short or long conidiophores or directly on the hyphae (Fig. 50.20B). Larger chlamydoconidia (7–18 μm) may also be produced.

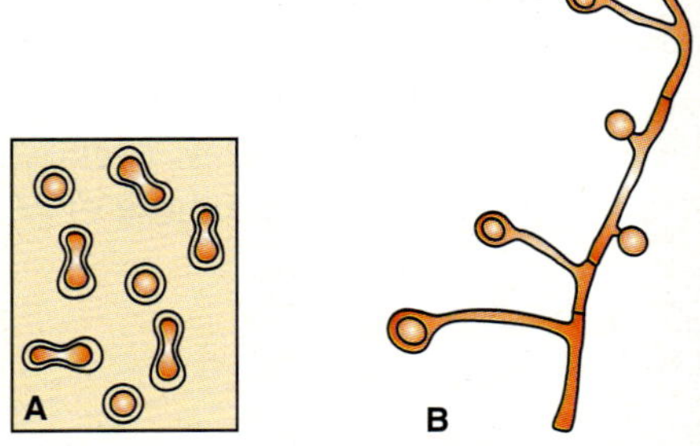

Fig. 50.20. *Blastomyces dermatitidis*: (A) yeast phase; and (B) mycelial phase.

Laboratory diagnosis

Diagnosis can be made by direct microscopy (calcofluor white, potassium hydroxide mount) and culture of sputum, pus and scrapings from skin lesions. An ELISA test that appears to be more than 90% specific has been developed.

Q. 18. Describe pathogenicity and laboratory diagnosis of paracoccidioidomycosis.

Ans. ### Pathogenicity

Paracoccidioidomycosis, formerly known as South American blastomycosis, is a chronic progressive granulomatous infection caused by *Paracoccidioides brasiliensis*, a dimorphic fungus. It is characterized by primary pulmonary infection that spreads by haematogenous route, to mucosa of the nose, mouth and the gastrointestinal tract, skin, lymphatic system, and the internal organs producing chronic granulomatous reaction. Infection is acquired usually via respiratory route by inhalation of spores from environmental sources. The fungus has been isolated from soil.

Laboratory diagnosis

- Microscopic examination of KOH wet mount of pus, crusts, sputum and biopsies from granulomatous lesions usually shows numerous yeast cells (10–60 μm) with multiple buds. The buds are attached to the mother cell (resembling 'pilot wheel') by very narrow necks (Fig. 50.21A).

- Tissue sections should be stained with H&E, PAS and GMS.
- The tissue form (yeast phase) may be obtained *in vitro* by inoculation of clinical material on enriched media such as brain-heart-infusion agar and incubating at 35–37°C.
- Mycelial (mold) phase of the fungus develops on SDA incubated at 25–30°C. It shows septate hyphae bearing intercalary and terminal chlamydoconidia. A few microconidia are sometimes observed along the hyphae (Fig. 50.21B).

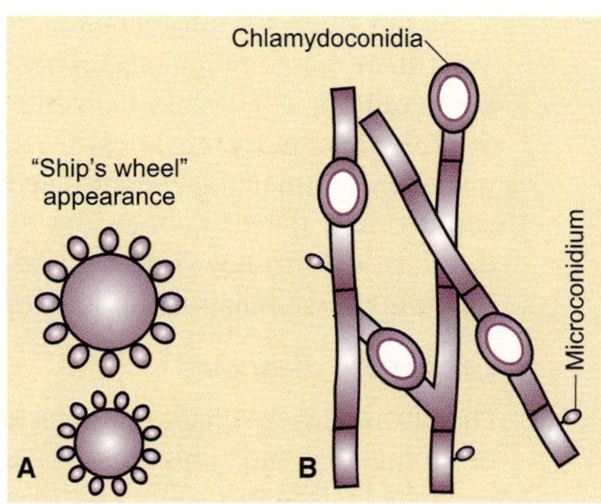

Fig. 50.21. *Paracoccidioides brasiliensis*: (A) yeast phase; and (B) mycelial phase.

- The tests for antibody detection like immunodiffusion, complement fixation and ELISA are useful for diagnosis and prognosis.

Q. 19. Describe pathogenicity, causative agent and laboratory diagnosis of coccidioidomycosis.

Ans. Coccidioidomycosis is primarily an infection of the lungs caused by *Coccidioides immitis*, a dimorphic fungus. It exists as a saprophyte in the soil. The arthroconidia of the saprophytic phase are carried by the wind and are inhaled by man and animals.

Patients with *C. immitis* infection may have chronic pneumonia, fungaemia, and extrapulmonary dissemination to skin, bones, meninges, and other body sites. The clinical features of coccidioidomycosis may mimic melioidosis, penicilliosis, and tuberculosis.

C. immitis differs from other dimorphic fungi because under standard laboratory conditions **it grows as a mold at 25°C as well as 37°C**. Only when grown on special Converse medium with increased CO_2 at 37–40°C is the spherule or tissue phase formed *in vitro* (Fig. 50.22A). The hyphae develop barrel-shaped arthroconidia measuring 2.5–4 × 3–6 µm. They characteristically alternate with smaller intervening empty cells (Fig. 50.22B). The walls of empty cells break easily and are characteristically present on either side of the freed conidia. The latter are highly infectious and are readily airborne, therefore, the handling of a well developed culture is hazardous. ***C. immitis* is probably the most virulent of all human mycotic agents. The inhalation of only a few arthroconidia produces primary coccidioidomycosis. It has been included as a select agent of bioterrorism.**

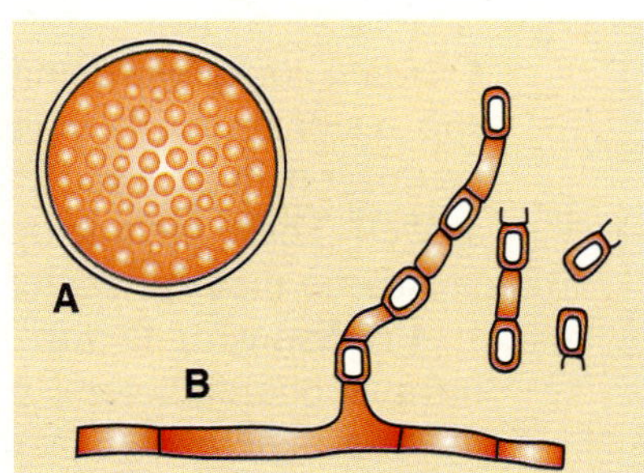

Fig. 50.22. *Coccidioides immitis*: (A) tissue phase; (B) mycelial phase.

In the lungs, the arthroconidia form **spherules** (30–100 μm or more in diameter). These contain numerous **endoconidia**, 2–4 μm in diameter (Figs. 50.22A and 50.23). The mature spherules have double wall measuring 2 μm in thickness. At maturity, the spherules rupture and their endoconidia are released which develop to form new spherules in adjacent tissue or following dissemination, in other organs of the body.

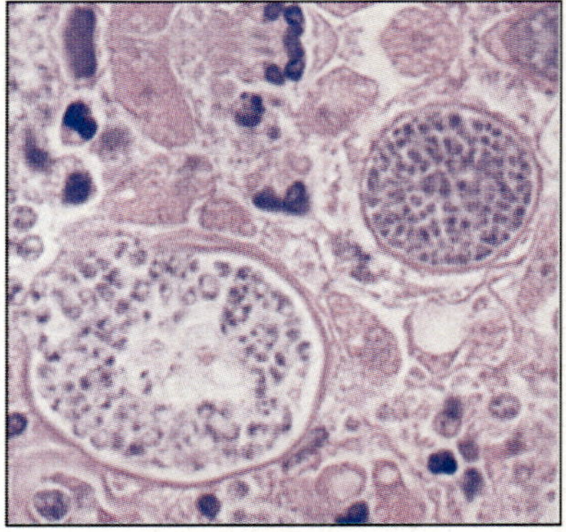

Fig. 50.23. Spherules of *Coccidioides immitis* containing endoconidia.

Laboratory diagnosis

Diagnosis may be made by microscopic examination of sputum, pus and biopsy material and culture on SDA incubated at 25–30°C. **Since arthroconidia are highly infectious and readily airborne, therefore, petri dish should not be used for isolation of *C. immitis* and all procedures should be carried out in a safety cabinet.**

IV. OPPORTUNISTIC MYCOSES

Q. 20. Describe causative agents, pathogenesis and clinical features of candidiasis.

Ans.

Causative agents

The genus *Candida* comprises about 200 species, of which about 20 have been associated with pathology in humans and animals. The major pathogenic species include *C. albicans*, *C. dubliniensis*, *C. glabrata*, *C. guilliermondii*, *C. kefyr*, *C. krusei*, *C. lusitaniae*, *C. parapsilosis* and *C. tropicalis*. *C. albicans* is round to oval yeast 3–6 μm in diameter. It produces budding cells, pseudohyphae, and true hyphae. This ability to simultaneously display several morphological forms is known as **polymorphism**.

Pathogenesis

Candida is a human commensal, so that the source of infection is mostly endogenous. *Candida* spp. reside primarily in the gastrointestinal tract, but they are also commensals in the vagina, urethra, on the skin and under fingernails. *Candida* can be introduced from exogenous sources as well. These include introduction through various catheters and lines, or other indwelling prosthetic medical devices.

Predisposing factors for candidiasis are AIDS, diabetes, iatrogenic immunosuppression, intravenous catheters, prolonged administration of antimicrobial agents, neutropenia, haematologic malignant diseases and burns. After *Candida* enters the blood stream, whether from exogenous or endogenous source, it adheres to the endothelial surface of the blood vessels, before dissemination into tissues.

Clinical features

Candida species can cause a range of clinical forms, from superficial manifestations involving skin, nails, and mucosal surfaces to deep-seated infections involving various internal organs and to disseminated disease (Table 50.3).

SUPERFICIAL INFECTIONS

Superficial infections result from invasion of the superficial layers of skin and/or mucosae by the microorganism. These infections are characterized by the formation of a grayish plaque, surrounded by edema, which on histopathological examination consists of the infecting microorganisms, neutrophils, and cell debris.

Table 50.3. Clinical forms of candidiasis

1. **SUPERFICIAL INFECTIONS**
   I. **Cutaneous infections**
   - Candidal intertrigo
   - Interdigital candidiasis
   - Perianal (diaper) rash
   - Candids
   - Chronic mucocutaneous candidiasis

   II. **Nail infections**
   - Paronychia
   - Onychomycosis

   III. **Mucosal infections**
   - Oral candidiasis
     - Acute pseudomembranous and acute atrophic candidiasis (oral thrush)
     - Denture stomatitis
     - Angular cheilitis
   - Vaginal candidiasis
2. **DEEP INFECTIONS**
   - Candidiasis of gastrointestinal tract
     - Esophagitis
     - Gastrointestinal candidiasis
   - Candidiasis of liver, spleen and other organs
   - Candidiasis of respiratory system
   - Candidiasis of cardiovascular system
   - Renal and urinary tract candidiasis
     - Lower urinary tract infection
     - Renal infection
   - Central nervous system candidiasis
   - Ocular *Candida* infection
3. **DISSEMINATED CANDIDIASIS AND CANDIDEMIA**

Cutaneous infections

The major symptoms discussed under this head are:

- Candidal intertrigo
- Interdigital candidiasis
- Perianal (diaper) rash
- Candids
- Chronic mucocutaneous candidiasis.

Candidal intertrigo

It is the most common clinical form of the cutaneous infection, as *Candida* spp. readily colonize skin folds, particularly in moist and macerated sites. These may include groin, perineum, gluteal folds, umbilicus, axillae, inframammary folds or interdigital spaces. Lesions may be erythematous, with vesicles and pustules, in combination with pruritis. Obesity, diabetes mellitus, various endocrine disturbances, HIV infection and steroid therapy are predisposing factors.

Interdigital candidiasis

In this form the skin folds between the fingers of the hand are macerated and itching. This condition is associated with excessive exposure to moisture, and thus seen particularly among dishwashers.

Perianal (diaper) rash

This occurs in infants wearing diapers. It causes rash in the perianal area and on the buttocks.

Candids

Sterile, grouped, vesicular lesions resembling dermatophytids may be found beyond the limits of infected lesions. They probably represent allergic responses to circulating fungal antigens.

Chronic mucocutaneous candidiasis (CMC)

It is a rare condition in which susceptible individuals develop superficial *Candida* infections as a result of variable defects in T lymphocyte responsiveness to the fungus. It is characterized by the presence of persistent lesions, with high rate of recurrence, starting in early childhood and possibly persisting throughout the individual's lifetime. Lesions can be seen on various skin sites. CMC may appear in a generalized form or may be localized and assume a form of hyperkeratotic lesions – *Candida* granuloma.

Nail infections

The syndromes discussed under this head are:

- Paronychia
- Onychomycosis

Paronychia

It is chronic swelling and inflammation of the nail fold usually affecting the nails of the hands and less frequently those of the feet.

Onychomycosis

It is an invasive infection of the fingernails. As in paronychia, it is more often seen in nails of the hands. Infected nails may become discoloured, eroded, brittle, detached from the nail bed, and painful.

Mucosal infections

Involvement of mucosal surfaces by *Candida* is the most frequent clinical manifestation of candidiasis. The syndromes discussed under this head are:

- Oral candidiasis
- Vaginal candidiasis

Oral candidiasis

Candidiasis of oral mucosa is a disease recognized since antiquity. Very old, very young and very ill persons are more susceptible to oral candidiasis. In the mouth, carbohydrate levels are important; food debris, likely to be present in the mouth of severely ill patients with inadequate oral hygiene may be as significant as diabetic saliva. It has gained renewed significance more recently as an infection frequently seen in AIDS patients and in other conditions. *C. albicans* is the most frequently isolated etiological agent of oral candidiasis. Additional *Candida* spp., such as *C. glabrata*, *C. tropicalis*, *C. parapsilosis* and *C. guilliermondii* are also implicated in oral candidiasis. Oral candidiasis can be clinically classified into:

- Acute pseudomembranous and acute atrophic candidiasis (oral thrush).
- Chronic atrophic and hyperplastic candidiasis (denture stomatitis).
- Angular cheilitis.

Acute pseudomembranous and acute atrophic candidiasis

Acute pseudomembranous candidiasis is also known as **oral thrush**. It occurs predominantly in patients with systemic or local immunosuppression. Immunosuppressed individuals at risk include newborns with birth asphyxia, malnourished or diabetic patients, patients with HIV infections, and those receiving corticosteroid or cytotoxic chemotherapy.

The tongue, soft palate, buccal mucosa and other oral surfaces are characteristically covered with discrete or confluent patches of a cream-white to gray pseudomembrane (Fig. 50.24) composed of hyphae and yeasts of *C. albicans*. The lesions, particularly when covering larger areas, may be painful. They may spread to the mucosa of esophagus (Fig. 50.25), as seen in significant number of AIDS patients, and cause dysphagia.

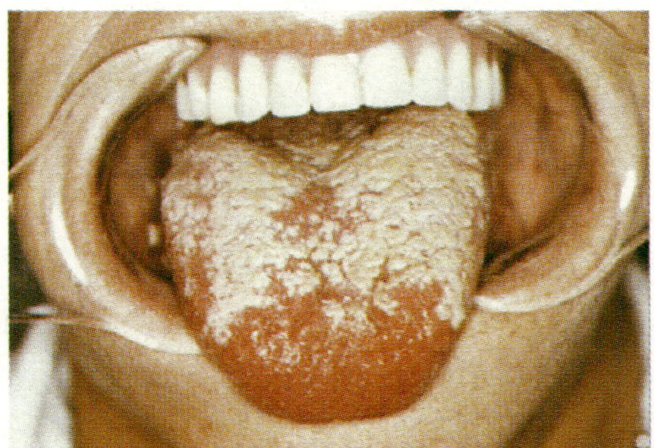

Fig. 50.24. Oral candidiasis (oral thrush).

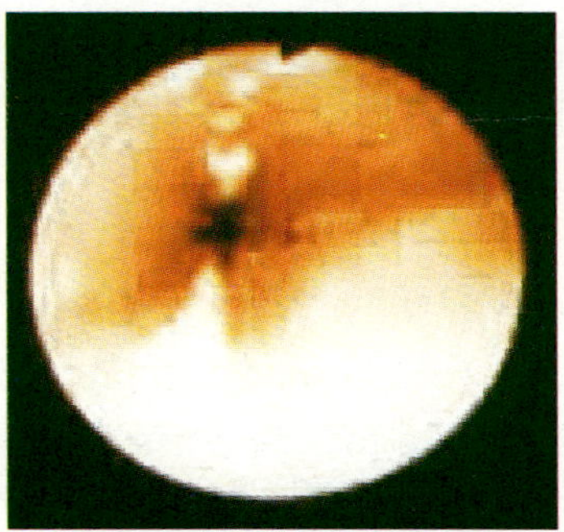

Fig. 50.25. Esophageal candidiasis.

Acute atrophic candidiasis is characterized by painful, erythematous mucosa, particularly on the tongue, which can be associated with loss of the tongue papillae, affecting food intake. It may follow the acute pseudomembranous form with the disappearance of the pseudomembranous lesions.

Denture stomatitis

Denture stomatitis has been well recognized as a complication of wearing dentures. It is a chronic inflammatory condition caused by the trauma of ill-fitting dentures or possibly by an allergic response to denture material with a superimposed *Candida* infection.

Angular cheilitis

Candida may cause red fissured lesions that crack and crust at the folds of the corners of the mouth. It may accompany other clinical forms of oral candidiasis, such as denture stomatitis or oral thrush.

Vaginal candidiasis

Candidal vulvovaginitis is a common genital complaint in women. This affects primarily young and middle-aged females, particularly during their active reproductive life. Around 75% experience at least one episode of this condition during their life-time. Severe forms of vaginal candidiasis may be associated with use of oral contraceptives, corticosteroids or antibiotics, diabetes and pregnancy. Besides *C. albicans*, *C. glabrata* and *C. tropicalis* are the most frequently isolated *Candida* spp. both from vulvovaginitis patients and from healthy carriers.

Patient complains of vulvovaginal pruritis, discharge which can be thick and curd-like or thin, and dyspareunia. The lesions on the mucosal surface are basically adherent plaques.

Sexual transmission to a male partner is known. In the male, infection presents as a balanitis and erythema on the penis.

DEEP INFECTIONS

Candida spp. may cause deep infections of several parenchymatous organs. These infections are characterized by microabscesses. Microscopically, these reveal blastoconidia, pseudohyphae, true hyphae (in case of *C. albicans*), neutrophils and mononuclear cells, and a necrotic centre. In chronic infections granulomata with giant cells and lymphocytes may be formed.

Q. 21. Describe laboratory diagnosis of candidiasis.

Ans. *Specimens*

Scrapings from mucosal, dermal or nail lesions, sputum, bronchial aspirate, pus, swabs, etc.

Direct examination

Place the specimen in a drop of 10% KOH, warm gently over a small flame and examine under microscope. All species of *Candida* form round to oval budding yeast cells, 3–6 μm in diameter.

They occur singly, in chains, or in small loose clusters. Some *Candida* species, when invading tissue, form both pseudohyphae and true hyphae. Pseudohyphae are actually chains of blastoconidia that have elongated and have not separated from one another. They can be recognized by distinct constrictions at the septa. True hyphae have no, or only slight constrictions at the septa. Blastoconidia develop along the sides of both types of hyphae (Figs. 50.26 and 50.27). *C. glabrata* is unique in that it is slightly smaller (2–5 μm in diameter) than the other species of *Candida*, and it does not produce hyphal forms. For species identification culture is required.

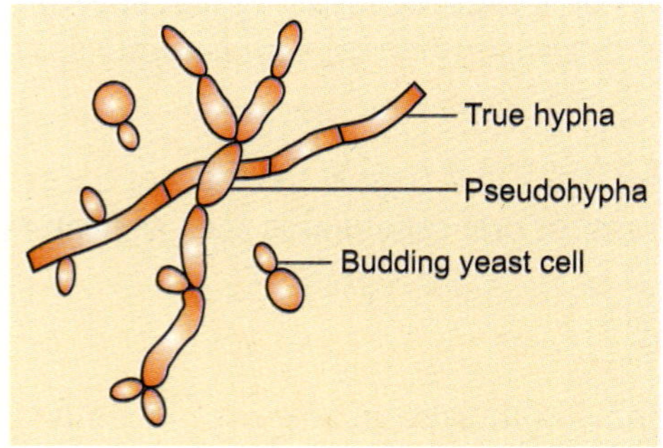

Fig. 50.26. Budding yeast cells, pseudohyphae and true hyphae of *Candida albicans*.

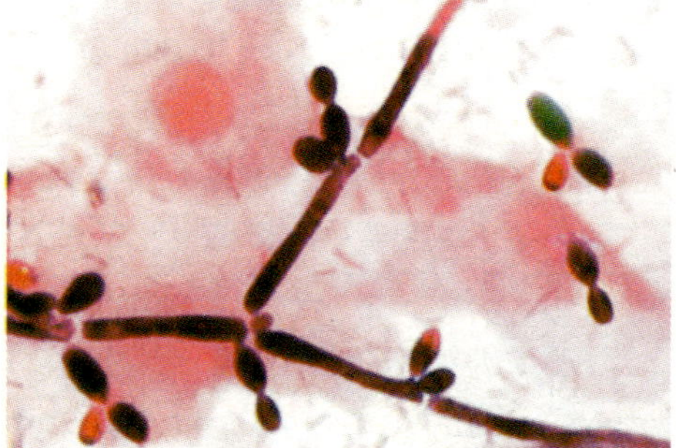

Fig. 50.27. Vaginal smear showing budding yeast cells, true hyphae and epithelial cells.

Histopathology

In systemic infections, *Candida* spp. most commonly elicit an acute suppurative inflammation composed of polymorphonuclear as well as mononuclear cells. Granulomas only rarely occur. *Candida* spp. are also known to invade blood vessels and produce infarcts.

Culture

Candida albicans: For isolation in culture spread pathological material on slants of SDA with chloramphenicol and incubate at 30°C. It grows rapidly. Growth matures in 3 days. Colonies are cream-coloured, pasty and smooth. On enriched media (e.g., blood agar or chocolate agar), extensions commonly called "feet" develop at the border of the colony. Lactophenol cotton blue preparation and Gram-stained smears show round to oval budding yeast cells (3.5–7 × 4–8 μm) and pseudohyphae. Rarely true hyphae may also be seen. On cornmeal-Tween 80 agar at 25°C for 72 hours, pseudohyphae form with clusters of round blastoconidia at the septa. Large thick-walled, usually single terminal chlamydoconidia are characteristically formed (Fig. 50.28). Chlamydoconidia formation is inhibited at 30–37°C.

After incubation in sheep, horse or normal human serum for about 90 minutes at 37°C yeast cells of *C. albicans* begin to form germ tubes (Fig. 50.29). Germ tube test is also positive in *C. dubliniensis*. All other species are negative for this test. **Germ tubes are the beginning of true hyphae and appear as filaments that are not constricted at their points of origin on the parent cell. If the filaments are constricted at their points of origin, they are pseudohyphae, not germ tubes** (Fig. 50.29).

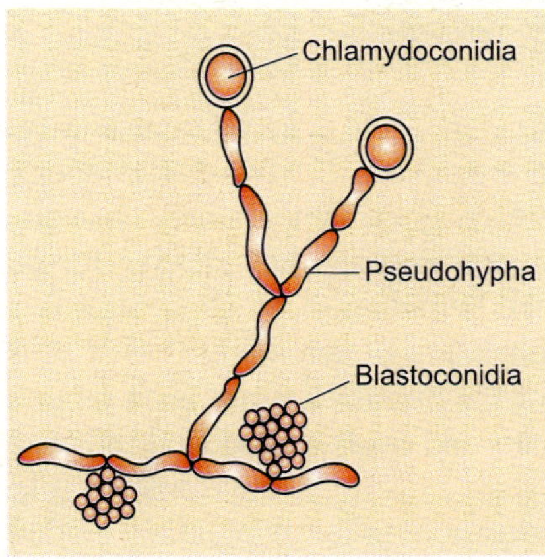

Fig. 50.28. Blastoconidia and chlamydoconidia of *Candida albicans*.

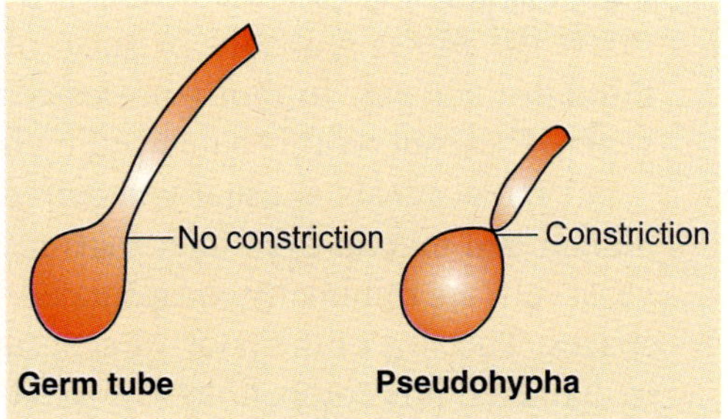

Fig. 50.29. Germ tube and pseudohypha of *Candida albicans*.

Candida dubliniensis: Cultural characteristics of *C. dubliniensis* are similar to those of *C. albicans*. However, in *C. dubliniensis* large, thick-walled terminal chlamydoconidia characteristically form in pairs or small clusters (as opposed to *C. albicans* which usually produces terminal chlamydoconidia singly).

Q. 22. Describe pathogenicity and mycology of *Cryptococcus neoformans.*

Ans. Cryptococcosis is an acute, subacute or chronic fungal infection caused by encapsulated **basidiomycetous yeast**, *Cryptococcus neoformans*. It is most frequently recognized as a disease of the central nervous system, although the primary site of infection is the lungs. The disease occurs sporadically throughout the world.

C. neoformans has become a major human pathogen and a common infection in immunocompromised hosts. It has emerged as an important cause of illness and death in human immunodeficiency virus-infected people. Cryptococcal meningitis is extremely common in AIDS patients.

Mycology

At least 19 species of genus *Cryptococcus* have been described, but few are recognized as causing infection in humans. The predominant pathogen is *C. neoformans*, but two other species, *C. albidus* and *C. laurentii* have been reported to rarely cause disease in humans. *C. neoformans* is a round or oval encapsulated yeast, measuring 4–10 µm in diameter in clinical specimens, and having a capsule ranging in size from 1 to > 30 µm. In specimens isolated from nature, organisms tend to be smaller and poorly encapsulated.

On the basis of antigenic differences in the capsular polysaccharide, five serotypes (A, B, C, D and an hybrid AD) have been identified which have been grouped in three varieties – var. *neoformans* (serotypes D and AD), var. *grubii* (serotype A) and var. *gattii* (serotypes B and C). *C. neoformans* var. *neoformans* and var. *grubii* are responsible for the majority of clinical infections in immunocompromised hosts while var. *gattii* causes disease primarily in immunocompetent hosts. Since there are considerable genetic differences among the varieties, it has been suggested that they should be considered separate species.

Pathogenicity

C. neoformans is ubiquitous in the soil and in avian faecal material, such as pigeon droppings which apparently provide a reservoir of the organisms. *C. neoformans* does not appear to infect the birds, probably because of their high body temperature, but survives passage through their gut. In moist or desiccated pigeon excreta, they survive for more than two years. Their survival is enhanced by increased humidity.

Cryptococcosis is usually acquired by inhalation of aerosolized yeast cells. Animal-to-human and human-to-human transmission of the disease has not been reported. In nature, yeast cells are minimally encapsulated, small dry and easily aerosolized and reach the alveolar spaces. The size of the poorly encapsulated yeast cells in the environment is less than 3 µm in diameter. It is compatible with alveolar deposition. In the alveoli they gradually rehydrate and acquire their characteristic polysaccharide capsule. Development of disease largely depends on the competence of the host's cellular defences, and the number and virulence of the inhaled yeast cells.

Most patients with cryptococcosis have evidence of some underlying immunocompromising condition. The most common of these underlying conditions worldwide is AIDS, followed by prolonged treatment with corticosteroids, organ transplantation, malignancies and sarcoidosis. The commonest form of the cryptococcosis is a mild, self-limiting pulmonary infection. Dissemination of infection may lead to the involvement of CNS, skin, mucosa, bone and other organs.

Q. 23. Describe laboratory diagnosis of cryptococcosis.

Ans. ***C. neoformans*** **is a true yeast. Both in tissues, and in culture at room temperature as well as at 37°C, only budding yeasts are seen.** Diagnosis is established by demonstration of budding yeast cells in CSF, sputum, pus, brain tissue, etc. by direct microscopy and culture, and by serological tests for capsular antigen.

Direct microscopy

The clinical specimens are collected as per the site involved particularly CSF, sputum, pus, brain tissue, etc. Place **a drop of India ink** on a clean glass slide, add and mix with it a drop of CSF or other body fluid and, under reduced light, look for the spherical cells of *C. neoformans* and their enveloping capsule (Fig. 50.30).

Sputum or pus should be mixed with **10% potassium hydroxide** before examination. In a properly prepared specimen, pus cells and partially digested cellular debris delineate the capsule which is resistant to potassium hydroxide.

Histopathology

The histopathological examination of biopsy specimen can be done **by staining with Mayer's mucicarmine, periodic acid-Schiff, Gomori methenamine silver, and haematoxylin and eosin staining**.

The yeast cells are round or oval with thin walls, 4–10 μm in diameter, vary in size within the microscopic field, bud on a narrow base and characteristically produce thick capsules. Tissue stained with Mayer's mucicarmine show the capsule as bright carmine red, often with a spiny or scalloped appearance (Fig. 50.31). Drying, fixing, and staining may cause the yeast cells to collapse or become crescent-shaped.

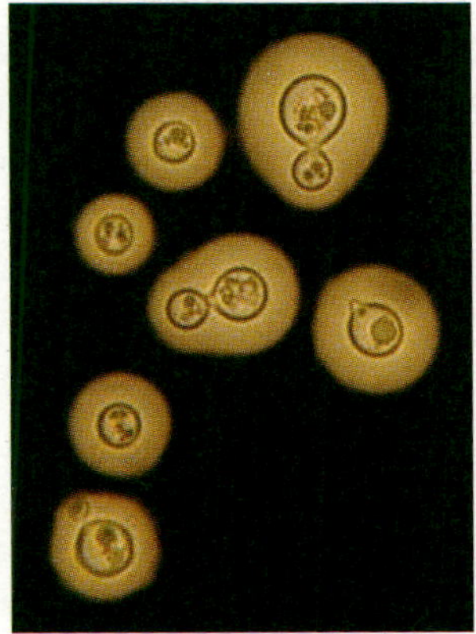

Fig. 50.30. An India ink wet mount of *Cryptococcus neoformans* showing encapsulated budding yeast cells.

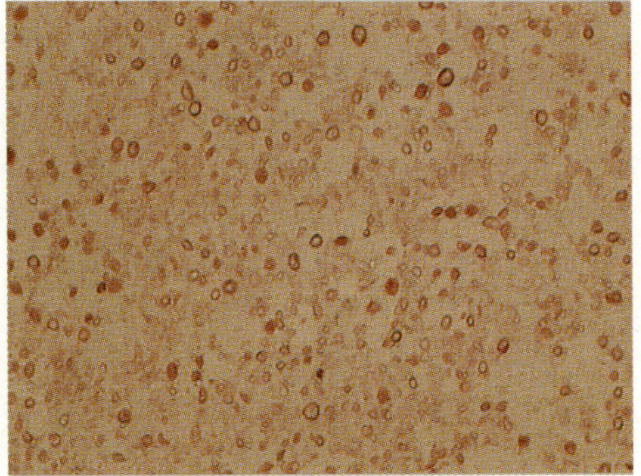

Fig. 50.31. Cryptococci stained with Mayer's mucicarmine stain. The capsule is stained bright carmine red in colour.

Culture

Cryptococci can be cultured from biologic samples on Sabouraud dextrose agar. Chloramphenicol (0.05 mg/ml) can be incorporated in the medium to inhibit growth of bacterial contaminants, but do not use cycloheximide because this inhibits *C. neoformans*. As only a few yeast cells may be present at the site of infection, pellets from centrifuged CSF and other biologic fluids should be cultured.

Colonies are flat or slightly heaped, shiny, moist, and usually mucoid with smooth edges. Colour is cream at first later becoming tannish. *C. neoformans* grows equally well at 25°C and 37°C, and incubation at 37°C inhibits other species of the genus.

C. neoformans possesses the enzyme phenol oxidase, and testing for its presence is another means of accurate identification. This can be done by culturing the suspected yeasts on special agars such as niger seed agar, bird seed agar and caffeic acid agar and looking for the black colonies. *C. neoformans* breaks down caffeic acid to melanin.

Serodiagnosis

Detection of polysaccharide antigen of *C. neoformans* in body fluids is highly effective for a rapid and accurate diagnosis. The titre is highest in serum, intermediate in CSF and lowest in urine. Bronchoalveolar lavage fluid may also be tested for cryptococcal antigen. The most frequently used test is the slide agglutination using latex particles coated with polyclonal or monoclonal antibodies. A positive serum antigen test at a dilution of 1 : 4 is strongly suggestive of cryptococcal infection. A titre of $\geq$ 1 : 8 is indicative of active disease. Higher antigen titres indicate more severe infections and a falling titre is a good prognostic sign.

Q. 24. Describe causative agents, pathogenicity and laboratory diagnosis of aspergillosis.

Ans. ***Causative agents***

There are more than 200 species of *Aspergillus* to which humans are constantly exposed. However, approximately 19 species have been implicated in human disease (aspergillosis), which is worldwide in occurrence. Of these *A. fumigatus* is most important. Other important pathogens in this group are *A. niger*, *A. flavus*, *A. terreus* and *A. nidulans*. Aspergilli are ubiquitous in nature. Aspergillosis is caused by inhalation of *Aspergillus* conidia or mycelial fragments which are present on vegetation (especially nuts and grains), decaying matter, soil and air. A high degree of natural resistance exists in healthy host, but when the host defence is compromised, as in AIDS and in patients on immunosuppressive therapy, aspergillosis may develop. It may cause:

Pathogenicity

1. Allergic bronchopulmonary aspergillosis (ABPA)

This is seen in atopic individuals with elevated IgE levels. Following inhalation of *Aspergillus* conidia or mycelial fragments, the fungus grows within the lumen of the bronchioles. Some patients may expectorate mucus plugs containing *Aspergillus* hyphae which may be seen in smear or may be isolated from sputum. Patient develops bronchial allergic reactions to inhaled *Aspergillus* conidia. Repeated allergic reactions in bronchi cause bronchiectasis. Patient suffers from breathlessness, fever and malaise after a few hours of exposure. ABPA may also occur in patients with cystic fibrosis.

2. Intracavitary aspergilloma (fungus ball)

Aspergilloma represents a non-invasive (saprophytic) form of aspergillosis. This usually develops in pre-existing pulmonary cavities such as in tuberculosis or cystic disease. Fungus balls are usually located in the upper lobes. Less frequently, they occur in the apical segments of the lower lobes. The inhaled conidia enter a cavity, germinate and produce abundant hyphae. It may also develop in maxillary sinus and occasionally in the ethmoid, sphenoid and frontal sinuses. It is only saprophytic colonization without invasion of the lung or sinus mucosa.

3. Acute invasive pulmonary aspergillosis

This occurs in severely immunocompromised individuals who are on immunosuppressive drugs, cytotoxic drugs, corticosteroids, broad spectrum antibiotics and AIDS patients. There is a widespread growth of the fungus in lung tissue that disseminates to involve other organs particularly kidneys and brain. The disease has poor prognosis.

4. Endocarditis

Aspergillus may sometimes cause endocarditis in immunosuppressed patients and those who have undergone open-heart surgery. This condition also has a poor prognosis.

5. Paranasal Aspergillus granuloma

In this condition, there is colonization of paranasal sinuses by *A. flavus* and *A. fumigatus*. There is no evidence of invasion of the sinus although pressure necrosis of the paranasal *Aspergillus* granuloma is a slowly progressive condition.

6. Cerebral aspergillosis

Brain is the most important organ affected in disseminated aspergillosis apart from lungs. It leads to focal neurological deficits including hemiparesis, focal seizures, and cranial nerve palsy.

7. Keratitis

Aspergillus spp. are an occasional etiologic agent of this locally invasive infection of the cornea following a penetrating injury or corneal surgery. *Aspergillus* keratitis is occupationally associated with agricultural workers. This infection is characterized by ocular pain and rapid loss of vision.

8. Otomycosis

Otomycosis refers to the growth of *Aspergillus* spp. (usually *A. niger* or *A. fumigatus*) within the external auditory canal. This causes irritation, pruritis and impairment of hearing.

Laboratory diagnosis

Direct examination and histopathology

Diagnosis may be made by microscopic examination and by culture. Ten per cent KOH preparation of sputum, bronchoalveolar lavage, transbronchial biopsy and other biopsies reveal non-pigmented septate hyphae, 3–5 μm in diameter with characteristic dichotomous branching. The hyphae have a tendency to branch repeatedly. The branches arise at an angle of approximately 45 degrees. In a majority of pulmonary and disseminated lesions, only hyphal forms are seen. Histological sections can be stained with H&E and GMS and examined for characteristic hyphae (Figs. 50.32 and 50.33). In allergic aspergillosis there is usually abundant fungus in the sputum and mycelial plugs may also be present. In aspergilloma, fungus may be difficult to find in sputum smear. In invasive aspergillosis, sputum smear is often negative.

Culture

For species identification, the clinical material is inoculated on SDA without cycloheximide and incubated at 25°C. Colonies appear after incubation for 1–2 days. The isolate is identified on the basis of growth characteristics and microscopic morphology. LCB mount shows

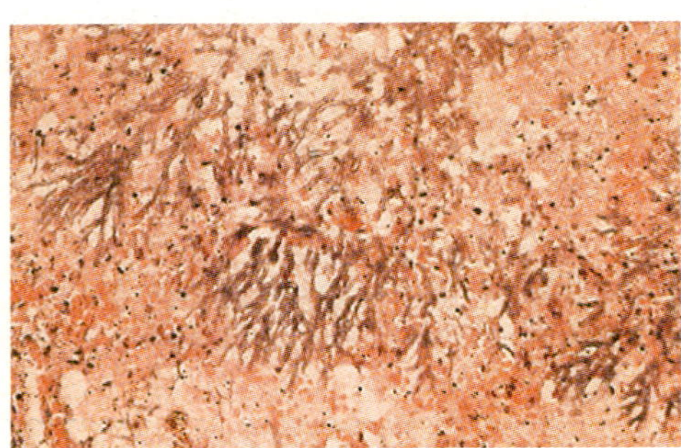

Fig. 50.32. *Aspergillus* showing septate hyphae with characteristic dichotomous branching.

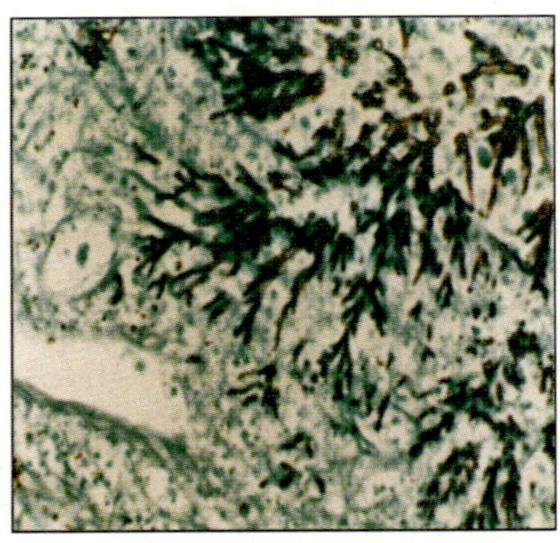

Fig. 50.33. Section similar to that in Fig. 50.32 but stained by Gomori's methanamine silver stain. The hyphae are stained black in colour.

branching and septate hyphae. From the latter arise conidiophores, the ends of which are expanded to form vesicles. The vesicle bears phialides which arise directly from the vesicle (uniseriate) or from sterile cells called metulae (biseriate) (Fig. 50.34).

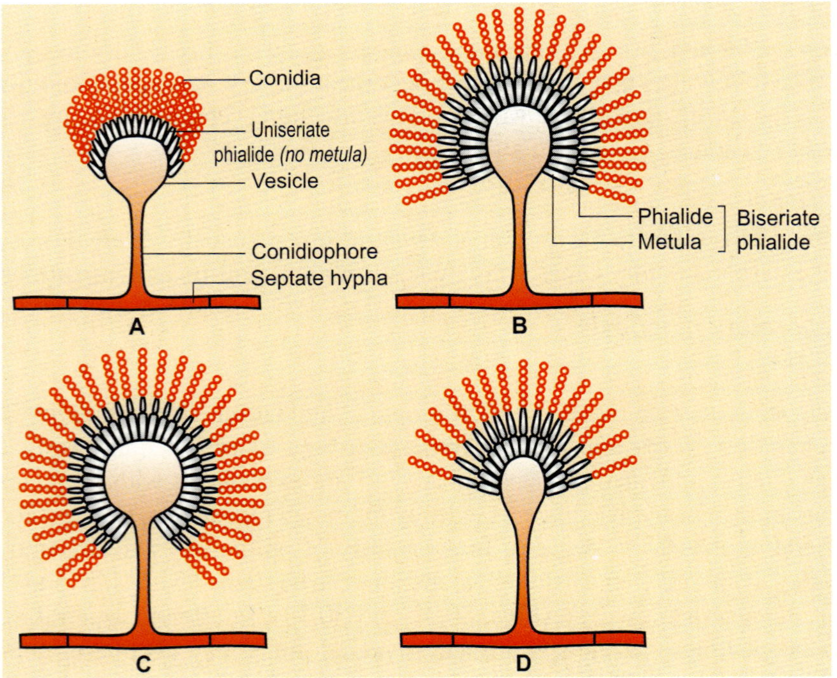

Fig. 50.34. *Aspergillus* spp.: (A) *A. fumigatus*; (B) *A. flavus*; (C) *A. niger*; (D) *A. terreus*.

Serological diagnosis

Immunodiffusion, CIE and ELISA are widely used for detection of antibodies in the diagnosis of all forms of aspergillosis, particularly aspergilloma and allergic bronchopulmonary aspergillosis. In invasive aspergillosis antigen can be detected by ELISA and latex agglutination.

Skin tests

Skin tests with *A. fumigatus* antigen are useful for the diagnosis of allergic aspergillosis. All patients give an immediate type-I reaction and 70% of those with pulmonary eosinophilia also give a delayed type-III Arthus reaction.

Q. 25. Describe briefly causative agents, predisposing factors, pathogenicity and laboratory diagnosis of mucormycosis.

Ans. Mucormycosis is an opportunistic infection caused by saprophytic fungi, notably species of *Mucor*, *Rhizopus* and *Lichtheimia* (formerly *Absidia*) of the family Mucoraceae, order Mucorales. These fungi are common saprophytes of soil, manure and decaying vegetables, and fruits. These are essentially opportunistic fungi. The major predisposing factors to mucormycosis are acute diabetes mellitus, metabolic acidosis, debilitating diseases such as leukaemia or lymphoma, immunosuppression, starvation, and widespread use of broad-spectrum antibiotics, steroids and antimetabolites. Mucormycosis may lead to:

1. Rhinocerebral mucormycosis

This is the most serious and fulminating type of disease. The infection begins in the mucosa of the nose or the hard palate and spreads to the paranasal sinuses, orbit and brain, where massive invasion of blood vessels causes thrombosis and ischaemic necrosis. If untreated, it is rapidly fatal.

2. Pulmonary mucormycosis

Inhalation of the sporangiospores may lead to pulmonary mucormycosis. The lesions may be focal or diffuse. Massive invasion of large pulmonary vessels produces pulmonary infarction.

3. Gastrointestinal mucormycosis

This is acquired by ingestion of food contaminated with the fungal spores. Ulceration of gastric mucosa with thrombosis of associated vessels has been observed. Involvement of intestinal tract is rare.

4. Subcutaneous mucormycosis

This leads to a chronic induration over the extremities, neck or pelvic region. There is chronic inflammation, eosinophilic infiltration and fibrosis.

5. Disseminated mucormycosis

Mucormycosis may be widely disseminated affecting the kidneys, gastrointestinal tract, heart, brain and lungs.

The characteristic pathological changes in mucormycosis are suppuration and necrosis. Invasion of thrombosed blood vessels by the fungus is a conspicuous feature. In tissues (Figs. 50.35 and 50.36), the organisms appear as irregularly branched, nonseptate, very broad hyphae (7–15 μm in diameter) which characteristically are deeply stained with routine H&E stain. On the other hand, the coloration by special fungus stains such as Gridley, PAS and in some cases GMS may be very poor. True septa are rarely seen in the hyphae but under low magnification, cross folds in the walls of the hyphae may resemble septa. In tissues,

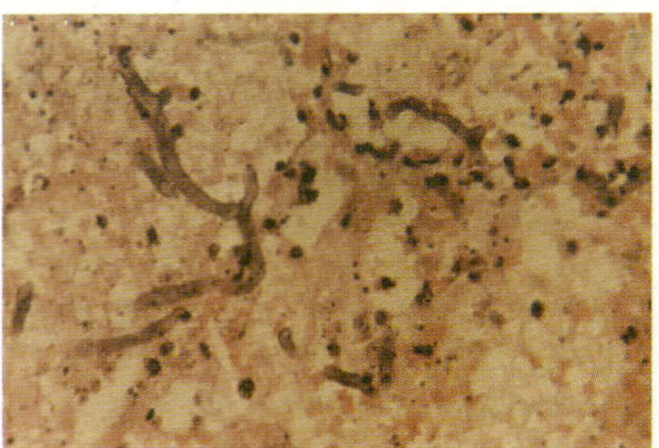

Fig. 50.35. Mucormycosis showing broad non-septate hyphae.

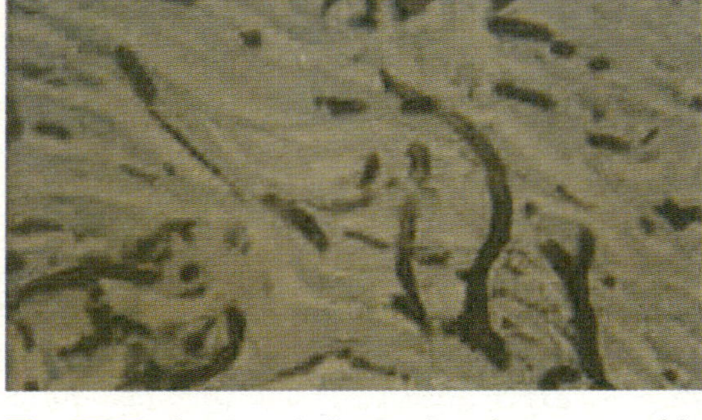

Fig. 50.36. Section similar to that demonstrated in Fig. 50.35 but stained by Gomori's methanamine silver stain. The hyphae are stained black in colour.

aspergillosis can be easily differentiated from mucormycosis in its uniform dichotomous pattern of branching, the presence of many septa and its much easier detection by the special stains than the routine H&E stain.

Subcutaneous mucormycosis shows chronic inflammatory reaction in which, sparse, thin-walled, broad hyphae are seen in the centre of the granulomas. **The hyphae are surrounded by eosinophilic Splendore-Hoeppli material.**

Laboratory diagnosis

Diagnosis can be made by examination of:

- KOH wet mounts of scrapings from the lesions, pus, sputum and nasal discharge shows characteristic hyphae.
- The fungi can be readily seen by histological sections stained with routine H&E stain.
- Fungi can be readily isolated on SDA at 37°C. *Rhizopus* has rhizoids and sporangiophores that arise in groups directly above the rhizoids. *Mucor* does not possess rhizoids and shows branched sporangiophores arising randomly along aerial mycelium. *Lichtheimia* has rhizoids and sporangiophores that arise from the aerial mycelium in between the rhizoids (Fig. 50.37).

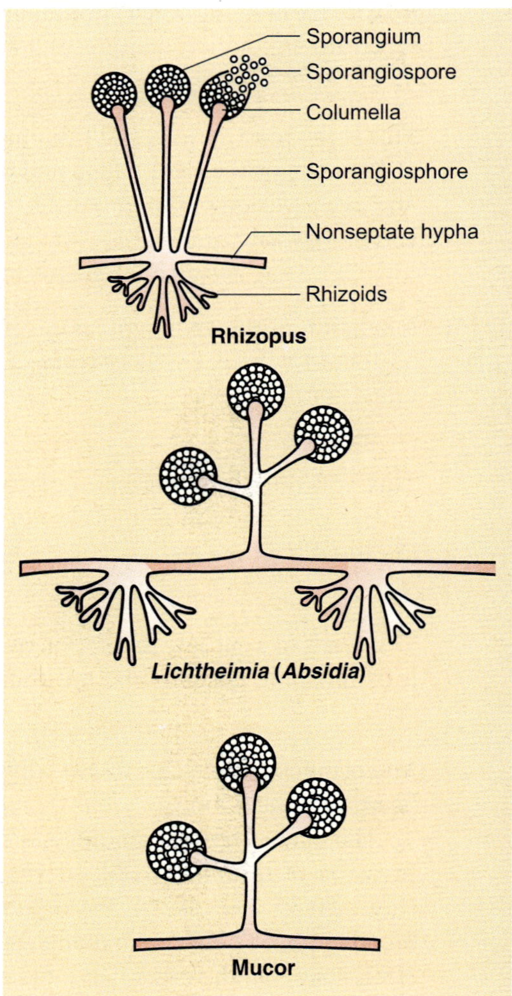

Fig. 50.37. *Rhizopus, Mucor* and *Lichtheimia*.

V. MISCELLANEOUS MYCOSES

Q. 26. Describe causative agent, pathogenicity and laboratory diagnosis of penicilliosis marneffei.

Ans. ***Causative agent***

There are more than 250 known species of the genus *Penicillium*. They occur as saprophytes in the soil and decomposing organic debris. ***P. marneffei* is the only species of genus *Penicillium* which is known to cause significant infection and is thermally dimorphic.** It exists in mycelial and yeast-like forms at two different temperatures, i.e., 25–30°C and 35–37°C, respectively. The mycelial form is similar to other species of the genus *Penicillium* but no other species of this genus has yeast-like morphology. Yeast-like form of *P. marneffei* is entirely different from other dimorphic fungi as it divides by fission with formation of transverse septum (schizogony) and not by budding.

Pathogenicity

The infection is thought to occur through inhalation of the conidia or through cutaneous inoculation. The organisms are engulfed by macrophages, in which they multiply intracellularly and transform into yeast. Melanin is produced by both conidia and yeast. It may act as a virulence factor.

The reticuloendothelial system is predominantly involved. It causes deep-seated infection that can be disseminated predominantly in immunocompromised (HIV-infected) patients. Most cases of penicilliosis marneffei are observed in patients who have CD4+ lymphocyte count < 100/μl. Disseminated disease is thought to be universally fatal, if untreated. In the immunocompetent host, the cell-mediated immune response is prominent with the formation of epithelioid granuloma.

Penicilliosis marneffei occurs mainly in adults. However, cases have also been reported in children with or without AIDS. Patient develops fever, anaemia, leucopenia, thrombocytopenia, weight loss, diarrhoea, hepatosplenomegaly, generalized lymphadenopathy, cough and pulmonary infiltrates, and a characteristic rash resembling molluscum contagiosum predominantly on face and trunk.

Laboratory diagnosis

Histopathology

Histologic sections of the affected organs reveal granulomatous inflammation, necrosis and oval to elliptical yeast-like cells 2–5 μm in length resembling *Histoplasma capsulatum*. These are packed within histiocytes. The presence of transverse septa and lack of budding distinguish these yeast-like forms from those of *H. capsulatum*. However, outside histiocytes, elongated cells 8–13 μm long may also be seen. They have blunt ends and are curved giving 'sausage-like' appearance, which has prominent cross-walls. The cells of *P. marneffei* are not stained by H&E, but are stained well by PAS and GMS.

Culture

The fungus can be readily isolated on SDA. It can be identified by the brush-like arrangement of conidia (Fig. 50.38).

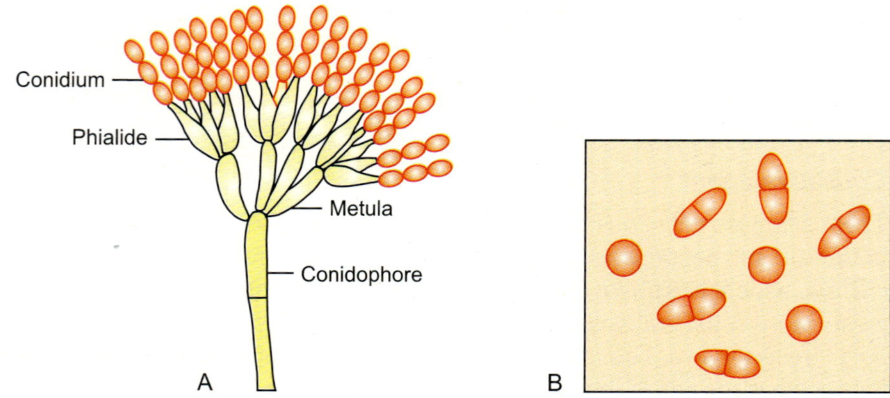

Fig. 50.38. *Penicillium marneffei*: mycelial phase (A) and yeast-like phase (B).

Q. 27. Write short note on otomycosis.

Ans. Otomycosis is a subacute or chronic superficial fungal infection of external auditory canal. It is more prevalent in warm and humid climate, particularly during rainy season as compared to cold climate. It is a common disease and is usually caused by *A. niger*, *A. fumigatus*, *Penicillium*, *Candida albicans*, *C. tropicalis* and *C. krusei*. The symptoms are itching, pain and deafness. Secondary bacterial infection, caused usually by *Pseudomonas* and *Proteus*, may develop. The diagnosis can be made by demonstration of the fungi in scrapings and by culture.

Q. 28. Write short note on keratomycosis.

Ans. Keratomycosis or mycotic or fungal keratitis is an invasive fungal infection of the cornea. It is most frequently caused by *A. fumigatus*, *A. flavus*, *A. glaucus* and *A. niger*. In addition, species of *Fusarium*, *Curvularia*, *Candida*, *Acremonium*, *Paecilomyces*, *Penicillium*, *Alternaria*, *Fonsecea*, *Pseudallescheria*, *Drechslera* and *Aureobasidium* may also cause keratomycosis. It usually follows trauma. Fungal spores colonize the injured tissue and initiate an inflammatory reaction leading to hypopyon, ulcer and endophthalmitis. If not recognized and treated early, enucleation may become necessary. Increased incidence of keratomycosis is due to widespread use of corticosteroids. Diagnosis can be made by microscopic examination and culture of scrapings taken from the base or edge of the ulcer.

Q. 29. Describe causative agent, pathogenicity and laboratory diagnosis of pneumocystosis.

Ans. ***Causative agent***

Pneumocystosis is caused by *Pneumocystis jirovecii*. Until recently, it was thought to be a protozoan, but molecular biologic studies have proved that it is a fungus, an **ascomycete**. Three developmental forms of *P. jirovecii* are generally recognized – trophozoite, pre-cyst and cyst.

Trophozoite

The trophozoite of *P. jirovecii* is the smallest of the life cycle stages of the organism. It ranges in size from 1–4 μm and is ellipsoidal in shape when unfixed preparations are viewed by light microscopy. After fixation it may appear amoeboid in form. It is thought to reproduce by binary fission.

Pre-cyst

The pre-cyst is recognized as an intermediate stage of the sexual phase of reproduction leading to cyst development. It is presumed that a mating event first occurs to provide a zygote that initiates sporogenesis.

Cyst

The cyst is the end product of sporogenesis. This form is spherical, 5–8 µm in diameter, and has a thick wall composed of three layers. Eight spores are commonly found within each cyst. The spores are 1–2 µm in diameter. The cysts can be stained with GMS stain, toluidine blue, Giemsa, and calcofluor white. With GMS stain the organisms appear deep blue-black (Fig. 50.39).

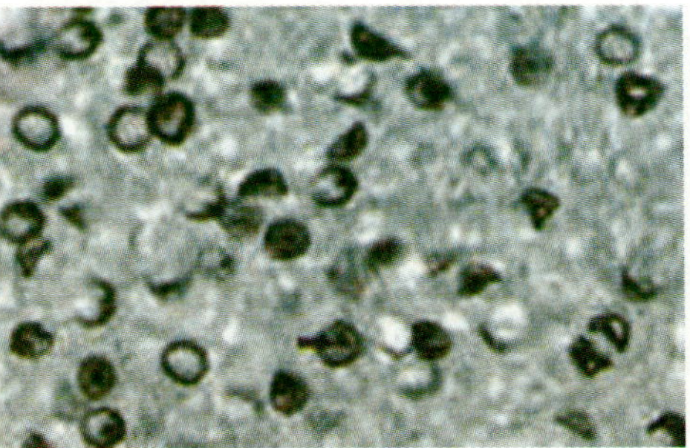

Fig. 50.39. Intra-alveolar clusters of non-budding cysts of *Pneumocystis jirovecii* stained by Gomori methanamine silver stain in an AIDS patient suffering from *Pneumocystis jirovecii* pneumonia.

Pathogenicity

P. jirovecii causes *Pneumocystis* pneumonia (PCP). It is the most important opportunistic infection in HIV-infected patients. *Pneumocystis* is also a significant cause of morbidity and mortality in non-HIV-associated immunosuppressed patients (transplantation, malignancy, connective tissue disease). Prior to introduction of effective chemoprophylactic regimens, it was a major cause of death among AIDS patients. Chemoprophylaxis has resulted in a dramatic decrease in the incidence of pneumonia.

Cell-mediated immunity presumably plays a dominant role in the resistance to disease. *P. jirovecii* pneumonia generally occurs in HIV-infected patients with CD4+ lymphocyte count < 200/µl.

Laboratory diagnosis

Histopathology

To establish the diagnosis of *P. jirovecii* pneumonia, specimens of bronchoalveolar lavage, lung biopsy or induced sputum (by administration of a saline mist to induce production of sputum) are stained by GMS, toluidine blue, Giemsa and calcofluor white and examined for the presence of cysts or trophozoites. The Papanicolaou stain, frequently used for staining cytopathological specimens, can demonstrate the foamy exudate surrounding the organisms, although the organisms stain poorly. With Giemsa stain, all forms of the organism are stained, which permits assessment of the total organism burden. The nuclei appear reddish-purple in contrast to the light blue cytoplasm. The cell wall excludes the dye and appears as a circumscribed clear zone around the cyst contents. Organisms can also be demonstrated by immunofluorescent techniques, using fluorescein-tagged monoclonal antibodies against surface antigens of both cysts and trophic forms. ***P. jirovecii* cannot be cultured.**

Polymerase chain reaction (PCR)

PCR-based detection of *P. jirovecii* DNA has been shown to have greater sensitivity and specificity for the diagnosis of PCP from respiratory specimens than conventional (Giemsa or GMS) microscopic methods.

Serology

A presumptive serodiagnosis can be made in suspected cases of *P. jirovecii* infections. Complement fixation titres of 1 : 4 or higher usually indicate active disease. Latex agglutination tests for *P. jirovecii* are positive in only about one third of patients with known disease.

Treatment

Acute cases of *P. jirovecii* pneumonia can be treated with trimethoprim-sulphamethoxazole or pentamidine isethionate. Prophylaxis can be achieved with daily trimethoprim-sulphamethoxazole or aerosolized pentamidine.

Q. 30. Write short note on mycotoxicoses.

Ans. Many fungi produce poisonous substances called mycotoxins that can cause acute or chronic intoxication and damage. The mycotoxins are secondary metabolites and their effects are not dependent on fungal infection or viability. The diseases that result from ingestion of food that contains mycotoxins are known as mycotoxicoses. Mycotoxins produced by various species of fungi are aflatoxin, ergot alkaloids, ochratoxin, fumonisins, gliotoxin, zearalenone and trichothecenes. Cooking has little effect on the potency of these toxins, which may cause severe or fatal damage to the liver and kidney.

Classic examples of human diseases caused by *Fusarium* mycotoxins include alimentary toxic aleukia, Urov or Kashin-Beck disease and Akakabi-byo (scabby grain intoxication). *Fusarium germinearum*, *F. poae* and *F. sporotrichoides* have been linked to human mycotoxicosis. T-2 toxin is produced by these fungi. T-2 toxin is a potent inhibitor of eukaryotic protein synthesis and inhibits platelet aggregation. It increases prothrombin time and causes cardiomyopathy.

Some fungi produce mutagenic and carcinogenic compounds that can be extremely toxic for experimental animals. One of the most potent is **aflatoxin** which is elaborated by *Aspergillus flavus* and related molds and is a frequent contaminant of peanuts, corn, grains, and other foods.

51

EMERGING AND REEMERGING INFECTIOUS DISEASES

Q. 1. Describe briefly emerging and reemerging infectious diseases. Enlist various factors which are responsible for emerging and reemerging infections.

Ans. **Emerging infectious diseases**

Emerging infectious diseases have been defined by WHO as those infections, the incidence of which in humans has either increased during the last two decades or threatens to increase in near future. *This term includes newly-appearing infectious diseases or those spreading to new geographical areas.* Surprisingly, 'new' agents of infectious diseases continue to be recognized (Table 51.1). The most notorious of these is undoubtedly the human immunodeficiency virus (HIV), the causative agent of acquired immunodeficiency syndrome (AIDS).

An emerging infectious disease may be a totally new disease with undescribed symptomatology as it was in case of **Kyasanur Forest disease in Karnataka**, but more often it is an introduction of a known or little known disease in an area where the disease did not occur earlier, e.g., **yellow fever in Kenya or Rift Valley fever in Egypt**.

Reemerging infectious diseases

Reemerging infectious diseases are those that have reappeared after a significant decline in their incidence. A breakdown of public health measures for previously controlled infections or the development of antimicrobial resistance in prevalent infections may lead them to reemerge as public health problems. Bacterial and parasitic re-emerging infections are given in Table 51.2.

Various factors responsible for the emergence and reemergence of communicable diseases are as under:

1. Weak public health system.
2. Unhygienic living conditions.
3. Rapid urbanization.

Table 51.1. Emerging infectious diseases

Year	Agent	Disease
BACTERIAL AGENTS		
1977	*Legionella pneumophila*	Legionnaires' disease
	Campylobacter jejuni	Enteritis
1981	Toxin-producing *Staphylococcus aureus*	Toxic shock syndrome
1982	*Escherichia coli* 0157:H7	Haemolytic uraemic syndrome and haemorrhagic colitis
	Borrelia burgdorferi	Lyme disease
1983	*Helicobacter pylori*	Gastritis
1989	*Ehrlichia chaffeensis*	Human ehrlichiosis
1992	*Vibrio cholerae* O139	Epidemic cholera
	Bartonella henselae	Cat-scratch disease and bacillary angiomatosis
	Mobiluncus spp.	Bacterial vaginosis
	Clostridium difficile	Pseudomembranous colitis
VIRAL AGENTS		
1973	*Rotavirus*	Infantile diarrhoea
1975	Parvovirus B19	Aplastic crisis in chronic haemolytic anaemia
1977	Ebola virus	Ebola haemorrhagic fever
1978	Hantaan virus	Haemorrhagic fever with renal syndrome
1980	Human T cell lymphotropic virus-1 (HTLV-1)	T cell lymphoma/leukaemia
1982	HTLV-2	Prevalent in intravenous drug users, not associated with disease
1983	Human immunodeficiency virus-1	AIDS
1985	Human immunodeficiency virus-2	AIDS
1986	Bovine spongiform encephalitis (BSE) agent	BSE in cattle
1988	Human herpesvirus 6 (HHV-6)	Exanthema subitum
	Hepatitis E virus	Hepatitis
1989	Hepatitis C virus	Hepatitis
1990	Sabia virus	Haemorrhagic fever
1991	Guanarito virus	Venezuelan haemorrhagic fever
1993	Sin Nombre virus	Hantavirus pulmonary syndrome
1995	Human herpesvirus 8 (HHV-8)	Kaposi's sarcoma
1996	Hepatitis G virus	Hepatitis
1997	H5N1	Avian flu
2003	*Coronavirus*	Severe acute respiratory syndrome
2009	H1N1	Swine flu
PARASITES		
1976	*Cryptosporidium parvum*	Acute and chronic diarrhoea
1985	*Enterocytozoon bieneusi*	Persistent diarrhoea
1986	*Cyclospora cayetanensis*	Persistent diarrhoea
1991	*Encephalitozoon hellem*	Conjunctivitis, disseminated disease
	New species of *Babesia*	Atypical babesiosis
1993	*Encephalitozoon cuniculi*	Disseminated disease

4. Industrial and other developmental activities.
5. Encroachment by humans to areas so far uninhabited leading to ecological changes.
6. Rapid means of transportation to and from any part of the world, resulting in geographical distribution of a pathogen.
7. Natural disasters.
8. Migration of population.
9. Increasing population density and poverty.
10. Overcrowding.
11. Proliferation of fast-food restaurants with uniform methods of preparation and frequent use of single source of food has expanded the opportunities for a large number of persons to be exposed to contaminated food.

Table 51.2. Reemerging infectious diseases

Disease	Causative agent
BACTERIAL	
Tuberculosis	Multidrug-resistant *Mycobacterium tuberculosis*
Typhoid fever	Multidrug-resistant *Salmonella* Typhi
Leptospirosis	*Leptospira interrogans*
Melioidosis	*Burkholderia* (*Pseudomonas*) *pseudomallei*
Anthrax	*Bacillus anthracis*
Plague	*Yersinia pestis*
PARASITIC	
Malaria	Drug-resistant *Plasmodium falciparum*
Leishmaniasis	*Leishmania donovani*
Lymphatic filariasis	*Wuchereria bancrofti*, *Brugia malayi* and *B. timori*

12. Individual host determinants such as specific risk behaviour. Behavioural influences include:
    (a) risk factors leading to sexually transmitted diseases (e.g., multiple sex partners, homosexual sex behaviour), and
    (b) risk factors pertaining to food preparation and storage in the home.
13. New pathogens may emerge as a result of mutation, recombination and reassortment leading to enhanced virulence.
14. The ability of animal viruses to cross the species barriers as a result of mutations. HIV-1 and HIV-2 may be examples of species cross-over.
15. Development of antimicrobial resistance as seen in *Mycobacterium tuberculosis* and *Plasmodium falciparum*.
16. Development of insecticide resistance in vectors as seen in DDT resistance in *Anopheles* mosquito, vector of *Plasmodium*.

In their fight for survival and supremacy, microorganisms have been developing and devising various methods to inactivate the action of antimicrobial agents or to circumvent immune response induced by the vaccine. The problem of drug resistance has assumed alarming proportions in various pathogens especially the causative agents of tuberculosis and the bacteria responsible for hospital-acquired (nosocomial) infections such as *Pseudomonas aeruginosa*, *Klebsiella pneumoniae* and *Staphylococcus aureus*.

The only way to combat the spread of these infectious diseases is to recognize these diseases early and take appropriate control measures rapidly.

52

INFECTIVE SYNDROMES

In this chapter important infective syndromes, caused by different microorganisms, have been discussed briefly, and the reader should refer back to the corresponding chapters for details including laboratory diagnosis.

Q. 1. Describe briefly sore throat. Enumerate its causative agents.

Ans. It is essentially an acute tonsillitis or pharyngitis. It is characterized by redness and oedema of mucosa, exudation of tonsils, pseudomembrane formation, oedema of uvula, grey coating of tongue and enlargement of cervical lymph nodes. Causative agents of sore throat are given in Table 52.1.

Of these, *Corynebacterium diphtheriae*, *Candida albicans*, β-haemolytic group A *Streptococcus*, *Borrelia vincentii* and *Leptotrichia buccalis* may lead to pseudomembrane formation.

Table 52.1. Causative agents of sore throat

BACTERIA

- *Streptococcus*, β-haemolytic group A and occasionally groups C and G
- *Corynebacterium diphtheriae*
- *Haemophilus influenzae*
- *Bordetella pertussis*
- *Neisseria gonorrhoeae*
- *Borrelia vincentii*
- *Leptotrichia buccalis*

FUNGI

- *Candida albicans*

VIRUSES

- Epstein-Barr virus
- Adenoviruses
- Coxsackievirus A

Q. 2. Define urinary tract infection. Name causative agents, and describe laboratory diagnosis of urinary tract infection.

Ans. Urinary tract infection (UTI) may be defined as the presence of bacteria undergoing multiplication in urine within the urinary drainage system. Kass (1956), gave a criterion of active bacterial infection of urinary tract according to which a count exceeding 10^5 organisms/ml denotes significant bacteriuria and indicates active UTI. Contamination accounts for less than 10^4 organisms/ml and usually less than 10^3/ml. UTI is generally caused by one species, while contaminants are generally of mixed species. However, in case of obstructive uropathy (bladder stones, prostate hypertrophy, spinal paralysis), it may be caused by more than one species of bacteria.

UTI is caused by *Escherichia coli* (70–80%), *Proteus mirabilis* and other spp. (10%), *Staphylococcus saprophyticus* (10–15%), *S. epidermidis* (1–5%), *S. aureus* (1–5%), *Enterococcus* spp. (1–5%), *Klebsiella* spp. (1–5%) and *Pseudomonas aeruginosa* (1–2%). Other organisms which may occasionally cause UTI include *Mycobacterium tuberculosis*, *Enterobacter*, *Citrobacter*, salmonellae, *Streptococcus pyogenes*, *S. agalactiae* and *Gardnerella vaginalis*. *Candida albicans* may cause UTI in diabetics and immunocompromised patients. *Ureaplasma urealyticum* accounts for some cases of urethritis and cystitis. *Mycoplasma pneumoniae* has been isolated from renal tissues of patients with acute pyelonephritis. Adenovirus causes acute haemorrhagic cystitis in children and in some young adults.

For the collection of specimen (urine), microscopy and culture, refer to the chapter on Enterobacteria. The isolates are identified on the basis of morphological and biochemical characters.

Q. 3. What do you understand by the term sexually transmitted diseases? Enumerate the causative agents of these and describe laboratory diagnosis of syphilis.

Ans. The sexually transmitted diseases (STD) are a group of communicable diseases that are transmitted predominantly by sexual contact and caused by a wide range of bacterial, viral, protozoal and fungal agents. STD may cause genital ulcers, genital discharge, or no genital lesion but only systemic manifestations. The organisms causing these infections are given in Table 52.2. For the laboratory diagnosis of syphilis refer to the corresponding chapter.

Q. 4. Define purulent and aseptic meningitis. Enumerate microorganisms causing these. Tabulate differentiating features of purulent meningitis and aseptic meningitis and describe laboratory diagnosis of meningococcal meningitis.

Ans. Meningitis is an inflammation of the membranes of the brain or spinal cord. It is of two types, purulent meningitis and aseptic meningitis. The causative agents of these types are given in Table 52.3.

Purulent meningitis

In purulent meningitis, the CSF is turbid due to the presence of a large number of leucocytes (from 100 to several thousands/µl) most of which are polymorphs. Bacteria causing acute purulent meningitis related to age are given in Table 52.4. *S. aureus*, streptococci, coliform bacilli and anaerobic cocci may be acquired during carelessly performed lumbar puncture. In patients with CSF-venous shunts, it may be caused by *S. epidermidis*.

Aseptic meningitis

In aseptic meningitis CSF is slightly turbid. It contains lesser number of leucocytes (10–500/µl), most of which are lymphocytes. Most of these cases are caused by viruses and a few cases are caused by bacteria, fungi and protozoa. In tuberculous meningitis also, cell count is usually 100–500 leucocytes/µl most of which are lymphocytes. When CSF is allowed

Table 52.2. Organisms causing sexually transmitted diseases

Disease	Causative agents
GENITAL ULCERS	
Painless ulcers	
• Syphilis	*Treponema pallidum*
• Lymphogranuloma venereum	*Chlamydia trachomatis*
• Donovanosis	*Klebsiella* (*Calymmatobacterium*) *granulomatis*
Painful ulcers	
• Chancroid	*Haemophilus ducreyi*
• Herpes genitalis	Herpes simplex virus types 2 and 1
GENITAL DISCHARGE	
• Gonorrhoea	*Neisseria gonorrhoeae*
• *Trichomonas* vaginitis	*Trichomonas vaginalis*
• Non-gonococcal urethritis	*C. trachomatis*, *Ureaplasma urealyticum*, *Mycoplasma genitalium*, *M. hominis*, *Acinetobacter lwoffii*, *Bacteroides urealyticus*, *Candida albicans*, *Torulopsis glabrata*
• Bacterial vaginosis	*Mobiluncus curtisii*, *M. mulieris*, *Mycoplasma hominis*, *Gardnerella vaginalis*, *Bacteroides* spp.
NO GENITAL LESIONS BUT ONLY SYSTEMIC MANIFESTATIONS	
• AIDS	HIV-1 and HIV-2
• Hepatitis B	HBV
• Hepatitis C	HCV
MISCELLANEOUS	
Shigella spp., *Campylobacter* spp., Group B streptococci, Human herpesvirus 5 (cytomegalovirus), Human papillomaviruses, Molluscum contagiosum virus, *Entamoeba histolytica*, *Giardia lamblia*	

Table 52.3. Causative agents of purulent and aseptic meningitis

PURULENT MENINGITIS

- *Haemophilus influenzae*
- *Streptococcus pneumoniae*
- *Neisseria meningitidis*
- *Escherichia coli*
- Group B streptococci
- *Pseudomonas*
- Salmonellae
- *Staphylococcus aureus*
- *S. epidermidis*
- *Listeria monocytogenes*
- *Klebsiella*
- Anaerobic cocci
- *Bacteroides*

ASEPTIC MENINGITIS

Viruses

- Enteroviruses (echoviruses, polioviruses, coxsackieviruses)
- Mumps
- Herpes simplex
- Varicella-zoster
- Measles
- Adenoviruses
- Arboviruses

Bacteria

- *Leptospira interrogans* serovars *icterohaemorrhagiae* and *canicola*
- *Treponema pallidum*
- *Mycobacterium tuberculosis*

Protozoa

- *Acanthamoeba*
- *Naegleria*
- *Toxoplasma gondii*

Fungi

- *Cryptococcus neoformans*

Table 52.4. Bacteria causing acute purulent meningitis related to age

PREMATURE NEWBORNS	INFANTS	ADOLESCENTS
• *Escherichia coli* • *Klebsiella* spp. • *Enterobacter* spp. • *Proteus* spp.	• *Streptococcus agalactiae* • *Listeria monocytogenes* • *Haemophilus influenzae* • *S. pneumoniae* **CHILDREN** • *Neisseria meningitidis* • *S. pneumoniae* • *H. influenzae*	• *N. meningitidis* **ADULTS** • *S. pneumoniae* **ELDERLY** • Gram-negative bacilli

to stand, a fibrin web (cobweb) often develops. In immunocompromised hosts, aseptic meningitis may be caused by *Listeria monocytogenes* and *Cryptococcus neoformans*. The latter is particularly seen in AIDS cases.

For laboratory diagnosis of meningitis, CSF is collected by lumbar puncture in three separate sterile vials, one each for cell count, chemical examination and culture. Differentiating features in CSF in purulent and aseptic meningitis are given in Table 52.5. For culture and identification of the causative agent refer to the corresponding chapters.

Table 52.5. Differentiating features in CSF in purulent and aseptic meningitis

Features	CSF values in		
	Normal	**Purulent meningitis**	**Aseptic meningitis**
Pressure	90–180 mm H_2O	Highly increased	Slightly to moderately increased
Total proteins	30–45 mg%	Highly increased (100–600 mg%)	Slightly increased (60–120 mg%)
Sugar	40–80 mg%	Diminished (10–20 mg%) or absent	Normal
Cell count	1–3/µl	100 to several thousands/µl	10–500/µl
Type of cells	Lymphocytes	Neutrophils 98%, Lymphocytes 2%	Lymphocytes
Smear from the centrifuged deposits			
Gram staining	—	Gram-negative or positve, cocci or bacilli depending on the causative agent	—
Ziehl-Neelsen staining	—	—	Acid-fast bacilli in case of tuberculous meningitis

Q. 5. Enumerate causes of pyrexia of unknown origin (PUO). Describe laboratory diagnosis of the same.

Ans. PUO may be defined as any febrile illness (body temperature greater than 38°C) lasting more than a few days, without an obvious cause. The causes of PUO are given in Table 52.6. Urinary tract infection, tuberculosis, infective endocarditis, osteomyelitis, and biliary tract infection are the commonest infectious causes of PUO. For diagnosis, refer to the chapters dealing with specific causative agents.

Q. 6. Enumerate causative agents of infective endocarditis. Describe laboratory diagnosis of the same.

Ans. Normal healthy endocardium of an immunocompetent host is generally not at risk when challenged transiently by a small number of organisms in the circulation. However, the heavy challenges that accompany intravenous drug use or the use of intravascular catheters in debilitated host or damage to the natural heart valve by rheumatic fever or atheroma and cardiac surgery, in particular prosthetic valve replacement may lead to infections of the endocardium. The important causative agents of infective endocarditis are given in Table 52.7.

Table 52.6. Causes of PUO

BACTERIAL
- Urinary tract infection
- Lung, subphrenic, appendix and other deep abscesses
- Septicaemia associated with pneumonia, pyelonephritis, biliary tract infection, infective endocarditis, osteomyelitis, etc.
- Enteric fever
- Tuberculosis
- Brucellosis
- Syphilis
- Relapsing fever
- Rheumatic fever
- Leptospirosis without jaundice or meningitis
- Typhus fever
- Non-meningitic meningococcal infection
- Q fever

PARASITIC
- Malaria
- Hepatic amoebiasis
- Leishmaniasis
- Trypanosomiasis
- Toxoplasmosis
- Filariasis

VIRAL
- EBV infection
- CMV infection
- HIV infection
- Rubella and other infectious fevers without typical rash

Table 52.7. Causative agents of infective endocarditis

Causative agent	Incidence
BACTERIA	
• Viridans group of streptococci	70%
– *Streptococcus sanguis*	
– *S. mutans*	
– *S. intermedius*	
– *S. mitis*	
• Groups F and G streptococci	10%
• *Staphylococcus epidermidis*	10%
• *Enterococcus faecalis*	5%
• *S. aureus*	5%
• Diphtheroids	Rare
• *Haemophilus* spp.	Rare
• Coliforms	Rare
• *Pseudomonas*	Rare
• *Coxiella burnetii*	Rare
• *Chlamydia psittaci*	Rare
FUNGI	
• *Candida* spp.	Rare
• *Aspergillus* spp.	Rare

Diagnosis of infective endocarditis can be established by isolation of the causative agent from the blood. Three to six samples of blood, 10 ml each should be collected from antecubital vein over 24 hours. Each sample should be inoculated into 50–100 ml of glucose broth.

Large amount of blood is required because the number of organisms in the blood may be very few. In addition, blood provides nutrition for the growth of organisms. Repeated blood cultures are made because the bacteraemia is intermittent. The blood is inoculated into large amount (50–100 ml) of culture medium so that bactericidal substances present in the blood are diluted. Cultures are incubated at 37°C for at least 3 weeks. Subcultures are made on blood agar and MacConkey agar after 24 hours, 48 hours and after one week. *Coxiella burnetii* and *Chlamydia* spp. cannot grow on cell free media. For the diagnosis of these agents, refer to corresponding chapters.

Q. 7. Define septicaemia, bacteraemia, pyaemia and endotoxaemia. Enumerate microorganisms causing septicaemia. How do they enter the blood stream?

Ans. *Septicaemia*

It is a condition in which bacteria circulate and actively multiply within the blood stream with clinical symptoms.

Bacteraemia

It may be defined as presence of bacteria in blood without overt disease.

Pyaemia

It is essentially septicaemia with metastatic infection.

Endotoxaemia

It is a condition in which bacterial endotoxin circulates in the blood.

Microorganisms causing septicaemia

These are given in Table 52.8.

Entry of bacteria into blood stream

Bacteria gain entry into blood stream:

- From breakages of blood vessels adjacent to skin or mucosal surfaces.
- By phagocytic cells carrying organisms into capillaries or the lymphatic system.

Table 52.8. Microorganisms causing septicaemia

GRAM-NEGATIVE BACILLI
• *Salmonella* Typhi
• *S.* Paratyphi A
• *S.* Paratyphi B
• *S.* Paratyphi C
• *Brucella* spp.
• *Haemophilus influenzae*
• *Escherichia coli*
• *Klebsiella pneumoniae*
• *Proteus* spp.
• *Enterobacter* spp.
• *Pseudomonas* spp.
GRAM-POSITIVE BACILLI
• *Listeria monocytogenes*
GRAM-NEGATIVE COCCI
• *Neisseria meningitidis*
GRAM-POSITIVE COCCI
• *Staphylococcus aureus*
• *S. epidermidis*
• *Streptococcus pyogenes*
• *S. pneumoniae*

Q. 8. What do you understand by the terms infective diarrhoea and dysentery? Enumerate microorganisms causing these. Tabulate differences between amoebic and bacillary dysentery.

Ans. Infective diarrhoea

Diarrhoea is the most common presenting symptom of an infection of the lower intestinal tract. Patient has bowel movements in excess of normal and the stool takes on a form that is softer or more liquid than usual. Infective diarrhoea may be caused by viruses, bacteria, parasites and fungi (Table 52.9).

Table 52.9. Causative agents of infective diarrhoea

VIRUSES • Rotavirus • Astrovirus • Calicivirus • Norwalk virus • Adenovirus **BACTERIA** • *Vibrio cholerae* • *V. parahaemolyticus* • *Escherichia coli* (ETEC, EPEC) • *Salmonella* Enteritidis • *S.* Typhimurium • Other *Salmonella* spp. • *Campylobacter* spp. • *Yersinia enterocolitica* • *Shigella* spp. • *Clostridium perfringens* • *C. difficile* • *Staphylococcus aureus* • *Bacillus cereus* • *Aeromonas hydrophila* • *Plesiomonas shigelloides*	**PROTOZOA** • *Entamoeba histolytica* • *Giardia lamblia* • *Cryptosporidium parvum* • *Isospora belli* **CESTODES** • *Hymenolepis nana* **NEMATODES** • *Trichuris trichiura* • *Strongyloides stercoralis* • *Ascaris lumbricoides* • Hookworms **TREMATODES** • *Schistosoma mansoni* **FUNGI** • *Candida albicans*

For the collection of specimen, enrichment and plating media, culture methods, morphological and biochemical characters, and other methods of identification, refer to corresponding chapters.

Dysentery

It is a disease marked by frequent watery stools, often with blood and mucus, and characterized clinically by cramping abdominal pain, tenesmus (painful straining when passing the stools), fever, and dehydration. Dysentery results from 'enteroinvasive' microorganisms (Table 52.10) that penetrate through the mucosa and cause inflammation of the intestinal wall. On the other hand, diarrhoea is nonpainful and is caused by *Vibrio cholerae* and other noninvasive 'enterotoxigenic' bacteria that produce vibrio-like toxins.

The differences between protozoal (amoebic) and bacterial (bacillary) dysentery are given in Table 52.11.

Table 52.10. Microorganisms causing dysentery
BACTERIA • *Shigella dysenteriae* • *S. flexneri* • *S. boydii* • *S. sonnei* • *Escherichia coli* (EIEC, EPEC, EHEC) **PROTOZOA** • *Entamoeba histolytica* • *Balantidium coli*

Q. 9. Define bacterial food-poisoning. Name different types of food-poisoning. Enumerate microorganisms causing these types of food-poisoning. Describe briefly laboratory diagnosis of food-poisoning.

Ans. The term bacterial food-poisoning is restricted to acute gastroenteritis due to the presence of bacteria, usually in large numbers, or their products in food. It is of three types:

Table 52.11. Differences between amoebic and bacillary dysentery

Character	Amoebic dysentery	Bacillary dysentery
MACROSCOPIC		
Number	6–8 motions a day	Over 10 motions a day
Amount	Copious	Small
Odour	Offensive	Odourless
Colour	Dark red	Bright red
Reaction	Acidic	Alkaline
Consistency	Not adherent to the container	Adherent to the container
MICROSCOPIC		
RBCs	In clumps	Discrete, sometimes in clumps due to rouleaux formation
Pus cells	Few	Numerous
Macrophages	Few	Numerous, many of them contain RBCs hence may be mistaken for *Entamoeba histolytica*
Eosinophils	Present	Scarce
Charcot-Leyden crystals	Present	Absent
Pyknotic bodies	Present	Absent
Ghost cells	Absent	Present
Parasites	Trophozoites of *E. histolytica*	Absent
Bacteria	Many motile bacteria	Few or absent

A. *Infective type:* In this type, multiplication of bacteria occurs *in vivo*.
B. *Toxic type:* In this type, the disease follows ingestion of food with preformed toxin.
C. *Infective-toxic type:* In this type, bacteria release the toxin in the bowel.

The causative agents of food poisoning are given in Table 52.12. For laboratory diagnosis refer to corresponding chapters.

Table 52.12. Causative agents of food-poisoning

INFECTIVE TYPE	**TOXIC TYPE**
• *Salmonella* Typhimurium • *S.* Enteritidis • *S.* Heidelberg • *S.* Indiana • *S.* Newport • *S.* Dublin • *Vibrio parahaemolyticus* • *Campylobacter jejuni*	• *Staphylococcus aureus* • *Bacillus cereus* • *Clostridum botulinum* **INFECTIVE-TOXIC TYPE** • *Clostridum perfringens*

53

Nosocomial Infections

Q. 1. Describe briefly nosocomial infections. Describe factors influencing nosocomial infections, nosocomial infection sites, microorganisms causing nosocomial infections, routes of transmission and prevention of nosocomial infections.

Ans. Healthcare-associated, hospital-acquired or nosocomial (*nosocomion* means hospital) infections represent one of the most common complications of healthcare delivery. A nosocomial infection is defined as infection developing in a patient after admission to the hospital, which was neither present nor in its incubation period when the subject entered the hospital. Such an infection may manifest during the stay in the hospital or sometime after the patient is discharged. Despite progress in public health and hospital care, infections continue to develop in hospitalized patients, and may also affect hospital staff. For most bacterial infections, an onset of symptoms more than 48 hours after admission is evidence of nosocomial acquisition. **To determine whether some infections, such as legionellosis, are hospital acquired, one must consider the usual incubation periods and determine whether the patient was hospitalized during that time period.**

Nosocomial infections occur worldwide and affect both developed and resource-poor countries. Infections acquired in healthcare settings are among the major causes of death and increased morbidity among hospitalized patients. They are a significant burden both for the patient and for the public health. Between 5 and 10% of patients admitted to acute care hospitals acquire an infection during hospitalization. At any time, over 1.4 million people worldwide suffer from infectious complications acquired in the hospital.

The most frequent nosocomial infections are infections of surgical wounds, urinary tract infections and lower respiratory tract infections. The vast majority of nosocomial infections are related to devices (e.g., urinary tract catheters, endotracheal tubes in ventilated patients, and venous catheters). Highest prevalence of nosocomial infections occurs in intensive care units and in acute surgical and orthopaedic wards. Infection rates are higher among patients with increased susceptibility because of old age, underlying disease or chemotherapy.

Factors influencing nosocomial infections

A large number of factors contribute towards the development of nosocomial infection. These include the following:

1. The hospital environment is heavily laden with a wide variety of pathogens. These may be present in air, dust, antiseptic lotions, water, food or may spread from shedding from the patients.
2. Due to injudicious use of antibiotics, the hospital microbial flora is usually multidrug resistant, thus limiting the choice of therapy.
3. Hospitalized patients with pre-existing diseases, such as diabetes, immunosuppression and patients with prosthetic implants are more susceptible to nosocomial infection.
4. Diagnostic or therapeutic intervention such as insertion of urethral or intravenous catheters may introduce the infection.
5. Blood and blood-products used for transfusion and also intravenous fluids, if not properly screened, can transmit many infections.

The source of the infecting organisms may be exogenous from another patient or a member of the staff or from the inanimate objects in the hospital like medical equipment (endoscopes, cystoscopes, catheters, needles, etc.), bed pans, food, water, hospital air and surfaces contaminated by patients' secretions, excretions, blood and body fluids. It may be endogenous from the patient's own flora which at the time of infection may invade the patient's tissues spontaneously or be introduced into them by surgical operation, instrumental manipulations or nursing procedure.

Nosocomial infection sites

Nosocomial infection sites include urinary infection, surgical site infection, nosocomial pneumonia, nosocomial bacteraemia, skin and soft tissue infections, gastroenteritis and endometritis.

Microorganisms causing nosocomial infections

The most important microorganisms causing nosocomial infections are given in Table 53.1. Presently, about 60% cases of nosocomial infections are caused by aerobic Gram-negative rods and about 30% by Gram-positive cocci. Remaining 10% are caused by viruses and fungi.

Routes of transmission of infection in hospitals

There are five main routes of spread of infection in hospitals.

1. Contact spread

It is the principal route of transmission of nosocomial infections. It may be by direct contact spread from person to person. *Staphylococcus aureus* and *Streptococcus pyogenes* are two important pathogens spread by hand contact. Certain equipment (endoscope, bronchoscope, cystoscope), if not properly disinfected, may transmit pathogenic organisms, e.g., *Pseudomonas aeruginosa*.

Table 53.1. Microorganisms causing nosocomial infections

Hospital infection	Causative agents
Urinary tract infections	*Escherichia coli*, *Klebsiella*, *Proteus*, *Serratia*, *Pseudomonas*, *Providencia*, coagulase-negative staphylococci, enterococci and *Candida albicans*
Respiratory infections	*Haemophilus influenzae*, *Streptococcus pneumoniae*, *Staphylococcus aureus*, *Klebsiella*, *Enterobacter*, *Serratia*, *Proteus*, *Escherichia*, *Pseudomonas aeruginosa*, *Acinetobacter*, *Legionella pneumophila*, respiratory viruses
Wound and skin sepsis	*Staphylococcus aureus*, *Escherichia coli*, *Proteus*, *Bacteroides*, enterococci, coagulase-negative staphylococci
Burn infections	*Staphylococcus aureus*, *Pseudomonas aeruginosa*, *Acinetobacter*, *Streptococcus pyogenes*
Gastrointestinal infections	*Salmonella* spp, *Shigella sonnei*, viruses
Eye infections	*Staphylococcus aureus*, *Pseudomonas aeruginosa*
Miscellaneous	Hepatitis B virus, human immunodeficiency viruses

2. Airborne spread

Hospital infection may be acquired by inhalation of droplets, droplet nuclei, dust from bedding and floors, and exudate dispersed from a wound during dressing.

Aerosols produced by nebulizers, humidifiers and air conditioning apparatus transmit certain pathogens like *Legionella* to the respiratory tract, because these organisms are widespread in water including potable water supplies. Occurrence of legionellae in hospital water supply and a number of persons with an impaired immune system has led to outbreaks of infection mainly with *Legionella pneumophila*, but also with *L. micdadei*, *L. bozmanii* and *L. longbeachae*. nosocomial infection occurs in patients rather than in staff who generally have circulating antibodies, which suggest exposure.

3. Oral route

Gastrointestinal pathogens may be transmitted by foods served to the patients. Hospital food may also be a source of antibiotic-resistant bacteria (*Pseudomonas aeruginosa*, *Escherichia coli*, *Klebsiella* spp. and others), which may colonize the gut and later cause infection in susceptible patients.

4. Parenteral route (inoculation)

With the use of single-use disposable needles, syringes and other devices and satisfactory procedure for the sterilization of surgical instruments, transmission of infection by parenteral route has been infrequent. However, certain infections may be transmitted by blood transfusion or tissue donation, contaminated blood-products (factor VIII), contaminated infusion fluids and from accidental injury with contaminated sharp instruments (AIDS, hepatitis B and C).

5. Self infection

Self infection may occur due to transfer into the wounds of staphylococci and streptococci carried by the patient in his nose and over his skin, or of coliform bacilli and anaerobes released from his bowel during surgery.

Prevention

Nosocomial infection can be prevented by:

1. The provision of sterile instruments, dressings, surgical gloves, face-masks, theatre clothing and fluids.
2. Thorough hand washing after any procedure involving nursing care or close contact with the patient.
3. Preoperative disinfection of the patient's skin.
4. The use of antiseptics for irrigation of the wound site at operation or for mucosal surfaces such as the bladder after urological surgery and peritoneum during dialysis.
5. Rational antibiotic prophylaxis.
6. Proper investigation of nosocomial infection and the treatment of the patients and the carriers.

Q. 2. Write short note on antibiotic policy.

Ans. Antibiotic policy constitutes one of the most important aspects of the infection control programme. Often, antibiotics are prescribed when there is no proof of infection. It has been seen that a wrong antibiotic has been chosen, or the timing of the antibiotic used is not in accordance with acceptable standards of practice. It is vital, therefore, that the Antibiotic Policy is properly framed and formulated. The prerequisites of an antibiotic policy are:

- Data of resistance among commonly encountered pathogens both in the community and in the hospital setting.
- Pattern of resistance to newer antimicrobial agents.
- Recognition of the trends of resistance.

The selection of the antimicrobial agent should be based on the sensitivity reports. Treatment of common infections should conform to standard regimen. In countries like ours where there is unrestricted sale "over the counter" of antibiotics, uncontrolled misuse of antibiotics is responsible for a general pool of resistant strains in the population. Sale of antibiotics should be restricted to medical prescription only.

Why an antibiotic policy?

- To retard the emergence of multiple antibiotic-resistant bacteria.
- To avoid wasteful expenditure of Government/non-Government organization.

Good practice

- Consider whether or not the patient actually requires an antibiotic.
- In general do not change antibiotic therapy if clinical condition indicates improvement.
- If there is no clinical response in 72 hours, the clinical diagnosis, the choice of antibiotics and a secondary infection should be reconsidered.
- Review the duration of antibiotic therapy after 7 days.
- For surgical prophylaxis start with induction of anaesthesia and continue for maximum of 24 hours only.
- Microbiology laboratory should provide antibiotic susceptibility of bacterial isolates from the local area.

- Do not use IV antibiotics without good cause.
- Do not give IV therapy for more than 3 days without review.
- Do not prescribe antibiotics for acute asthma without strong evidence of bacterial infection.
- Do not use multiple antibiotics without good indications.

When prescribing antibiotics ask following questions from yourself.

- What is most likely anatomical site of infection?
- What is the clinical, radiological and laboratory evidence of infection?
- Have bacteriological investigations been requested?
- Has the organism responsible for the infection been isolated?
- If not, then what is the suspected organism?
- Are there any underlying or predisposing conditions relevant to the diagnosis of infection?
- Should the patient have received an antibiotic?
- Was the antibiotic an appropriate choice?
- Was the dose appropriate?
- Was the route of administration appropriate?
- Was the treatment cost-effective?

Q. 3. Write short note on hospital disinfection policy.

Ans. In most hospitals no disinfection policy exists and a number of different disinfectants are used at many different strengths, with particular disinfectant often used for quite unsuitable purposes. The irrational use of disinfectants has both safety and cost implications. The choice of disinfectant for a particular purpose is important because an inappropriate product may be either inherently unsuitable or unnecessarily expensive. The correct-use dilution is important because too low a concentration will be ineffective, and too high a concentration uneconomic and possibly hazardous.

Q. 4. Write short note on infection control committee.

Ans. Every hospital should have an infection control committee (ICC) with responsibilities that include the production and implementation of a disinfection policy. List of suggested infection control committee members is given in Table 53.2. Infection control personnel should review microbiology records regularly to identify unusual clusters or a greater-than-usual incidence of certain species or strains of microorganisms. All healthcare facilities must have access to the services of personnel trained and experienced in conducting outbreak investigations. When an outbreak occurs, the infection control team must have adequate resources and authority to ensure a comprehensive and timely investigation and the implementation of appropriate control

Table 53.2. Suggested infection control committee members

Member	Role
1. Hospital Director/Dean/Principal	Chairman
2. Microbiologist/Epidemiologist	Infection Control Officer
3. Chief of medical services	Member
4. Quality control/assurance officer	Member
5. Heads of various clinical departments	Members
6. Head of pharmacy	Member
7. Head of support services	Member
8. Chief nurse	Member
9. Infection control nurses	Members

measures. The ICC should meet regularly, at least once a month and as often as required, to formulate and update policy for the whole hospital matters having implications for infection control and to manage outbreaks of nosocomial infection.

The functions of ICC include surveillance and control of infection and monitoring of hygiene practices and the education of all staff in the microbiologically safe performance of procedures. Close working links between the microbiology laboratory and the different clinical specialities and support services (including sterile services, laundry, pharmacy and engineering) are important to establish and maintain the infection control policy, and to ensure that it is rationally based and that the recommended procedures are practicable.

54

Antimicrobial Sensitivity Testing

Q. 1. Describe briefly antimicrobial sensitivity testing. In which situations it should and should not be done?

Ans. Antimicrobial sensitivity tests are performed on bacteria isolated from clinical specimens. Sensitivity tests are not performed on bacteria that are predictably sensitive to the antimicrobial agents commonly used to treat infections caused by these bacteria. Group A β-haemolytic *Streptococcus*, for example, is not routinely tested because it is universally sensitive to penicillin, the drug of choice in treating infections caused by this bacterium. In contrast, the recommended agent for treating *Staphylococcus aureus* infections is oxacillin, and *S. aureus* may or may not be sensitive to oxacillin. Consequently, sensitivity testing is indicated for *S. aureus* isolates.

Sensitivity tests are not performed on bacteria that are isolated from the anatomic site of which they are normal inhabitants. For example, *Escherichia coli* is normal flora in the lower gastrointestinal tract and, therefore, would not be tested when isolated from stool; however, *E. coli* from a blood culture would be tested because blood is normally sterile. Similarly, viridans streptococci represent normal flora in throat specimens and would not be routinely tested. Because coagulase-negative staphylococci are commonly found on skin surfaces, these organisms should not be tested when isolated from superficial wound specimens. Coagulase-negative staphylococci isolated from multiple blood culture bottles should be tested. Testing of normal flora isolates or isolates likely to represent contamination or colonization should be avoided.

Q. 2. Describe methods of antimicrobial sensitivity testing.

Ans. Antimicrobial sensitivity tests are of two types – diffusion methods and dilution methods (Table 54.1).

Disc diffusion tests are most widely used and are satisfactory for pathogenic aerobes and facultative as well as rapidly growing anaerobes. These methods have, however, been found to be unsuitable for slow growing microbes.

Table 54.1. Antibiotic sensitivity tests

Diffusion methods
• Kirby-Bauer disc diffusion method
• Stokes disc diffusion method
Dilution methods
• Broth dilution method
• Agar dilution method

Medium

The medium must support good overnight growth of test and control organisms. Mueller-Hinton broth and agar may be used for testing aerobic and facultative anaerobic isolates.

Inoculum

The ideal inoculum after overnight incubation gives even semi-confluent growth. Too heavy an inoculum reduces the size of inhibition zones produced by many antibiotics. Isolation of organisms in pure culture is of utmost importance. Using a straight wire, touch the tops of 5–10 similar appearing well isolated colonies on an agar plate. Inoculate them in a suitable broth medium. Incubate at 35–37°C for 4–6 hours when the growth is considered to be in logarithmic phase. Five to ten colonies rather than a single colony, are selected to minimize the possibility of testing a colony that might have been derived from a suspected mutant. The density of the organisms is adjusted to approximately 10^8 colony-forming units (cfu)/ml by comparing its turbidity with that of 0.5 McFarland opacity standard.

Control strains

Control strains for Kirby-Bauer and Stokes disc diffusion methods are given in Table 54.2.

Antibiotic discs

Commercially prepared discs 6 mm in diameter may be used. Manufacturers produce discs with accurate antibiotic content. If discs are prepared locally in the laboratory, then pure antimicrobial agents obtained from the manufacturers and not the ones for clinical use should be used. Disc contents of antimicrobial agents are given in Table 54.3. Discs and disc dispensers should be stored in sealed container with a desiccant. Bulk stock should be stored at –20°C and working ones at <8°C. These should be warmed slowly to room temperature to overcome hydrolysis. Therefore, they should be taken out from refrigerator 1–2 hours before applying on the culture medium.

Kirby-Bauer disc diffusion method

Within 15 minutes after adjusting the turbidity of the inoculum suspension to that of standard, dip a sterile nontoxic cotton swab into the inoculum and rotate the swab several times with firm pressure on the inside wall of the tube to remove excess fluid. Inoculate the dried surface of Mueller-Hinton agar plate that has been brought to room temperature by streaking the swab three times over the entire agar surface. Replace the lid of the dish. Allow 3–5 minutes but no longer than 15 minutes for surface of the agar to dry before applying the antibiotic discs.

Place the appropriate antimicrobial-impregnated discs on the surface of the agar, using either sterile forceps or multidisc dispenser. After placement, press the disc on the surface of

Table 54.2. Control strains for Kirby-Bauer and Stokes disc diffusion methods

Test bacteria	Control strain	
	Kirby-Bauer	Stokes
Coliform organisms	*E. coli* ATCC 25922	*E. coli* NCTC 10418
Pseudomonas	*P. aeruginosa* ATCC 27853	*P. aeruginosa* NCTC 10662
Haemophilus spp.	*H. influenzae* ATCC 49247	*H. influenzae* NCTC 11931
Gonococci	*N. gonorrhoeae* ATCC 49226	*N. gonorrhoeae* (sensitive strain)
Enterococci	*E. faecalis* ATCC 29212	*E. faecalis* NCTC 12697
Other organisms that can grow aerobically	*S. aureus* ATCC 25923	*S. aureus* NCTC 6571

Table 54.3. Disc contents of various antimicrobial agents

Antimicrobial agent	Disc content	Antimicrobial agent	Disc content
Benzyl penicillin		Methicillin	5 µg
– Staphylococci	1.2 µg	Carbenicillin	100 µg
– Pneumococci and meningococci	0.15 µg	Ticarcillin	75 µg
		Imipenem	10 µg
Ampicillin		Gentamicin	10 µg
– Enterobacteriaceae and enterococci	10 µg	Amikacin	30 µg
		Tobramycin	10 µg
– *Haemophilus* and *Moraxella* spp.	2 µg	Neomycin	30 µg
		Netilmicin	10 µg
Amoxicillin/clavulanic acid		Erythromycin	15 µg
– Enterobacteriaceae and enterococci	20 µg/10 µg	Clindamycin	2 µg
		Tetracycline	30 µg
– *Haemophilus* spp., *Moraxella* spp. and staphylococci	2 µg/1 µg	Fusidic acid	30 µg
		Chloramphenicol	
		– Enterobacteriaceae	30 µg
Piperacillin	100 µg	– Haemophili, pneumococci and meningococci	10 µg
Mezlocillin	30 µg		
Azlocillin	30 µg	Colistin	10 µg
Cephalothin	30 µg	Nalidixic acid	30 µg
Cephalexin	30 µg	Nitrofurantoin	300 µg
Cephadroxil	30 µg	Trimethoprim	5 µg
Cephradine	30 µg	Trimethoprim/ sulphamethoxazole	1.2 µg/23.8 µg
Cefuroxime	30 µg		
Ceftazidime	10 µg	Vancomycin	30 µg
Cefotaxime	10 µg	Rifampicin	5 µg
Cefsulodin	30 µg	Ciprofloxacin	1 µg

the medium to provide uniform contact. Do not move the disc once it has contacted the agar, because some of the drug diffuses almost immediately. The discs must be evenly distributed on the agar so that they are not closer than 24 mm centre to centre. On a plate of 100 mm diameter, seven discs may be placed one in the centre and six in the periphery (Fig. 54.1).

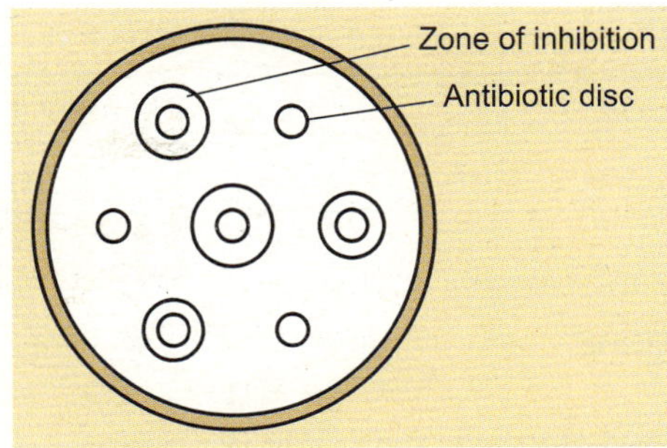

Fig. 54.1. Kirby-Bauer disc diffusion method.

As soon as the antibiotic impregnated disc comes in contact with the moist agar surface, it absorbs moisture from the agar and the antibiotic diffuses into the surrounding medium (Fig. 54.2). The rate of extraction of the antibiotic out of the disc is greater than outward diffusion into the medium, so that the concentration immediately adjacent to the disc may exceed that in the disc itself. However, as the distance from the disc increases, there is logarithmic reduction in the antibiotic concentration. The extent of antibiotic diffusion is also affected by the depth of the agar. The plates are then incubated at 35–37°C for 16–18 hours.

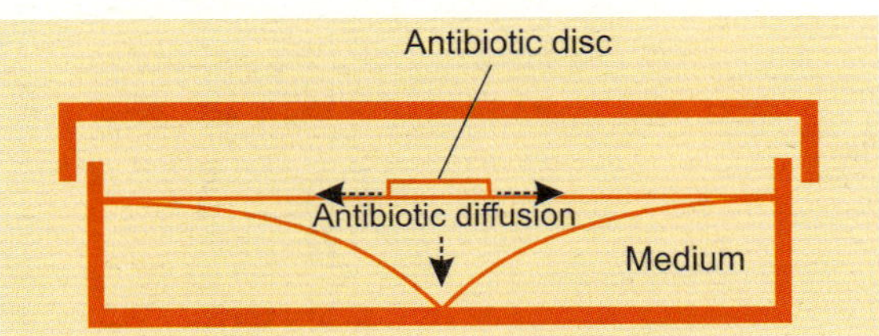

Fig. 54.2. The principle of antibiotic diffusion in agar. The concentration of antibiotic decreases as the distance from the disc increases.

Visible growth of the bacteria occurs on the surface of the agar where the concentration of the antibiotic has fallen below its inhibitory level for the test strain. Bacterial growth occurs in the form of a circle with middle of the disc forming the centre of the circle. The concentration of diffused antibiotic at the interface of growing and inhibited bacteria approximates to the minimum inhibitory concentration (MIC) obtained in dilution tests.

By using caliper or a transparent plastic ruler, the zones of complete growth inhibition around each of the discs are carefully measured. The diameter of the disc is included in this measurement. The zone size that is observed in a disc diffusion test has no meaning by itself. The interpretation of zone size into susceptible (infection treatable with normal dosage), moderately susceptible (infection that may respond to therapy with higher dosage) or resistant (not treatable with this agent) is based on the interpretation chart (Table 54.4). Reference strains of *S. aureus*, *E. coli*, *P. aeruginosa*, etc. should be tested each time a new batch of discs or agar is used.

Stokes disc diffusion method

The plate is divided into three parts. The test organism is inoculated on central one third and control on upper and lower thirds of the plate. However, in modified Stokes disc diffusion

Table 54.4. Interpretation chart of zone size in Kirby-Bauer disc diffusion method

Antimicrobial agent	**Diameter of zone of inhibition (mm)**		
	Resistant	**Moderately susceptible**	**Susceptible**
Benzyl penicillin	≤ 28	—	≥ 29
Ampicillin			
– Enterobacteriaceae	≤ 13	14–16	≥ 17
– Enterococci	≤ 16	—	≥ 17
– *Haemophilus* and *Moraxella* spp.	≤ 19	—	≥ 20
Cephalothin	≤ 14	15–17	≥ 18
Cefuroxime	≤ 14	15–17	≥ 18
Ceftazidime	≤ 14	15–17	≥ 18
Cefotaxime	≤ 14	15–22	≥ 23
Methicillin	≤ 9	10–13	≥ 14
Carbenicillin			
– *E. coli* and *Proteus* spp.	≤ 17	18–22	≥ 23
– *P. aeruginosa*	≤ 13	14–17	≥ 18
Gentamicin	≤ 12	–	≥ 13
Amikacin	≤ 14	15–16	≥ 17
Tobramycin	≤ 12	13–14	≥ 15
Erythromycin	≤ 13	14–17	≥ 18
Clindamycin	≤ 14	15–20	≥ 21
Tetracycline	≤ 14	15–18	≥ 19
Fusidic acid	≤ 14	15–18	≥ 19
Chloramphenicol	≤ 12	13–17	≥ 18
Colistin	≤ 8	9–10	≥ 11
Nalidixic acid	≤ 13	14–18	≥ 19
Nitrofurantoin	≤ 14	15–16	≥ 17
Trimethoprim	≤ 10	11–15	≥ 16
Trimethoprim/ sulphamethoxazole	≤ 10	11–15	≥16
Ciprofloxacin	≤ 15	16–20	≥ 21
Piperacillin			
– Enterobacteriaceae	≤ 17	18–20	≥ 21
– *Pseudomonas*	≤ 14	15–17	≥ 18

method, the test organism is inoculated in the upper and lower thirds and control on central one third. An uninoculated gap 2–3 mm wide should separate the test and control areas on which antibiotic discs are applied (Fig. 54.3). A maximum of six antibiotic discs can be accommodated on a single 100 mm diameter plate. The plates are then incubated at 35–37°C for 16–18 hours.

For reading and reporting of results, discard any plate on which growth is not semi-confluent and repeat the test. Measure the zone size, i.e., the distance in mm from edge of the disc to the zone edge, if that is obvious, if it is not, measure to the point of 80% or more inhibition of growth. However, if the test zones are obviously larger than the control or give no zone of inhibition at all, it is not necessary to perform any measurement. Each zone size is interpreted as follows:

1. ***Sensitive:*** The zone size is equal to, larger than or not more than 3 mm smaller than the control.
2. ***Intermediate:*** The zone size of the test strain is at least 2 mm, but also at least 3 mm smaller than that of the control strain.
3. ***Resistant:*** The zone size of the test strain is smaller than 2 mm.

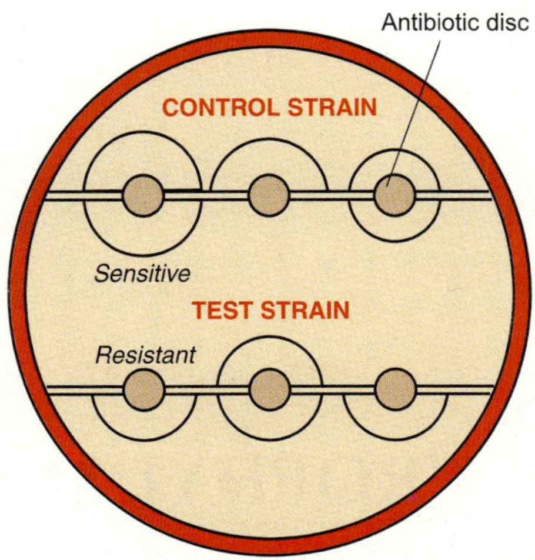

Fig. 54.3. Stokes disc diffusion test.

55

PROPHYLACTIC IMMUNIZATION

Q. 1. Describe briefly prophylactic immunization.

Ans. Immunization against infectious diseases is one of the greatest successes of modern medicine. During the last 200 years, since the time of Edward Jenner, vaccination has controlled nine major diseases, namely, smallpox, diphtheria, pertussis, tetanus, poliomyelitis, mumps, measles, rubella and yellow fever. Major headway has been made against influenza, hepatitis B, pneumococci and *Haemophilus influenzae* type b infections, at least in some parts of the world. Of the major scourges of mankind, malaria, leprosy, helminthic diseases and human immunodeficiency virus infections have remained without useful vaccines. Immunization is of three types – active immunization, passive immunization and combined passive and active immunization.

Q. 2. Tabulate national immunization schedule and describe briefly WHO EPI immunization schedule.

Ans. ***National immunization schedule***

The national immunization schedule is given in Table 55.1.

Table 55.1. National Immunization schedule

Age	Vaccine
For infants	
• At birth (for institutional deliveries)	BCG and OPV-0 dose
• 6 weeks	BCG (if not given at birth), DPT-1, OPV-1 and hepatitis B-1
• 10 weeks	DPT-2 and OPV-2 and hepatitis B-2
• 14 weeks	DPT-3 and OPV-3 and hepatitis B-3
• 9 months	Measles

(*Contd.*)

Age	Vaccine
16–24 months	DPT and OPV
5–6 years	DT*
10 years	TT**
16 years	TT**
For pregnant women	
• Early in pregnancy	TT-1 or booster
• One month after TT-1	TT-2

* The second dose of DT should be given at an interval of one month if there is no clear history or documented evidence of previous immunization with DPT.

** The second dose of TT should be given at an interval of one month if there is no clear history or documented evidence of previous immunization with DPT, DT or TT.

WHO EPI immunization schedule

In May 1974, the WHO officially launched a global immunization programme known as *Expanded Programme of Immunization* (EPI) to protect all children of the world against six vaccine-preventable diseases, namely diphtheria, whooping cough, tetanus, poliomyelitis, tuberculosis and measles by the year 2000. EPI was launched in India in January 1978. WHO EPI immunization schedule is given in Table 55.2. This programme is now called Universal Child Immunization, 1990.

Table 55.2. WHO EPI immunization schedule

Age	Vaccine
Birth	BCG, OPV
6 weeks	DPT, OPV
10 weeks	DPT, OPV
14 weeks	DPT, OPV
9 months	Measles

In addition, hepatitis B vaccine may be given at birth, 1 month and 6 months of age and booster dose at the age of 10 years. Children of the age of 15 months may be given MMR vaccine, followed by a booster at the age of 4–6 years.

Q. 3. Write short note on passive immunization.

Ans. Passive immunization is used when it is considered necessary to protect a patient at short notice and for a limited period. Three types of preparations are available for passive immunization – homologous and heterologous sera, pooled immunoglobulins and specific immunoglobulins.

Q. 4. Write short note on homologous and heterologous sera.

Ans. Antitoxic, antibacterial or antiviral antibodies in human (homologous) or animal (heterologous) serum are injected to give temporary protection. Homologous sera confer protection for 3–6 months, whereas protection afforded by a heterologous serum is likely to last for only a few weeks.

Q. 5. Write short note on pooled normal human serum and specific immunoglobulins.

Ans. ***Pooled immunoglobulins***

Pooled normal human serum contains protective levels of antibodies to a range of diseases. It may be used for short-term prophylaxis of hepatitis A in contacts or travellers who intend to visit countries where hepatitis A is common. It also protects an immunocompromised child temporarily against measles if given promptly after contact with a case.

Specific immunoglobulins

Specific immunoglobulins are available for passive immunization against tetanus (human tetanus immunoglobulin, HTIG), hepatitis B (HBIG), rabies (HRIG) and varicella-zoster (ZIG).

Q. 6. Write short note on combined passive and active immunization.

Ans. In some diseases (e.g., tetanus, diphtheria, rabies) passive immunization is often undertaken in conjunction with inactivated vaccine products, to provide both immediate (but temporary) passive immunity and slowly developing active immunity. Both injections should be given at separate sites.

Q. 7. What measures are taken for the prevention of nutritional blindness?

Ans. For the prevention of nutritional blindness massive doses of vitamin A are given to the children up to the age of 5 years. First dose of 100,000 IU of vitamin A is given with measles vaccination at nine months of age. Subsequent doses of 200,000 IU each are given every six months up to the age of 5 years.

Bacteriology of Water, Milk and Air

Q. 1. What are natural water, soil and sewage bacteria? Enumerate organisms in these categories.

Ans. 1. ***Natural water bacteria:*** This group includes those organisms that are commonly found in water free from gross pollution.

2. ***Soil bacteria:*** These organisms are not normal inhabitants of water, but are frequently washed into it during heavy rains.
3. ***Sewage bacteria:*** Many of the bacteria in this group are normal inhabitants of the intestine of man and animals. Others live mainly on decomposing organic matter of either animal or vegetable origin. Bacterial flora in water is given in Table 56.1.

Table 56.1. Bacterial flora in water

Natural water bacteria	*Micrococcus*, *Pseudomonas*, *Serratia*, *Flavobacterium*, *Chromobacterium*, *Acinetobacter* and *Alcaligenes*
Soil bacteria	*Bacillus subtilis*, *B. megaterium*, *B. mycoides*, *Enterobacter aerogenes* and *E. cloacae*
Sewage bacteria	
• Intestinal bacteria	*Escherichia coli*, *Enterococcus faecalis*, *Clostridium perfringens*, *Salmonella* Typhi and *Vibrio cholerae*
• Sewage bacteria proper	*Proteus vulgaris*, *Clostridium sporogenes*, *Zoogloea ramigera*, *Sphaerotilus natans*, *Haliscomenobacter hydrossis*, *Nostocoida limicola*, *Microthrix parvicella*, *Flexibacter*, *Microscilla* and *Nocardia*

Q. 2. Describe briefly factors determining number of bacteria in water.

Ans. Following are the factors determining number of bacteria in water:

1. ***Surface or deep water:*** Surface water is more likely to be contaminated.

2. ***Salinity:*** Number of bacteria is less in saline water as compared to fresh water. However, halophilic bacteria can survive in saline water.
3. ***Mineral springs:*** These are usually pure and most of the organisms found in water derived from them come from imperfectly sterilized bottles.
4. ***Nutrition:*** When organic matter is plentiful, organisms are abundant, when it is scarce they are few, and tend to die out.
5. ***Temperature:*** When nutrition is available, rise in temperature leads to multiplication, otherwise, the number decreases. Low temperature favours survival of bacteria.
6. ***Light:*** Day light with the wavelength of 300–400 nm is bactericidal. However, this effect is reduced by opacity and movement in water.
7. ***Acidity:*** Acidity of water has a bactericidal action, thus purifying water.
8. ***Dissolved oxygen:*** It is essential for survival of aerobes.
9. ***Protozoal content:*** Certain flagellates exterminate bacteria in water and bring down their number.
10. ***Rain:*** Early rain washes large number of bacteria from the soil which may contaminate water sources. Subsequent rains dilute the bacterial population.
11. ***Storage:*** Storage of water decreases bacterial count due to sedimentation and devitalization.

Q. 3. Tabulate water-borne pathogens.

Ans. Faecal pollution of drinking water may introduce a variety of intestinal viral, bacterial, protozoal and helminthic pathogens (Table 56.2).

Table 56.2. Water-borne pathogens

Viruses	Hepatitis A virus, hepatitis E virus, poliovirus, rotavirus.
Bacteria	*Vibrio cholerae*, *Salmonella* Typhi, *S.* Paratyphi A, B and C, *Escherichia coli*, *Shigella* spp., *Yersinia enterocolitica*, *Campylobacter jejuni* and *C. coli*
Protozoa	*Entamoeba histolytica*, *Giardia lamblia*, *Balantidium coli*, *Cryptosporidium parvum*, *Isospora belli*
Helminths	*Ascaris lumbricoides*, *Enterobius vermicularis*, *Trichuris trichiura*, *Echinococcus granulosus*
Pathogens borne by aquatic hosts	*Dracunculus medinensis* and *Diphylobothrium latum* through cyclops and schistosomes through snail

Q. 4. Describe bacteriological analysis of water.

Ans. **Collection of water samples**

Water sample should be collected in heat-sterilized glass bottle of 230 ml with ground glass stopper. To neutralize the bactericidal effect of chlorine in water, it should contain 0.23 ml of a fresh 1.8% aqueous solution of sodium thiosulphate.

1. Sampling from a tap or pump outlet

Clean the tap or pump outlet from outside. Turn on the tap at maximum flow rate and let the water flow for 2–3 minutes. Then open the stopper, fill the bottle, replace the stopper and wrap the bottle in a kraft paper.

2. Sampling from reservoir (streams, rivers, lakes and tanks)

Fill the bottle by holding it at its lower part, submerge it to a depth of about 30 cm below the surface of water. The bottle is then turned so that the mouth is directed to the current and water flows into the bottle without coming in contact with the hand. If there is no current the bottle should be moved horizontally, the mouth foremost, so that water flows into it. Thereafter, stopper the bottle and wrap it in a kraft paper.

3. Sampling from a dug well

A stone of suitable size is tied with the bottle. Then a clean cord of suitable length is tied with the bottle and lowered into the well. Immerse the bottle completely in the water. When the bottle is filled, pull it out, stopper it and wrap it in a kraft paper. The bottle should not touch the sides of the well any time.

The water sample should be properly labelled with full details of the source, time and date of collection and it should be delivered to the laboratory as quickly as possible, at least within 6 hours, in a cool container and protected from light.

Bacteriological examination

The standard tests usually employed for water bacteriology are given in Table 56.3.

Table 56.3. Standard tests usually employed for water bacteriology

MULTIPLE TUBE TEST
• Total coliform (presumptive coliform) count
• Faecal coliform and confirmed *Escherichia coli* count: Eijkman test
• Count of faecal streptococci
• Count of *Clostridium perfringens*
MEMBRANE FILTRATION TESTS

Total coliform (presumptive coliform) count

This test is called presumptive coliform count because the reaction observed may occasionally be due to the presence of some other organisms. Double strength and single strength MacConkey broth containing bromocresol purple indicator in bottles or tubes containing inverted Durham tubes for indication of gas production is used. Measured amount of water sample is added by sterile graduated pipettes as under:

1. One, 50 ml volume of water to 50 ml double strength medium.
2. Five, 10 ml volumes of water each to 10 ml double strength medium.
3. Five, 1 ml volumes of water each to 5 ml single strength medium.
4. Five, 0.1 ml volumes of water each to 5 ml single strength medium.

The inoculated tubes/bottles are incubated at 37°C for 48 hours. The presumptive coliform count per 100 ml is determined from the tubes/bottles showing acid and gas production using the probability table. The probability table with one 50 ml and five each of 10 ml and 1 ml of water is given in Table 56.4. The presumptive coliform count of water 0, 1–3, 4–10 and more than 10 per 100 ml is interpreted as excellent, satisfactory, suspicious and unsatisfactory for human consumption respectively.

Faecal coliform and confirmed Escherichia coli count

Eijkman test

Some spore-bearing bacteria give false positive reactions in the presumptive coliform test. Therefore, it is necessary to confirm the presence of true (faecal) coliform bacilli. After the usual presumptive test, subcultures are made from all the tubes/bottles showing acid and gas to fresh tubes of single strength MacConkey broth warmed to 44°C. These are incubated at 44°C in thermostatically controlled water bath and examined after 24 hours. Those tubes showing gas in Durham tube contain *E. coli*. It can be further confirmed by plating on solid media and testing for indole production and citrate utilization.

Count of faecal streptococci (enterococci)

Subcultures are made from all positive tubes/bottles in the presumptive coliform count into the tube containing 5 ml glucose azide broth. The presence of *Enterococcus faecalis* is indicated by the production of acid in the medium within 18 hours at 45°C. Further confirmation can be done by plating onto MacConkey agar medium. Alternatively, the membrane filtration method may be used, the membranes being cultured on well dried plates of glucose azide agar.

Count of Clostridium perfringens

Varying quantities of water sample are inoculated in litmus milk medium, and incubated at 37°C for 5 days. A typical stormy clot reaction together with acidity confirms the presence of *C. perfringens*. Further confirmation may be made by motility and nitrate reduction test.

Membrane filtration tests

In this method, a measured volume of water is filtered through a membrane which retains the bacteria on its surface. The membrane is then placed and incubated on a selective indicator medium, so that the indicator bacteria grow into colonies on its upper surface. The number of the colonies is counted and the bacteriological content of water calculated.

Examination for specific pathogens

Specific pathogens such as *Salmonella* Typhi and *Vibrio cholerae* may be isolated from water

Table 56.4. McCrady probability table

Quantity of water			
50 ml	10 ml	1 ml	
No. of samples of each quantity tested			
1	5	5	
Number giving positive reaction (acid and gas)			Probable number of coliform bacilli in 100 ml of water
0	0	0	0
0	0	1	1
0	0	2	2
0	1	0	1
0	1	1	2
0	1	2	3
0	2	0	2
0	2	1	3
0	2	2	4
0	3	0	3
0	3	1	5
0	4	0	5
1	0	0	1
1	0	1	3
1	0	2	4
1	0	3	6
1	1	0	3
1	1	1	5
1	1	2	7
1	1	3	9
1	2	0	5
1	2	1	7
1	2	2	10
1	2	3	12
1	3	0	8
1	3	1	11
1	3	2	14
1	3	3	18
1	3	4	20
1	4	0	13
1	4	1	17
1	4	2	20
1	4	3	30
1	4	4	35
1	4	5	40
1	5	0	25
1	5	1	35
1	5	2	50
1	5	3	90
1	5	4	160
1	5	5	180 +

by employing enrichment and selective media. For isolation of *S.* Typhi, equal volume of water is added to double strength selenite broth followed by incubation and subculture on Wilson and Blair's medium. For isolation of *V. cholerae*, alkaline peptone water (10X) is mixed with nine times its volume of water, incubated and subcultured on bile salt agar. Pathogenic organisms may also be isolated by membrane filtration method already described.

Q. 5. Enumerate microorganisms likely to be present in milk.

Ans. Table 56.5 shows microorganisms likely to be present in milk.

Table 56.5. Microorganisms likely to be present in milk

Microorganisms likely to be present in hygienically produced raw milk

- Coagulase-negative staphylococci
- Micrococci
- Streptococci

Microorganisms likely to be present in milk if the cow has mastitis

- *Staphylococcus aureus*
- *Streptococcus agalactiae* (Lancefield group B)
- *S. dysgalactiae* (Lancefield group C)
- *S. uberis*
- *S. pyogenes* (Lancefield group A)
- *Mycobacterium bovis*
- *Escherichia coli*
- *Leptospira interrogans* serovar *hardjo*
- *S. zooepidemicus* (Lancefield group C)
- *Listeria monocytogenes*
- *Bacillus cereus*
- *Pasteurella multocida*
- *Clostridium perfringens*
- *Nocardia* spp.
- *Actinomyces* spp.
- *Corynebacterium ulcerans*
- *Salmonella* spp.
- *Campylobacter jejuni*
- *Cryptococcus neoformans*

Q. 6. Describe methods of bacteriological examination of milk.

Ans. Bacteriological examination of milk can be carried out by following methods:

1. Viable count

This is done by plate dilution method. Raw milk may contain 500 to several million bacteria per ml.

2. Coliform count

Varying dilutions of milk are inoculated into 3 tubes of MacConkey broth with Durham tube and incubated at 37°C for 48 hours. Look for the production of acid and gas as the evidence of presence of coliform bacilli. All coliforms are killed by adequate pasteurization and their presence in pasteurized milk indicates faults in pasteurizer or postpasteurization contamination.

3. Methylene blue test

This test is a simple substitute for the viable count. It depends on the reduction of methylene blue by bacteria in milk when incubated at 37°C in complete darkness. The rate of reduction is related to the degree of bacterial contamination. The test is performed by adding 1 ml of standard methylene blue solution to 10 ml of milk in a test tube. The tube is closed with a sterile rubber stopper, inverted twice and incubated in the dark at 37–38°C. The milk is considered satisfactory, if it fails to reduce the dye in 30 minutes.

4. Phosphatase test

Alkaline phosphatase is a normal constituent of raw milk and is inactivated if pasteurization has been carried out properly. The test depends upon the ability of the enzyme to liberate *p*-nitrophenol from disodium *p*-nitrophenyl phosphate and thereby produce a yellow colour that can be quantitated by a colorimeter.

5. Turbidity test

This is a check on the sterilization of milk. If milk has been boiled, all heat coagulable proteins are precipitated. If ammonium sulphate is then added to the milk, filtered and boiled for 5 minutes, no turbidity results. Absence of turbidity indicates that the milk has been heated to at least 100°C for at least 5 minutes.

6. Examination for specific pathogens

(a) **Tubercle bacilli:** Centrifuge 100 ml of milk at 3,000 rpm for 30 minutes and inoculate two guinea-pigs and two slants of Lowenstein-Jensen medium. If the milk contains tubercle bacilli, growth of these organisms, in the animals and culture media, can be seen.

(b) **Brucella:** *Brucella* may be isolated by inoculating cream from the milk sample on serum dextrose agar. It may also be injected intramuscularly into guinea-pigs. The animals are sacrificed after six weeks and serum is tested for agglutinins and spleen is used for culture of brucellae. Brucellosis in animals can also be detected by demonstrating antibodies against brucellae, by milk ring test and whey agglutination test.

Q. 7. Describe indications and methods of bacteriological examination of air.

Ans. ***Indications***

- In hospital wards in which there is an outbreak of cross-infection.
- Surgical operation theatre.
- Premises where food articles are prepared and packed.
- Premises where pharmaceutical preparations are made.

Methods

1. Those that measure the rate at which bacteria-carrying particles, chiefly the larger particles, settle by gravity from the air onto exposed surface, e.g., the settle plate method.
2. Those that count the number of bacteria-carrying particles contained in a given volume of the air, e.g., the slit sampler method.

Each bacteria-carrying particle or droplet nucleus may contain from 1 to 100 or more bacteria.

Settle plate method

Petri dishes containing an agar medium of known surface area are left open for a measured period of time. Large bacteria-carrying dust particles settle onto the medium. The plates are incubated at 37°C for 24 hours and a count of the colonies formed shows the number of settled particles. Blood agar medium may be used for the count of the pathogenic, commensal and saprophytic bacteria in the air and is used for testing air in surgical operation theatres and hospital wards. However, this method measures only the rate of deposition of large particles from air and not the total number of large and small bacteria-carrying dust particles suspended in it.

Slit sampler method

By this method, the number of bacteria in a measured volume of air is determined. One $foot^3$ of air is directed onto a plate of culture medium through a slit 0.25 mm wide. The plate is rotated mechanically so as to allow the organisms to spread out on the medium. The culture medium is incubated and colonies counted which gives the number of bacteria present in the air.

Bacterial count should not exceed 50 per $foot^3$ in factories, offices and homes, 10 per $foot^3$ in general operation theatre and 1 per $foot^3$ in theatre for neurosurgery.

INDEX

B

C

D

E

I

J

K

U

V

W

Y

Z